Common haematology values if outside this range, consult.

Haemoglobin	men:	13–18g/dL
	women:	11.5–16g/dL
Mean cell volume, MCV	76–96fL	
Platelets	150–400 × 10⁹/L	
White cells (total)	4–11 × 10⁹/L	
Neutrophils	40–75%	
Lymphocytes	20–45%	
Eosinophils	1–6%	

Blood gases	*kPa*	*mmHg*
pH 7.35–7.45		
PaO₂	>10.6	75–100
PaCO₂	4.7–6	35–45
Base excess ±2 mmol/L		

U&E etc *If outside this range, consult:*

Sodium	135–145mmol/L
Potassium	3.5–5mmol/L
Creatinine	70–150µmol/L
Urea	2.5–6.7mmol/L
Calcium	2.12–2.65mmol/L
Albumin	35–50g/L
Proteins	60–80g/L

LFTs

Bilirubin	3–17µmol/L
Alanine aminotransferase, ALT	3–35U/L
Aspartate transaminase, AST	3–35U/L
Alkaline phosphatase	30–35U/L (*adults*)

'Cardiac enzymes'

Creatine kinase	25–195U/L
Lactate dehydrogenase, LDH	70–250U/L

Lipids and other biochemical values

Cholesterol	<6mmol/L *desired*
Triglycerides	0.5–1.9mmol/L
Amylase	0–180*somorgyi* U/dL
C-reactive protein, CRP	<10mg/L
Glucose, fasting	3.5–5.5mmol/L
Prostate specific antigen, PSA	0–4ng/mL
T4 (total thyroxine)	70–140mmol/L
TSH	0.5–~5mu/L

Keele

OXFORD MEDICAL PUBLICATIONS

Oxford Handbook of
Clinical Surgery

WITHDRAWN

Published and forthcoming Oxford Handbooks

Oxford Handbook for the Foundation Programme 3e
Oxford Handbook of Acute Medicine 3e
Oxford Handbook of Anaesthesia 3e
Oxford Handbook of Applied Dental Sciences
Oxford Handbook of Cardiology 2e
Oxford Handbook of Clinical and Laboratory Investigation 3e
Oxford Handbook of Clinical Dentistry 5e
Oxford Handbook of Clinical Diagnosis 2e
Oxford Handbook of Clinical Examination and Practical Skills
Oxford Handbook of Clinical Haematology 3e
Oxford Handbook of Clinical Immunology and Allergy 3e
Oxford Handbook of Clinical Medicine – Mini Edition 8e
Oxford Handbook of Clinical Medicine 8e
Oxford Handbook of Clinical Pathology
Oxford Handbook of Clinical Pharmacy 2e
Oxford Handbook of Clinical Rehabilitation 2e
Oxford Handbook of Clinical Specialties 9e
Oxford Handbook of Clinical Surgery 4e
Oxford Handbook of Complementary Medicine
Oxford Handbook of Critical Care 3e
Oxford Handbook of Dental Patient Care 2e
Oxford Handbook of Dialysis 3e
Oxford Handbook of Emergency Medicine 4e
Oxford Handbook of Endocrinology and Diabetes 2e
Oxford Handbook of ENT and Head and Neck Surgery
Oxford Handbook of Epidemiology for Clinicians
Oxford Handbook of Expedition and Wilderness Medicine
Oxford Handbook of Gastroenterology & Hepatology 2e
Oxford Handbook of General Practice 3e
Oxford Handbook of Genetics
Oxford Handbook of Genitourinary Medicine, HIV and AIDS 2e
Oxford Handbook of Geriatric Medicine
Oxford Handbook of Infectious Diseases and Microbiology
Oxford Handbook of Key Clinical Evidence
Oxford Handbook of Medical Dermatology
Oxford Handbook of Medical Imaging
Oxford Handbook of Medical Sciences 2e
Oxford Handbook of Medical Statistics
Oxford Handbook of Nephrology and Hypertension
Oxford Handbook of Neurology
Oxford Handbook of Nutrition and Dietetics 2e
Oxford Handbook of Obstetrics and Gynaecology 2e
Oxford Handbook of Occupational Health 2e
Oxford Handbook of Oncology 3e
Oxford Handbook of Ophthalmology 2e
Oxford Handbook of Oral and Maxillofacial Surgery
Oxford Handbook of Paediatrics 2e
Oxford Handbook of Pain Management
Oxford Handbook of Palliative Care 2e
Oxford Handbook of Practical Drug Therapy 2e
Oxford Handbook of Pre-Hospital Care
Oxford Handbook of Psychiatry 3e
Oxford Handbook of Public Health Practice 2e
Oxford Handbook of Reproductive Medicine & Family Planning
Oxford Handbook of Respiratory Medicine 2e
Oxford Handbook of Rheumatology 3e
Oxford Handbook of Sport and Exercise Medicine 2e
Oxford Handbook of Tropical Medicine 3e
Oxford Handbook of Urology 3e

Oxford Handbook of
Clinical
Surgery

Fourth edition

Edited by

Greg McLatchie

Consultant Surgeon,
Hartlepool General Hospital,
Hartlepool, UK

Neil Borley

Consultant Colorectal Surgeon,
Cheltenham General Hospital,
Cheltenham, UK

Joanna Chikwe

Associate Professor, Department of Cardiothoracic
Surgery, Mount Sinai Medical Center,
New York, United States

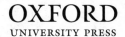

OXFORD
UNIVERSITY PRESS

OXFORD
UNIVERSITY PRESS

Great Clarendon Street, Oxford, OX2 6DP,
United Kingdom

Oxford University Press is a department of the University of Oxford.
It furthers the University's objective of excellence in research, scholarship,
and education by publishing worldwide. Oxford is a registered trade mark of
Oxford University Press in the UK and in certain other countries

© Oxford University Press, 2013

The moral rights of the authors have been asserted

First Edition published 1990
Second Edition published 2002
Third Edition published 2007
Fourth Edition published 2013
Reprinted 2013

Impression: 5

British Library Cataloguing in Publication Data
Data available

ISBN 978–0–19–969947–6 (flexicover: alk.paper)

Printed in China by
C&C Offset Printing Co. Ltd.

Preface to the fourth edition

Sometimes we have to look backward to look forward. Since 1990, surgery has witnessed cataclysmic changes. In our Trust, the first laparoscopic cholecystectomy was performed in 1992, and has now become the procedure of choice for most gall bladder disease and many other surgical operations in the western world. With the expansion of laparoscopic surgery, we have encountered a whole new range of complications with an escalation in the demise of general surgery as the result of hyperspecialization. There are many surgical trainees who have scant experience of open surgery and who have, due to European directives, limited time exposure to surgical procedures. In fact, most technical training is now obtained from emergency on call such that a new speciality of emergency surgery is developing. A recent *British Medical Journal* (BMJ) article recommended a training programme for surgeons wishing to work in remote and rural surgery—not only in the Developing World, but in remote and isolated communities in the United Kingdom! General surgery may largely have gone, but it should not be forgotten. Most countries in the world do not have access to these recent innovations and there is still a case in the developed world for experience in open and general surgery to be incorporated in the formal training programmes of junior surgeons.

G. R. McLatchie
Hartlepool, September 2012

Preface to the third edition

This, the third edition of the *Oxford Handbook of Clinical Surgery*, reflects the changes which have occurred in general surgery over the 17 years since the first edition was published.

Firstly, we have recruited the services of two new editors, a stark contrast to the original, which was written by a single author with the assistance of a surgical registrar.

Secondly, each chapter has been written by a specialist consultant or registrar in the subject and, therefore, presents a modern, state-of-the-art treatise on each topic.

Again, each condition is covered in the original two-page format with blank pages for accompanying notes.

I am particularly grateful for the commitment that Jo Chikwe and Neil Borley have made, and also wish to thank staff at Oxford University Press for their support and patience. I am also grateful for the contribution and support given by many colleagues.

G. R. McLatchie
Hartlepool, March 2007

Preface to the first edition

The idea of this book was first suggested by Mr Gordon McBain, consultant surgeon at the Southern General Hospital, Glasgow. We have received considerable support from the staff of Oxford University Press, and are also indebted to Mr J. Rhind and Dr J. Daniel for their contributions and our surgical teachers, especially Mr J. S. F. Hutchison, Mr M. K. Browne, Mr J. Neilson, Mr D. Young, Mr A. Young, and the late Mr I. McLennan whose practical advice and anecdotes pepper the pages....

G. R. McLatchie
S. Parameswaran
1990

Dedications

For Ross, Cameron, Ailidh, Claire, and Calum
GRM

For Alexander, Christopher, and Jennifer
NB

Acknowledgements

We are grateful to the support of our colleagues and Oxford University Press and to Mrs Pamela Lines for her diligent support in the final editing of the manuscript.

Contents

Detailed contents

Contributors

Alex Acornley
Consultant Orthopaedic
Surgeon,
Airedale Hospital NHS
Foundation Trust, West
Yorkshire, UK

Anil Agarwal
Consultant General and Colorectal
Surgeon,
North Tees and Hartlepool NHS
Trust, University Hospital of
Hartlepool, UK

Khalid A. Al-Hureibi
Specialist Registrar,
Department of General Surgery,
Lister Hospital, Stevenage, UK

John Asher
Consultant Transplant Surgeon,
Transplant Unit, Western
Infirmary, Glasgow, UK

David Chadwick
Consultant Urological Surgeon,
The James Cook University
Hospital, Middlesbrough, UK

Lucy Cogswell
Specialist Registrar,
Department of Plastic &
Reconstructive Surgery, John
Radcliffe Hospital, Oxford, UK

J. H. Dark
Consultant Cardiothoracic
Surgeon,
Freeman Hospital, Newcastle upon
Tyne, UK

Richard P. Jeavons
Specialist Registrar,
Trauma and Orthopaedics
(Northern Deanery), Department
of Trauma and Orthopaedics,
University Hospital of North Tees,
Stockton, UK

Vijay Kurup
Consultant Breast and Endocrine
Surgeon,
University Hospital of North Tees,
Stockton on Tees, UK

Jamie Lyall
Consultant Head and Neck
Surgeon (Maxillofacial),
Surgical Division, James Cook
University Hospital Trust,
Middlesbrough, Queen Margaret
Hospital, Dunfermline, UK

Alan Middleton
Consultant Orthopaedic Surgeon,
Department of Hand and Wrist
Surgery, University Hospital of
North Tees, Stockton, UK

Rob Milligan
ST3 General Surgery, Northern
Deanery, UK

**Sandrasekeram
Parameswaran**
General Surgeon,
Cold Lake Healthcare Centre,
Visiting Surgeon, Canadian forces
base, 4 Wing, Cold Lake, Alberta,
Canada

Lakshmi Parameswaran
Senior House Officer,
Mater Misericordiae University
Hospital, Dublin, Ireland

Saumitra Rawat
Consultant Laparoscopic and GI
surgeon, and surgical tutor,
East Cheshire NHS Trust; Member,
Court of Examiners,
Royal College of Surgeons of
England, London, UK

Andreas Rehm
Consultant Paediatric Orthopaedic
and Trauma Surgeon,
Depatment of Orthopaedic and
Trauma Surgery, Addenbrooke's
Hospital, Cambridge University
Hospitals NHS Trust, Cambridge,
UK

David Talbot
Consultant Transplant and
Hepatobiliary Surgeon,
Transplant Institute, Freeman
Hospital, Newcastle. Visiting
Professor, University of Sunderland.
Reader, University of Newcastle
upon Tyne, UK

Mark Whyman
Consultant General and Vascular
Surgeon,
Department of Surgery,
Cheltenham General Hospital,
Cheltenham, UK

Symbols and abbreviations

↓	decreased
↑	increased
↔	normal
→	leading to
⚠	warning
▶	important
▶▶	don't dawdle
📖	cross reference
♀	female
♂	male
1°	primary
2°	secondary
<	less than
>	more than
≥	equal to or greater than
≤	equal to or less than
%	per cent
~	approximately
≈	approximately equals to
α,	alpha
β	beta
°C	degree Celsius
AAA	abdominal aortic aneurysm
ABG	arterial blood gas
A&E	Accident and Emergency Department
ABPI	ankle–brachial pressure index
ACAS	Asymptomatic Carotid Artery Stenosis Study
ACE	angiotensin-converting enzyme
ACh	acetylcholine
AChE	acetylcholinesterase
ACJ	acromioclavicular joint
ACL	anterior cruciate ligament
ACST	Asymptomatic Carotid Surgery Trial
ACTH	adrenocorticotropic hormone
ADH	antidiuretic hormone
ADP	adenosine diphosphate

AF	atrial fibrillation
AFP	alpha-fetoprotein
AIDS	acquired immunodeficiency syndrome
AIN	anal intraepithelial neoplasia
AKA	above-knee amputation
ALI	acute lung injury
ALS	advanced life support
a.m.	*ante meridiem*
amp	ampere
AMPLE	allergy/medication/past medical history/last meal/events of the incident
ANDI	abnormalities of normal development and involution (of breast)
ANF	antinuclear factor
APA	aldosterone-producing adenoma
APACHE	Acute Physiology And Chronic Health Evaluation
APC	antigen-presenting cell *or* argon plasma coagulation
APER	abdominoperineal resection
APTR	activated partial thromboplastin time ratio
APTT	activated partial thromboplastin time
AR	aortic regurgitation
ARDS	acute respiratory distress syndrome
ARR	absolute risk reduction *or* aldosterone/renin ratio
5-ASA	5-aminosalicyclic acid
ASB	assisted spontaneous breathing
ATG	anti-thymocyte globulin
ATLS	advanced trauma life support
ATP	adenosine triphosphate
AUR	acute urinary retention
AV	arteriovenous *or* atrioventricular
AVM	arteriovenous malformation
AVN	avascular necrosis
AVS	adrenal venous sampling
AXR	abdominal X-ray
BCC	basal cell carcinoma
BCG	Bacillus Calmette–Guérin
BCR	B-cell receptor
β-HCG	beta-human chorionic gonadotrophin
BiPAP	biphasic positive airway pressure
BKA	below-knee amputation

BMI	body mass index
BMJ	*British Medical Journal*
BNF	British National Formulary
BP	blood pressure
BPH	benign prostatic hyperplasia
BS	blood sugar
BSA	body surface area
BXO	balanitis xerotica obliterans
Ca	calcium
CABG	coronary artery bypass graft
CAD	coronary artery disease
CAPD	continuous ambulatory peritoneal dialysis
CAVH	continuous arteriovenous haemofiltration
CBP	cardiopulmonary bypass
CCF	congestive cardiac failure
CD	cellular differentiation (molecule)
CDH	congenital dysplasia of the hip
CDT	*Clostridium difficile* toxin
CEA	carcinoembryonic antigen or carotid endarterectomy
CF	cystic fibrosis
CFU	colony-forming unit
CI	confidence interval
Cl	chloride
CLI	critical limb ischaemia
cm	centimetre
CMI	cell-mediated immune (reaction)
CMV	cytomegalovirus or controlled mechanical ventilation
CNI	calcineurin inhibitor
CNS	central nervous system
CNST	criminal negligence scheme for Trusts
CO	cardiac output
CO_2	carbon dioxide
COAD	chronic obstructive airway disease
COC	combined oral contraceptive
COPD	chronic obstructive pulmonary disease
CPAP	continuous positive airway pressure
CPB	cardiopulmonary bypass
C,P,&O	cysts, parasites, and ova
CPR	cardiopulmonary resuscitation
Cr	creatinine

CRCa	colorectal cancer
CRP	C-reactive protein
CSF	cerebrospinal fluid
C-spine	cervical spine
CT	computerized tomography
CTA	CT angiography
CTPA	computerized tomography pulmonary angiography
Cu	copper
CV	central venous
CVA	cerebrovascular accident
CVP	central venous pressure
CVVH	continuous venovenous haemofiltration
Cx	circumflex
CXR	chest X-ray
2D	two-dimensional
3D	three-dimensional
DA	dopamine
DALM	dysplasia-associated lesion or mass
DBD	donor after brainstem death
DC	direct current
DCD	donor after circulatory death
DCIS	ductal carcinoma *in situ*
DDAVP	1-deamino-8-D-arginine vasopressin
DDH	developmental dysplasia of the hip
DHS	dynamic hip screw
DHT	dihydrotestosterone
DIC	disseminated intravascular coagulation
DIEP	deep inferior epigastric perforator (flap)
DIPJ	distal interphalangeal joint
dL	decilitre
DM	diabetes mellitus
DMSA	dimercaptosuccinate
DNA	deoxyribonucleic acid
DNR	do not resuscitate
DOH	Department of Health
DP	distal phalanx *or* diastolic pressure
2,3-DPG	2,3-diphosphoglycerate
DPL	diagnostic peritoneal lavage
DRUJ	distal radioulnar joint
DSA	digital subtraction angiography

DTPA	diethylene triamine pentaacetic acid
DVT	deep venous thrombosis
EBV	Epstein–Barr virus
ECF	extracelllular fluid
ECG	electrocardiogram
ECST	European Cardiac Surgery Trial
ED	erectile dysfunction
e.g.	*exempli gratia* (for example)
ELISA	enzyme-linked immunosorbent assay
EMD	electromechanical delay
EMG	electromyography
EMR	endocospic mucosal resection
EOCP	(o)estrogen-containing contraceptive pill
EPL	extensor pollicis longus
EPO	erythropoietin
ER	(o)estrogen receptor
ERAS	enhanced recovery after surgery
ERCP	endoscopic retrograde cholangiopancreatography
ES	endoscopic sphincterotomy
ESD	endoscopic submucosal dissection
ESR	erythrocyte sedimentation rate
ESWL	extracorporeal shock wave lithotripsy
ET	endotracheal tube
EUA	examination under anaesthetic
EUS	endoscopic ultrasound
EVAR	endovascular aneurysm repair
EVLT	endovenous laser therapy
FAP	familial adenomatous polyposis
FAST	focused abdominal sonography for trauma
FBC	full blood count
FDP	flexor digitorum profundus
FDS	flexor digitorum superficialis
FEV_1	forced expiratory volume in 1 second
FFP	fresh frozen plasma
FiO_2	fraction of oxygen in inspired air
FLC	fibrolamellar carcinoma
FNAB	fine needle aspiration biopsy
FNAC	fine needle aspiration cytology
FPL	flexor pollicis longus
FSH	follicle-stimulating hormone

5-FU	5-fluorouracil
g	gram
G	gauge
GA	general anaesthetic
GANT	gastrointestinal autonomic nerve tumour
GCS	Glasgow coma scale
GFR	glomerular filtration rate
GGT	gamma glutamyl transferase
GH	growth hormone
GI	gastrointestinal
GIP	gastric inhibitory polypeptide
GIST	gastrointestinal stromal tumour
GMC	General Medical Council
GORD	gastro-oesophageal reflux
GP	general practitioner
GTN	glyceryl trinitrate
Gy	gray
h	hour
HAT	hepatic artery thrombosis
Hb	haemoglobin
HCC	hepatocellular carcinoma
HCG	human chorionic gonadotrophin
HCO_3	bicarbonate
HCV	hepatitis C virus
HDU	high dependency unit
HES	hydroxyethyl starch
HGV	heavy goods vehicle
HHD	handheld Doppler
HIDA	hepatobiliary iminodiacetic acid
HIT	heparin-induced thrombocytopenia
HITT	heparin-induced thrombocytopenia and thrombosis
HIV	human immunodeficiency virus
HLA	human leucocyte antigen
HMMA	4-hydroxy-3-methoxymandelic acid
HNPCC	hereditary non-polyposis colorectal cancer
H_2O	water
HPV	human papilloma virus
HR	heart rate
HRT	hormone replacement therapy
HSV	herpes simplex virus

5-HT	5-hydroxytryptamine (serotonin)
HTLV	human T-cell lymphocytotrophic virus
HVA	homovanillic acid
IABP	intra-aortic balloon pump
IC	intermittent claudication
ICA	internal carotid artery
ICD	intracardiac defibrillator
ICP	intracranial pressure
ICU	intensive care unit
i.e.	*id est* (that is)
IF	intrinsic factor
IGF	insulin growth factor
IHD	ischaemic heart disease
IM	intramuscular
IMA	inferior mesenteric artery
IMHS	intramedullary hip screw
in	inch
INPV	intermittent negative pressure ventilation
INR	international normalized ratio
IPJ	interphalangeal joint
IPPV	intermittent positive pressure ventilation
IPSS	international prostate symptom score
ITA	internal thoracic artery
ITU	intensive treatment unit
IU	international unit
IV	intravenous
IVU	intravenous urogram
J	joule
JCHST	Joint Committee on Higher Surgical Training
JVP	jugular venous pressure
K	potassium
kcal	kilocalorie
KCl	potassium chloride
kg	kilogram
kPa	kilopascal
KUB	kidneys/ureters/bladder
L	litre
LA	local anaesthetic *or* left atrium/atrial
LAD	left anterior descending (artery)
LAP	left atrial pressure

LatexAT	latex agglutination test
lb	pound
LDH	lactate dehydrogenase
LDL	low density lipid
LESS	laparoscopic and endoscopic single site (surgery)
LFT	liver function test
LH	luteinizing hormone
LHRH	luteinizing hormone releasing hormone
Li	lithium
LIF	left iliac fossa
LITA	left internal thoracic artery
LMS	left main stem
LMWH	low molecular weight heparin
LOS	lower oesophageal sphincter
LSV	long saphenous vein
LUQ	left upper quadrant
LUTS	lower urinary tract symptoms
LV	left ventricle
LVEDP	left ventricular end-diastolic pressure
LVEDV	left ventricular end-diastolic volume
LVF	left ventricular failure
m	metre
MAG3	^{99m}Tc-mercaptoacetyltriglycine
MALT	mucosa-associated lymphoid tissue
MAO	monoamine oxidase
MAP	mean arterial pressure
MCPJ	metacarpophalangeal joint
MCRP	magnetic resonance cholangiopancreatography
M,C,&S	microscopy, culture, and sensitivity
MCV	mean cell volume
MDT	multidisciplinary team
MEN	multiple endocrine neoplasia
mEq	milliequivalent
mg	milligram
Mg	magnesium
MHC	major histocompatibility complex
MHz	megahertz
MI	myocardial infarction
MIBG	meta-iodo-benzyl-guanidine
min	minute

MIP	minimally invasive parathyroidectomy
MIST	mechanism of injury/injuries identified/(vital)signs at scene/treatment administered
mL	millilitre
MMF	mycophenolate mofetil
mmHg	millimetre mercury
mmol	millimole
MMR	mismatch repair (genes)
MMV	mandatory minute ventilation
Mn	manganese
MODS	multiple organ dysfunction syndrome
mph	mile per hour
MR	mitral regurgitation
MRA	magnetic resonance angiography
MRC	Medical Research Council (scale)
MRCP	magnetic resonance cholangiopancreatogram
MRI	magnetic resonance imaging
ms	millisecond
MRSA	methicillin (or multiply) resistant *Staphylococcus aureus*
MSU	midstream urine
MTC	medullary thyroid carcinoma
mTOR	mammalian target of rapamycin
MTP	mid-thigh perforator
MTPJ	metatarsophalangeal joint
MUA	manipulation under anaesthesia
MV	mitral valve
Na	sodium
NA	noradrenaline (norepinephrine)
NaHCO$_3$	sodium bicarbonate
NAI	non-accidental injury
NASCET	North American Symptomatic Carotid Endarterectomy Trial
NBM	nil by mouth
NCEPOD	National Confidential Enquiry into Patient Outcomes and Death
NEC	necrotizing enterocolitis
ng	nanogram
NG	nasogastric
NGT	nasogastric tube
NHS	National Health Service
NICE	National Institute for Health and Clinical Excellence

NIPPV	non-invasive intermittent positive pressure ventilation
NK	natural killer (cell)
NNT	number needed to treat
N_2O	nitrous oxide
NSAID	non-steroidal anti-inflammatory drug
NSF	National Service Framework
NSGCT	non-seminomatous germ cell tumour
NSPCC	National Society for the Prevention of Cruelty to Children
NSTEMI	non-ST segment elevation myocardial infarction
NVB	neurovascular bundle
nvCJD	new variant Creutzfeldt–Jakob disease
NYHA	New York Heart Association
O_2	oxygen
OCP	oral contraceptive pill
od	*omne in die* (once a day)
OGD	oesophago-gastro-duodenoscopy
OM	obtuse marginal
OPT	orthopantomogram
ORIF	open reduction with internal fixation
PA	pulmonary artery *or* posterior-anterior
PAC	plasma aldosterone concentration
$PaCO_2$	arterial carbon dioxide tension
PAF	platelet-activating factor
PAL	primary hyperaldosteronism
PaO_2	arterial oxygen tension
PAP	pulmonary artery pressure *or* placental alkaline phosphatase
PAS	patient administration system
PAWP	pulmonary artery wedge pressure
PCA	patient-controlled analgesia
PCI	percutaneous coronary intervention
PCNL	percutaneous nephrolithotomy
pCO_2	carbon dioxide tension
PCR	polymerase chain reaction
PCV	packed cell volume *or* pressure control ventilation
PDA	posterior descending artery
PDGF	platelet-derived growth factor
PE	pulmonary embolism
PEEP	positive end-expiratory pressure
PEFR	peak expiratory flow rate
PEG	percutaneous endoscopic gastrostomy

PEP	post-exposure prophylaxis
PET	positron emission tomography
PGME	Postgraduate medical education
PH	portal hypertension
PHPT	primary hyperparathyroidism
PICC	peripherally inserted central venous catheter
PID	pelvic inflammatory disease
PIPJ	proximal interphalangeal joint
PLL	posterior longitudinal ligament
PMETB	Postgraduate Medical Education and Training Board
PMN	polymorphonuclear neutrophil
PO	orally (*per os*)
PO_2	oxygen tension
PO_4	phosphate
POSSUM	Physiologic and Operative Severity Score for the enumeration of Mortality and morbidity
PPH	procedure for prolapse and haemorrhoids
PPI	proton pump inhibitor
PPN	peripheral parenteral nutrition
PR	per rectum
prn	*pro re rata* (as required)
PS	pressure support
PSA	prostate-specific antigen
PSARP	posterior sagittal anorectoplasty
PT	prothrombin time
PTC	percutaneous transhepatic cholangiogram
PTE	pulmonary thromboembolism
PTEF	polytetrafluoroethylene
PTH	parathyroid hormone
PTLD	post-transplant lymphoproliferative disorder
PTT	partial prothrombin time
PUJ	pelviureteric junction
PV	per vagina
PVD	peripheral vascular disease
PVR	pulmonary vascular resistance
PVRI	pulmonary vascular resistance index
qds	*quater die sumandus* (four times a day)
RA	right atrial *or* rheumatoid arthritis
RAP	right atrial pressure
RCA	right coronary artery

RCT	randomized controlled trial
Rh	rhesus
rhTSH	recombinant human thyroid-stimulating hormone
RIF	right iliac fossa
RLN	recurrent laryngeal nerve
RNA	ribonucleic acid
RR	relative risk or risk ratio
RRR	relative risk reduction
RSTL	relaxed skin tension line
RTA	road traffic accident
RUQ	right upper quadrant
RV	right ventricle
s	second
SA	sinoatrial (node)
SAC	specialist advisory committee
SaO_2	arterial oxygen saturation
SBE	subacute bacterial endocarditis
SC	subcutaneous
SCAT	sheep cell agglutination test
SCC	squamous cell carcinoma
SCI	spinal cord injury
SCM	sternocleidomastoid
SD	standard deviation
SEMS	self-expanding metal stenting
SEPL	subfascial endoscopic perforator ligation
SFA	superficial femoral artery
SFJ	saphenofemoral junction
SILS	single incision laparoscopic surgery
SIMV	synchronized intermittent mandatory ventilation
SIRS	systemic inflammatory response syndrome
SL	sublingual
SLE	systemic lupus erythematosus
SMA	superior mesenteric artery
SNP	sodium nitroprusside
SPJ	saphenopopliteal junction
spp	species
STD	sodium tetradecyl sulphate
STEMI	ST segment elevation myocardial infarction
STI	sexually transmitted infection
SUFE	slipped upper femoral epiphysis

SV	stroke volume
SVC	superior vena cava
SVI	stroke volume index
SvO_2	percentage oxygen saturation of mixed venous haemoglobin
SVR	systemic vascular resistance
SVRI	systemic vascular resistance index
SVT	supraventricular tachycardia
T_3	triiodothyronine
T_4	thyroxine
TAP	transversus abdominis percutaneous
TAPS	transabdominal pre-peritoneal surgery
TB	tuberculosis
TBSA	total body surface area
TCC	transitional cell carcinoma
TCR	T-cell receptor
TCT	transitional cell tumour
tds	*ter die sumendus* (three times a day)
TEDS	thromboembolic deterrent stockings
TEMS	transanal endoscopic microsurgery
TEPS	totally extra-peritoneal surgery
TFCC	triangular fibrocartilage complex
TFT	thyroid function test
TGF	transforming growth factor
THR	total hip replacement
TIA	transient ischaemic attack
TIBC	total iron binding capacity
TIPS	transjugular intraparenchymal portosystemic shunt/stent
TKA	through-knee amputation
TKR	total knee replacement
TLSO	thoracolumbar spine orthosis
TMT	tarsometatarsal
TNF	tumour necrosis factor
TNM	tumour nodes metastasis (cancer staging)
tPA	tissue plasminogen activator
TPN	total parenteral nutrition
TRAM	transverse rectus abdominis myocutaneous (flap)
TRUS	transrectal ultrasound
H	thyroid-stimulating hormone
TT	thrombin time *or* total thyroidectomy
TTE	transthoracic echocardiogram

TUIP	transurethral incision in the prostate
TURP	transurethral resection of the prostate
TVF	transversalis fascia
U	(international) units
UADT	upper aerodigestive tract
U&E	urea and electrolytes
UC	ulcerative colitis
UCL	ulnar collateral ligament
UFH	unfractionated heparin
UK	United Kingdom
UOS	upper oesophageal sphincter
USA	United States of America
UTI	urinary tract infection
UV	ultraviolet
V	volts
VACTERL	vertebral defects/anorectal atresia/cardiac defects/ tracheo-oesophageal fistula ± (o)esophageal atresia/ renal anomalies/limb defects
VAD	ventricular assist device
VATS	video-assisted thoracoscopic surgery
VF	ventricular fibrillation
VHL	von Hippel–Lindau (disease)
VIP	vasoactive inhibitory polypeptide
VMA	vanillylmandelic acid
VQ	ventilation/perfusion (scan)
VRE	vancomycin-resistant *Enterococcus*
VT	ventricular tachycardia
VTE	venous thromboembolism
VWF	von Willebrand factor
WCC	white cell count
WHO	World Health Organization
y	year

Good surgical practice

Duties of a doctor

The General Medical Council (GMC) lists the duties of a doctor in its document *Good medical practice*.[1] The duties can be thought of under three headings (the 3 Cs): competency, communication, correctness (or probity).

Competency

- Keep your professional knowledge and skills up to date.
- Recognize the limits of your professional competence.
  - Perform an adequate assessment of the patient's conditions, based on the history and symptoms and, if necessary, an examination.
  - Arrange investigations or treatment where necessary.
  - Take suitable and prompt action when necessary.
  - Refer the patient to another practitioner when indicated.
  - Be willing to consult colleagues.
  - Keep clear, accurate, legible, and contemporaneous patient records that report relevant clinical findings, decisions made, information given to patients, and any drugs or other treatment prescribed.
  - Keep colleagues well informed when sharing the care of patients.
  - Provide the necessary care to alleviate pain and distress whether or not curative treatment is possible.
  - Prescribe drugs or treatment, including repeat prescriptions, only where you have adequate knowledge of the patient's health and medical needs. You must neither give or recommend to patients any investigation or treatment that you know is not in their best interests, nor withhold appropriate treatments or referral.
  - Report adverse drug reactions as required under the relevant reporting scheme and cooperate with requests for information from organizations monitoring the public health.
  - Take part in regular and systematic medical and clinical audit, recording data honestly, and respond to the results of audit to improve your practice, e.g. by undertaking further training.

Communication

- Treat every patient politely and considerately.
- Respect patients' dignity and privacy.
- Listen to patients and respect their views.
- Give patients information in a way they can understand.

Correctness (or probity)

- Make the care of your patient your first concern.
- Respect the rights of patients to be involved in decisions.
- Be honest and trustworthy.
- Respect and protect confidential information.
- Make sure your personal beliefs do not prejudice your patients' care.
- Act quickly to protect patients from risk if you have good reason to believe that you or a colleague may not be fit to practise.
- Avoid abusing your position as a doctor.
- Work with colleagues in the ways that best serve patients' interests.
- In an emergency, wherever it may arise, you must offer anyone at risk the assistance you could reasonably be expected to provide.

Confidentiality

Patients have a right to expect that information about them will be held in confidence by their doctors. Confidentiality is central to trust between doctors and patients. Without assurances about confidentiality, patients may be reluctant to give doctors the information they need in order to provide good care. The GMC states that if you are asked to provide information about patients, you must:

- Inform patients about the disclosure or check that they have already received information about it.
- Anonymize data where unidentifiable data will serve the purpose (this includes your surgical logbook).
- Keep disclosures to the minimum necessary.
- Keep up to date with and observe the requirements of statute and common law, including data protection legislation.

Daily practice

- When you are responsible for personal information about patients, you must make sure that it is effectively protected against improper disclosure at all times (e.g. password-protected electronic files).
- Many improper disclosures are unintentional. You should not discuss patients where you can be overheard or leave patients' records, either on paper or on screen, where they can be seen by other patients, unauthorized health care staff, or the public. You should take all reasonable steps to ensure your consultations with patients are private.
- Patients have a right to information about the health care services available to them presented in a way that is easy to follow and use.

Special circumstances

If in any doubt, contact your medical defence union for advice.

- You must disclose information to satisfy a specific statutory requirement, such as notification of a known or suspected communicable disease. Inform patients about such disclosures, wherever that is practicable, but their consent is not required.
- You must also disclose information if ordered to do so by a judge or presiding officer of a court. You should object if attempts are made to compel you to disclose what appear to you to be irrelevant matters.
- You must not disclose personal information to a third party, such as a solicitor, police officer, or officer of a court, without the patient's express consent, except when:
  - The patient is not competent to give consent.
  - Reasonable efforts to trace patients are unlikely to be successful.
  - The patient has been or may be violent, or obtaining consent would undermine the purpose of the disclosure (e.g. disclosures in relation to crime).
  - Action must be taken quickly (e.g. in the detection or control of outbreaks of some communicable diseases) and there is insufficient time to contact patients.

Reference

1 GMC (2012). Good medical practice. Available at: ℛ http://www.gmcuk.org/guidance/good_medical_practice.asp

Communication skills

Communicating with patients and relatives

When

- During admission and before discharge.
- On ward rounds.
- During clinical examinations and procedures.
- When the results of treatments are known and management changes.
- In outpatient clinics.

Where

▶ Maintain the patient's privacy. This is particularly important on an open ward. Knock on doors and close them after you. Draw the curtains round the bed. Ask a nurse to accompany you, particularly if you are explaining something complex or breaking bad news. They will have to answer the patients' and relatives' questions when you have left the ward or clinic room.

How

- Know your facts. Are you giving the right diagnosis to the right patient? Are you equipped to consent a patient for the surgical procedure?
- Sit at the same level as the person to whom you are talking, maintain appropriate eye contact, and introduce yourself.
- Find out what the patient knows and what they are expecting.
- Listen. The patient's own knowledge, state of mind, and ability to grasp concepts will dictate both how and how much you explain.
- Tell the truth. Know your facts, be sensitive to what the patient may not want to know at this stage, and do not lie.
- Avoid jargon. 'Chronic' may simply mean 'longstanding' to you; to most patients, it means 'severe'.
- Avoid vague terms. Try to describe risk quantitatively, 'a 1 in a hundred chance', rather than qualitatively, 'a small risk'.
- Check that the patient understands. Don't assume that they do.
- Help the patient to remember. Use information booklets, draw diagrams, write instructions down.
- Maintain a professional relationship. Never allow your personal likes, dislikes, and prejudices to hamper your clinical skills.

Breaking bad news

- Is there a relative or friend whom the patient might wish to have with them, who may be a source of emotional support as well as being better able to retain information?
- Know what options, if any, are available. If a cancer is inoperable, is chemotherapy planned? If an operation is cancelled, when is the next date?
- Do not be afraid to stop to allow the patient time to gather their thoughts and emotions, and recommence at a later time.
- Do not mistake numbness for calm acceptance and try not to take anger personally unless the bad news is actually your fault.

Communicating with nurses

- Introduce yourself on arrival to the staff nurse in charge.
- Establish early on which nurses are experienced. The help you get from them will be different from the questions you get from others.
- In theatre, scrub nurses are not the enemy. Your inexperience is.
- Try to remember all their names as they will remember yours.
- Do ward work efficiently. Recognize how important it is for the smooth running of the ward that your ward rounds, note-keeping, prescriptions, and discharge letters are timely and accurate.
- Let the nurses know when you are going for lunch, teaching, or sleep. If they can discuss problems now, it will save you being paged later.
- Do an evening ward round to check on problem patients and drug requirements—your sleep is less likely to be constantly interrupted.

Communication with hospital doctors

- Don't refer without first asking your consultant or registrar.
- When making requests for clinical consultations, write a concise, but clear letter in the notes to the appropriate clinician.
- When asked to see a patient, go the same day, write your opinion in the case notes, stating clearly what you recommend, and always discuss it with the seniors on your own firm.
- If a preoperative patient is complex or has significant comorbidity, contact the appropriate anaesthetist. They will help you ensure that the patient is adequately prepared for surgery.

Communication with general practitioners (GPs)

The GP has usually looked after your patient for years and, however inspired your diagnostic or operating skills, they will be there to sort out all the complications that are hidden from you once the patient is discharged. They often know your consultant well. So think!

- *Telephone the GP* in the case of a death of a patient, if you unexpectedly admit a patient, or to help with a difficult discharge.
- *Write useful, legible discharge summaries.* What would you want to know if you were going to have to wait 4 weeks for the typed discharge letter to arrive—at an absolute minimum, the date and name of the operation, post-operative complications, and plan.
- *Keep clinic letters clear and concise.*

Radiology and laboratory colleagues

- Know exactly how the investigation will change your management.
- If there is doubt about the correct investigation, telephone for advice.
- Complete request forms correctly and include clinical data. It can make a big difference, particularly if you have requested the wrong test.

Administration

- Introduce yourself to your consultant's secretary early, find out how they like things run, and then run things their way: they will usually have more than typing input on your reference.
- Produce GMC, defence union, occupational health, holiday, and study leave paperwork with good grace. They are mostly legal requirements and being rude won't change that.

Evidence-based surgery

Summarizing simple data

Table 1.1 Auditing preoperative Hb in 100 patients

Hb (g/dL)	No. of patients	Hb (g/dL)	No. of patients
7–7.9	1	11–11.9	36
8–8.9	3	12–12.9	9
9–9.9	9	13–13.9	4
10–10.9	37	14–14.9	2

This pattern of results is called a *normal* or *Gaussian distribution*: the curve is a symmetrical *bell-shaped curve*. Height, weight, age, serum sodium, and blood pressure (BP) are other examples of normally distributed data (see Table 1.1).
- The *mean* is the same as the *average*: add up every result and divide by the number of results. The average Hb here is 11.1g/dL.
- The *standard deviation* (SD) is a measure of how spread out the values are: result − mean = its deviation.

  $\sqrt{(\text{sum of deviations}^2/(\text{sample size} - 1))}$ = SD. Here SD = 1.6g/dL.
- With normally distributed data, the mean ± 1 SD includes 68% of observations; ± 2 SD includes 95%; ± 3 SD includes 99%.

This pattern of results is called a *skewed* distribution. Post-operative blood loss (see Table 1.2), length of stay, and survival all show skewed distributions.
- ▶ Don't use mean and SD to summarize skewed data.
- The mean blood requirement, which is skewed to 8U of blood because of one outlier (*), is useful for planning budgets.
- The best summary statistic for skewed data is the *median* (2U of blood) which is the value exactly halfway through the sample.
- The *interquartile range* is what the middle 50% of observations were (1–2U here) and should be used instead of SD when summarizing skewed data.

Table 1.2 Auditing post-operative blood transfusions in 100 patients

Units of blood	No. of patients	Units of blood	No. of patients
0	1	4	5
1	34	5–10	1
2	41	10–20	0
3	17	20–30	1*

* Outlier.

Tests (see Table 1.3)

Table 1.3 Sensitivity

	Disease present	No disease
Test is positive	a	b
Test is negative	c	d

Sensitivity (a/(a+c)) A measure of how good the test is at correctly identifying a positive result (>98% is very sensitive). If a very **sen**sitive test is negative, it rules the condition *out (sign out)*.

Specificity (d/(b+d)) A measure of how good the test is at correctly identifying a negative result (>98% is very sensitive). If a very **sp**ecific test is negative, it rules the condition *in (spin)*.

Likelihood ratio This is the chance that a person testing positive has the disease, divided by the chance that a person testing positive doesn't have the disease, or *sensitivity/(1 – specificity)*. A likelihood ratio >10 is large and represents an almost conclusive increase in the likelihood of disease, <0.1 is an almost conclusive decrease, and 1 signifies no change.

Treatments and hazards (see Table 1.4)

Table 1.4 Risk Assessment

	Outcome event	No outcome event
Exposure	a	b
No exposure (control)	c	d

Absolute risk reduction (ARR) a/(a+b) – c/(c+d) This is the difference in the event rate between the control and the exposed group. It reflects the prevalence of a disease and the potency of a treatment or hazard.

Relative risk or risk ratio (RR) a/(a+b)/c/(c+d) The event rate in the exposed group divided by the event rate in the control group. Used in randomized controlled trials (RCTs) and cohort studies. It is not affected by the prevalence of a disease.

Relative risk reduction (RRR) (a/(a + b) – c/(c + d))/(c/c + d) ARR divided by the control event rate. It reflects disease prevalence.

Number needed to treat (NNT) 1/ARR The number of people who must be treated to prevent one event.

Odds ratio This is the odds of an exposed person having the condition divided by the odds of the control group having the condition. If the event is rare, it approximates to relative risk. Odds ratios are less intuitive than relative risk, but they are used because they are:
• Usually larger.
• Mathematically versatile.

- Always used in case control studies and appear in meta-analyses of case control studies.
- The basis of logistic regression analysis.

Statistical significance

- Studies are designed to disprove the *null hypothesis* that findings are due to chance.
- The *p-value* is the probability of a study rejecting the null hypothesis if it were true (a *type I error*), i.e. finding a difference where none exists.
- *Statistical significance* is commonly taken as a less than 1 in 20 chance of this happening, i.e. p <0.05.
- *Power* is the probability of detecting an association if one exists. Underpowered trials contain too few patients and may make *type II errors*, accepting the null hypothesis when it is false, i.e. finding no difference where one does exist.
- *95% confidence intervals*, derived from the mean and SD, are the range of results predicted if the study were repeated 95 times.

Other useful terms

Censored data Essentially incomplete data, usually due to variable lengths of follow-up. Common in surgical studies because 1) some patients will have been lost to follow-up and 2) patients will have shorter follow-up where they had operations more recently in a study.

Actuarial and Kaplan–Meier survival Two methods used to calculate the percentage of study patients that survive a specified time after an operation when a study provides *censored data*.

Survival curves Usually not curves. A linear graph, with percentage survival (or freedom from a complication) on the x-axis and time on the y-axis, which drops as each study patient dies (or gets the complication). If there are thousands of patients in the study, the curve is smooth. If there are very few, it is possible to see individual deaths/events as steps in the graph. Ideally, these graphs should have *confidence intervals*.

Confidence intervals These reflect the precision of the study results. Narrow confidence intervals are better than wide ones because the confidence interval provides a range of values for the percentage survival (or odds ratio or other proportion) that has a specified probability (usually 95%) of containing the true value for the entire population from which the study patients were recruited. Always look for confidence intervals; they give you a 'best case and worst case' snapshot.

Regression analysis Essentially looking back from a group of patients with a known outcome (e.g. dead/alive) to see whether there were any predictors (e.g. age, recent myocardial infarction (MI)). *Univariate analysis* looks at single variables in turn. *Multivariate analysis* looks at a group of variables together; it is used to identify *independent risk factors* for an outcome. For example, age may be found to be a risk factor for post-operative death in univariate analysis, but that is because elderly patients are more likely to have other risk factors for post-operative death (e.g. recent MI). If age is not found to be an independent risk factor in multivariate analysis, it suggests that elderly people without other risk factors (e.g. recent MI) are not at higher risk of post-operative death.

Critical appraisal

Types of study
Studies appraising treatments can take several forms.

Randomized controlled trial (RCT) Prospective study in which participants are allocated to control or treatment groups on a random basis. Gold standard for assessing treatment efficacy, but time-consuming and expensive to run.

Cohort study Partly prospective study in which two cohorts of patients are identified, one of which was exposed to the treatment and one is the control group. They are followed over time to see the outcome. Cheaper and quicker than RCT and suitable for looking at prognosis, but prone to bias or false associations.

Case control study Retrospective study in which patients with the outcome of interest are identified and paired with patients without the outcome of interest, and the exposure rates are compared. Cheapest and quickest way of looking for causation. Bias arises when patients are misclassified as cases or controls.

Case series A collection of anecdotes or case reports.

Systematic review Differs from the traditional literature review by applying explicit, systematic, and reproducible methods to retrieve and appraise literature to answer a clearly formulated question. Large amounts of data are summarized and conclusions are more accurate.

Meta-analysis A mathematical synthesis of the results of two or more primary studies, increasing the statistical significance of positive overall results. However, it reduces the ability of studies to demonstrate local effects.

Levels of evidence
Studies of treatment/hazard can be arranged in order of decreasing statistical validity.
- Level 1a. Systematic review of RCTs.
- Level 1b. High quality RCT with narrow confidence intervals.
- Level 1c. All-or-none case series (either *all* patients died before treatment became available, but some now survive *or* some used to die, but now with treatment, *all* survive).
- Level 2a. Systematic review with homogeneity of cohort studies.
- Level 2b. Cohort study or low quality RCT.
- Level 2c. 'Outcomes' research.
- Level 3a. Systematic review with homogeneity of case control studies.
- Level 3b. Individual case control study.
- Level 4. Case series and poor quality cohort and case control studies.
- Level 5. Expert opinion without explicit critical appraisal or based on physiology, bench research, or first principles.

How to appraise a paper
Answer these questions systematically. This information should all be stated explicitly within the manuscript.

How relevant is the paper?
Does the paper address a clearly focused, important, and answerable clinical question that is relevant to my patients?

How valid are the findings?
- Was the paper published in an independent peer-reviewed journal?
- Does the paper define the condition to be treated, the patients to be included, the interventions to be compared, and the outcomes to be examined?
- Was a power calculation performed and is the power adequate?
- Were all clinically relevant outcomes reported?
- Was follow-up adequate?
- Were all patients accounted for at the end of the study?
- Was the appropriate study type selected and was the design appropriate?
- Were the statistical methods described and were they appropriate?
- Were the sources of error discussed?

Systematic reviews
- Is the clinical question clearly defined and an acceptable basis for including or excluding papers?
- Was the literature search thorough and were other potentially important sources explored?
- Were trials appropriately included and excluded?
- Was the methodological quality assessed and trials appropriately weighted?

RCTs
- Were patients properly randomized?
- Were patients treated equally apart from the intervention being studied?
- Was analysis on an intention-to-treat basis?
- Are confidence intervals narrow and not overlapping?

Case control studies
- Were patients correctly classified as case or control?
- Were all patients accounted for at the end of the study?

How important are the results?
- Were the results statistically significant?
- Were the results expressed in terms of numbers needed to treat and are they clinically important?

How applicable are the findings?
- Were the study patients similar to mine?
- Is the treatment feasible within my practice: is information on safety, tolerability, efficacy, and price presented?

Audit

What is audit?

National Institute for Health and Clinical Excellence (NICE) defines clinical audit as 'a quality improvement process that seeks to improve patient care and outcomes through systematic review of care against explicit criteria and the implementation of change. Aspects of the structure, processes, and outcomes of care are selected and systematically evaluated against explicit criteria. Where indicated, changes are implemented … and further monitoring is used to confirm improvement in health care delivery.'

Why do it?

Clinical audit is currently seen as the most effective way of assessing routine health care delivery and the basis of improving outcomes.
- All hospital doctors are required to fully participate in clinical audit (*NHS Plan*, Department of Health, 2000).[1]
- The GMC advises that all doctors 'must take part in regular and systematic medical and clinical audit … Where necessary, you must respond to the results of audit to improve your practice'.

How to do it

Audit of outcome or process can be divided into five stages: each stage needs to be carefully planned to produce a clinically effective audit.

Preparing for audit Choose a topic and define the purpose of the audit. One option is to identify (by consulting patients and clinicians) a potential problem that may involve high costs or risks for which there is good evidence to inform standards and that may be amenable to change. NICE stresses the importance of identifying skills and resources to carry out the audit.

Selecting audit criteria Audit can assess *process* or *outcome*.
- Define the patients to be included.
- Criteria to assess performance should be derived from the available evidence, e.g. trials, systematic reviews, society guidelines, or clinician consensus.
- Benchmarking prevents unrealistically high or low targets.

Measuring performance This is about collecting data. Identify patients or episodes from several sources (e.g. operating room logbooks and patient administration system (PAS)) to avoid missing patients because of incomplete data. Electronic information systems can improve data collection. Training dedicated audit personnel can improve the process further.

Making improvements Identify local barriers to change, develop a practical implementation plan, which should involve several interventions (practice guidelines, education, and training). Clinical governance programmes should provide the structure.

Sustaining improvements Repeating the audit to assess improvements is also called closing the audit loop. Alternatives such as critical incident review may be effective.

Measuring surgical performance

Rationale *The Kennedy report* on the enquiry into perioperative deaths in paediatric cardiac surgery at Bristol Royal Infirmary stated that 'Patients must be able to obtain information as to the relative performance of the Trust...and consultant units within the Trust'. The idea that every patient has the right to expect their surgery to be performed by a surgeon whose results are not statistically worse than average is widely held.

- League tables ranking cardiothoracic surgeons on the basis of surgeon-specific mortality data have been published by the government.
- Surgeons can be ranked using a number of other outcomes.
- Ranking should incorporate a system that accounts for differences in case mix, i.e. *risk stratification*, so that surgeons who operate on sicker or more complicated patients are not unfairly penalized.

Risk scoring systems Examples include:
- Euroscore and Parsonnet scores for predicting operative mortality in cardiac surgical patients.
- Apache II scores for intensive care patients.
- POSSUM (Physiologic and Operative Severity Score for the enUmeration of Mortality and morbidity)—variants exist for vascular and colorectal surgery.

Presenting results The aim of presenting performance data is to distinguish between normal variation between surgeons or institutions and significant divergence. There are three main ways of doing this:
- Average outcome over a given time frame.
  - Ranking or league tables of surgical mortality or other complications; the data may be crude or risk-stratified (i.e. taking into account the case mix).
  - Survival plots which may also be crude or risk-stratified.
  - Standardized mortality ratio plots.
- Volume and outcome control charts.
  - Funnel plots (see Fig. 1.1).
  - Spectrum plots.
- Performance trends over time.
  - Cumulative summation charts (CUSUM).
  - Variable life-adjusted display charts (VLAD), risk-adjusted CUSUM.

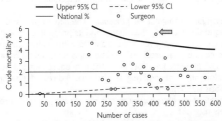

Fig. 1.1 Funnel plot of mortality data for 50 cardiac surgeons. The arrow marks an outlier with mortality outside 95% confidence intervals (CI).

Reference

1 Department of Health. (2000). The NHS Plan: a plan for investment, a plan for reform. Available at: ℘ http://www.dh.gov.uk/en/Publicationsandstatistics/Publications/PublicationsPolicyAndGuidance/ DH_4002960

Consent

Legal aspects

Successful surgery depends on a relationship of trust between the patient and doctor. The patient's right to autonomy must be respected, even if their decision results in harm or death. This right is protected by law.

- A doctor performing a procedure on a patient without their consent can be found guilty of *battery*.
- A doctor who has failed to give the patient adequate information to allow them to give informed consent can be found guilty of *negligence*.
- *No adult in the United Kingdom (UK) can legally consent to surgery on behalf of another adult.* It is important to involve relatives, particularly where patients are unable to consent, but their wishes are *not* legally binding and do not form part of the legal consent.

Obtaining consent

The key to good consenting is good communication (see 📖 p. 4). It may be necessary to use a translator and some Trusts will not accept consent gained by using patients' relatives as translators. GMC guidelines state 'If you are the doctor providing treatment or undertaking an investigation, it is your responsibility to discuss it with the patient and obtain consent'. In practice, this may be done verbally by the consultant or registrar in clinic, or on a ward round with a house officer obtaining written confirmation later. Consent must be given freely: patients may not be put under duress by clinicians, employers, police, or others to undergo tests or treatment. Declare any potential conflicts of interest. The *amount* of information should be sufficient to allow a mentally competent patient to make an informed decision. It will vary according to the individual, the nature of the condition, the complexity of treatment, and risks involved. It is unacceptable to limit the amount of information on the basis that it may cause distress, but be sympathetic to the patients' needs. Consent must be obtained for taking photographs for teaching or publication, and taking samples for research.

Informed consent

There are five aspects that the patient must understand to give informed consent:

- *The reason for carrying out the procedure.* The patient needs to understand the nature of their illness and its prognosis.
- *What the procedure involves.* Where and how long is the scar; what is being removed; what prosthesis will be implanted; will there be drains?
- *The risks of the procedure.* Specific to the procedure (e.g. stoma, limb dysfunction) and in general (e.g. anaesthesia, bed rest, deep vein thrombosis (DVT)).
- *The benefits of the procedure.* Improvement in symptoms or prognosis or purely diagnostic.
- *Alternatives.* Including conservative treatment, with their advantages and disadvantages.

Modes of consent

- *Implied consent.* The patient is presumed to consent to minor procedures, e.g. X-rays, phlebotomy, by cooperating with ward procedures.
- *Express written consent.* Whenever possible, this should be obtained for all patients undergoing procedures involving an anaesthetic, complex treatments with significant risks and side effects, or as part of research. *Written consent is not legal proof that adequate consent was obtained* at the time the document was signed.
- *Express verbal consent.* Should be obtained when it is not possible to get written consent, witnessed by an independent health care professional, and documented in the notes accordingly, or for simple procedures with minimal risk of harm.

Special considerations

Emergencies When consent cannot be obtained, you may provide emergency medical treatment, provided it is limited to what is needed to preserve life. However, you must respect any valid advance refusals that you know about or that are drawn to your attention.

Mentally incapable patients No adult in the UK can legally consent to surgery on behalf of another adult. Assess the patient's competence to make an informed decision. If unable to decide, and provided they comply, treatment may be instigated that is judged to be in their best interests. Otherwise, treatment may be carried out under the Mental Health Act 1989. Controversial and non-therapeutic treatments (e.g. sterilizations) require court approval.

Advance statements/living wills Advance statements made by patients before losing the capacity of informed consent must be respected, provided the decision is applicable to the present circumstances and there is no reason to believe that they may have changed their minds. The known wishes of the patient should be taken into consideration if an advance statement is unavailable.

Children
- Over 16s are regarded as young adults and have capacity to decide.
- Under 16s may give their own consent if they are judged to understand what is involved.
- Unlike adults, where a competent child refuses treatment, a person with parental responsibility (except in Scotland) or a court may authorize treatment if deemed in the child's best interests.
- If the parents refuse treatment deemed in the child's best interests, you are not bound by this and may seek a ruling from the court.
- Emergency treatment may be instigated without consent in a similar manner to that in adults.

Pregnancy The right to autonomy applies equally to pregnant women. It includes the right to refuse treatment that is intended to benefit the unborn child.

Death

Confirming death

There is no legal definition of death in the UK. It is generally regarded as the cessation of circulation and respiration.

- Clinically, there is:
  - No respiratory effort, denoted by the absence of breath sounds on auscultation over 1min.
  - Absence of a palpable pulse and heart sounds over 1min.
  - No response to painful stimuli, e.g. sternal or supraorbital rub.
  - Fixed dilated pupils (beware drugs such as atropine).
- If there is doubt, perform an electrocardiogram (ECG).
- Hypothermia (core temperature <34°C) must have been corrected.

Brain death/brainstem death

The concept of *brain death* has arisen from the advances in intensive therapy, and the ability to maintain cardiac and respiratory function artificially in patients who have sustained severe irreversible brain damage. Brain death is defined as the 'irreversible cessation of all functions of the entire brain, including the brainstem'.[1] This, alongside the traditional definition, is taken to equate to death in the UK, United States of America (USA), Australia, and many other countries. In order to diagnose brain death, a number of strict criteria must be met.

- An identifiable cause for the brain death must be established, e.g. severe head injury/intracerebral bleed, *and*
- Other causes, including central nervous system (CNS) depressants, hypothermia, metabolic and endocrine disturbance, need to be excluded, *and*
- The patient is unable to breathe spontaneously despite adequate CO_2 drive (i.e. $PaCO_2$ >6.7kPa), *and*
- The following brainstem reflex tests, performed by the consultant in charge (or deputy of 5y registration) and another suitably experienced doctor, have been failed on two separate occasions, usually 24h apart:
  - Both pupils are fixed and unresponsive to light (oculomotor nerve).
  - Corneal reflexes are absent (trigeminal nerve).
  - Vestibulo-ocular reflexes are absent (absent eye movements when 20mL of ice-cold water is injected into each ear with tympanic membranes visualized beforehand) (vestibulo-cochlear nerve).
  - Absent motor responses to painful stimuli in the distribution of the cranial nerves in the absence of neuromuscular blockade (spinal cord injury may ablate peripheral motor responses).
  - Absence of respiratory effort when disconnected from the ventilator despite a $PaCO_2$ >6.7kPa (↑ in chronic obstructive pulmonary disease (COPD)).
  - Absent gag and cough reflex upon pharyngeal and endotracheal stimulation.

Coroners

It is always wise to discuss with the consultants involved if there is any reason to discuss cases with the coroner's officer. Poor quality information can lead to death certificates being returned or the coroner becoming involved unnecessarily.

In-hospital deaths must be discussed with the coroner's officer if:
- Death has occurred during an operation.
- Death occurred before recovery from anaesthetic.
- More than 14 days have elapsed since the patient last saw a doctor.
- There is doubt about the cause of death.
- Death is thought to be suspicious (e.g. caused by overdoses of prescribed substances, medical error, suicide).

Certifying death

Documenting in the medical notes

If you are asked to 'certify' a patient, first confirm death (see 📖 p. 16):
- Document the date and time that death was pronounced.
- Document your examination.
- Document the causes of death as they will appear on the death certificate *if* these have been decided. ▶ If in doubt, always speak to the consultant.

The death certificate

This can be issued by anyone with full medical qualifications who looked after the patient during their last illness, or where referral to the coroner has been made and permission to issue the certificate has been granted.
- Write legibly. The record is retained by the relatives and illegible or incomplete certificates may be rejected by the funeral director.
- *Part I*. The cause of death. Events leading to Ia are listed in Ib and Ic.
- *Part II*. Conditions that *contributed to*, but did not directly cause death.
- General terms like heart failure and sepsis may not be accepted.

Cremation forms

These forms vary slightly between regions, but certain rules always apply.
- There are two parts. The first is filled in by a doctor who attended the patient during the illness leading up to death, the second by an independent clinician who has been fully registered for at least 5y.
- They should not be issued if the cause of death is not established.
- It is the responsibility of the issuing doctor to ensure that they have seen and identified the person after death, and that there are no radioactive implants or pacemakers present.

Post-mortems

- A *coroner's post-mortem* is required for suspicious deaths, but is most commonly performed where the Coroner's Office has 'taken' a case where the cause of death is uncertain, or may be related to surgery or interventions. The consent of relatives is not necessary to proceed.
- A *hospital post-mortem* may be carried out with the consent of relatives to investigate other deaths. In 60% of post-mortems in one series, new diagnoses that would have substantially changed management were found—they are a vital part of audit.

Reference

1 (1981). Guidelines for the determination of death: report of the medical consultants on the diagnosis of death to the president's commission for the study of ethical problems in medicine and biomedical and behavioral research. *J Am Med Assoc* **246**, 2184–6.

End-of-life issues

Do not resuscitate (DNR) orders

A DNR order should be considered when the frailty, comorbidity (e.g. inoperable disseminated malignancy, multiple organ failure), maximal medical treatment, or advanced age of a patient means that any attempt at cardiopulmonary resuscitation (CPR) in the event of a cardiac or respiratory arrest will be futile. DNR decisions should be reached on a case by case basis: a blanket 'do not resuscitate' policy based on a specific patient group, such as elderly patients, is unacceptable. An 84-y-old patient who was an appropriate candidate for cardiac surgery is an appropriate candidate for CPR post-operatively, whereas a 72-y-old patient undergoing palliative care for end-stage hepatorenal failure is probably not.

- Never make a DNR decision without discussing it with a consultant.
- Patients and, where appropriate, their relatives must be involved.
- Document the clinical reasons for the DNR order and state explicitly whether 'full active medical management' is to be continued: DNR orders do not always include withdrawing treatment. Discuss each case with the nurses involved.
- Complete the appropriate documentation and review process, which varies from Trust to Trust, and make sure the nursing staff are fully aware so that they do not call the arrest team when the patient dies.

Euthanasia

Euthanasia is the painless termination of life at the request of the patient concerned. In the UK, *it is illegal to administer any drug to accelerate death*, irrespective of how compassionate the motive may be. Withdrawing futile treatment is not euthanasia. UK law states that the intention to kill is malicious and such action would be classified as murder. Terminally ill people and the parents of terminally ill or severely disabled children may have several reasons for requesting euthanasia. Effective palliative care, counselling, and multidisciplinary support should be able to address most of these reasons, which include:

- Pain.
- Disability.
- Disfigurement.
- Depression.
- Fear of being a burden, being unable to cope.

Palliative care

Palliative care is surgical, medical, and nursing care aimed specifically at relieving the problems associated with terminal conditions when the possibility of cure has been abandoned. Palliative care is delivered by palliative medicine and nursing specialists and can take place in the community or in residential care settings. Refer early: palliative care beds are limited and acute surgical wards are rarely the best places for dying patients. Palliative care physicians specialize in:

- Control of symptoms, including pain, anorexia, nausea and vomiting, confusion, dysphagia, dyspnoea, incontinence.

- Psychological aspects of terminal illness.
- Bereavement.

Suicide The suicide rate in the UK is currently 12.5 per 100 000.
Patients at risk
- The recently bereaved.
- Cancer patients have a five times increased risk.
- Men over 55y with oral cancer and a history of alcohol abuse.
- Women of any age, often suffering from gynaecological or breast cancer. (In both of these latter groups, the treatment of the disease involves disfigurement and a change of body image.)

Action
Patients about to undergo disfiguring surgery for any reason should be counselled carefully in the period after confirmation of the diagnosis and before surgery. Doctors should discuss all treatment options and implications clearly. The support of a 'mastectomy counsellor' or 'stoma therapist' is invaluable. Post-operatively:
- Look for symptoms of depression, including low mood, tearfulness, anorexia, early morning waking, suicidal thoughts, especially in long-term patients.
- Do not discontinue antidepressant medication.
- Ensure that arrangements for discharge include community nursing support and that the GP is aware of the patient's state of mind.

Organ donation
- When brain death is established, organ donation should be considered for all patients who are under 75y of age with no history of malignant disease or major untreated sepsis.
- All donors should be tested for human immunodeficiency virus (HIV), hepatitis B and C, herpes simplex virus (HSV), and cytomegalovirus (CMV).
- Organ donation is usually coordinated by regional transplant teams.
- The body should be identified and next of kin contacted.
- If, despite reasonable attempts, the identity of the corpse or next of kin remains unknown, the body becomes the property of the health authority.
- If a donor card is present, it is reasonable to assume that the deceased wished to donate his organs and the transplant team can proceed.
- If relatives are identified and do not wish organ donation to proceed, even though there is a donor card, their wishes must be respected.
- Relatives should be asked to act as agents in expressing what they believe to be the wishes of the patient. Ideally, the person seeking permission should be someone whom they already know. This may be the consultant in charge, but, on occasion, a senior staff nurse, chaplain (or other religious figure), or the family GP may be more appropriate.
- In the case of accidental deaths, the coroner's permission should be sought before proceeding.

Clinical governance

Clinical governance is the system through which National Health Service (NHS) organizations are accountable for continuously improving the quality of their services. Clinical governance involves setting standards, performance monitoring, and reporting systems at national, institutional, and personal levels. *Risk management* is an integral part of clinical governance: it is the systematic identification and avoidance of risks associated with any procedure.

Setting standards

In addition to conventional clinical evidence and guidelines, the following organizations have a responsibility for setting standards in health care.

National Service Frameworks (NSFs)

NSFs are long-term national strategies for improving specific areas of care, produced by government after consultation with clinicians. They set standards and establish methods of delivering them. NSFs have been published for coronary heart disease and cancer.

National Institute for Health and Clinical Excellence (NICE)

NICE is the governmental organization responsible for setting standards by reviewing the best available evidence and publishing guidelines. Local authorities are obliged to fund interventions recommended by NICE, but NICE guidance does not overrule individual clinical decision-making. Currently, NICE produces three kinds of guidance:
- *Technology appraisals.* Guidance on the use of new and existing medicines and treatments within the NHS in England and Wales.
- *Clinical guidelines.* Guidance on the appropriate treatment and care of people with specific conditions within the NHS in England and Wales.
- Guidance on whether *interventional procedures* used for diagnosis or treatment are safe enough and work well enough for routine use in England, Wales, and Scotland.

Postgraduate Medical Education and Training Board (PMETB) and professional organizations

The PMETB was set up in 2003 to develop a single, unifying framework for postgraduate medical education (PGME) and training across the UK.
- Medical ethics, undergraduate and pre-registration medical education, and fitness to practise remain the responsibility of the GMC.
- Accreditation and the approval of basic surgical training remain the responsibility of the Royal Colleges of Surgeons.
- Higher surgical training is supervised by the Joint Committee on Higher Surgical Training (JCHST) and the specialist advisory committees (SACs).

Performance monitoring

Healthcare Commission (replaces CHI and the Audit Commission)

The Healthcare Commission is a new body that has been set up to help improve the quality of health care. It will do this by providing an independent assessment of the standards of services, whether they are provided by the NHS, independent health services, or voluntary organizations. It provides an independent second stage of complaints assessment, assesses the arrangements in place to promote public health, and acts as the coordinating inspectorate in relation to health care.

National Confidential Enquiry into Patient Outcomes and Death (NCEPOD)

NCEPOD (which used to be the National Confidential Enquiry into PeriOperative Deaths) is an organization independent of the Department of Health (DOH) and the professional associations, although it receives over 85% of its funding from the DOH via NICE. It stopped collecting data on all deaths within 30 days of surgery in 2002 when its remit was extended to cover all medical and surgical deaths. Data is now collected by local reporters in response to specific areas of research.

National Patient and User Survey The Healthcare Commission has carried out five national surveys involving over 500 institutions and 300 000 patients. The results are disseminated to health care providers and governmental agencies to inform strategy.

Audit See 📖 p. 12.

Revalidation The purpose of revalidation will be to create public confidence that all licensed doctors are up to date and fit to practise. Currently, consultants and general practitioners undergo regular appraisal: this will be included within revalidation which is yet to be introduced.

Reporting systems

Critical incident reporting Critical incident reporting was initially voluntary and anonymous. Incidents perceived to have exposed patients or staff to actual or potential risk were reported on forms that would be sent to responsible individuals in each directorate, serious adverse events being discussed at regular meetings with the clinical director. Now effective critical incident reporting systems are a requirement for CNST (criminal negligence scheme for Trusts) insurance and are assessed by the Healthcare Commission on Trust visits.

Complaints Patients make formal complaints about treatment or clinicians to the hospital concerned: the new NHS complaints procedure, which was reformed in 2002 to address concerns that it was fragmented, complex, and insufficiently independent, still stresses that wherever possible, issues should be resolved locally. Effective use of the patient advice and liaison services (PALS) and independent complaints advocacy service (ICAS) should mean that only serious complaints are referred to the second level, which is handled by the Healthcare Commission which currently handles 3000–5000 complaints per annum.

Whistle-blowing Trusts are required to have a whistle-blowing policy to enable individual staff members to express concerns about treatment and to protect them from reprisals. The policy must include a mechanism for investigating and acting on such claims.

Principles of surgery

Terminology in surgery

How to describe an operation

The terminology used to describe all operations is a composite of basic Latin or Greek terms.

First describe the organ to be operated on

Examples:
- lapar-, abdomen (*laparus* = flank);
- nephro-, kidney;
- pyelo-, renal pelvis;
- cysto-, bladder;
- chole-, bile/the biliary system;
- ileo-, small bowel (distal)
- col(on)-, large bowel;
- hystero-, uterus;
- thoraco-, chest;
- rhino-, nose;
- masto/mammo-, breast.

Second describe any other organs or things involved in the procedure

Examples:
- docho-, duct;
- angio-, vessel (blood- or bile-carrying);
- litho-, stone.

Third describe what is to be done

Examples:
- -otomy, to cut (open);
- -ectomy, to remove;
- -plasty, to change shape or size;
- -pexy, to change position;
- -raphy, to sew together;
- -oscopy, to look into;
- -ostomy, to create an opening in (*stoma* = mouth);
- -paxy, to crush;
- -graphy/gram, image (of).

Lastly add any terms to qualify how or where the procedure is done

Examples:
- percutaneous, via the skin;
- trans-, across;
- antegrade, forward;
- retrograde, backward;
- ventral, anterior surface of.

Examples of terms

- *Choledochoduodenostomy*. An opening between the bile duct and the duodenum.
- *Rhinoplasty*. Nose reshaping.
- *Pyelolithopaxy*. Destruction of pelvicalyceal stones.

- *Bilateral mastopexy.* Breast lifts.
- *Percutaneous arteriogram.* Arterial tree imaging by direct puncture injection.
- *Loop ileostomy.* External opening in the small bowel with two sides.
- *Flexible cystourethroscopy.* Internal bladder and urethral inspection.

History taking and making notes

Making medical notes

All medical and paramedical professionals have a duty to record their input and care of patients in the case notes. These form a permanent legal and medical document. There are some basic rules.

- Write in blue or black ink; other colours do not photocopy well.
- Date, time, and sign all entries; always identify retrospective entries.
- Be accurate.
- Make it clear which diagnoses are provisional.
- Abbreviations are lazy and open to misinterpretation; avoid them.
- Clearly document information given to patients and relatives.
- Avoid non-medical judgements of patients or relatives.

Basics

- Always record name, age, occupation, and method of presentation.
- Cover all the principal areas of medical history:
  - Presenting complaint and past history relevant to it.
  - Other past medical history, drug history, and systematic enquiry.
  - Previous operations/allergies/drugs.
  - Family history, social history, and environment.

Presenting complaint

This is a one- or two-word summary of the patient's main symptoms, e.g. abdominal pain, nausea and vomiting, swollen leg, PR bleeding.

- In emergency admissions, do not write a diagnosis here (e.g. ischaemic leg). The diagnosis of referral may well turn out to be wrong.
- In elective admissions, it is reasonable to write: 'elective admission for varicose vein surgery'.

History of presenting complaint

- This is a detailed description of the main symptom and should include the relevant systems enquiry.
- Try to put the important positives first, e.g. right-sided lower abdominal pain, sharp, worse with moving, and coughing, anorexia 24h.
- Include the relevant negatives, e.g. no vomiting, no PR bleeding.
- Be very clear about the chronology of events.
- In a complicated history or with multiple symptoms, use headings, e.g. 'Current episode', 'Previous operations for this problem', 'Results of investigations'.
- Summarize the results of investigations performed prior to admission systematically: bedside tests, blood tests, histology or cytology, X-rays, cross-sectional imaging, specialized tests.

Past medical history

- Ask about thyroid problems, tuberculosis (TB), hypertension, rheumatic fever, epilepsy, asthma, diabetes, ischaemic heart disease, stroke, and previous surgery, specifically.
- List and date all previous operations.
- Ask about previous problems with an anaesthetic.
- Asking 'Have you *ever* had any medical problem or been to hospital for anything?' at the end often produces additional information.

Systematic enquiry

This is extremely important and often neglected. A genitourinary history is highly relevant in young females with pelvic pain. A good cardiovascular and respiratory systems enquiry will help avoid patients being cancelled because they have undiagnosed anaesthetic risks. Older patients may have pathology in other systems that may change management, e.g. the patient with prostatism should be warned about urinary retention.

- *Cardiovascular.* Chest pain, effort dyspnoea, orthopnoea, nocturnal dyspnoea (see 🕮 p. 58), palpitations, swollen ankles, strokes, transient ischaemic attacks, claudication.
- *Respiratory.* Dyspnoea, cough, sputum, wheeze, haemoptysis.
- *Gastrointestinal.* Anorexia, change in appetite, weight loss (quantify how much, over how long).
- *Genitourinary.* Sexual activity, dyspareunia (pain on intercourse), abnormal discharge, last menstrual period.
- *Neurological.* 3 Fs: fits; faints; funny turns.

Social history

- At what time did they last eat or drink?
- Ask who will look after the patient. Do they need help to mobilize?
- Smoking and alcohol history.

▶ Tips for case presentation

- *Practise.* Every case is a possible presentation to someone!
- *Always 'set the scene' properly.* Start with name, age, occupation, and any key medical facts together with the main presenting complaint(s).
- *Be chronological.* Start at the beginning of any relevant prodrome or associated symptoms; they are likely to be an important part of the presenting history.
- *Be concise with the past medical history.* Only expand on things that you really feel may be relevant either to the diagnosis or management, e.g. risks of general anaesthesia.
- For systematic examination techniques, see the relevant following pages.
- Always summarize the general appearance and vital signs first.
- Describe the most significant systemic findings first, but be systematic—'inspection, palpation, percussion, and auscultation'.
- *Briefly summarize other systemic findings.* Only expand on them if they may be directly relevant to the diagnosis or management.
- Finally, *summarize and synthesize*—don't repeat. Try to group symptoms and signs together into clinical patterns and recognized scenarios.
- Finish with a proposed diagnosis or differential list and be prepared to discuss what diagnostic or further evaluation tests might be necessary.

Common surgical symptoms

Pain

Pain anywhere should have the same features elicited. These can be summarized by the acronym SOCRATES.

- **S**ite. Where is the pain, is it localized, in a region, or generalized?
- **O**nset. Gradual, rapid, or sudden? Intermittent or constant?
- **C**haracter. Sharp, stabbing, dull, aching, tight, sore?
- **R**adiation. Does it spread to other areas? (From loin to groin in ureteric pain, to shoulder tip in diaphragmatic irritation, to back in retroperitoneal pain, to jaw and neck in myocardial pain.)
- **A**ssociated symptoms. Nausea, vomiting, dysuria, jaundice?
- **T**iming. Does it occur at any particular time?
- **E**xacerbating or relieving factors. Worse with deep breathing, moving, or coughing suggests irritation of somatic nerves either in the pleura or peritoneum; relief with hot water bottles suggests deep inflammatory or infiltrative pain.
- **S**urgical history. Does the pain relate to surgical interventions?

Dyspepsia (epigastric discomfort or pain, usually after eating) What is the frequency? Is it always precipitated by food or is it spontaneous in onset? Is there any relief, especially with milky drinks or food? Is it positional?

Dysphagia (difficulty during swallowing) Is the symptom new or long-standing? Is it rapidly worsening or relatively constant? Is it worse with solid food or fluids? (Worse with fluids suggests a motility problem, rather than a stenosis.) Can it be relieved by anything, e.g. warm drinks? Can the patient point to a 'level' of hold-up on the surface (usually related to the sternum)? This often accurately relates to the level of an obstructing lesion. Is it associated with 'spluttering' (suggests tracheo-oesophageal fistula or inhalation of food/fluid).

Oesophageal reflux (bitter or acidic tasting fluid in the pharynx or mouth) How frequently? What colour is it? (Green suggests bile whereas white suggests only stomach contents). When does it occur (lying only, on bending, spontaneously when standing)? Is it associated with coughing?

Haematemesis (the presence of blood in vomit) What colour is the blood (dark red-brown 'coffee grounds' is old or small-volume stomach bleeding; dark red may be venous from the oesophagus; bright red is arterial and often from major gastric or duodenal arterial bleeding)? What volume has occurred over what period? Did the blood appear with the initial vomits or only after a period of prolonged vomiting (suggests a traumatic oesophageal cause).

Abdominal distension Symmetrical distension suggests one of the '5 Fs' (fluid ascites, flatus due to ileus or obstruction, fetus of pregnancy, fat, or a 'flipping big mass'). Asymmetrical distension suggests a localized mass. What is the time course? Does it vary? It is changed by vomiting, passing stool/flatus?

Change in bowel habit May be change in frequency or looser or more constipated stools. Increased frequency and looser stools is more likely than isolated constipation to be due to a pathological cause. Is it a persistent or transient? Are there associated symptoms? Is it variable?

Frequency and urgency of defecation New urgency of defecation is almost always pathological. What is the degree of urgency—how long can the patient delay? Is there associated discomfort? What is passed—is the stool normal?

Bleeding per rectum What colour is the blood? Is it pink-red and only on the paper when wiping? Does it splash in the pan? (Both suggest a case from the anal canal.) Is it bright red on the surface of the stool (suggests a lower rectal cause)? Is the blood darker with clots or marbled into the stools (suggests a colonic cause)? Is the blood fully mixed with the stool or altered (suggests a proximal colonic cause)?

Tenesmus (desire to pass stools with either no result or incomplete satisfaction of defecation) Suggests rectal pathology.

Jaundice (yellow discoloration due to hyperbilirubinaemia; 📖 p. 312) How quickly did the jaundice develop? Is there associated pruritus? Are there any symptoms of pain, fever, or malaise (suggests infection)?

Haemoptysis (the presence of blood in expectorate) What colour is the blood? (Light pink froth suggests pulmonary oedema.) Are there clots or dark blood (infection or endobronchial lesion)? How much blood? Moderate bleeds quickly threaten airways: get help quickly.

Dyspnoea (difficulty in or increased awareness of breathing) When does the dyspnoea occur—quantify the amount of effort. Is it positional?
- *Orthopnoea.* Difficulty in breathing that occurs on lying flat; quantify it by asking how many pillows the patient needs at night to remain symptom-free.
- *Paroxysmal nocturnal dyspnoea.* Intermittent breathlessness at night. Both orthopnoea and paroxysmal nocturnal dyspnoea suggest cardiac failure.

Claudication (the presence of pain in the muscles of the calf, thigh, or buttock precipitated by exercise and relieved by rest) After what degree of exercise does the pain occur (both distance on the flat and gradients)? How quickly is the pain relieved by rest?

Rest pain (pain in a limb at rest without significant exercise) How long has the pain been present? Is it intermittent? Does it occur mainly at night? Is it relieved by dependency of the limb involved?

Dysuria (pain on passing urine) When does the pain occur (beginning, end, or throughout the stream)? Is it felt in the penis or suprapubically? Is it associated with frequency? Is the urine discoloured or does it contain debris?

Haematuria (blood in the urine) Does the blood occur at the start (suggests bladder origin), during, or end (suggests prostatic or penile origin) of the stream? Is there associated pain (suggests infection or stone disease)?

Evaluation of breast disease

Positioning and inspection

Breasts are best examined semi-recumbent and then sitting upright. Initially, the arms are by the side, semi-recumbent. After initial inspection, they should be positioned 'hands on hips', sitting upright (initially relaxed and then with forced pressure on the hips to tense the pectoral muscles), and finally abducted slowly above the head. For palpation, the hands should return to the hips and the patient may lie back semi-recumbent again.

Inspection is critical and should concentrate on the following.

• *Overall symmetry and position.* Are the breasts the same size? Is there deformity due to underlying disease? Is the position normal?
• *Skin appearance.* Is the skin erythematous or oedematous? Is there fixed lymphoedema of the skin ('peau d'orange')? Are there scars from previous surgery?
• *Skin tethering.* Does the skin move freely as the arms are raised? (Tethering is suggestive of underlying intraparenchymal scarring or tumour.)
• *Nipples.* Are the nipples indrawn, deviated, or ulcerated (suggestive of retroareolar tumour or infection)? Is there any evidence of discharge?

Palpation

Use the flat of the fingers and use all four fingers at once. Palpate the 'normal' breast first. Be methodical and don't 'knead' the breast. A common routine is: upper outer quadrant; lower outer; lower inner; upper inner; central (retroareolar); supraclavicular fossa; axilla. Features to look for include the following:

• *Palpable mass.* Is it hard, irregular, and tethered (cancer) or smooth, rounded, and mobile (cysts or fibroadenoma)?
• *Diffuse nodularity.* Typical of benign disease.
• *Nipple discharge.* On palpation of the central area. Blood suggests tumour; pus suggests infection; serous or milky may not be relevant.
• *Axillary and supraclavicular lymphadenopathy.* Is it multiple and tethered (cancer)?

Investigations

Ultrasound

• Easy to perform and painless—often done in breast outpatient clinic.
• Avoids radiation dose in young women.
• Highly sensitive for differentiating between solid tumours and cysts.

Mammography

• Used both for population screening and diagnostic testing.
• Uncomfortable for most women and involves a low radiation dose.
• Able to identify impalpable lesions.
• Able to identify premalignant lesions (e.g. ductal carcinoma *in situ*).
• Mammographic features of malignancy include: spiculated microcalcification; irregularity; stellate outline.

Aspiration cytology
- Well tolerated, easy to perform, and quick to report on—often done in one half day during breast outpatient clinic.
- Does not provide histology: provides only cellular information and relies upon cellular atypia for a diagnosis of malignancy.
- Does not differentiate between invasive and *in situ* carcinoma.
- Occasionally therapeutic for cysts.
- Good sensitivity and specificity.

Guided core biopsy
- Performed under ultrasound or mammographic guidance using a Trucut® needle or similar device.
- Can be done under general or local anaesthetic.
- Provides actual histology information—allows cancers to be graded.
- Able to differentiate between invasive and carcinoma *in situ*.
- Highly sensitive and specific.

Computerized tomography (CT) scanning
- Relatively non-specific for local breast pathology.
- Useful for assessment of extensive local invasion and regional and systemic staging.

CT positron emission tomography (PET) scanning
- Occasionally used to assess indeterminate lesions identified on plain CT and identify unsuspected metastatic disease.

Magnetic resonance imaging (MRI) scanning
- Occasionally used for the assessment of local breast pathology.

Key revision points—anatomy of the breast
- Breast comprises epithelial ductal tissue, epithelial secretory lobules, fat, and connective tissue.
- It is divided into four 'quadrants' and a peri/retroareaolar central zone for clinical description of abnormalities.
- The **areola** is the pigmented area around each nipple.
- The **arterial supply** is from segmental perforators from the **internal thoracic artery** (ITA).
- **Lymphatic drainage**—important in breast cancer management.
  - Non-pathological lymph drainage is almost entirely to the axillary nodes.
  - Medial half can occasionally drain to internal mammary nodes.
  - Lymph nodes are divided into three levels (1, below; 2, behind; 3, above pectoralis minor).

Evaluation of the neck

Evaluation of carotid artery disease is described on 📖 p. 658.

Positioning and inspection

- Sit the patient upright at rest with the head looking straight ahead. Inspect the neck from the front, side, and, if necessary, behind.
- Observe the neck at rest and during swallowing (a glass of water). If necessary, inspect rotation left and right.
- Observe the neck while asking the patient to protrude the tongue.

Inspection includes looking for the following.

- *Overall symmetry and lumps.* Are there obvious lumps? Are they single or multiple? Is the lump lying in or close to the midline? Does the lump move with swallowing (suggests thyroid-related lesion)?
- *Skin abnormalities.* Are there any ulcers of sinuses (suggests chronic infection such as TB)?
- *Associated structures.* Is there evidence of venous engorgement or collateral vessels visible?

Palpation

Be systematic; palpate the regions of the neck in order. Use both hands with the flats of the fingers to compare each side, but move only one hand at once to prevent 'cross-palpation'. A typical sequence of palpation is: anterior triangle (bottom to top); submental area; submandibular area; posterior triangle (top to bottom); supraclavicular fossae; parotid, pre-auricular and post-auricular areas. Repalpate the neck with the patient swallowing a mouthful of water—particularly the anterior triangle (see Fig. 2.1). Lastly, feel specifically for the carotid arteries.

- *Lumps.* Is it single or multiple (multiple strongly suggests lymphadenopathy)? Is it strictly in the midline (likely to be related to the thyroid)? Does it move with swallowing (almost always thyroid-related)? What are the general features (see 📖 p. 42)?
- *Thyroid lumps.* Is it unilateral or bilateral? Does it move with tongue protrusion?
- *Carotid arteries.* Are they normal, ecstatic, or aneurysmal?
- *Supraclavicular fossae.* Is there associated lymphadenopathy (suggests malignancy)?

Auscultation Listen to the carotid arteries and any large masses for bruits, suggesting a hypervascular local circulation or stenosis.

Investigations

Ultrasound

- Easy to perform and painless.
- Avoids radiation dose.
- Highly sensitive for the differentiation between solid tumours and cysts.

Aspiration cytology

- Easy to perform and quick to report on—often done in one half day during outpatients.

- Usually well tolerated in outpatients.
- Provides only cellular information and relies upon cellular atypia for a diagnosis of malignancy.
- Does not provide histological information.
- Occasionally therapeutic for cysts.
- Good sensitivity and specificity.
- Contraindicated where there is a suspicion the lesion may be vascular.

CT scanning
- Useful for assessment of extensive local invasion and regional and systemic staging of tumours.
- Allows evaluation of the thorax in some thyroid tumours.

CT PET scanning
Occasionally used to assess indeterminate lesions identified on plain CT and identify unsuspected metastatic disease.

MRI scanning
Useful for detailed assessment of local invasion of tumours.

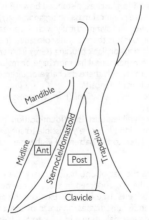

Fig. 2.1 Key revision points—triangle of the neck.

Evaluation of the abdomen

Positioning

- Lie the patient supine with the head slightly raised with adequate support for the head to ensure the abdominal muscles are relaxed.
- Arms should be by the sides to relax the lateral abdominal muscles.
- The patient may be rolled into left or right lateral positions during palpation and percussion.
- Ask the patient to cough during inspection; it may reveal hernias.
- Stand the patient up to examine the groin only if necessary; most hernias and groin pathology can be fully assessed in supine position.

Inspection

- Perform during normal and deep respiration.
- *General features.* Is there evidence of jaundice or signs of anaemia? Does the patient looked underweight, malnourished, or cachectic?
- *Scars.* Where are they? How old do they appear? Is there evidence of herniation on coughing?
- *Is there a stoma?* What type? Does it look healthy or abnormal? What is the content in the stoma appliance?
- *Overall appearance.* Is the abdomen symmetrical? Is there evidence of global distension (e.g. ascites, distended bowel)? Is there evidence of local distortion (e.g. a local mass or organomegaly)? Does the abdomen move well and symmetrically with deep respiration (reduced in peritoneal irritation)? Is there any discoloration (periumbilical bruising (Cullen's sign) or flank bruising (Grey Turner's sign), where either suggests retroperitoneal haemorrhage or major inflammation)?
- *Umbilicus.* Is it herniated? Is there discharge or ulceration suggestive of infection or a malignant deposit?
- *Pulsation.* Is there visible pulsation? (Further assessment requires palpation.)
- *Peristalsis.* Is there visible peristalsis? (Identification may take several minutes of observation.) It is rarely possible to suggest a cause or level of obstruction related to the pattern of visible peristalsis.

Palpation

Be methodical. Use the flat of one hand (usually the right). It is usual to examine and describe the abdomen in areas. It can be divided into nine regions or five 'quadrants' (see Fig. 2.2). Examine the areas lightly at first in a set order. Identify any masses or areas of tenderness. Repeat the examination with deeper palpation. Go back to any identified masses and try to ascertain their key features.

- *Signs of peritoneal irritation.* Are there signs of local visceral peritoneal irritation (tenderness and pain on palpation)? Are there signs of mild parietal peritoneal irritation (guarding) or signs of marked parietal peritoneal irritation (rigidity)? Rigidity may be localized or generalized. Rebound tenderness is an unnecessary test; it merely confirms the presence of guarding and is often excessively painful for the patient.
- *Masses.* Assess their surface, edge, consistency, movement with respiration, and overall mobility.

- *Organs.*
  - *Liver.* Palpate from right lower quadrant into right upper quadrant, feeling for the liver edge during inspiration every few cm upwards until it is found. Assess the edge. Is it smooth/nodular/craggy? Assess any palpable surface. Is it smooth/nodular/craggy?
  - *Spleen.* Palpate from right lower quadrant into left upper quadrant, feeling for the spleen edge during inspiration as for the liver. Assess the edge and any palpable surface.
  - *Kidneys.* Palpate bimanually in each loin. 'Ballotting' (bouncing the kidneys between each hand) is of little additional value.

Percussion

Percussion identifies the presence of excessive amounts of gas or fluid. It is also useful, when done carefully, in the confirmation of the presence of mild to moderate parietal peritoneal irritation ('percussion tenderness').

- *Gas* (hyperresonance). Is it generalized or localized? Is there evidence of loss of dullness over the liver (suggestive of copious free intraperitoneal gas)?
- *Fluid* (ascites). Usually identified as 'shifting dullness'; dullness in the flanks in the supine position moves to the lower portion of the abdomen on turning to the lateral position.

Auscultation

To fully assess bowel sounds, it is necessary to listen for at least 1min, but they are a notoriously unreliable sign of either intra-abdominal pathology or bowel function. If commented on, bowel sounds should broadly be divided into: absent, normal, active, or obstructive (characterized by high-pitched, frequent sounds often with crescendos of activity, e.g. 'tinkling', 'bouncing marbles').

Abdominal assessment should always include a rectal examination in adults; this is very rarely useful and should usually be avoided in children.

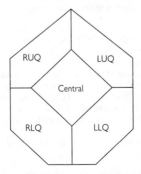

Fig. 2.2 The five quadrants: RUQ, right upper quadrant; LUQ, left upper quadrant; LLQ, left lower quadrant; RLQ, right lower quadrant.

Abdominal investigations

Faecal occult blood testing
- May be chemical or immunological.
- Commonest use is as the primary community test for colorectal carcinoma (see 📖 p. 400) as part of the National Bowel Cancer Screening Programme.

Rigid proctoscopy and sigmoidoscopy (see 📖 p. 216).

Flexible sigmoidoscopy
- Very low risk (perforation 1 in 5000) outpatient procedure, usually performed without sedation.
- Should visualize up to the descending colon.
- Allows minor therapeutic procedures (polypectomy, biopsy, injection).

Colonoscopy
- Low risk (perforation 1 in 1000) outpatient procedure, usually performed with sedation; requires bowel preparation.
- Should visualize the entire colon (>95% of the time).
- Allows minor therapeutic procedures (polypectomy, including 'advanced' endoscopic mucosal resection (EMR) and endoscopic submucosal dissection (ESD), injection, marking by tattoo, and biopsy).
- Typically used for: assessment of (suspected) colitis, diagnosis and assessment of colonic neoplasia, investigation of rectal bleeding.

Transabdominal ultrasound
- Easy, safe, non-invasive, and avoids radiation dose.
- Typical uses include:
  - Identification of ovarian disease, e.g. in suspected acute appendicitis.
  - Primary investigation of the biliary tree for gallstones, bile duct size, and liver parenchymal texture.
  - Investigation of suspected subphrenic or pelvic collections.
  - Assessment of the liver/splenic parenchyma.
  - Identifying free fluid in abdominal trauma.

CT scanning
- Easy, non-invasive; requires significant radiation exposure and intravenous (IV)/oral (PO) contrast.
- Typical uses include:
  - Primary assessment of all intra-abdominal masses.
  - Staging of intra-abdominal and pelvic malignancy.
  - Investigation of acute abdominal pain of unknown origin.
  - Investigation of suspected intestinal obstruction.
  - May be specifically tailored for pancreatic, biliary, visceral vessel assessment.
  - Investigation of suspected post-operative complications.

MRI scanning
- Conventional body scanner with external coils.
- Avoids radiation dose.

- May be performed with specialized 'contrast' agents (e.g. ferumoxides).
- Typically used for:
  - Investigation of suspected bile duct disease.
  - Assessment of liver disease/possible metastases.
  - Assessment of pancreas.
  - Assessment of pelvic and retroperitoneal soft tissue disease, e.g. pelvic cancers.

Plain abdominal radiograph

- Limited use.
- May identify intestinal obstruction, urinary tract stones, free intra-abdominal air, intra-abdominal fluid.

Barium enema (double contrast, single contrast)

- May be single contrast (contrast material filling the colon) or double contrast (dilute contrast and air to coat the mucosal surface of the colon).
- Requires bowel preparation and relatively mobile patient.
- Single contrast used to identify strictures and obstructions (used to assess colorectal anastomoses in dilute or water-soluble form).
- Double contrast typically used to identify colonic neoplasia, assess colonic anatomy.

Intestinal transit studies

- Serial abdominal X-rays to identify the progress of ingested radio-opaque markers.
- Used to assess intestinal motility and transit time.

PET scanning

- Injection of radioactive metabolic substrate to identify metabolically active tissue.
- Combined with high resolution CT scanning to co-locate 'hot spots'.
- Typically used to:
  - Identify unsuspected metastatic tumour deposits.
  - Differentiate fibrosis from tumour post-surgery.

Physiological testing

- Manometry testing of the oesophagus, including lower oesophageal sphincter and the anal canal.
- Pressure sensitivities of the oesophagus and anal canal.
- pH testing of the contents of the oesophagus (isolated or continuously for 24h).
- Used to assess anorectal function, oesophageal motility and function, and gastro-oesophageal reflux.

Evaluation of pelvic disease

Positioning and inspection

Examination is performed in up to three positions: supine (for transabdominal palpation of the 'false' pelvis); supine with hips flexed and abducted (for vaginal and bimanual palpation which may be performed to help assess rectal disease); and left lateral position with hips flexed (for rectal palpation and rigid endoscopy). *Any* intimate examination should always have a chaperone present and particularly so for pelvic examinations.

- *Anus.* Is the anus deformed? Is there evidence of mucosal or rectal prolapse? Does the vaginal introitus look normal? Is there vaginal prolapse or evidence of a cystocele? Are there scars from previous surgery, sinuses, or evidence of sepsis?
- *Look for additional or abnormal tissue.* Are there skin tags, external haemorrhoids, warts, or abnormal areas of skin (such as anal intraepithelial neoplasia (AIN))? Is there an external punctum (as may be seen in a fistula) or the outer limit of a fissure visible?

Palpation

- Palpate the lower abdominal quadrants.
- *Rectal examination.* Is anal tone normal and the sphincter symmetrical? Is the prostate normal size with a normal central sulcus? Does the rectal mucosa feel normal? Is there any mass or tenderness anterior to the upper rectum (pouch of Douglas)? The latter may be due to sigmoid disease, small bowel in the pelvis, a pelvic appendix, or ovarian disease.
- *Vaginal examination* (often omitted unless there is a clear indication that valuable information may be gained from it). Is the cervix present and normal? Is the vagina of normal calibre and feel? Is there tenderness in either vaginal fornix?

Investigations

Rigid proctoscopy ('anoscopy')

- Performed in outpatients without sedation.
- Only visualizes the very lowermost rectum and anal canal (referred to as anoscopy in USA). Views may not be good if done without enema preparation.
- May be combined with therapy (banding, injection, or cryotherapy) for anorectal disorders.

Rigid sigmoidoscopy

- Performed in outpatients without sedation.
- Aims to visualize the rectum to the recto-sigmoid junction. The sigmoid colon is NOT adequately seen with this (referred to as proctoscopy in USA). Views may not be good if done without enema preparation.

Flexible sigmoidoscopy

- Low risk, outpatient procedure, usually performed without sedation.
- Should visualize up to the descending colon.
- Allows minor therapeutic procedures (polypectomy, tattoo, injection).

Transabdominal/transvaginal ultrasound
- Easy, safe, and avoids radiation dose.
- Good for identification of ovarian disease (e.g. in right iliac fossa pain).

Endoanal/transrectal ultrasound
- A 360° scanning endoanal/endorectal probe without sedation.
- Endoanal scans. For assessment of anal sphincter integrity.
- Transrectal scans. For assessment of some rectal tumours, prostatic disease (including biopsy), pre-sacral lesions.

CT scanning
- Easy, safe, but significant radiation exposure and IV contrast.
- Investigation of choice for undiagnosed pelvic symptoms and post-operative complications.

MRI scanning
- Usually via conventional body scanner with external coils (occasionally performed with endorectal coil).
- Investigation of choice for the assessment of advanced rectal, gynaecological, and urological cancer, or complex pelvic sepsis.
- Investigation of choice for complex pelvic and anal sepsis.

Key revision points—pelvic anatomy
- The true pelvis lies between the pelvic inlet (sacral promontory, illiopectineal lines, symphisis pubis) and outlet (coccyx, ischial tuberosities, pubic arch).
- Pelvic floor muscles (such as levator ani) support and are integral to the function of the anorectum, vagina, and bladder. They are innervated by anterior primary rami of S2, 3, 4.
- Anterior relations of the rectum (palpable during PR exam) are (from below up):
  - Women—vagina, cervix, pouch of Douglas.
  - Men—prostate, seminal vesicals, recto-vesical pouch.

Evaluation of peripheral vascular disease

Positioning and inspection

Ideally, the patient should be examined in a warm environment at rest. Remember first to take the pulse and blood pressure, and examine the abdomen (aneurysm, scars). Inspect the limb in the supine position, then elevated (passively), and finally dependent. Expose the entire limb, including the foot or hand to allow thorough inspection. If necessary, take any dressings down (or ask for them to be removed if you are not happy to). For venous disease, the patient should also be examined standing.

During supine inspection, look for the following.

- *Appearance*. Are there any areas of established skin necrosis (dry gangrene, e.g. apex of digits, between digits, heel of the foot)? Are there changes of chronic venous stasis (flare veins, venous eczema, lipodermatosclerosis, leg ulceration)?
- *Colour*. Waxy white suggests severe acute ischaemia; blue and mottled suggests potentially irreversible acute ischaemia; dark red/purple suggests chronic ischaemia.
- *Colour changes during position*. Note the angle at which the skin of the limb blanches when passively elevated (Buerger's test). Normal limbs may not blanch at all. An angle of 15° or less suggests severe ischaemia. Note the presence and delay in change in colour when the limb is dependent. Ischaemic limbs slowly turn deep purple.
- *Ulcers*. What is the location (digital or foot suggests arterial disease)? Be sure to inspect between the toes/fingers and on the plantar surface of the foot (especially for diabetic disease).
- *Venous inspection*. Stand the patient up. Inspect for varicose veins. Are they in the long saphenous or short saphenous distribution?

Palpation

- *Temperature*. Does the skin feel cold or warm? Is there a transition level?
- *Skin capillary compression and refill*. Normal is 2s or less. A delay of greater than 5s suggests significant ischaemia.
- *Peripheral pulses*. Start with the most proximal (major) vessels and work distally. Record if the pulse is normal, reduced, or absent. Record if there are any thrills palpable.
- In venous disease, tests of *venous competence* may be performed (see 📖 p. 666).
- *Surgical grafts*. Palpate the course of any surgical grafts and record the presence or absence of pulses.

Auscultation

Listen for bruits. Are there bruits in the proximal vessels (suggestive of stenosis)?

Investigations

Doppler ultrasound
- Straightforward and portable.
- May be used to confirm or refute the presence of flow in a vessel or graft.
- May be used to evaluate the relative flow in vessels by measuring the pressure at which detectable flow ceases using a compression cuff. The commonest example is ankle–brachial pressure index (ABPI).
- May be used to evaluate the presence of reflux in veins.

Colour flow duplex
- Combined two-dimensional (2D) ultrasound image with Doppler-derived flow represented using colour, superimposed in real time.
- May be used for assessment of stenosis/occlusion in vessels or grafts.
- May be used for assessment of reflux or occlusion in deep and superficial veins.

Direct angiography
- Most commonly, digital subtraction angiography (DSA; used to reduce background image 'noise' and convert the arterial images to black for easier viewing).
- Invasive, requiring direct arterial puncture with the associated risks.
- Requires IV contrast with the small risk of allergy (relatively contraindicated in renal dysfunction or where renal blood flow is poor).
- Gives direct views of arterial tree, but lumen only so not good for aneurysm sizing.

Magnetic resonance angiography
- Provides images of an arterial tree based on the presence of arterial flow during scanning.
- Safe and non-invasive; requires no 'contrast', but commonly gadolinium used to highlight flowing blood.
- Tends to overestimate degree of stenosis due to very low flow being underrepresented.

CT angiography
- Requires multislice rapid acquisition ('helical'/'spiral') scanner.
- Images acquired in arterial phase after IV injection of contrast.
- Three-dimensional (3D) reconstruction allows 'virtual angiogram' images to be produced.
- Fast and relatively safe, especially where direct angiogram is difficult, e.g. visceral vessels.
- Requires dose of IV contrast, so caution with allergy and renal dysfunction.

Evaluation of the skin and subcutaneous tissue disease

Assessment and description of a lump

Key features in the history include the following:

- *Speed of development.* Rapid increase in size is suspicious of malignancy (primary or secondary).
- *Recent change in size.* Suggests malignant change or infection in a previously benign lesion.
- *Associated symptoms.* Paraesthesia or weakness suggests involvement of nerves; reduced movement suggests involvement of muscle.
- *History of local trauma.* May indicate a cause, although a previously undiagnosed underlying lump should always be suspected.

The following features should all be considered when examining the lump.

Basic facts
- Position.
- Size.
- Shape.

Features of infection or inflammation
- Temperature.
- Tenderness.
- Colour.

Features of malignancy
- Surface (e.g. craggy).
- Edge (e.g. irregular).
- Consistency (e.g. hard).

Features of fluid or vascular lesions
- Fluctuant (fluid-filled).
- Presence of thrill (fluid-filled connected to the vascular tree).
- Transilluminance (fluid-filled).
- Pulsatile (arterial lesion).
- Presence of a bruit (arterial lesion).
- Presence of expansility (indicative of an arterial aneurysm).
- Presence of compressibility (e.g. venous lesion or arteriovenous malformation).

Features of locoregional invasion
- Tethering to surrounding structures.
- Involvement of surrounding structures (e.g. nerves).
- Regional lymphadenopathy.

Lumps in detail
- Superficial lumps, see 📖 pp. 600–603.
- Neck lumps, see 📖 pp. 222, 224.
- Abdominal lumps and herniae, see 📖 p. 336.
- Scrotal lumps, see 📖 p. 366.

Assessment and description of an ulcer

Key features in the history include the following:

• Is it painful (venous, diabetic, and neuropathic ulcers are painless)?
• Did it start as an ulcer or did a lump become ulcerated (suggests a malignancy in/of the skin)?
• Is there a history of underlying infection, e.g. of bone?

Describe the basic morphology of the ulcer:

• *Location.*
  • Over pressure points and bony prominences suggests pressure sore.
  • Medial shin suggests venous ulcer.
  • Lateral shin, dorsum of foot, toes suggest arterial ulcer.
• *Edge.*
  • Sloping edge suggests conventional ulcer (can be many aetiologies).
  • Rolled edge is typical of basal cell or squamous carcinomas.
  • Everted edge suggests squamous or metastatic carcinomas.
  • Vertical edge (punched out) suggests syphilis or chronic infection.
• *Base.*
  • Friable, red, and bleeding suggests venous or traumatic.
  • Green slough suggests infected.
  • Black hard eschar suggests chronic ischaemia.
• *Discharge.* May suggest an underlying cause, e.g. intestinal fistula with enteric content, golden pus in chronic actinomycosis.
• *Surrounding tissue.* Erythema and swelling suggest secondary infection.

Ulcers in detail

• Cutaneous malignancy, see 📖 p. 647.
• Ischaemic ulcers, see 📖 p. 647.
• Venous ulcers, see 📖 pp. 148, 666.
• Fistulas, see 📖 p. 150.
• Wound infections, see 📖 p. 104.

Surgery at the extremes of age

Surgery is increasingly used in older and older patients and the range of procedures available to surgeons for both the very elderly and the very young and neonates is increasing. Minimally invasive surgery is increasingly being offered to older patients at risk from open surgery. Both these groups need particular attention and have specific potential problems.

Surgery and the elderly

Common misconceptions corrected

- Elderly patients benefit just as much from potentially curative cancer surgery as younger patients. Cancers demonstrate the same range of behaviours in all ages and are neither more 'benign' nor less responsive to treatment in the elderly.
- Minimally invasive procedures in the elderly can offer all the benefits available to younger patients.
- 'Palliative' procedures for benign disease (e.g. cholecystectomy, joint surgery, eye surgery) are just as important in the elderly as they may allow preservation of independence and offer just as much improvement in quality of life as in the young.

Common problems in the elderly

- Multiple comorbidities and polypharmacy increase the scope for potential complications and drug interactions.
- Comorbidities are often 'silent', either due to atypical presentation or underreporting of symptoms (e.g. angina may not be manifest due to reduced mobility).
- Social, family, nursing, and medical support structures are often complex and easily lost during a hospital admission.
- Reduced or acutely impaired mental faculties may make history taking and consent taking difficult.
- Reduced or abnormal immune responses may reduce or impair some physical signs (e.g. clinically detectable peritonism may be absent).
- The elderly are particularly prone to mild or moderate chronic malnutrition, increasing general complication rates, and the risk of pressure sores, etc.

Strategies for the management of the elderly

- Involve all the necessary specialities as soon as possible (prior to admission for elective surgery), e.g. elderly care, anaesthetists, physicians.
- Consider pre-optimization in critical care (high dependency unit (HDU)), especially in urgent or emergency surgery.
- Start to plan for discharge on the day of admission and liaise with the GP and family, if necessary.
- Consider nutrition as soon as possible after surgery. Is hyper-alimentation necessary?

Surgery and the young

Although most surgery undertaken in neonates and very young children is done so by specialist paediatric surgical and nursing teams, most surgeons will care for young children at some time and the principles of care used in paediatric surgery can be usefully applied to older children.

Common problems in children

- Young children may not be able to accurately report symptoms and illness behaviour is often non-specific.
- Cardiovascular responses in the young are excellent. Tachycardia and particularly hypotension are (very) late signs of hypovolaemia.

▶ *Tips for managing children*

- Take the history from the parents or carers *and* the child.
- Remember infections are common and often present with non-specific signs.
- Consider non-surgical diagnoses at all times, e.g. meningitis, urinary sepsis, systemic viral infections.
- Examine the child as much as possible while they are sitting on a parent's lap. Use the same position for phlebotomy and siting cannulae.
- Put local anaesthetic cream on phlebotomy sites 30min in advance.
- Some children are simply too young to cooperate with procedures under local anaesthetic and will require general anaesthesia for relatively trivial procedures.
- Make sure all prescriptions for drugs and fluids are written according to weight to avoid inadvertent adult dosing—if in doubt, *ask*.
- Fluid balance may be critical since small volume changes are highly significant in small children. Pay close attention to fluid resuscitation.

Paediatric surgery

- Conversion tables, see 📖 p. 424.
- Paediatric surgery, see 📖 pp. 424–474.
- Consent and children, see 📖 p. 14.

Day case and minimally invasive surgery

Day surgery procedures

An increasing number of procedures in all aspects of surgery are being performed as day surgery. The key features that make a procedure suitable include:

- Low risk of major complications.
- Predictable recovery period not requiring specialist post-operative therapy or treatment.
- Post-operative analgesia that does not need routine opiates.
- Anaesthetic technique not requiring invasive monitoring, prolonged muscle relaxation, or epidural/spinal anaesthesia.
- Low risk of difficult or unpredictable anaesthetic technique.

Many areas of surgery are now performed routinely as day surgery, including minor and intermediate anorectal surgery, hernia surgery, minor laparoscopic surgery, arthroscopy, and minor endoscopic bladder surgery.

Selection of patients for day case surgery

Most hospitals have well defined protocols to select patients for suitability for day surgery and most day surgery units conduct their own pre-admission assessment either by telephone or questionnaire. Typical criteria might include:

- Maximum age of 75y (this upper limit has gradually increased as familiarity with the procedures has grown).
- Appropriate social support for the patient at home, including transport and a responsible adult to monitor progress.
- No history of more than mild to moderate cardiac or respiratory disease (e.g. uncomplicated asthma or controlled angina).
- Non-insulin dependent diabetes only (unless for local anaesthetic (LA) procedures).
- Body mass index (BMI) below 35 (typically)—higher than this is associated with increased risk of anaesthetic and surgical complications.

Minimally invasive surgical procedures

Minimally invasive surgery is becoming more common in many areas of surgery. It is a broad term that includes many types of procedure and there is much overlap with conventional 'open' surgery and, at the other end of the spectrum, interventional radiological procedures. A useful definition of minimally invasive surgery is a procedure that can be performed by a technique involving fewer or smaller incisions than alternative 'conventional' surgery or under less invasive anaesthetic techniques. This includes most laparoscopic and thoracoscopic surgery (cholecystectomy, gastric fundoplication, colectomy, lobectomy, nephrectomy, adrenalectomy). It also includes flexible and rigid endoscopic procedures (diagnostic and therapeutic colonoscopy, cystoscopy, transurethral prostate surgery, hysteroscopic surgery), and several procedures using specific techniques or equipment (e.g. transanal endoscopic microsurgery, subfascial endoscopic venous surgery).

Advantages of minimally invasive surgery

Many minimally invasive surgical techniques require specific training to perform and utilize expensive equipment and consumables so surgeons and managers look to minimally invasive surgery to provide benefits to both patients and hospitals. Although some benefits can be achieved by modern post-surgical management, there are demonstrable benefits in different areas.

Patient benefits
- Smaller, fewer, or absent scars.
- Reduced time in hospital.
- Fewer post-operative complications (particularly wound and respiratory-related).

Surgeon benefits
- Reduced post-operative stay.
- Possible avoidance of the need for interventional anaesthetic techniques such as epidurals.

Hospital benefits
- Increased bed use efficiency.
- Reduced post-operative complications.

To whom should minimally invasive surgery be offered?

The advantages of minimally invasive surgery give it a wide application.
- *Young patients.* Small scars and short hospital stays are ideal.
- *Elderly.* Reduced post-operative complications and shortened hospital stay are vital in patients who often have multiple comorbidities.
- *Unfit patient.* Easier anaesthetic techniques and reduced surgical stress may reduce the perioperative risk.

Surgery in pregnancy

Pregnancy testing

- Urinary dipstick β-HCG is 91% sensitive (even lower for women self-testing). Specificity ranges from 61% to 100% if tested from the first day of the first missed period (2 weeks after ovulation).
- Blood β-HCG is almost 100% sensitive and specific and able to detect pregnancy 6–8 days after ovulation.
- False negatives and positives are most commonly due to user error.

Changes in anatomy and physiology

Pregnancy results in several changes relevant to surgery.

First trimester

- Drugs may have teratogenic effect (see Box 2.1).
- Reduced lower oesophageal sphincter tone, increasing the risk of gastro-oesophageal reflux and aspiration when supine.

Second trimester

- Drugs may have adverse effect in fetal development or metabolism without causing gross malformation.
- Increased susceptibility to urinary tract infections, particularly ascending renal infections and pyelonephritis.
- Increased risk of venous thromboembolism rises in the second trimester and remains constantly raised in the third.
- Increased susceptibility to superficial infections.

Third trimester

- Drugs may induce labour.
- Displacement of the mobile abdominal viscera superiorly and behind the enlarging uterus. In particular, the appendix comes to lie in the right upper quadrant.
- Risk of hypotension in the supine position due to inferior vena caval compression by the gravid uterus: this can be avoided by positioning the sedated or unconscious patient in slight lateral decubitus.

Risks of miscarriage

The risk of miscarriage related to surgical pathology and surgery varies according to trimester. It is highest in the first. The risk of a viable premature labour rises in the third trimester. The risk of miscarriage induced by general anaesthetic (GA) is always balanced against the risk induced by sepsis from untreated surgical pathology, particularly acute appendicitis. It is a common dilemma in surgical practice. Ultrasound imaging may be less useful due to poor views and CT scanning is contraindicated due to radiation dose. Diagnostic laparoscopy is contraindicated due to the effects of pneumoperitoneum on the pregnancy. The only way to a diagnosis may be surgery, once important differential diagnoses have been excluded.

Common differential diagnoses of appendicitis in pregnancy
- Ectopic pregnancy complications.
- Pyelonephritis.
- Threatened miscarriage/placental abruption.

Box 2.1 Prescribing drugs in pregnancy

It is clearly unethical to screen drugs for harmful effects on the human fetus; many new and commonly used drugs have, therefore, never been used in pregnancy. Some older drugs have been used in pregnancy and are regarded as 'safe' in the absence of any reports of fetal harm. There is an important balance to maintain between treating serious illness in the mother and potentially harming the fetus. Generally:
- Avoid prescribing drugs, if at all possible.
- Know the stage of the pregnancy; many drugs are only approved in particular trimesters.

▶ Check every drug that you prescribe in Appendix 4 of the *British National Formulary (BNF)*.
- If in doubt, seek specialist advice.
- Important teratogens include:
  - Thalidomide (an antiemetic).
  - Carbamazepine and sodium valproate.
  - Isotretinoin (Roaccutane®).
  - Tetracycline.
  - Warfarin.
  - Angiotensin-converting enzyme (ACE)-inhibitors.
  - Lithium.
  - Methotrexate, cyclophosphamide.

Surgery and the contraceptive pill

(O)estrogen-containing contraceptive pills (EOCP) increase the risk of thromboembolic disease in women taking them prior to surgery. Progesterone-only contraceptives appear to pose little or no additional risk and may be continued during surgery. The increase in risk is related to the size of the operative procedure and the existing comorbidity; the advice is adjusted accordingly.

- *Low risk procedures.* Dental, day case, minor laparoscopic. EOCP may be continued.
- *Medium risk.* Abdominal, orthopaedic, major breast surgery.
  - EOCP should be discontinued at least 1 month prior to elective surgery.
  - Urgent or emergency surgery should be conducted with full thromboprophylaxis (see p. 72).
- *High risk.* Pelvic, lower limb orthopaedic surgery, cancer.
  - EOCP should be discontinued at least 1 month prior to elective surgery.
  - Urgent or emergency surgery should be conducted with extended thromboprophylaxis (see p. 72).

Surgery in endocrine disease

Diabetes

Specific perioperative risks

- Hypoglycaemia, hyperglycaemia, or ketoacidosis.
- Underlying diabetes-related comorbidity is often unrecognized (e.g. mild renal impairment, small-vessel coronary and cerebrovascular disease, mild autonomic neuropathy with associated reduced cardiovascular homeostasis responses).
- Increased susceptibility to infection, poor wound healing.
- Increased susceptibility to skin pressure necrosis.

Management of the diabetic patient

- Inform the anaesthetist, the diabetologist, and any specialists involved in the patient's ongoing care, e.g. nephrologists.
- Clarify if the patient is oral-controlled, insulin-dependent (low or high requirement), or brittle insulin-dependent since the risk of perioperative problems increases with each group.
- Diabetics should be first on operating lists to ensure timings can be as predictable as possible for blood sugar management.
- Check preoperative investigations for signs of underlying comorbidity.
- Ketoacidosis in the perioperative period is associated with a very high morbidity and mortality and should be avoided at all costs.

Minor surgery

- *Oral-controlled.* Give normal regimen.
- *Insulin-controlled.* Omit preoperative insulin on day of surgery; monitor blood sugar (BS) every 4h; restart normal insulin once oral diet is established.

Major surgery

- *Oral-controlled.* Omit long-acting hypoglycaemics preoperatively. Monitor BS every 4h. If BS exceeds 15mmol/L, start IV insulin regimen.
- *Insulin-controlled.* Commence on IV insulin sliding scale preoperatively once nil by mouth (NBM) and continue until normal diet is re-established. Check BS every 4h. Restart normal insulin regimen (initially at half dose) once oral diet is established.

Emergency surgery

- Check for existing ketoacidosis. If present, use medical treatment algorithm to control BS and postpone surgery until BS <20mmol/L unless the condition is life-threatening.
- Use IV insulin sliding scale for all patients to optimize BS control. A typical IV sliding scale (Actrapid® with 5% dextrose) is:
  - BS <4mmol/L, infusion 0.5U/h + consider medical review.
  - BS 4–15mmol/L, infusion 2.0U/h.
  - BS 15–20mmol/L, infusion 4.0U/h.
  - BS >20mmol/L, infusion 4.0U/h + consult diabetology team and consider treatment as for ketoacidosis.

Steroids

Specific perioperative risks

Oral steroids are used to treat a number of common illnesses, including rheumatoid arthritis, severe asthma, and COPD, temporal arteritis, and polymyalgia rheumatica. Steroids reduce neutrophil and fibroblast function and immune response and lead to irreversible changes in connective tissue. Long-term use of systemic steroids results in adrenal suppression. The following problems are associated with chronic steroid use.

Addisonian (hypoadrenal) crisis (see Box 2.2)
- Increased susceptibility to infection.
- Poor wound healing, including anastomotic leaks, pressure areas.
- Osteoporosis.
- Patients on long-term inhaled steroids, e.g. for asthma and COPD, are not high risk as there is minimal systemic absorption.

Box 2.2 Addisonian (hypoadrenal) crisis

Stresses such as surgery and sepsis require increased adrenal secretion of corticosteroids; failure to mount this response can result in an Addisonian (hypoadrenal) crisis. The following groups of patients are at high risk:
- Any patient currently taking >5mg prednisolone for >2 weeks.
- Any patient who reduced their long-term steroids within 2–4 weeks.
- Patients who have undergone adrenalectomy.

Clinical features
- Lethargy and malaise.
- Abdominal pain, often poorly localized (may present as an acute abdomen).
- Nausea and vomiting.
- Hypotension.
- Hypoglycaemia, hyponatraemia.
- Coma, death.

Management
- Treat with IV hydrocortisone 100mg qds or 400mg infusion over 24h as long as the patient is NBM.
- Fluid resuscitation with normal saline.
- 50% dextrose IV to treat hypoglycaemia (titrate against BS).

Management of the patient on steroids
- If the steroid dose can be weaned preoperatively, this should be done.
- Prescribe IV hydrocortisone 25–100mg qds (roughly corresponding to 2.5–20mg od of prednisolone) to start on the morning of surgery and continuing until the patient is able to go back to their oral steroids.

Thyroid disease (see pp. 250–256).

Surgery and heart disease

Ischaemic heart disease

Risk factors include age ($\male$ >45y; $\female$ >55y), family history of early MI, current or treated ↑ BP, smoking, diabetes, ↑ cholesterol.

- Assess severity: quantify exercise tolerance; enquire about palpitations, orthopnoea, use of anti-anginals, previous MI, percutaneous coronary intervention (PCI), or coronary artery bypass graft (CABG).
- The ECG is the most important routine screening test, but it is normal in about one-third of patients with proven ischaemia.
- Symptomatic patients undergoing major surgery should be discussed with a cardiologist with a view to optimizing anti-anginal medications.

Myocardial infarction

The risk of a perioperative MI relates to past history and risk factors.

- Overall population incidence after abdominal surgery, 0.5%.
- Incidence with pre-existing cardiovascular symptoms, 2%.
- Incidence with previous MI (old), 5–10%.
- Incidence after recent MI, 25% (70% will die with re-infarction).

Strategies to reduce risk

- Non-urgent surgery should be delayed for at least 6 months following acute MI and, possibly, acute ischaemia. Cancer surgery may be undertaken if the risk of disease progression is felt to outweigh the increased perioperative mortality rate.
- Ensure all normal cardiovascular medication is continued up to and through surgery. Control any new symptoms of angina if surgery is urgent.
- Continue antiplatelet medication if not contraindicated.
- Consider involving the critical care services (HDU) for the perioperative period.

Valvular heart disease

Cardiac murmurs are common. Request a transthoracic echo to evaluate the lesion and discuss abnormalities with a cardiologist.

- Severe *aortic stenosis* carries a high risk of mortality (see 🕮 p. 630). Elective surgery should be postponed: high gradient aortic stenosis carries an associated mortality of 10% with non-cardiac surgery.
- Severe *mitral stenosis* can lead to pulmonary oedema and heart failure. Major elective surgery should be postponed until lesion corrected.
- *Aortic regurgitation* requires attention to fluid and rate control. Antibiotic prophylaxis should be given, but surgery can go ahead.
- *Mitral regurgitation* (MR) should be managed with diuretics and vasodilators. Beware: left ventricular function is frequently overestimated in MR.
- *Prosthetic valves* have several associated issues.
  - *Mechanical valves* require anticoagulation. Stop warfarin 5 days preoperatively and admit early for IV heparinization.

- Do not heparinize if the international normalized ratio (INR) will be only briefly subtherapeutic.
- Stop IV heparin 6h pre-surgery and resume as soon as surgical bleeding is no longer a problem until INR therapeutic.
- Thrombosis is most likely in mechanical mitral valves, atrial fibrillation (AF), poor left ventricle (LV), previous embolus, ball-and-cage valves.
- In surgery for life-threatening bleeding, e.g. bleeding peptic ulcer, intracranial haemorrhage, it may be necessary to reverse anticoagulation for several days. Liaise closely with cardiology.
  ▶ Prosthetic valves no longer require antibiotic prophylaxis for procedures that cause bacteraemias[1]; if in doubt, discuss with cardiology.

Arterial hypertension

Control of BP preoperatively may reduce the tendency to perioperative ischaemia. Always note BP and, if severe (>180mmHg), surgery should be delayed until control is obtained.
- Review existing antihypertensive management or start treatment:
  - Beta-blockers (e.g. metoprolol 25–50mg PO tds) reduce BP and perioperative ischaemia and mortality.
  - Calcium channel blockers are often used, e.g. nifedipine 10mg sublingual (SL).
- Look for evidence of end-organ damage and associated heart disease.
- Look for rare, but important causes: phaeochromocytoma, hyperaldosteronism, coarctation of the aorta, renal artery stenosis.

Congestive cardiac failure

Heart failure is associated with a poorer outcome in non-cardiac surgery. Risk factors include ischaemic and valvular heart disease.
- Listen for S_3 as well as pedal oedema, raised jugular venous pressure (JVP), bibasal crepitations.
- Chest X-ray may show cardiomegaly or pulmonary oedema.

Cardiac arrhythmias

Arrhythmias and conduction defects are common. Asymptomatic arrhythmias are not associated with an increase in cardiac complications, but look for underlying problems, e.g. ischaemic heart disease, drug toxicity, metabolic derangements.
- High grade conduction abnormalities, e.g. complete heart block, should be discussed with a cardiologist. Pacing may be indicated.
- Patients with known AF and either a history of embolic stroke or associated structural cardiac defect normally take warfarin.
- Request a cardiology review preoperatively if rate control is poor.
- Beware of the patient with the *permanent pacemaker or intracardiac defibrillator (ICD)*. Diathermy may cause the pacemaker to reset or completely inhibit pacing and trigger ICD discharge.
  - Pacemakers and ICDs should be evaluated by a cardiac technician preoperatively and post-operatively.
  - Pacemakers should be changed to fixed-rate pacing for surgery and then reprogrammed after surgery.

- ICDs should be switched off to prevent discharge and external fibrillator pads positioned on the patient.
- If defibrillation or synchronized cardioversion is required, place the paddles as far from the pacemaker or ICD as possible.
- Type of diathermy used should be considered. Monopolar is not absolutely contraindicated, but bipolar may be preferable.

Reference

1 http://publications.nice.org.uk/prophylaxis-against-infective-endocarditis-cg64

Surgery and respiratory disease

Surgery and smoking
Smoking tobacco increases the risks of anaesthesia and many of the risks of surgery. There is a six-fold increase in post-operative respiratory complications among patients smoking in excess of ten cigarettes per day.

Effects of smoking
- Reduction in general and specific immune function via reduced neutrophil chemotaxis and reduced natural killer (NK) cell efficacy.
- Increased platelet aggregation (probably explaining the increased risk of perioperative acute MI and cerebrovascular accident in smokers).
- Reduced oxygen-carrying capacity of blood per unit volume due to the presence of carboxyhaemoglobin increasing the risk of tissue hypoxia in susceptible organs.
- Increased upper aerodigestive mucosal secretions. This worsens initially after stopping smoking until the chronic effects on the mucosa wear off.
- Reduced mucociliary escalator function.
- Reduced lung compliance and increased 'closing volume' of the small airways, increasing the risk of air trapping, especially whilst supine in the post-operative period.

Stopping smoking
- Within 48h: carboxyhaemoglobin is cleared from the blood, platelet aggregation begins to return to normal.
- Within 7 days: neutrophil, macrophage, and NK cell function improve. Mucus production temporarily increases, but mucociliary escalator function takes up to 6 weeks to recover, leading to a 'rebound' effect.
- Within 6 weeks: upper aerodigestive function returns to underlying level, lung dynamics improve to 'normal' levels (depending on the extent of fixed parenchymal disease).

The optimal time for stopping smoking is at least 6 weeks prior to surgery, but a minimum of 7 days is required to reduce the 'rebound' effects of stopping on upper aerodigestive tract function.

▶ *Mitigating the effects of smoking in the post-operative period*
Active and recently stopped smokers should receive extra attention to prevent the risks associated with smoking and surgery.
- Ensure patients remain well hydrated until oral intake is restored.
- Use thromboembolic prophylaxis in most cases.
- Use preoperative chest physiotherapy and education on breathing and coughing techniques.
- Mobilize as soon as possible post-operatively.
- Consider the use of epidural anaesthesia to improve compliance with post-operative physiotherapy.
- Use preoperative and post-operative saline nebulizers 5mL qds.
- Ensure post-operative analgesia is effective.

Respiratory conditions

Respiratory tract infection

An active respiratory tract infection may be sufficient reason to cancel elective patients, so ask about cough, fevers, and sputum, but minor colds and nasal discharge may not prevent GA.

- If you suspect the patient has a respiratory tract infection, check their temperature, C-reactive protein (CRP), and white cell count (WCC) early.
- Elective patients should be cancelled and asked to return in 2 weeks if their symptoms are better.
- Reserve antibiotics for patients with suspected bacterial infections; most acute respiratory tract infections are viral.

Asthma

- Assess severity of asthma by asking about hospital admissions, inhalers, nebulizers, peak expiratory flow rates (PEFR), and home oxygen.
- Elective surgery should ideally coincide with remission of symptoms.
- Identify patients on long-term steroid therapy.
  - Sometimes it is possible to time surgery to coincide with a reduction in steroids, but this requires several weeks' notice.
  - Any patient taking more than 5mg daily prednisolone and undergoing inpatient surgery or presenting with sepsis should be started on an equivalent dose of IV hydrocortisone; adrenal suppression may otherwise result in an Addisonian crisis (see 📖 p. 52).
- Patients receiving a general anaesthetic generally experience deterioration in their lung function (see 📖 p. 108). Prophylactically increase their normal therapy by converting inhalers to nebulizers and increasing frequency.

Chronic obstructive pulmonary disease (COPD)

- If dyspnoea is the prominent symptom and the patient has COPD, get lung function tests, including blood gases.
- Admitting these patients a few days early for physiotherapy, education, and nebulizers can reduce the length of hospital stay.
- Patients receiving a general anaesthetic generally experience deterioration in their lung function (see 📖 p. 108). Prophylactically increase their normal therapy by converting inhalers to nebulizers and increasing the frequency.
- Prescribe 6-hourly 5mL nebulized saline and give humidified oxygen wherever possible (to prevent mucus plugging).
- Ensure the patient gets twice daily chest physiotherapy.
- Ensure the patient is on their usual inhalers and consider converting these to nebulizers for major surgery (see 📖 p. 108).

Surgery in renal and hepatic disease

Renal impairment

Renal impairment covers a spectrum, ranging from patients with subclinical dysfunction (normal serum creatinine and urea, but borderline creatinine clearance) to patients with end-stage renal failure. It is helpful to consider these patients in two main groups: patients with chronic renal impairment and dialysis-dependent patients. Post-operative management of renal impairment is discussed on 🕮 p. 110; dialysis is discussed on 🕮 p. 134.

Chronic renal impairment

Surgery may precipitate acute renal failure in patients with chronic renal impairment.

- Avoid hypovolaemia and hypotension. Ensure these patients receive adequate IV hydration if they are to be NBM for any length of time.
- Avoid nephrotoxic drugs wherever possible, including non-steroidal anti-inflammatory drugs (NSAIDs), aminoglycosides, ACE-inhibitors, and radiological contrast.
- Reduce doses of drugs with renal elimination, e.g. morphine, low molecular weight heparin (LMWH), digoxin, and request appropriate levels frequently.

Patients with established renal failure, on dialysis

- Discuss post-operative management of patients undergoing major surgery with the anaesthetist and intensive care unit (ICU) as early as possible.
- Dialysis should be performed the day before surgery.
- Patients must have full blood count (FBC) and urea and electrolytes (U&E) on admission, pre- and post-dialysis, and twice daily U&E post-major surgery until the patient is stabilized on their normal dialysis regime.
- Reduce doses of drugs with renal elimination, e.g. morphine, LMWH, digoxin, and request appropriate levels frequently.
- If the patient is normally anuric, there is little point in inserting a urinary catheter which exposes them to unnecessary infection risk.
- Note the sites of arteriovenous fistulas. *Never* use them for phlebotomy or cannulation and avoid using BP cuffs on that side.
- These patients are prone to several problems. ▶ Hyperkalaemia, acidosis, and pulmonary oedema are potential life-threatening emergencies. Management is described on 🕮 p. 110.
  - Infection.
  - Anaemia and coagulopathy.
  - Fluid and electrolyte disturbances.
  - Metabolic acidosis.
  - Systemic hypertension, pericarditis.

Hepatic impairment

The risk posed by liver disease to patients undergoing general surgery was graded by Child and Turcotte (see Box 2.3). Child grade C is associated with high perioperative mortality.

Box 2.3 Child's classification of surgical risk in hepatic dysfunction

A (minimal risk)	B (moderate risk)	C (advanced risk)
• Serum bilirubin <20mg/L	• Serum bilirubin 20–30mg/L	• Serum bilirubin >30mg/L
• Serum albumin >35g/L	• Serum albumin 30–35g/L	• Serum albumin <30g/L
• No ascites	• Controlled ascites	• Uncontrolled ascites
• No focal neurology	• Minimal neurological dysfunction	• Coma
• Excellent nutrition	• Good nutrition	• Cachexia

• Liver failure causes the following problems:
  • Hypoglycaemia.
  • Hepatic encephalopathy.
  • Coagulopathy.
  • Ascites.
  • Infection.
• Several factors may cause acute decompensation of mild hepatic impairment and should be avoided or treated aggressively in this group:
  • Infection, especially bacterial peritonitis.
  • Sedation.
  • Diuretics.
  • Constipation.
  • Electrolyte imbalance.
  • Dehydration and hypotension.
• Preoperatively:
  • Check hepatitis serology.
  • Request liver ultrasound in newly diagnosed hepatic impairment.
  • Discuss requesting additional blood products with haematology.
  • Discuss doses of standard medication with a specialist.

Jaundice

Patients with obstructive jaundice are at risk of developing renal failure post-operatively (hepatorenal syndrome). This is thought to be due to the nephrotoxic effect of toxins normally eliminated by the liver as well as circulatory changes.

• Ensure adequate hydration. When the patient is NBM, prescribe IV normal saline 1L over 6–8h.
• Insert a urinary catheter and start an hourly fluid balance chart.
• Measure U&E and liver function tests (LFTs) daily.
• Coagulopathy in longstanding cholestatic jaundice may be improved with vitamin K 1mg IV: discuss with haematology.
• Avoid or reduce the doses of hepatotoxic drugs and drugs with hepatic elimination.

Surgery in neurological disease

Cerebrovascular accidents (stroke)
- Ischaemic events are associated with a risk of re-infarction or extension of the infarct area due to interference with cerebrovascular autoregulation by anaesthetic agents. Autoregulation is re-established in around 6 weeks.
- Haemorrhagic infarcts are associated with a small increased risk of further bleeding, especially if the patient is given thromboprophylaxis. Penumbral oedema also interferes with autoregulation as for ischaemic events.

Strategies to reduce risk
- Delay all non-essential surgery for 6 weeks following infarcts, especially ischaemic ones.
- Consider omitting thromboprophylaxis in patients with a recent haemorrhagic event.
- Ensure BP is well controlled (the prevention of both hypotension and hypertension) in the perioperative period to reduce fluctuations in cerebral blood flow.
- Avoid positioning the patient head down on the operating table as this increases cerebral venous pressure.

Epilepsy
Paroxysmal neuronal discharge from various areas of the brain causes a range of disturbances that may affect consciousness (grand mal seizures, and petit mal or absences), movement, or sensory perception. In addition to epilepsy, cerebral space-occupying lesions, uraemia, cerebral oedema, drug toxicity, and hypercalcaemia may cause the same problems. In patients with known epilepsy, the following measures are advised.
- Try to establish the normal frequency and severity of seizures, what form they take, and features, if any, of the prodrome.
- Ensure that normal anticonvulsant medication is continued while the patient is NBM preoperatively and immediately post-operatively.
- If this is not possible, phenytoin and sodium valproate may be given IV: check the BNF for equivalent dosing regimes.
- Phenytoin interacts with a number of drugs used perioperatively.
  - Phenytoin induces monoamine oxidase, increasing elimination of the following commonly used drugs: prednisolone, warfarin, lignocaine.
  - The following drugs increase oral absorption of phenytoin: amiodarone, fluconazole, omeprazole, paroxetine.
  - The following drugs reduce oral absorption of phenytoin: antacids containing magnesium, calcium carbonate, or aluminium, and enteral tube feeding.
- Management of status epilepticus (uncontrolled fitting).
  - *Airway.* Remove dentures; insert Guedel or nasophayngeal airway if unable to open jaw.
  - *Breathing.* Give high flow oxygen (O_2); get Yankauer sucker and wall suction.

- Give diazepam 10mg IV over 2min (PR if no IV access); repeat once if seizures do not stop.
- Check blood sugar and give 50mL 50% dextrose IV if BS <5mmol/L.
- If seizures persist start, phenytoin 18mg/kg IV at a maximum rate of 50mg/min in a separate line to the diazepam.
- Seizures should resolve quickly. If they do not:
  — Get expert help.
  — Discuss with anaesthetist.
  — Consider pseudoseizures (pelvic thrusts, flailing limbs, resistance to attempts to open eyes).

Myasthenia gravis

An antibody-mediated autoimmune disease with insufficient muscle ace-tylcholine receptors, leading to muscle weakness. Usually found in young adults, the disease presents with extraocular (ptosis, diplopia), bulbar (weak voice), neck, limb girdle, distal limb, and finally trunk weakness. Patients may present for thymectomy as specific treatment or for inciden-tal surgery. Management includes the following:

- Continue normal medication.
- Elective post-operative ventilation is indicated in major thoracic or upper abdominal surgery or if the patient's vital capacity <2L. Discuss with an anaesthetist and ICU.
- If ventilation is prolonged post-operatively, a tracheostomy may be required. This should be discussed with the patient at time of consent.
- Post-operative respiratory failure may occur as a result of muscle weakness. Precipitants include:
  - Hypokalaemia.
  - Infection.
  - Over- or undertreatment.
  - Emotion, exertion.

Fluid optimization

▶ Identifying patients in need of fluid optimization

Any patient may be in need of preoperative fluid resuscitation, but several groups are typically affected. Remember to think of less obvious cases of fluid depletion—there are typically more patients who would benefit from fluid optimization than get it.

- Acute presentations with vomiting or diarrhoea, including intestinal obstruction, biliary colic, gastroenteritis.
- Acute presentations where the patient has been immobile or debilitated for a period before presentation, causing reduced fluid intake, e.g. pancreatitis, chest infections, acute-on-chronic vascular insufficiency, prolonged sepsis with pyrexia.
- Elderly patients in whom reduced renal reserve makes fluid balance control less effective.
- Drugs that impair renal responses to fluid changes, e.g. diuretics.
- Patients with low body weight with overall lower total body fluid volume in whom similar losses have a greater effect.
- Children are more susceptible to fluid depletion and may not show such obvious physical signs.

Fluids used for optimization

The most important aspects of fluid optimization are using the correct volumes at the correct rate. Other than exceptional circumstances, isotonic crystalloids are the fluid of choice to correct imbalances.

- Isotonic ('normal') 0.9% saline—the most widely used fluid. Provided there is adequate renal function, isotonic saline prevents rapid cellular fluid shifts during rehydration and excess Na^+ is excreted via the kidney. K^+ should usually be added only if ↓ K^+ is present or likely (e.g. prolonged vomiting, pancreatic or small bowel fistula).
- Dextrose (4%) saline (0.18%).
- Hartmann's solution.
- Ringer's lactate solution—technically, the closest fluid to serum composition although theoretical advantages are of limited practical value.

Fluids that should only be used in very specific circumstances include hypertonic (1.8%) or hypotonic (0.45%) saline since they risk causing significant fluid shifts in and out of cells, which can cause cellular injury, particularly to neurons. If there is a significant disorder of sodium balance that may require non-isotonic fluid optimization, the patient is likely to require optimization in HDU.

How to give the fluids

Before giving fluid, it is important to assess the volume of depletion. It is rarely possible to use estimates of losses due to vomiting or diarrhoea as these are wholly inaccurate. Useful calculations include the following:

- Body weight on admission (provided a recent, accurate body weight during normal health is known) since acute weight loss is mostly water.

- Haematocrit on admission (provided a recent haematocrit during normal health is known) since the degree of haemoconcentration is due to fluid depletion. An approximate calculation is given by:

Fluid depletion (L) = $((PCV_1 - PCV_2)/PCV_1) \times 0.7 \times$ weight in kg

PCV_1 = normal haematocrit; PCV_2 = current haematocrit

- Serum urea is raised disproportionately more than serum creatinine in dehydration, renal disease, gastrointestinal (GI) bleeds, and acute proteolysis.
- Signs of extracellular fluid depletion (lax skin tone, reduced sweating, dry mucosae) are often misleading and can be affected by age and underlying diseases, including pyrexia and tachypnoea.
- Signs of intravascular volume depletion (hypotension, tachycardia) may be unreliable and usually only occur with loss of 10–15% of body water.

Once the volume of fluid required is assessed, it can be given. There are some broad rules on how to give fluid resuscitation.

- Young, fit patients with normal renal and cardiac function can usually be given up to 15% of body fluid volume by rapid infusion. A typical regimen might include: 1000mL 0.9% saline over 2h, further 1000mL infusions of 0.9% saline over 4h each until corrected.
- Elderly patients and patients with renal or cardiac impairment should have infusions more slowly to prevent acute intravascular volume overload. A typical regimen might include: 1000mL 0.9% saline over 4h, 500mL infusion of 0.9% saline over 3–4h with regular review of vital signs, including chest auscultation. Patients requiring more fluid volume more rapidly than this should be monitored closely in critical care during resuscitation.

Monitoring fluid optimization

Methods of assessing the progress of fluid optimization include the following:

- Skin turgor and mucosal hydration change slowly after optimization and are unreliable guides.
- 1-hourly urine output measurement is a good guide to renal blood flow, which indirectly relates to intravascular fluid volume and cardiac output. It is an easy and reliable indicator of adequate blood volume repletion. It is not a good indicator of total body water and there may be significant intra- and extracellular depletion in the presence of an acceptable urine output. A commonly used minimum is 0.5mL/kg/h.
- Monitoring of serum urea is an approximate guide provided renal function is adequate and there is no acute GI bleeding or proteolysis.

In the emergency situation, particularly where patients require urgent surgery and require fluid optimization prior to anaesthesia, more rapid fluid infusions may be required and it may be appropriate for this to be monitored on HDU.

Nutrition in surgical patients

Nutrition is critical to the well-being of surgical patients and timely nutritional support helps reduce acute catabolism and resultant skeletal muscle weakness due to increased metabolic demands.

- It is common and amenable to effective intervention that influences the outcome of surgical patients.
- Incidence of pre-existing malnutrition is substantial and rises with age.
- Anticipate those patients with higher than normal nutritional requirements (e.g. severe burns, severe sepsis, intestinal fistulas, advanced malignancy, immunosuppression); even if they are well nourished prior to illness, they may need nutritional support to prevent excessive acute catabolism due to increased metabolic demands.

Assessment of nutritional status

All patients should be considered for nutritional assessment. Many methods can be used:

- *BMI* (weight/height^2 in kg/m^2). Relatively insensitive for all but major malnutrition, but easy to perform. A BMI of 18–25 is normal, <18 is underweight, >30 is obese.
- *Triceps skinfold thickness.* Easy to perform and a good measure of body fat as a marker of chronic nutritional status.
- *Grip strength.* Easy repeatable index of lean skeletal muscle.
- *Serum albumin.* Poor indicator of acute nutritional status. Responds slowly to nutritional supplementation and is affected by many other diseases and conditions.
- *Serum transferrin.* Accurate responsive indicator of acute status and response to treatment. Not commonly used.

Effects of protein–calorie malnutrition

- Reduced neutrophil and lymphocyte function.
- Impaired albumin production.
- Impaired wound healing and collagen deposition.
- Skeletal muscle weakness ('critical illness myopathy') with resultant increase in respiratory and abdominal complications.
- Micronutrient deficiencies may cause specific clinical syndromes.

Types of nutritional support

- *Oral supplementation.* High calorie, high protein nutritional supplements (e.g. Fortisip®, Calshakes®, Ensures®/Enlives®). May be used in addition to promotion of conventional oral intake.
- *Nasogastric (NG)/nasojejunal feeding.* Often used in addition to oral supplementation. Sometimes given overnight to reduce the impact on appetite suppression during the day.
- *Feeding gastrostomy/jejunostomy* (via a surgically implanted tube). Not routinely used. Reserved for patients where the GI tract is functioning, but food cannot be taken via the oropharyngeal route.
- *Parenteral nutrition.* May be central or peripheral. (See 📖 p. 67.)

The oral route is always to be preferred in nutritional supplementation. It promotes the normal health of the GI flora and has been shown to reduce the risk of complications after GI surgery.

Total parenteral nutrition (TPN)

TPN is commonly encountered in surgical wards. It is a major advance in the treatment of surgical malnutrition, but has serious side effects and both long- and short-term potential complications.

Routes of administration for TPN

- *Peripheral (PPN)*. Given via a medium calibre cannula in a peripheral vein. Maximum calorie input limited by the maximum osmolarity of the solution. Avoids the risks of central venous cannulation. Usually used for short-term supplementation.
- *Central (TPN)*. Given into a central vein (superior vena cava (SVC) or brachiocephalic). May be via a dedicated tunnelled line (e.g. Hickman line), a conventional central venous (CV) cannula, or a peripherally inserted central venous catheter (PICC line). Maximum calorie input only limited by volume of fluid that can be infused. Carries risks of central venous catheterization.

General risks of TPN/PPN

- Hyperosmolarity.
- Lack of glycaemic control.
- Micronutrient deficiencies.
- Liver cell dysfunction, cholestasis, and pancreatic atrophy.
- Fluid volume overload.

Specific catheter-related risks of TPN

- Complications of insertion (air embolism, pneumothorax, vascular injury, dysrhythmias).
- Catheter thrombosis and thromboembolism.
- Central line infection, infective endocarditis, and bacteraemia.

Care of TPN patients

Patients on TPN require regular review and monitoring, including:
- U&E (initially daily, then twice weekly once established).
- Glucose (initially od, then twice weekly unless signs of abnormal glucose levels).
- LFTs (twice weekly).
- Micronutrients, including magnesium (Mg), phosphate (PO_4), manganese (Mn), copper (Cu) (weekly).

CV catheters require specific attention. They should not be used for non-TPN infusions and/or phlebotomy unless in exceptional circumstances as this increases the risk of catheter sepsis dramatically. Dressings should be dated, changed regularly, and the catheter entry site kept clean.

Common indications for TPN

Short term

- Prolonged post-operative 'ileus' (unresolved GI tract dysfunction).
- Acute abdominal sepsis with ITU likely (possibly slow oral route).

Long term

Inability for GI tract to absorb adequate nutrition (e.g. extensive resection, extensive radiotherapy damage, extensive disease such as Crohn's).

Enhanced recovery after surgery

Enhanced recovery after surgery (ERAS) is one of many similar approaches to patient recovery after major surgery, which aims to coordinate many aspects of patient care to minimize the perioperative physiological derangement of the patient, reduce the stress response to surgery, optimize speed of recovery and reduce complication rates. It is usually applied to otherwise healthy individuals who do not need particular preoperative correction or adjustments.

The major areas of consideration are the following.

Nutrition

- *Preoperative carbohydrate loading.* Often given as oral solutions over the 24h prior to surgery, including up to 4h prior to anaesthetic. Has been shown to reduce the early catabolic response to major surgery.
- *Early re-introduction of carbohydrate rich fluids.* Given from 6h post-surgery and encouraged from first post-operative day.
- *Early re-introduction of full nutrition.* Nutritional supplements and 'light diet' components from 48h post-op to encourage 'immediate' return of GI tract function.

Anaesthetic technique

- *Avoidance of the use of opiates* (e.g. IV/PO morphine, opiate patient-controlled analgesia (PCA), opiate epidurals). Aims to prevent reduction in GI tract motility and nausea associated with opiates.
- *Avoidance of the use of epidurals* (some regimens use LA epidurals). Aims to improve early mobilization and reduce cardiovascular and GI effects of autonomic spinal blockade.
- *Use of regional LA-based techniques* (e.g. transversus abdominis percutaneous (TAP) block, regional LA infiltration, regional LA infusional catheters). Aims to minimize central nociceptor input, which may enhance the systemic stress response to surgery.

Surgical technique

- *Laparoscopic or other minimally invasive techniques* are often, but not always a feature of ERAS type programmes. Aim to reduce the metabolic response to surgery, aid early mobilization, and reduce GI tract exposure (and associated impact on function) in abdominal surgery.
- *Avoidance of bowel preparation* for abdominal surgery where possible. Reduces the risk of fluid and electrolyte imbalances, reduces disruption to GI tract flora and has been associated with lower GI tract-related complications (e.g. anastomotic leakage).

Physiotherapy

- *Early mobilization.* Specific exercises, including sitting out within 12h of surgery, walking within 48h of surgery.
- *Perioperative respiratory exercises.*

Nursing
- *Intensive patient preparation.* Preoperative leaflets and education on what to expect.
- *Intensive perioperative and post-operative nursing.* Encouraging early re-establishment of diet, early mobilization and early self-care.

Although intensive and demanding, ERAS type protocols are as effective in the elderly as the young.

They are not suitable for:
- Some insulin-dependent diabetics.
- Patients with pre-existing significant nutritional compromise.
- Patients with cognitive impairment.

Getting the patient to theatre

Preparing the patient for a surgical procedure is all about organization and routine. If the preparation is not good, much can go wrong with major consequences for the patient.

Background paperwork

Ensure the theatre or endoscopy list is correctly filled in and available well in advance. The list should specify the patient's name, hospital number, location, operation details as well as the operating surgeon and anaesthetist.

Patient paperwork

- Make sure the medical notes are available and contain the most up-to-date history and examination for this admission.
- Check the blood results are up to date and specific blood results, e.g. clotting function in anticoagulated patients, K^+ in patients with renal failure, Ca^{2+} in parathyroidectomy patients, have been collected.
- If they are not available in digital format, ensure imaging results that might be needed in theatre are available with the notes (e.g. arteriograms, staging CT scans, barium enema films).
- Check that the consent form has been completed and is on the medical notes even though you may not be responsible for seeing the form signed.
- The drug chart should be completed and include any specific prescriptions for drugs to be administered in theatre or the anaesthetic room. It is the job of the surgical team to prescribe prophylactic antibiotics, etc.

Patient preparation

- Check that the side is marked on the patient for any operation that might involve an organ or tissue that is bilateral. This *must* be done with the patient awake and verified by the nursing staff.
- If necessary, check that the patient has been assessed and marked by any relevant specialists (stoma care if a stoma is possible; prosthetist for amputees).
- Ensure that if the patient requires any blood or blood products, these are available or requested from the transfusion department. Most hospitals have protocols to ensure that the correct number of units of blood is requested for major surgery.
- Find out well in advance if any specific preparation is required. Examples follow.

Bowel preparation

Bowel preparation is sometimes used for operations on or around the large bowel. Types of preparation include the following.

- Stimulant mechanical bowel preparation, e.g. Picolax® (piccosulphate), two sachets taken with plenty of fluid at least 8h prior to surgery. Should be avoided whenever there is a risk of obstruction present. Commonly used for barium enemas.

- Osmotic mechanical bowel preparation, e.g. Citramag® (Mg citrate), Kleen Prep®, two or four sachets taken dissolved in water up to 8h prior to surgery. Used for most colonic operations where bowel preparation is required, colonoscopy, and CT colonography.
- Stimulant left colon preparation, e.g. phosphate enema. Used for operations on the rectum/anus or for flexible sigmoidoscopy.
- Mechanical bowel preparation is less commonly used than previously. There is evidence that it may actually increase the septic complication rates following bowel surgery and has well recognized side effects. These include the risks of:
  - Electrolyte imbalances.
  - Hypovolaemia, especially in the elderly.
  - Nausea and vomiting (particularly with the large volume osmotic preparations).

Anaesthetic premedication

Principles

Anaesthetic premedication is used for the following reasons:
- Relaxing the patient to reduce anxiety during preparation for anaesthesia.
- Relaxation of the patient decreases the amount of anaesthetic agent required for induction of anaesthesia.

Typical agents used for premedication

- *Benzodiazepines.* Often given 1–2h preoperatively on the ward (e.g. diazepam PO). May be given shortly before some procedures (e.g. midazolam 5mg IV).
- *Buscopan®.* Rarely given, but sometimes used to reduce upper aerodigestive tract secretions.

Prophylaxis—antibiotics and thromboprophylaxis

Antibiotic prophylaxis
- Prophylactic antibiotics are used to reduce the risk of surgical site infection and are usually of very short course (one to three doses).
- Active antibiotic treatment for established infections encountered during surgery may be for 5 or more days.
- Most prophylaxis is directed at prevention of infection of the surgical wound or to counter the effect of potential spillage of organisms from colonized organs such as the bowel once it has been opened.

The broad principles of prophylaxis are the following:
- It is most important to have a high circulating serum level of antibiotics at the time of potential tissue contamination, i.e. administered around the time of induction of anaesthesia.
- Prophylaxis rarely needs to continue beyond the time of the procedure unless there are high risk factors or specific indications, i.e. most prophylaxis is one or occasionally three doses on the day of surgery.
- Many clean wounds, e.g. skin lesion excision, do not require prophylaxis.
- High risk patients who may warrant an extended prophylactic course (e.g. up to 3 days) or specific prophylaxis include:
  • Neutropenic or immunosuppressed patients.
  • Severely malnourished patients.

Prophylactic regimens
Most hospitals have established guidelines for prophylaxis and these should be consulted for prescribing. See Table 2.1 for an example of a regimen.

Thromboprophylaxis
Types of thromboprophylaxis
Mechanical devices
- *Thromboembolic deterrent stockings (TEDS).* Reduce stasis in infrapopliteal veins by continuous direct compression.
- *Pneumatic compression boots.* Reduce stasis in infrapopliteal veins by intermittent compression emptying of foot and lower leg veins, promoting venous flow.

Drugs acting on the clotting cascade
- *Heparin.* Activates antithrombin III.
  • Prophylaxis: 5000U SC od.
  • Treatment: IV 2000U loading dose, 2000U/h (usually 1000U/mL of normal saline). Check APTT 6h after starting and 6–12h thereafter. Titrate to maintain APTT 50–70.
- *LMWH.* Activates antithrombin III. Given by SC injection.
  • Prophylaxis: 20–40mg SC Clexane® od.
  • Treatment: 2mg/kg SC in two divided doses.

Table 2.1 An example of an antibiotic prophylactic regimen

Indication	Typical prophylaxis (single dose on induction)
'Clean' bowel surgery, e.g. acute non-perforated appendicitis, elective colonic resection	Cefuroxime, 1.5g IV + metronidazole 500mg IV or gentamicin 120mg IV Amoxicillin 500mg IV + metronidazole 500mg IV
'Clean' hepatobiliary surgery, e.g. ERCP, open biliary surgery	Gentamicin 120mg IV + amoxicillin 500mg IV + metronidazole 500mg
'Clean' gynaecological surgery	Metronidazole 500mg IV or 1g PR
Elective orthopaedic surgery	Flucloxacillin 1g IV
'Clean' vascular surgery	Flucloxacillin 500mg IV + gentamicin 120mg IV + amoxicillin 500mg IV

Antiplatelet drugs (not used as venous thromboembolism (VTE) prophylaxis)
- Aspirin (300mg PO od).
- Dipyridamole (75mg PO qds).
- Clopidogrel (75mg PO od).

Drugs indirectly affecting clot formation
- *Dextran 70*. Interferes with clot formation. Given as regular bolus infusions (500mL over 1h od).

At risk groups
▶ All patients are 'at risk' of developing deep vein thrombosis just as is the general population. National requirements for VTE prophylaxis require all patients to be assessed for risk factors on admission and after 24h in hospital.[1] Risk is judged according to:
- *Procedure factors*. Prolonged anaesthetic time, lower limb or pelvic surgery.
- *Patient factors*. Immobility, malignancy, age, dehydration, obesity, diabetes, cardiorespiratory disease, inflammatory pathologies, oral contraceptive pill or hormone replacement therapy (HRT), past or family history of thromboembolic disease.

Balanced against:
- *Bleeding risks*. Active bleeding, stroke, invasive procedures, bleeding disorders (liver disease, thrombocytopenia, inherited disorders).
- *Risks of compression devices*. Peripheral vascular disease (PVD).

The risks should be recorded on the patient's drug chart or VTE documentation and mechanical devices (e.g. TEDS) and/or chemical thromboprophylaxis (e.g. LMWH) prescribed according to local policy.

Reference
1 🖉 http://publications.nice.org.uk/venous-thromboembolism-reducing-the-risk-cg92

In-theatre preparation

Theatre is a potentially dangerous place for patients; many of these dangers arise directly as a result of poor preparation and checking of basic facts. For example:

- Wrong side surgery (e.g. healthy kidney removed, wrong hip joint replaced).
- Wrong site surgery (e.g. inguinal, not femoral, hernia repaired; hip, not knee, arthroscoped).
- Allergic reaction to medication.
- Vital material not available, if required (e.g. blood not cross-matched).
- Vital equipment required for surgery not available (e.g. image intensifier, specialist joint replacement jig).
- Retained swabs or instruments.

Experience from other high risk industries (e.g. the airline industry) has shown that strict adherence to a checklist can minimize the risk of these 'never events' happening. The World Health Organization (WHO) recommends a standardized checklist approach.

WHO checklist[1]

The WHO checklist is a basic template that sets out a series of steps, which can be modified or adapted in different organizations, but has four areas of focus.

Before commencement of the list

- Confirm surgical, anaesthetic, and nursing team present and identified.
- Confirm patients on the list and the order of the procedures to be performed.
- Check anaesthetic requirements are correct and functioning (machine, medication, monitoring).
- Confirm vital imaging/equipment required for the list.

Before induction of anaesthesia

- Check patient identity and consent valid.
- Check site and side marked, if appropriate.
- Check anaesthetic requirements are correct and functioning (machine, medication, monitoring).
- Check allergies, anticipated blood loss.

Before skin incision

- Check all team members present and known.
- Check the procedure to be performed.
- Confirm any surgical/anaesthetic/nursing concerns.
- Confirm vital imaging/equipment available.

Before the patient leaves the theatre

- Check the correct name for the procedure actually performed is known and recorded.
- Check the swab and instrument count correct.

- Confirm any surgical specimens collected, 'potted', and labelled correctly.
- Confirm any specific instructions, either surgical or anaesthetic, which apply to the patient in recovery or on transfer to the ward.

Reference

1 🖗 http://www.who.int/patientsafety/safesurgery/ss_checklist/en/index.html

Positioning the patient

Getting the patient on to the operating table

The surgical team is partly responsible for the safety of the patient all the way onto and off the operating table. Be sure the basic rules of safety are being observed. See Fig. 2.3 for some typical patient positions in surgery.

- The anaesthetist is responsible for the patient's airway and should coordinate all moves of the patient to ensure it is maintained.
- Be sure not to dislodge IV cannulae, epidural sites, or existing drains.
- Use approved manual handling techniques (e.g. a 'Patslide' or similar device, rather than lifting the patient).
- Be aware if extra care needs to be taken, e.g. prosthetic joints that may dislocate once protective muscle tone is lost during relaxation, unstable fractures, potentially unstable joints due to rheumatoid arthritis, existing ulcers or skin lesions.

Once in position

- Ensure that no points on the patient are in contact with the metal of the operating table to prevent diathermy exit point burns.
- Make sure bony prominences and areas of thin skin are well padded, e.g. the neck of the fibula in leg stirrups.
- Ensure any diathermy pad is correctly applied and not liable to be affected by skin preparation.
- Ensure there are appropriate supports for the patient to secure the position, particularly if the table may be moved, tilted, or rotated during the procedure (e.g. arm, thoracic, and abdominal supports for lateral positions; shoulder bolsters if the patient will be head down).
- For procedures requiring access to the perineum, be sure that the pelvis is properly supported, but that the perineum is exposed over the end of the operating table.
- Consider the positioning of ancillary equipment (e.g. where will video stacks be positioned? Is more than one energy source required and where will the generators be located? Is there access of mobile imaging equipment or on-table radiography?). All equipment positioning needs to allow enough access to the patient for the surgical team.

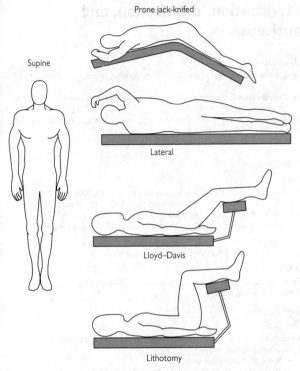

Fig. 2.3 Typical positions for surgery. Supine (most abdominal surgery); prone jackknifed (some rectal or vaginal procedures); lateral (thoracotomy); Lloyd–Davis (pelvic surgery); lithotomy (most perineal procedures).

Sterilization, disinfection, and antisepsis

Definitions
- **Sterilization** is removal of all viable microorganisms, vegetative, and spores.
- **Disinfection** is the removal of actively dividing vegetative microorganisms.
- **Antisepsis** is the process whereby the risk of medical cross-infection by microorganisms is reduced.

Sterilization
Heat
- Dry heat (e.g. incineration, flaming to red hot) is effective, but rarely useful. Dry heat requires temperatures of 160°C for at least 60min.
- Moist heat (e.g. autoclave heating using pressurized steam 121°C at 15lb/in², 15min) is effective and useful, especially in operating theatres.

Irradiation
Gamma radiation. Effective for inorganic materials.

Filtration
Air or fluids can be sterilized by ultrafine membrane filters, but are rarely useful in hospital practice.

Disinfection
Chemical
- Acids/alkalis, e.g. bleach. Effective for non-human contact use.
- Alcohols/phenols, e.g.
  - Ethyl alcohol—skin swabs.
  - Alcohol solutions (Aqagel®)—hand disinfection.
  - Carbolic.
  - Chloroxylenols (Dettol®).
  - Phenol (Clearsol®).
- Oxidizers, e.g.
  - Povidone–iodine (Betadine®)—skin disinfection/surgical scrubbing.
  - Hydrogen peroxide (H_2O_2)—superficial wound cleansing.
  - Aldehydes (Cidex®)—surgical instruments such as endoscopes.
- Cationic solutions, e.g. Chlorhexidine®—antiseptic washes.
- Organic dyes, e.g. Proflavine®.

Antisepsis
Principles of antisepsis include the following.
- Always remove gross contamination with simple soap first.
- Use high potency acid/alkali disinfection on inert surfaces.
- Use less corrosive oxidizers on delicate inert materials.
- Use weak alcohols, oxidizers for skin cleansing.

Scrubbing up

Scrubbing up is designed to reduce the risk of infection from the surgeon to the patient. A thorough clean with bactericidal soaps reduces the number of organisms that can be cultured from skin swabs, but the skin (particularly sweat glands and hair follicles) cannot be sterilized. Moisture and heat occurring under surgical gloves quickly raise the bacterial count again and despite modern cleaning agents, significant growth can be achieved within 2h. Common bactericidal soaps include:

- Hibiscrub® (chlorhexidine).
- Betadine® (povidone–iodine).

Protocol

The first time you come to theatre, ensure that the senior scrub nurses know who you are. It is polite and safe. Everybody should know who the people in theatre are and what they are there for/can do.

How to scrub

- Wet your hands and arms first.
- Lather well with disinfectant soap and wash off.
- 'Scrub' under the nails and heavily soiled areas with a sterile brush and more disinfectant soap. Don't scrub too vigorously, especially on clean skin as this causes irritation without any increased bactericidal effect.
- Wash again with soap, being sure to cover the commonly missed areas—between the fingers, back of the hands, under fingernails, base of the thumbs.
- Rinse thoroughly to remove all soap to reduce the chance of skin irritation.
- Rinse off, trying to ensure the water runs off the arms at the elbows.
- Dry the hands completely first and do not go back to them once drying the arms. Be sure your hands are completely dry before trying to put on gloves—there's nothing worse than gloves that aren't on properly due to wet hands!

How to gown and glove

- Be sure to open the gown without touching the outer 'face'.
- Don't push your hands through the cuffs.
- Pick up the right glove with your right hand 'through' the cuff of the gown, holding it by the edge of the glove on the palm side with the fingers pointing down your forearm.
- With your left hand, fold the other side of the edge of the glove 'over' your right hand.
- Slide your right hand into the glove.
- Once on, pick up the left glove, holding it by the edge and pull it over the cuff of the left hand.
- Slide your left hand into the glove and adjust glove positions.

It is becoming common practice to wear eye protection and two pairs of gloves to reduce the risk of exposure to infectious agents (see p. 178).

Surgical instruments

See Fig. 2.4.

'Sharps'

- *Scalpels.* Two sizes of handle (4 and 6). Types of blade and uses include: no. 11 (used for stab incisions), no. 10 (most skin incisions), no. 15 (fine incisions), no. 22 (adhesiolysis).
- *Scissors.* May be dissecting or stitch cutting. Dissecting scissors may be straight (e.g. Mayo) or curved (e.g. curved Mayo, McIndoe, Metzenbaum, Nelson's).

Forceps

- *Non-toothed.* Fine non-toothed (e.g. DeBakey, Adson's forceps) used for handling delicate tissues such as vessels, bowel. Heavy non-toothed used for general handling, including specimens and sutures.
- *Toothed.* Fine toothed (e.g. Gillie's, McIndoe's forceps) used for handling skin, fine fascia, and occasionally for precise holds on delicate tissues. Heavy toothed (e.g. Lane's forceps) used for holding heavy tissues such as fascia and scar tissue.
- *Ring-tipped and microforceps.* Used in microvascular anastomoses.

Clips and clamps

- Artery clips (e.g. Spencer–Wells, Robert's (large), Dunhill's, Mosquito (small)) have serrated jaws. Used for vascular clamps and tissue/suture holding.
- Tissue clamps, for example:
  - *Lahey clamp.* Similar to a curved arterial clip.
  - *Doyen bowel clamp.* Non-crushing atraumatic.
  - *Babcock/Duval clamp.* Non-toothed semi-atraumatic tissue-holding clamp.
  - *Lane's/Allis's/'Littlewood' clamp.* Heavy toothed traumatic tissue-holding clamps.

Retractors

- Self-retaining retractors:
  - Large (e.g. Goligher retractor for abdominal incisions, Finichetto retractor for thoracic incisions).
  - Small (e.g. Travers/Norfolk and Norwich retractors for small skin and abdominal incisions).
- Handheld retractors:
  - Large (e.g. Deaver, Kelly, Morris).
  - Small (e.g. Kilner 'Catspaw', Langenbeck).

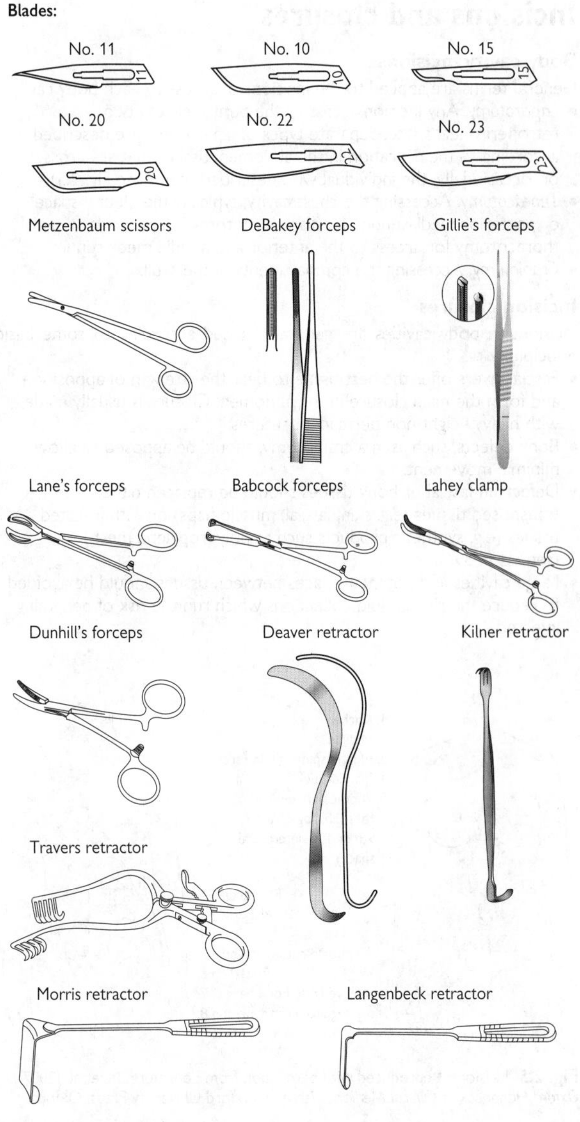
Blades:
No. 11
No. 10
No. 15
No. 20
No. 22
No. 23
11
10
15
20
22
23
Metzenbaum scissors
DeBakey forceps
Gillie's forceps
Lane's forceps
Babcock forceps
Lahey clamp
Dunhill's forceps
Deaver retractor
Kilner retractor
Travers retractor
Morris retractor
Langenbeck retractor

Fig. 2.4 Commonly used surgical instruments.

Incisions and closures

Body cavity incisions

General terms are applied to the incisions of access to each body cavity.

- *Laparotomy.* Any incision accessing the peritoneal cavity or retroperitoneal space. Separate types of laparotomy are described according to their location in the abdomen, tissues that are crossed, or, occasionally, the individual who described them (see Fig. 2.5).
- *Thoracotomy.* Accessing the chest cavity, typically the pleural space or posterior mediastinum. Median sternotomy is a particular type of thoracotomy for access to the anterior and middle mediastinum.
- *Craniotomy.* Accessing the compartments of the skull.

Incision closures

Incisions in body cavities are generally closed according to some basic principles.

- Fascial layers offer the best tissue to bear the strength of apposition and form the main closure in the abdomen. Closure is usually made with heavyweight non-permanent sutures.
- Bony defects, such as in a craniotomy, should be apposed to allow minimal movement.
- Defects in fascial or bony tissues should be replaced either with transposed tissues (e.g. skin, fascial, muscle flaps) or with inserted tissues (e.g. synthetic products such as polypropylene mesh) (see 📖 p. 596).
- Large cavities and potential spaces between tissues should be avoided to reduce the risk of fluid collections which run the risk of becoming infected.

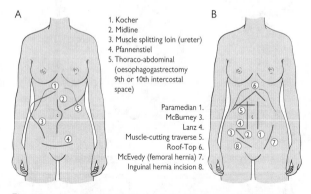

A
1. Kocher
2. Midline
3. Muscle splitting loin (ureter)
4. Pfannenstiel
5. Thoraco-abdominal (oesophagogastrectomy 9th or 10th intercostal space)

B
Paramedian 1.
McBurney 3.
Lanz 4.
Muscle-cutting traverse 5.
Roof-Top 6.
McEvedy (femoral hernia) 7.
Inguinal hernia incision 8.

Fig. 2.5 Incisions. Reproduced with permission from Longmore, M. et al. (2007). *Oxford Handbook of Clinical Medicine*, 7th edn. Oxford University Press, Oxford.

Drains

Uses and complications

Drains may be used for several reasons (see also 🕮 p. 93).

- To remove existing abnormal collections of fluid, blood, pus, air (e.g. drainage of a subphrenic abscess, removal of a pneumothorax).
- To prevent the build-up of either normal bodily fluids (e.g. bile after surgery to the bile duct) or potential abnormal fluids or air (e.g. bloody fluid in the pelvis after rectal surgery).
- Occasionally used to prevent or 'warn' of potentially serious or life-threatening complications (e.g. neck drains after thyroid surgery, chest drains after chest trauma in patients undergoing GA).

Potential complications should be balanced against drain use.

- Damage to structures during insertion, even if under CT or ultrasound guidance (e.g. risk of injury to spleen in subphrenic abscess drainage, haemorrhage from abdominal vessels in operative drains).
- Drains provide a potential route of introduction of infection, especially external drains that remain for longer than a few days.
- Damage to structures close to the drain, e.g. pressure injury to bowel if subjected to high pressure suction drainage.
- Drains do not always drain the substance expected and may give a false 'sense of security', e.g. failure to drain bleeding after thyroid surgery or failure to drain faecal fluid after anastomotic leakage.

There is no place for 'routine' use of drains after surgery unless there is a clear indication—'Better no drainage than ignorant use of it.' (Halstead).

Types of drain (see Box 2.4)

Materials used include latex rubber (e.g. T tubes), silastic rubber (e.g. long-term urinary catheters), polypropylene (e.g. abdominal drains), polyurethane (e.g. NGT).

Box 2.4 Types of drains

Open passive drains

These provide a conduit around which secretions may flow.

- Yates corrugated drain (after subcutaneous abscess drainage).
- Penrose tube drain.
- Drainage setons placed in anal fistulas.

Closed passive drains

These drain fluid by gravity ('siphon effect') or by capillary flow.

- Robinson tube drain (after intra-abdominal abscess drainage).
- NGT.
- Ventriculoperitoneal shunt.
- Chest drain (tube thoracostomy).

Closed active drains

These generate active suction (low or high pressure).

- Exudrains®, Redivac drains®, Minivac®, Jackson Pratt drains (after pelvic or breast surgery).

Stomas

Terminology and types

The term stoma is usually applied to an external opening (temporary or permanent) in a lumenated organ.

- *Ileostomy*. Formed from any part of the mid- or distal small bowel. May be loop (often to 'rest' the distal bowel) or end (usually as a result of surgical removal of distal bowel).
- *Colostomy*. Formed from any part of the large bowel. May be loop (to rest distally) or end (because of surgical resection).
- *Urostomy*. Formed from a short length of disconnected ileum into which one or both ureters are diverted (usually after radical lower urinary tract surgery).
- *Gastrostomy*. Either a surgically created or endoscopically formed connection between anterior stomach and anterior abdominal wall. Often for stomach drainage or direct feeding.
- *Jejunostomy*. Either a surgically created or endoscopically formed connection between proximal jejunum and anterior abdominal wall. Often for direct feeding.

Identifying stomas

Any stoma may have many different appearances. Typical features that help in identifying stomas are the following:

- Ileostomies (loop or end) are usually spouted, have prominent mucosal folds, tend to be dark pink/red in colour, and are most common in the right side of the abdomen.
- Colostomies (loop or end) are usually flush, have flat mucosal folds, tend to be light pink in colour, and are most common in the left side of the abdomen.
- Urostomies (end) are usually spouted, have prominent mucosal folds, tend to be dark pink/red in colour, and are most common in the right side of the abdomen. They are indistinguishable from end ileostomies unless the output can be seen.
- Gastrostomies and jejunostomies are usually narrow calibre, flush with little visible mucosa, and are most common in the left upper quadrant of the abdomen. They are usually fitted with indwelling tubes or access devices.

Knots and sutures

Types of suture

See Fig. 2.6 and Table 2.2.

- Non-absorbable sutures tend to be used where any loss of strength might compromise the future integrity of the tissues being joined, e.g. vascular anastomoses, hernia mesh fixation, tendon repairs, sternal wiring.
- Absorbable sutures tend to be used where the persistence of foreign material would cause unnecessary tissue reaction or increased risk of infection, e.g. bowel anastomoses, skin and subcutaneous tissues.
- Monofilaments have the advantage of smooth tissue passage and minimal tissue reaction, but tend to have a crystalline structure that increases the 'memory' effect of the suture, making knotting less secure and increasing the risk of suture 'fracture'.
- Braided polyfilaments exert more tissue friction during the passage through, but are intrinsically more flexible and knot securely more easily.

Sizes of suture

Size is denoted by imperial sizes from 10/0 (smallest—invisible to naked eye) through 4/0 (typical size for fine vascular anastomoses), 2/0 (typical size for bowel anastomoses), and 1 (typical size for abdominal closure), to 4 (largest available—size of sternal wires).

Types of needle

Needles may be curved (anything from half round to shallow curved) or straight.

- *Blunt-ended, round-bodied* (often used for closing major incisions). Relatively safe as it has low tissue penetrance.
- *Round-bodied* (sharp-pointed, but smooth, round, cross-sectional profile). 'Pushes' tissue apart so often used for delicate tissues such as bowel, blood vessels, etc.
- *Cutting point* (sharp point with triangular cross-section giving a specific cutting edge). Slices through tissues so often used for dense structures such as fascia and tendons (also reverse cutting point).

Table 2.2 Types of suture material

	Natural fibre	Synthetic fibre
Non-absorbable monofilament	Silver wire Steel wire	Polypropylene nylon
Non-absorbable braided polyfilament	Silk (eventually does decay)	Ethilon®
Absorbable monofilament		Monocryl® PDS®
Absorbable braided polyfilament		Vicryl® Dexon®

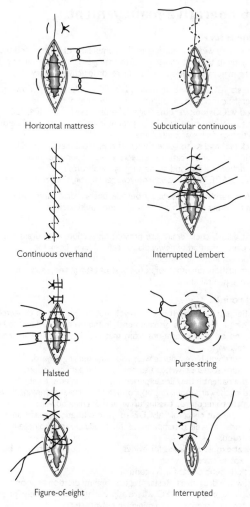

Horizontal mattress

Subcuticular continuous

Continuous overhand

Interrupted Lembert

Halsted

Purse-string

Figure-of-eight

Interrupted

Fig. 2.6 Types of suturing used (illustrated as skin sutures).

Post-operative management

Routine tests

Protocols vary widely according to the complexity of surgery and the age of the patient: this is a rough guide to management of the older patient following major abdominal, cardiac, or reconstructive surgery.

Blood tests FBC and U&E on days 1, 2, and 5. Look for the following.
- Anaemia: consider haemodilution or slow surgical bleeding.
- Raised WCC: look for other signs of sepsis (see ☐ pp. 104, 138).
- Monitor INR/clotting daily if the patient is anticoagulated and before insertion of drains or central lines.
- Check Na^+ and K^+ to guide choice of crystalloid (see ☐ p. 92).
- Monitor urea and creatinine, especially in preoperative renal dysfunction, cardiac and aortic surgery, nephrotoxic drugs (e.g. NSAIDs, ACE-inhibitors, vancomycin/gentamicin, fluid restriction).

ECG Very rarely used routinely outside post-cardiac surgery. Look for: rhythm disturbances such as AF or evidence of ischaemia.

CXR

Request daily if chest drains are present on suction, after drain removal, and to check position of newly placed central lines. Look for:
- Position of indwelling lines;
- Consolidation, pneumothorax (on side of central line), pulmonary oedema, pleural effusion.

Ward rounds

See patients once a day (twice if unwell, not progressing as expected, or undergoing investigations or treatment). In the evening, review the blood results and other investigations from that day. For formal ward rounds, do the following:
- Make sure you have a nurse with you—the nursing record.
- Make sure someone writes a summary in the patient's notes.
- Ask the patient if they are experiencing any problems: establish whether they are mobilizing appropriately, eating and drinking, have adequate pain control, passing urine, and opening bowels.
- Check the obs chart for 'ABCDE' (oxygen saturations, pulse, and BP trends), as well as temperature, fluid balance, and drainage if monitored.
- Look at exposed wounds for evidence of infection or seromas, but do not expose covered wounds.
- Check diabetic charts for BS control.
- Review the drug chart. Restart regular oral medication as soon as possible. Convert IV to PO where appropriate. Look actively for drugs that can be discontinued to minimize polypharmacy.
- Review the most recent blood results.
- Review the nutritional status of the patient—what is the best route?
- Make a clear problem list and a clear plan.

Special cases
Surgery for malignancy

Liaise with specialist nurses; they will know the overall plan from the multi-disciplinary team (MDT). Don't discuss results without consulting them first. Breaking bad news is discussed on 📖 pp. 4 and 16.

Plastic and reconstructive surgery
- Check perfusion of flaps daily.
- Check take of split-skin grafts on day 5.
- Book post-operative medical illustration for photos prior to discharge.

Orthopaedic surgery

Check X-rays of prosthesis to assess position, fraction reduction.

Vascular surgery
- Check distal pulses and capillary refill in patients after reconstructive surgery.
- Perform neurological examination to evaluate patients post-carotid endarterectomy.
- Arrange prosthesis fitting for amputees.

Cardiac surgery
- Check sternal stability daily (ask the patient to cough while you feel for abnormal sternal movement).
- Request transthoracic echo for day 4–5 post-operatively in valve repair patients and auscultate daily.

Discharge
- Plan discharge from the day of admission. Use the hospital discharge team and identify patients requiring special facilities, such as rehabilitation as soon as possible.
- Make sure the patient understands what operation they have had.
- Tell them how to look out for common problems like wound infections, what is normal, and who to contact if they are worried.
- Tell them when they will be seen in clinic.
- Tell them when they can expect to go back to work.
- Ensure an informative, but concise, discharge summary for the GP (see 📖 p. 5).

Rehabilitation
The average times for patients to be fit to go back to work are as follows:
- Two to six weeks after abdominal or thoracic surgery, depending on size and approach (e.g. laparoscopic or open).
- Weight bearing takes up to 2 months after lower limb arthroplasties and 3 months after lower limb fractures.
- Patients can usually drive once they are fully mobile as long as they have not experienced blackouts or fits.
- There are detailed rules for heavy goods vehicle (HGV) drivers and pilots available online.[1]

Reference
1 🔗 http://www.dvla.gov.uk/medical.aspx

Drain management

Uses and types of abdominal drains are covered on 📖 p. 83. A summary follows:

- Drains may remove collections of fluid or gas from body cavities.
- They can be inserted as *prophylaxis or treatment*.
- Effluent can be collected in *closed or open containers*.
- Closed containers may have a *simple or an underwater seal*.
- Drainage can be *suction or non-suction*.
- Drains may be made of latex, PVC, polyurethane, or silicone.

Chest drains

Indications for chest drains and insertion are described on 📖 p. 194. Chest drainage should always be into an underwater sealed container.

Management of chest drains inserted for pneumothorax

- Put the drain on low pressure, high volume wall suction (−3–5kPa) initially (*not* the high pressure wall suction used for tracheal toilet).
- Request and review CXRs daily.
- Bubbling in the underwater seal, either continuously or only when the patient coughs, indicates an air leak and implies that the lung parenchyma has not healed. ▶ You can only remove the drain when there is no air leak; otherwise a pneumothorax will rapidly re-form.
- When the air leak stops, take the drain off suction for 12h and repeat the CXR: if the lung is fully up, the drain can be removed.
- Get a CXR after drain removal to check for a pneumothorax.

Management of chest drains inserted to drain collections

Management of chest trauma is described on 📖 p. 480.

- There is no evidence that suction improves outcome.
- Make sure that the nursing staff measures the drainage: hourly in the post-operative patient, every 24h in longer-term drains.
- A haemodynamically unstable post-operative patient or one who is draining more than 200mL blood/h should be discussed urgently with the thoracic surgeons.
- Post-operative thoracic drains are normally removed when they drain nothing for 2 consecutive hours unless there is an air leak.
- Drains for pleural effusions can be removed when they drain less than 250mL in 24h.
- Drains for empyemas can be removed when they stop draining.
- Always request and review a CXR after drain removal to check for pneumothorax.

Clamping chest drains

Clamping drains when transferring patients stems from the days of TB treatment with caustic solutions and was aimed to prevent drain effluent draining back into the chest. In modern practice, the *only* indications to clamp a drain are: (1) in the trauma setting if the patient is exsanguinating through it; (2) under specialist supervision in patients with chronic air leaks or pneumonectomy.

• Clamping a thoracic drain in a patient with an air leak may rapidly result in a **tension pneumothorax**.
• Clamping a mediastinal drain in a patient who is bleeding may rapidly result in **cardiac tamponade**.
• The safest mode is an **unclamped** drain connected to an underwater seal that is kept **below** the level of the patient at **all** times.
• If you connect the drain to wall suction, but do not put the wall suction on, this is effectively clamping the drain; if you and the nurses do not know what you are doing, *ask for help*.
• If you press in the one-way valve on the top of the underwater seal too tightly, this effectively clamps the drain. If in doubt, leave it alone!

Fluid management

Fluid management is aimed at making sure the patient is neither fluid depleted nor fluid overloaded. The principle is to replace whatever is lost. Success can make the difference between a short, uncomplicated post-operative course and the patient ending up on ICU.

Maintenance crystalloid

The principle is to replace Na^+, K^+, and water loss from urine, vomiting, diarrhoea, high output fistulae and stomas, and fluid 'third-spaced' (e.g. ascites, tissue oedema). For fluid management in burns, see 📖 pp. 604–7.

Approximate average daily loss of fluid and electrolytes

- *Water loss 2500mL/day* (insensible loss from skin, respiratory and GI tract, and in urine). ↑ loss in sepsis, ventilation, diarrhoea, vomiting, high output fistulas, polyuric renal failure.
- *Na^+ 100mmol/day* (in urine). ↑ loss in pyrexia, diarrhoea, vomiting, high output fistulas. Urine concentration is less effective in elderly patients and dextrose infusions may cause hyponatraemia.
- *K^+ 80mmol/day* (in urine). ↑ loss in pyrexia, diarrhoea, vomiting, high output fistulas.

Regime 1

This gives 3L of fluid, 200mmol Na, and 80mmol KCl in 24h. It is only suited to adult patients with no significant comorbidity. It takes no account of patient age, size, cardiac function, or fluid loss.
- 1L normal saline with 40mmol KCl over 8h.
- 1L normal saline with 40mmol KCl over 8h.
- 1L 5% dextrose over 8h.

Regime 2

This adjusts fluid given to fluid lost, but needs the nursing resources to run an hourly fluid balance chart and infusion pumps. It is more suited to patients on HDU.
- 1mL/kg/h normal saline.
- Gelofusine or 5% dextrose fluid challenges to maintain central venous pressure (CVP) 8–12cmH$_2$O or BP >120mmHg.
- 10–40mmol KCl in 100mL 5% dextrose via central line if K^+ <3.0.

Regime 3—Alder Hey paediatric regimen

Useful in all ages and all body weights, except extreme starvation.
- *Fluid volume/24h.* 100mL/kg for each kg 0–10kg; 50mL/kg for each kg 10–20kg; 20mL/kg for each kg over 20kg.
- *Electrolytes.* Na^+ 2mmol/kg/24h; K^+ 1mmol/kg/24h.

Colloid

Colloids (especially blood) produce a more lasting expansion of intravascular volume than crystalloid which rapidly enters the interstitial tissues.
- Gelofusine is succinylated gelatin (a bovine collagen) which has a half-life of about 2h in plasma and is associated with increased bleeding times in post-operative patients.

- Dextran is a glucose polymer mixture that has a plasma half-life of about 2h; it has been associated with anaphylactic reactions and profound coagulopathy.
- HES preparations are derived from hydroxyethyl starch; they have widely differing plasma half-lives and effects on plasma expansion.
- Albumin is a naturally occurring plasma protein, sterilized by ultrafiltration: 5% albumin is isotonic; 20% albumin is hypertonic. Indications for use of albumin as a volume expander are very limited.
- Blood, platelets, fresh frozen plasma (FFP), and cryoprecipitate (see 📖 p. 96).

Assessing volume status This is usually straightforward, but in the HDU patient 24h post-complex surgery, you need information from several sources.

History and examination
- *The dry patient.* May have been NBM several days preoperatively and feels thirsty, complains of a dry mouth, may be dehydrated because of diarrhoea or vomiting, has a low JVP, dry mucous membranes, and reduced skin turgor.
- *The overfilled patient.* Usually doesn't feel thirsty, has a raised JVP, normal skin turgor, and may have dependent oedema and evidence of pulmonary oedema on auscultation.

Observations chart
- *The dry patient.* May have falling BP, rising pulse rate, low CVP that does not rise with fluid challenges, weight is several kg below preoperative weight.
- *The overfilled patient.* Is not usually tachycardic and has a high CVP that rises and plateaus with fluid challenges. BP may fall with fluid challenges; weight is several kg above preoperative weight.

Fluid balance chart
In sick patients, ask the nurses to start an hourly fluid balance chart. Add up all fluid loss (urine output, wound, stoma, and fistula drainage) and subtract from all IV, NG, and oral fluids given.
- *The dry patient.* Will usually be in several litres of negative fluid balance, possibly over a few days, with a urine output <1mL/kg/h.
- *The overfilled patient.* Will be in several litres of positive fluid balance, possibly over a few days. Urine output may be low because of heart failure or renal dysfunction.

Blood results
- *The dry patient.* Has high Na, K, creatinine, and urea, with the urea often disproportionately raised.
- *The overfilled patient.* May have low Na.

CXR
- *The dry patient.* Has no evidence of pulmonary oedema or effusions.
- *The overfilled patient.* May have both pulmonary oedema and effusions.

Acid–base balance

The pH of arterial blood is maintained at 7.35–7.45. Normal functioning of the body's complex enzyme systems depends on this stability. Derrangements may be primarily due to *respiratory or metabolic* dysfunction (see Box 2.5). Compensatory mechanisms are also divided into metabolic and respiratory. The true clinical picture is mixed.

Box 2.5 Diagnosing acid–base abnormalities

pH <7.35 is an acidaemia; pH >7.45 is an alkalaemia

- Look at the pH—is there an acidaemia or an alkalaemia?
- Look at the $PaCO_2$—is there a change *in keeping with* the pH derangement? If so, the derangement is a respiratory one.
- Look at the base deficit (or anion gap). This will tell you if there is a metabolic derangement; if pH is normal, it is fully compensated.

The *Flenley nomogram* (see Fig. 2.7) is a useful diagnostic aid where mixed metabolic and respiratory derangements are present.

Base excess, base deficit, and anion gap

These are derived numbers, calculated by blood gas analysers, quantifying changes in metabolic or fixed acids, but because they depend on several assumptions, they do not always reflect the true acid–base balance.

- *Base excess* is defined as the mmol/L of acid that would be required to titrate the blood pH back to 7.4 if the pCO_2 were normal.
- *Base deficit* (negative base excess) is defined as the mmol/L of base to titrate the blood pH back to 7.4 if the pCO_2 were normal.
- A base deficit is negative and a base excess is positive by convention. Normal values are −2mmol/L to +2mmol/L. A base deficit greater than this (e.g. −6mmol/L) indicates a metabolic acidosis.
- The *anion gap* is the difference between measured cations and measured anions ($= K^+ + Na^+ − Cl^- + HCO_3^-$). This is made up of metabolic acids: ketones, lactate, and phosphates. The anion gap is normally 8–16mmol/L; an increase in anion gap indicates a metabolic acidosis.

Metabolic acidosis

- Uncompensated: $\downarrow$pH, $\leftrightarrow$$pCO_2$, $\downarrow$$HCO_3^-$.
- Compensated: $\downarrow\leftrightarrow$pH, $\downarrow$$pCO_2$, $\downarrow$$HCO_3^-$.

Metabolic acidosis due to increased metabolic acids ($\uparrow$ anion gap)

- Lactic acid (global and/or regional hypoperfusion, hypoxia, sepsis, hepatic failure as the liver normally metabolizes lactate).
- Uric acid (renal failure).
- Ketones (diabetic ketoacidosis, alcoholic and starvation ketoacidosis).
- Drugs/toxins (salicylates, sodium nitroprusside overdose).

Due to loss of bicarbonate or hyperchloraemia (normal anion gap)

- Renal tubular acidosis (loss of bicarbonate).
- Diarrhoea, high output ileostomy (loss of bicarbonate).

- Pancreatic fistulas (loss of bicarbonate).
- Hyperchloraemic acidosis (excessive saline administration).

Metabolic alkalosis
- Uncompensated: ↑ pH, ↔ pCO_2, ↑ HCO_3^-.
- Compensated: ↑↔ pH, ↑ pCO_2, ↑ HCO_3^-.
- Loss of H^+ from gut (vomiting, NG tube suction).
- Renal loss of H^+ (diuretics), ↑ reabsorption of HCO_3^- (hypochloraemia).
- Administration of base (NaHCO₃, citrate in blood transfusions).

Respiratory acidosis
- Uncompensated: ↓ pH, ↑ pCO_2, ↔ HCO_3^-.
- Compensated: ↓↔ pH, ↑ pCO_2, ↑ HCO_3^-.
- Any cause of respiratory failure or hypoventilation.
- Increased production of CO_2, e.g. sepsis, malignant hyperpyrexia.
- Rebreathing CO_2 (circuit misconnections, soda lime exhaustion).

Respiratory alkalosis
- Uncompensated: ↑ pH, ↓ pCO_2, ↔ HCO_3^-.
- Compensated: ↔↑ pH, ↓ pCO_2, ↓ HCO_3^-.
- Hyperventilation: deliberate, inadvertent, or in non-ventilated patients caused by stroke, anxiety, pulmonary embolism (PE), pneumonia, asthma, pulmonary oedema.

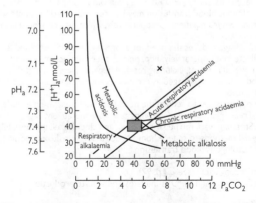

Fig. 2.7 Flenley nonogram. Reproduced with permission from Longmore M. et al. (2007). *Oxford Handbook of Clinical Medicine*, 7th edn. Oxford University Press, Oxford.

Blood products and procoagulants

Indications for blood products

- Young, fit patients tolerate haemodilution much better than elderly patients with multiple comorbidities (particularly cardiovascular and respiratory disease).
- There is a higher threshold for giving blood products in the patient who is not actively bleeding or about to undergo a procedure.
- **Blood.** In general, aim to maintain Hb at 7–9.0g/dL; in older patients, in those with cardiorespiratory disease, maintain Hb >9.0g/dL.
- **FFP.** Patient's circulating blood volume replaced or activated partial thromboplastin time ratio (APTR) >1.5 with active bleeding.
- **Platelets.** Platelets <50 x 10^9/L or <100 x 10^9/L with active bleeding (lower threshold if patient was on aspirin or clopidogrel within 5 days and is actively bleeding).
- **Cryoprecipitate.** Patient's circulating blood volume replaced or fibrinogen <1g/L with active bleeding.

Blood

- One unit of blood increases Hb by about 1g/dL in a 70kg adult.
- Blood is normally provided as packed red cells (1U ≈ 350mL).
- Cross-matched blood can normally be provided within 20min; it contains blood from a single donor.
- In dire emergencies, O-negative blood (universal donor) can be given to recipients of any ABO Rh group without incompatibility reaction.
- Autologous blood transfusion may be used with up to 2U of blood withdrawn from patients preoperatively, which may be stored for up to 5 weeks.
- Cell salvage reduces the need for allogeneic blood. Shed blood is collected intraoperatively, heparinized, spun with normal saline to remove all material, including residual heparin, platelets, and clotting products, and repackaged as red blood cells suspended in saline for transfusion.
- Simple measures to reduce the need for blood transfusion include:
  - Treating anaemia and coagulopathies preoperatively.
  - Stopping warfarin, heparin, aspirin, and clopidogrel appropriately.
- Special methods to reduce homologous blood transfusion include:
  - Autologous blood transfusion.
  - Cell salvage.
  - Procoagulants (see 📖 p. 97).
  - Erythropoietin (EPO) stimulates erythrocyte production.

Platelets

- One unit of platelets increases platelet count by 10^9/L in a 70kg adult.
- Platelets are provided as units (1U ≈ 50mL).
- Platelets do not need to be cross-matched, but they should be ABO-compatible (and rhesus-matched in females of childbearing age).
- One unit contains platelets from a single donor.
- They are stored at 22°C and have a shelf life of 5 days.

Fresh frozen plasma (FFP)

- One unit of FFP contains all the coagulation factors except platelets.
- 1mL of FFP per kg will raise most clotting factors by 1% in a 70kg adult.
- One unit of FFP = 150–250mL and 5–10mL/kg is normally given.
- One unit of FFP usually contains product from a single donor, but is sometimes pooled, in which case it may be from several donors.
- FFP does not need to be cross-matched, but should be ABO compatible (and rhesus-matched in females of childbearing age).
- FFP must be stored at <–18°C. It must be thawed, usually over 20min, before giving and discarded if not used within 2h.

Cryoprecipitate

- One bag of 'cryo' contains 150–250mg fibrinogen and factors VII and VIII.
- If cryopreciptate is unavailable, 5U of FFP contain the same amount of fibrinogen as 10U of cryoprecipitate.
- Ten bags of 'cryo' raises the fibrinogen 0.6–0.7mg/L in a 70kg adult.
- One bag of cryoprecipitate = 20mL; 5–10 pooled bags are normally given.
- ABO and rhesus compatibility are not relevant.

Antifibrinolytics (e.g. aprotinin and tranexamic acid)

- *Action.* Inhibit plasminogen and plasmin; reduce active fibrinolysis.
- *Indications.* Prophylaxis against bleeding in cardiovascular surgery, especially high risk (e.g. redo surgery). Some studies suggest they are useful in 'high risk' orthopaedic surgery. Treatment of excessive bleeding post-operatively (liver surgery; very rarely, radical pelvic resections).

Key revision points—physiology of blood groups

- **ABO antigens** pre-exist on red cells. **ABO antibodies** pre-exist in the circulation and will cause immediate reaction if incompatible.
- **Anti-rhesus (D/E) antibodies** only develop following exposure to the RhD antigen, e.g. during blood transfusion or delivery.
- O Rh negative are **universal donors** (red cells carry no ABO/Rh antigens).
- AB Rh positive are **universal recipients** (serum contains no A, B, RhD antibodies).
- **Blood grouping** involves adding A, B, RhD agglutinins to donated blood to determine blood type; it takes less than 5min.
- **Cross-matching** involves mixing donated blood with the intended recipient serum; assessing compatibility takes about 20min.

Transfusion reactions

▶▶ **Acute haemolytic reaction**

ABO incompatibility as a result of clerical, bedside, sampling, or laboratory error is the most common cause. It may also be caused by incompatibility within other antigen systems (Duffy/Kidd). Donor erythrocytes carrying either A and/or B erythrocyte antigens bind to the recipient's anti-A or anti-B antibodies, resulting in complement formation, membrane attack complex, and immediate haemolysis. Cytokine and chemokine release mediates sympathetic inflammatory response characterized by sudden onset of hypotension, tachycardia, pyrexia, breathlessness, tachypnoea, and back pain. Bilirubinaemia, anaemia, and haemoglobinuria as a result of haemolysis ensue.

- Stop the transfusion immediately and give basic life support if required.
- Keep the bag and giving set for analysis; inform haematology.
- Give crystalloid and furosemide to encourage diuresis.
- Dialysis may be required.

▶▶ **Anaphylaxis and allergic reactions**

Normally, IgE-mediated histamine release reactions to plasma, platelets, and red blood cells. Mild allergic reactions are relatively common and are characterized by erythematous papular rashes, wheals, pruritus, and pyrexia. These are treated by stopping the transfusion and administering chlorpheniramine (10mg IV). Anaphylaxis characterized by hypotension, bronchospasm, and angioedema occasionally occurs.

- Stop the transfusion immediately and disconnect connection tubing.
- Basic life support may be required.
- Treat bronchospasm and angioedema with adrenaline (1mL of 1:10 000 IV), chlorpheniramine (10mg IV), and hydrocortisone (100mg IV).

Non-haemolytic febrile reaction

These common and normally mild reactions are caused by recipient antibodies directed against donor human leucocyte antigen (HLA) and leucocyte-specific antigen on leucocytes and platelets. Cytokine release mediates mild pyrexia, typically over an hour after transfusion is started. Antipyrogens such as paracetamol 1g PO/PR limit pyrexia, but antihistamines are not helpful. Severe reactions feature high grade fever, rigors, nausea, and vomiting. The severity of symptoms is proportional to the number of leucocytes in the transfused blood and the rate of transfusion. Leucocyte-depleted blood helps prevent these reactions.

Delayed extravascular haemolytic reaction

Although pre-transfusion antibody testing is negative (a satisfactory cross-match), these patients experience accelerated destruction of transfused red blood cells 7–10 days following transfusion. This is an antibody-mediated reaction, usually by a patient's antibody (commonly Rh E, Kell, Duffy, and Kidd), present in levels too low to be detected clinically until produced in larger amounts on exposure to circulating antigen. As haemolysis is extravascular, haemoglobinaemia and haemoglobinuria are uncommon:

it is characterized by an unexpected fall in haematocrit a few days post-transfusion, hyperbilirubinaemia, and positive Coombs' test.

Transfusion-related acute lung injury

Non-cardiogenic pulmonary oedema, typically within 6h of transfusion, is mediated by recipient antibodies against donor HLA. Activated recipient leucocytes migrate to the lung, releasing proteolytic enzymes that cause a localized capillary leak syndrome and pulmonary oedema.

Infection

Bacterial

Serious bacterial contamination of stored blood may occur although platelets, which are usually stored at room temperature, are at greater risk of this. Common organisms include *Staphylococcus* spp., *Enterobacter*, *Yersinia*, and *Pseudomonas* spp. Contamination is difficult to detect. The recipient becomes pyrexial at >40°C and hypotensive. This may occur during the transfusion or hours after completion and unlike febrile transfusion reactions, is not self-limiting.

• Volume resuscitation.
• Culture the patient and send bag and giving sets to microbiology.
• Start empirical broad-spectrum antibiotics.

Non-bacterial

Pre-transfusion testing includes screening for hepatitis B (HbsAg, anti-HBc), hepatitis C (anti-HCV), HIV (anti-HIV-1/2, HIV-1 p24 antigen), HTLV (anti-TLC-1/2), and syphilis. HIV can be transmitted by an infective, but seronegative, donor for about 15 days after infection. The HCV window is 20 days. CMV is common in the donor population (40–60%) and immunocompromised donors must receive leucocyte-depleted or CMV-negative blood. Malaria may be transmitted by blood transfusion as may new variant Creutzfeldt–Jakob disease (nvCJD).

Fluid overload

Characterized by hypotension, acute dyspnoea, high CVP, and hypoxia.
• Stop the transfusion.
• Give high flow O_2 and loop diuretics (40mg furosemide IV).

Massive transfusion

• Replacement of the patient's circulating volume within 24h.
• Stored red cells are depleted of ATP and 2,3-DPG and leak K^+ and the fluid contains citrate.
• Large volumes of this blood lead to a blood volume that has poor O_2 carrying capacity, ↑ K^+, hypothermic (if blood is not warmed), and coagulopathic due to Ca^{2+} sequestration.

Reduce the effect of massive transfusion by the following.
• Use infusion warmers and a warming blanket.
• Monitor central circulation and respiratory function closely.
• Consider giving Ca^{2+} supplements (with care!).
• Check platelets, APTT, and fibrinogen: replace if needed.
• Check potassium regularly.

Shock

Definition

Inadequate end-organ perfusion and tissue oxygenation. 'Cellular shock' is a term describing failure of normal cellular processes, including oxygen processing.

3 Recognizing shock

- ↓ BP, ↑ pulse, and *usually* cold, clammy, pale, sweating.
- Confused—may be agitated *or* drowsy.
- Young patients will compensate, with the only signs being decreased pulse pressure, tachycardia, and decreased urine output.

Emergency management

- Assess the airway. If patent, give high flow O_2 by non-rebreathing mask.
- Check carotid or femoral pulse.
- Secure IV access and start giving 500mL crystalloid rapidly.
- Recheck BP. If low and falling fast, call crash team.
- Take a rapid history and examine patient to differentiate between the following types of shock.

Hypovolaemic shock

- *Causes*. Trauma, ruptured abdominal aortic aneurysm (AAA), ruptured ectopic, post-operative haemorrhage, profound dehydration, burns, pancreatitis.
- *Clinical features*. As above with history of trauma/surgery/illness.
- *Treatment*.
  - Lie patient flat; high flow O_2; lift legs to autotransfuse if no IV access.
  - Repeat fluid infusion 500mL IV rapidly: you should see rise in BP.
  - Take blood and send for FBC, U&E, clotting, and cross-match.
  - Take arterial blood gas (ABG): estimate Hb, K^+ as well as ABG.
  - Treat ↑ K^+.
  - If no rapid improvement in BP, look for other causes.

Anaphylactic shock

- *Causes*. Drug allergy, blood product reaction, latex allergy.
- *Clinical features*. History of sudden onset after administration of drug. Stridor or bronchospasm, angioedema, urticaria, pruritus, rash.
- *Treatment*.
  - Sit patient up; give high flow O_2; call anaesthetist if stridor.
  - If IV access: give 1mL of 1:10 000 adrenaline bolus; flush; then 100mg hydrocortisone bolus; flush; then 10mg chlorpheniramine IV.
  - Repeat again in 5–10min if no improvement.
  - If no IV access: give 1mL 1:1000 adrenaline IM. Then secure IV access.
  - If wheezy, give 5mL nebulized salbutamol.

Septic shock

- *Cause*. Overwhelming sepsis (see 🕮 p. 138).

- *Clinical features.* May be the same as hypovolaemic shock or, if established, with circulatory collapse. Earlier in the evolution, the patient may look 'septic'—pyrexial, flushed, bounding pulses.
- *Treatment.*
  - As for hypovolaemic shock.
  - Take blood cultures; then give IV cefuroxime 750mg tds.

Cardiogenic shock

- *Rapidly reversible causes.* cardiac tamponade (trauma, post-cardiac surgery), arrhythmias, tension pneumothorax.
- *Other causes.* Fluid overload and congestive cardiac failure (CCF), MI, PE, subacute bacterial endocarditis (SBE), aortic dissection, decompensated valvular heart disease.
- *Clinical features.* History of recent surgery/trauma, chest pain, dyspnoea, palpitations.
- *Treatment.*
  - Give high flow O_2.
  - Give 2.5mg morphine IV (anxiolytic, venodilator, analgesic, anti-arrhythmic).
  - Put patient on cardiac and sats monitors; request 12-lead ECG.
  - Treat arrhythmias (see advanced life support (ALS) algorithm on inside back cover).
  - Treat myocardial ischaemia with 0.1mg GTN, 300mg aspirin.
  - Auscultate heart sounds and lung fields.
  - Treat tension pneumothorax (see 📖 p. 636), cardiac tamponade (see 📖 p. 638).
  - Discuss with ITU.
  - Consider central venous and peripheral arterial monitoring.
  - Send blood for ABGs, FBC, U&E, clotting, troponin.
  - Catheterize the patient.
  - Request CXR—look for pulmonary oedema.
  - Treat fluid overload with diuretics: furosemide 40mg IV.
  - Consider transthoracic echo to exclude pericardial effusion and valvular lesions, and to assess LV function.

Post-operative haemorrhage

Post-operative haemorrhage may be arterial or venous. Significant arterial haemorrhage is rare and usually occurs from vascular anastomoses. Very rarely, it arises from solid organ injury or loosening of arterial ties. It is rapid, bright red in colour, and often pulsatile. Venous bleeding is a more common cause of post-operative haemorrhage and is usually due to the opening up of unsecured venous channels, or from damage to the liver or spleen at surgery. Although it is non-pulsatile, low pressure, and dark in colour, it can be very large volume and is every bit as life-threatening as arterial bleeding. Most post-operative bleeding is not overt and is contained within body cavities. Drains, even correctly placed, are an unreliable sign of bleeding. Rely on your clinical instincts even if the drains are empty.

Causes and features

- *Primary haemorrhage*. Occurs immediately after surgery or as a continuation of intraoperative bleeding. Usually due to unsecured blood vessels (e.g. liver bleeding following trauma).
- *Reactionary haemorrhage*. Occurs within the first 24h. Usually due to venous bleeding and is commonly thought to be due to improved post-operative circulation and fluid volume, exposing unsecured vessels that bleed (e.g. delayed splenic bleeding following minor trauma at laparotomy).
- *Secondary haemorrhage*. Occurs up to 10 days post-operatively. Usually due to infection of operative wounds or raw surfaces, causing clot disintegration and bleeding from exposed tissue.

Symptoms

Confusion and agitation (due to cerebral hypoxia secondary to hypotension).

Signs

- Soaked dressings, acute wound swelling, blood in drains.
- Pallor, sweaty, tachypnoea, tachycardia, hypotension (a late sign in children and young adults).

Emergency management

Resuscitation

- Establish large calibre IV access. Give crystalloid fluid up to 1000mL bolus if tachycardic or hypotensive. Do not waste time trying to insert a CV catheter. They are unreliable measures of CVP at the bedside in acute situations and are too long and too fine calibre to be of use for rapid volume resuscitation.
- Attempt to control superficial bleeding with direct compression. Do not use tourniquets on limb wounds.
- Take blood for emergency cross-match if serum is not already available. Detail an assistant to telephone blood transfusion for emergency cross-match of a minimum of 2U of blood.
- Inform senior help immediately if significant blood loss. Consider alerting theatres and/or ITU.

- Do not use O Rh negative blood for resuscitation unless the patient is *in extremis*. In these cases, the patient should already be being transferred to theatre or ITU.
- Catheterize and place on a fluid balance chart if hypotensive, but stable.

Establish a diagnosis

The cause may be obvious from the bleeding or the operation.

- Read the operation notes. Is there any potential cause mentioned?
- If the bleeding is severe, the only way to establish a diagnosis may be at re-operation.

If the patient is stable and re-operation is undesirable, consider imaging.

- CT scanning may reveal intra-abdominal or intrathoracic blood.
- Angiography may reveal active bleeding sites and may be therapeutic (coil embolization).

Definitive management

Most post-operative bleeding does not require re-operation, but if it does, it should always be done by a senior surgeon. If this is not the surgeon who performed the original surgery, it may be wise to try to contact them in case they can give useful information about the original procedure.

If re-operation is highly undesirable, e.g. rebleeding after solid organ trauma, then definitive conservative management might include:

- Radiologically guided embolization;
- FFP infusions (see 📖 p. 96);
- Controlled, permissive hypotension;
- Monitoring on ITU.

Wound haematoma

A localized collection of blood beneath the wound or at the site of surgery, usually characterized by swelling and discoloration.

- ▶ If this occurs after vascular surgery, flap surgery, or procedures on the limbs or neck, get senior help as urgent surgical exploration and evacuation may be indicated to avoid ischaemia, compartment syndromes, airway obstruction, flap failure, or ongoing haemorrhage.
- Apply firm pressure followed by a pressure dressing.
- Check clotting and FBC and treat appropriately (see 📖 p. 96).
- Withhold heparin.
- Surgical management is the same as for haemorrhage.

Wound emergencies

Infection
Causes
Most wound infections are acquired from the patient's own flora. The majority are skin organisms (e.g. *Staphylococcus aureus, Staphylococcus epidermidis*), although the second commonest cause is contamination from opened viscera during surgery (e.g. *Escherichia coli* from the GI tract, *Pseudomonas* from the biliary tree).

Symptoms
- Pain and discharge in the wound.
- Malaise, anorexia, and fever (systemic inflammatory features).

Signs
- Fever, tachycardia.
- Red, swollen, tender wound (may be discharging pus or fluctuant due to contained pus).

Complications
- Bacteraemia is common, but rarely significant.
- Septicaemia is rare unless the organism is resistant or the patient is immunosuppressed.

Emergency management
Resuscitation
Ensure there is IV access. Give crystalloid fluid up to 1000mL if tachycardic or hypotensive.

Establish a diagnosis
- Send any discharging pus for microscopy, culture and sensitivities (M,C,&S).
- Send blood for FBC (Hb, WCC) and blood cultures.

Early treatment
- Give IV antibiotics if there are any systemic features. If there is no pre-existing infection, use anti-staphylococcals: flucloxacillin 1g + 500mg qds. If the patient is immunosuppressed or very unwell, add in broad-spectrum cover to include anaerobic cover: metronidazole 500mg IV + 500mg IV tds and cefuroxime 1.5g IV + 500mg IV tds.
- If there is real concern about MRSA infection, consult microbiology and consider adding IV vancomycin 500mg. If so, monitor drug plasma concentration.
- Open or aspirate the wound if there is contained pus. Wash the wound.

Dehiscence
Wound dehiscence may be superficial (including skin and subcutaneous tissue) or full thickness/deep (involving fascial closures or bony closures). Full thickness dehiscence may expose deep structures. In the abdomen, this includes the viscera which may protrude through the wound (evisceration).

Causes

Most wound dehiscences are secondary to wound infection. Contributory factors include immunosuppression, malnutrition, steroid use, poor surgical technique, previous surgery or procedures. Occasionally, the dehiscence is due to intracavity pathology causing wound breakdown from within (e.g. anastomotic leakage causing enteric fistulation).

Symptoms

Usually painless.

Signs

- Open wound, visible fat and fascia if superficial; visible viscera if full thickness.
- Occasionally associated organ dysfunction if involved by the accompanying wound infection (e.g. pericarditis/anterior mediastinitis in sternal dehiscence).

Emergency management

Resuscitation

- Ensure there is IV access.
- Calm the patient, particularly if there is any degree of evisceration.

Early treatment

- If there are exposed viscera, cover these with saline soaked dressings.
- Give IV antibiotics if there are features of wound infection (see 📖 p. 104).
- If the dehiscence is superficial, ensure the wound is open and any pus is fully drained. Lightly pack the wound with absorbent dressing (e.g. Sorbsan®).

Definitive management

Superficial

- Continue regular wound lavage and dressings.
- For large defects, consider vacuum-assisted closure.

Full thickness

- Resuturing/closure of the defect in theatre may be appropriate.
- For some deep defects, re-closure may be inappropriate (e.g. the presence of infection, intestinal contents/fistulas, severe immunocompromise, physiologically unstable, intracavity pathology causing the dehiscence). In these cases, the wound should be allowed to form a chronic wound and close by secondary intention (e.g. called a laparostomy in the abdomen). This may be assisted by vacuum closure devices.

Bleeding (see 📖 p. 102).

Cardiac complications

Chest pain

Taking a careful pain history should help differentiate between the causes of chest discomfort listed in Box 2.6 below.

Box 2.6 Causes of post-operative chest pain

Dull, central ache
- Myocardial ischaemia.
- Gastric distension.

Central pain radiating through to back
- Thoracic aneurysm or dissection.
- Peptic ulcer disease, oesophagitis, rarely pancreatitis.

Pain on movement
- Musculoskeletal pain.
- Chest drains.

Pleuritic pain
- Chest infection.
- Pneumothorax.
- Haemothorax, pleural effusion, empyema.
- Chest drain *in situ*.
- PE.

Diagnosis
- Take a careful history and examine the patient.
- A CXR will demonstrate most lung pathology.
- 12-lead ECG should help exclude myocardial ischaemia.
- Recent WCC and CRP help identify sepsis.
- Review previous medical history for peptic ulcer disease and the drug chart for NSAID use.

Myocardial ischaemia

Patients, particularly in vascular surgery, may have pre-existing ischaemic heart disease. Surgery can precipitate ischaemia through:
- Stress response to major surgery (endogenous catecholamine release triggered by anxiety, pain).
- Fluid overload post-operatively.
- Profound hypotension.
- Failing to restart anti-anginal medication post-operatively.

Diagnosis

Take a history, particularly of chest discomfort brought on by exertion and relieved by GTN. Check that the patient is back on any regular cardiac medication. The physiotherapists may report bradycardia on exercising. A 12-lead ECG will confirm the presence of myocardial ischaemia (see Box 2.7). Cardiac enzymes (troponin T (and I) or CK^{MB}) may be slightly raised post-operatively, but a high level or serial measurements showing a continued rise would suggest ongoing myocardial damage.

Management
- Sit patient up; give high flow O_2.
- Ensure the patient is on aspirin 75mg od PO and LMWH, e.g. 40mg enoxaparin (Clexane®) SC.
- Give GTN sublingually.
- Restart preoperative anti-anginal medication.
- Discuss urgently with a cardiologist.

Perioperative MI

Perioperative MI may be difficult to diagnose because the patient may be unable to give a good history or to distinguish between chest and upper abdominal pain.
- The presentation is similar to that of myocardial ischaemia, but the duration is longer (>20min) and may be associated with haemodynamic instability, nausea, vomiting, confusion, and distress.
- The patient will often be cold, clammy, and may be hypoxic.

Box 2.7 Diagnostic criteria for MI

In the setting of symptoms suggestive of acute coronary syndrome:
- ECG shows ST segment elevation—ST segment elevation MI (STEMI).
- No ST elevation, but elevated CK^{MB} (2 x normal) or troponin T-positive—non-Q wave or non-ST segment elevation MI (NSTEMI).

Management
- Attach an ECG monitor and a sats probe and get a 12-lead ECG.
- Make sure the defibrillator trolley is close at hand.
- Give high flow O_2.
- Get IV access.
- Give morphine 5mg IV and metoclopramide 10mg IV.
- Give aspirin 300mg PO/PR and GTN 0.5mg SL.
- Contact cardiologists urgently for consideration of acute intervention.

Key revision points—physiology of coronary blood flow
- Myocardial cells extract up to 70% of O_2 from blood.
- Coronary blood flow occurs during diastole.
- Tachycardia reduces diastolic interval and increases O_2 demand, which may reveal occult ischaemia.
- Coronary vasodilatation is mediated by adenosine, K^+, hypoxia, and β_2 stimulants and the N_2O pathway.

Respiratory complications

These are common after surgery as a result of the effect of general anaesthetic, post-operative pain, and immobility.

Respiratory failure

> **Definitions of respiratory failure**
> - **Hypoxia.** PaO_2 <10.5kPa.
> - **Hypercapnia.** $PaCO_2$ >6.5kPa. **Hypocapnia.** $PaCO_2$ <3.5kPa.
> - **Type I respiratory failure.** PaO_2 <8.0kPa on air.
> - **Type II respiratory failure.** PaO_2 <8kPa *and* $PaCO_2$ >6.0kPa.

Basic assessment and management
- Sit the patient up and give high flow O_2 through a tight fitting mask.
- Assess the airway. Is chest expansion asymmetrical?
- Auscultate the chest. Listen for bilateral breath sounds, poor air entry, wheeze, bronchial breathing, crepitations.
- Assess circulation and treat shock which causes hypoxaemia (see 📖 p. 100).
- Treat bronchospasm with nebulized salbutamol 5mg.
- Get a CXR. Look for consolidation, oedema, effusions, and pneumothoraces.

Chest infection

Diagnosis
- Cough with purulent sputum.
- Pyrexia.
- Bronchial breath sounds and reduced air entry on auscultation.
- Leucocyte neutrophilia, raised CRP.
- Consolidation on CXR.
- Culture of sputum may yield sensitivities of causative organisms.
- In the dyspnoeic, hypoxic patient perform ABGs to guide immediate management.

Prevention
There is no good evidence that prophylactic physiotherapy helps to prevent chest infection after surgery. The single most important intervention is to prevent patients with active chest infections undergoing surgery. Any elective patient with a current cough (dry or productive), temperature, clinical signs of chest infection, neutrophilia, or suspicious CXR should be deferred for a fortnight and then reassessed. Other risk factors include active smokers or those who have stopped smoking within the last 6 weeks; patients with COPD, obesity; patients requiring prolonged ventilation post-operatively; and patients who aspirate.

Management
- Physiotherapy helps the patient with a cough to expectorate sputum and prevent mucus plugging.
- Effective analgesia is important to allow patients to cough.

- Definitive treatment is antibiotics: ciprofloxacin 500mg bd PO provides good Gram −ve and +ve cover until organism sensitivities are known.
- Suspected aspiration pneumonia should be treated (e.g. IV cefuroxime 1g tds and IV metronidazole 500mg tds).
- If the patient requires oxygen (PaO_2 <8.0kPa on room air), humidify it reduces the risk of mucus plugs and makes secretions easier to shift.
- Continuous positive airway pressure (CPAP) can be used to improve basal collapse.
- The hypoxic, tachypnoeic, tiring patient on respiratory support should be reviewed urgently by the critical care team.

Exacerbation of COPD

The incidence of moderate to severe COPD in surgical patients is 5%.

- Most studies show that moderate COPD is not associated with an increase in post-operative complications, mortality, or length of stay.
- Severe COPD and preoperative steroid use are associated with increased morbidity and mortality after surgery.
- Ensure that all patients on preoperative β-agonist inhalers are routinely prescribed regular post-operative nebulizers (saline 5mL prn, salbutamol 2.5–5mg qds prn, and becotide 500 micrograms qds prn).
- In hypoxic patients with COPD, give maximal O_2 by CPAP and titrate against $PaCO_2$ and PO_2: do *not* restrict O_2 empirically.

Key revision points—monitoring/measuring lung function

- Pulse oximetry estimates the percentage of saturated Hb present in capillary blood by the change in wavelength ratios of absorbed red light. It is inaccurate in carbon monoxide poisoning, cold peripheries, low flow states, and tachydysrhythmias.
- PaO_2 can be approximately *estimated* from the SaO_2.
  - 95%, >12kPa.
  - 85%, ~10kPa.
  - 75%, <6kPa.
- Capnography works on similar principles; different gases (e.g. CO_2) absorb different amounts of infrared light.

Renal complications

Renal dysfunction
- Creatinine: >126μmol/L in males; >102μmol/L in females.
- Urea: >7.0mmol/L.
- Creatinine clearance: <90mL/min.

Aetiology of renal failure
- *Preoperative risk factors.* Age >75y; creatinine >150μmol/L; LV dysfunction; hypertension; diabetes; peripheral vascular disease; hypoperfusion as a result of diuretic therapy and vasodilators; sepsis; CCF; intrinsic renal damage caused by NSAIDs, contrast, aminoglycosides, diuretics; endocarditis; obstructive uropathy.
- *Intraoperative risk factors.* Cardiac surgery, aortic surgery.
- *Post-operative risk factors.*
  - *Pre-renal.* Shock, e.g. hypovolaemic, septic, cardiogenic (see p. 106).
  - *Renal.* Sepsis, hypoxia, drugs (NSAIDs, gentamicin, vancomycin, teicoplanin), haemoglobinuria, myoglobinuria.
  - *Post-renal.* Obstructive uropathy, obstructed Foley catheter, prostatic hypertrophy.

Preventing renal failure
There are a number of measures that reduce the risk of renal dysfunction.
- Preoperatively, *ensure adequate hydration*, particularly before undergoing procedures involving contrast.
- Identify and *eliminate nephrotoxic medications* where possible, particularly NSAIDs and ACE-inhibitors.
- Consider whether the patient would benefit from HDU preoperatively.
- Avoid intraoperative hypotension.
- Post-operatively maintaining satisfactory cardiac output and optimizing intravascular volume are the most important factors in avoiding renal dysfunction.

Management of renal failure
The management of oliguria is described on pp. 112–3. This section deals with the management of established oliguric renal failure. The aim is firstly to avoid the potentially lethal complications of renal failure (hyperkalaemia, acidosis, pulmonary and cerebral oedema, severe uraemia, and drug toxicity) and secondly to avoid exacerbating the renal insult. Investigation of the underlying causes of renal failure is also important.
- Aim for higher BP (stop antihypertensives; optimize fluid balance), except in established anuria.
- Treat hypoxia aggressively.
- Aim for daily fluid balance of even to negative 500mL to avoid pulmonary oedema in anuric patients.

- Monitor electrolytes daily, and potassium and acid–base balance every few hours. Avoid potassium supplements and medication that increases potassium levels (ACE-inhibitors).
- Avoid nephrotoxic drugs (aminoglycosides, NSAIDs, ACE-inhibitors) and monitor serum levels of drugs dependent on renal excretion (digoxin, antibiotics such as vancomycin and gentamicin).
- Essential amino acid diets are recommended for patients who are able to eat. Patients on dialysis require high protein content (1.5g/kg/day) as dialysis results in negative nitrogen balance.
- Enteral and parenteral feeds can be similarly adjusted.
- Renal ultrasound, renal angiography may be indicated.

Hyperkalaemia

Hyperkalaemia (K^+ >5.0) is seen in the setting of renal failure, tissue necrosis, and potassium-sparing diuretics and supplements. Acute hyperkalemia (K^+ >6.0) can cause life-threatening ventricular arrhythmias. ECG changes that herald myocardial dysfunction are *flattened P waves, wide QRS complexes, tenting of T waves*, and, in peri-arrest, a sine wave.
- ▶ Treat the patient with ECG changes as an emergency.
- Treat the underlying cause.
- Give *50mL of 50% dextrose containing 15U of Actrapid*® as an IV infusion over 10–20min, repeating as necessary, monitoring BS after each infusion. If inadequate response:
- Give *10mL calcium gluconate 10% IV over 2min*; repeat as necessary.
- Calcium resonium enema binds K^+ and removes it from the body.
- *Dialysis* should be urgently considered in patients with refractory hyperkalemia despite these measures, irrespective of renal function.

Hypokalaemia

Hypokalaemia (K^+ <3.0) is common. It predisposes patients to dysrhythmias. It is normally related to diuretic therapy, insulin sliding scales, diarrhoea and vomiting, steroids, and poor nutrition. Acute severe hypokalaemia (K^+ <2.5) may result in life-threatening arrhythmias. It can be recognized by small or inverted T waves, depressed ST segments, prolonged PR interval, and U waves on the ECG.
- Educate the patient about which foods are rich in potassium (bananas, prunes, apricots, tomatoes, orange juice) and ensure availability.
- Change furosemide to co-amilofruse 5/40 or 2.5/20 which contains furosemide (either 40mg or 20mg) and amiloride (5mg or 2.5mg).
- Add oral potassium supplements up to 160mmol daily (1 tablet of Sando K^+ contains 20mmol of K^+, 1 tablet of Slow K^+, which is better tolerated by most patients, contains 12.5mmol KCl).
- If a central line is in place, give 20mmol KCl in 50–100mL of 5% dextrose over 20min to 1h.
- If it is necessary to use a peripheral line, place a maximum of 40mmol of potassium in 1L 5% dextrose running at a maximum of 125mL/h.
- Monitor K^+ daily and avoid discharging the patient home on a combination of potassium supplements and potassium-sparing diuretics.

Urinary complications

Oliguria

> ### Terminology
> • Oliguria—urine output <0.5mL/kg/h.
> • Anuria—no measurable urine output.

Urine ouput is an indicator of glomerular filtration rate which is an indicator of renal plasma flow and renal perfusion. Hence, *urine output is an indirect measure of renal (and hence systemic) blood flow as well as renal function.* Patients with normal renal function usually maintain a urine output of at least 0.5mL/kg/h.

Management of oliguria
• *Check that the Foley catheter is not the problem.*
• The urine catheter may be obstructed, bypassing, or malpositioned. Is the bed wet? Flush with 60mL saline—can you draw this amount back without difficulty? If not, or if the urine is bypassing the catheter, or if the bladder is palpable, change the catheter.

Optimize cardiac function
• Patients who were markedly hypertensive (see 📖 pp. 92, 132) preoperatively may require high BPs to maintain a satisfactory urine output.
• *Is the patient overfilled or underfilled?*
• *Make sure the patient is adequately filled* by giving careful fluid challenges to achieve CVP of 14–16mmHg or raise the JVP moderately.
• *But not too filled.* If the CVP rises to >16mmHg and stays up with a fluid challenge or if the BP falls, the patient may be overfilled and need diuretics (see below).
• *Invasive monitoring.* If the patient does not rapidly respond to basic measures, need CVP line insertion and monitoring (see 📖 p. 198).

Loop diuretics
Furosemide will *not* prevent acute tubular necrosis, *but* it does have a useful role in offloading fluid from the overfilled patient. It converts oliguric renal failure to polyuric renal failure.
• If the patient is adequately filled and mean arterial pressures are satisfactory, give a loop diuretic: 20mg of furosemide IV. If there is no response, give a further 40mg furosemide IV.
• If the urine produced in response to diuretic challenges is concentrated, the patient is probably inadequately filled.

Important problems associated with oliguria of any cause
• Pulmonary and cerebral oedema.
• CCF (see 📖 p. 106).
• Hyperkalaemia (see 📖 p. 110).
• Acidosis.
• Drug toxicity.

Further assessment and management
Haemodialysis is indicated in the oliguric patient to avoid pulmonary oedema indicated by deteriorating blood gases despite increasing respiratory support, hyperkalaemia, and acidosis. It is not indicated purely for rising serum creatinine and urea in the first instance (📖 p. 134).

Acute urinary retention
Common post-operatively, especially in elderly males, after abdomino-pelvic or groin surgery and after anticholinergics.

Clinical features
- Suprapubic discomfort, inability to initiate micturition, or dribbling.
- History of prostatic disease or symptoms preoperatively (see 📖 p. 362).
- Percussable bladder on examination.

Management
- Conservative. Improve analgesia, treat constipation, mobilize, warm bath to encourage micturition, restart preoperative tamsulosin.
- Insert urethral catheter if conservative measures fail and patient in great discomfort or renal dysfunction is suspected.

Urinary tract infection
Common in females and patients catheterized for prolonged periods.

Clinical features
- Dysuria, frequency, dribbling, offensive smell, pyrexia, ↑ WCC.
- Dipstick urine to confirm (dipstick should test nitrites and leucocytes).
- Send specimen for microbiology to identify organism and sensitivities.

Management
- Remove catheters as soon as possible.
- Encourage drinking or increase fluid infusion if safe to increase urine flow.
- Treat empirically with trimethoprim 400mg bd until sensitivities known.

Key revision points—physiology of diuretics
- **Osmotic diuretics**, e.g. mannitol, are not well reabsorbed in the distal tubules. Increased osmotic pressure reduces H_2O reabsorption.
- **Loop diuretics** inhibit $Na^+K^+Cl^-$ exchange in the ascending loop of Henle, decreasing osmolality in the medulla and water reabsorption.
- **Aldosterone antagonists**, e.g. spironalactone, and **sodium channel blockers**, e.g. amiloride, reduce Na^+ reabsorption and K^+ and H^+ secretion in the distal tubule.
- **Alcohol** inhibits antidiuretic hormone (ADH) release.

Gastrointestinal complications

Paralytic ileus
This is the cessation of GI tract motility.

Causes
- Prolonged surgery, exposure and handling of the bowel.
- Peritonitis and abdominal trauma.
- Electrolyte disturbances (most can affect GI function!!).
- Anticholinergics or opiates.
- Prolonged hypotension or hypoxia.
- Immobilization.

Clinical features
- Nausea, vomiting and hiccoughs.
- Abdominal distension, tympanic or dull on percussion.
- Air-/fluid-filled loops of small and/or large bowel on abdominal X-ray (AXR).

Prognosis
Intestinal ileus usually settles with appropriate treatment.

Treatment
- Pass an NGT to empty the stomach of fluid and gas if the patient is nauseated or vomiting. Small volumes of tolerated oral intake may help mild ileus to resolve.
- Ensure adequate hydration by IV infusion ('drip and suck').
- Maintain the electrolyte balance.
- Reduce opiate analgesia and encourage the patient to mobilize.
- Consider other causes (e.g. occult intra-abdominal sepsis) and consider nutritional status.

Post-operative mechanical small bowel obstruction
It is important to distinguish between mechanical obstruction and ileus since management may be different.

Causes
- Early adhesions (usually self-limiting).
- Internal, external, parastomal, or wound herniation.
- Intra-abdominal sepsis (usually slightly later presentation).

Clinical features
- Nausea and vomiting.
- Colicky abdominal pain.
- Abdominal distension, tympanic on percussion.
- Examine hernial orifices and stoma, if any, for incarcerated hernias.
- High-pitched 'tinkling' bowel sounds MAY be present.
- Dilated loops of small bowel (relative paucity of gas in colon).

Treatment
- As for paralytic ileus with strict bowel rest.
- Consider CT scan to define diagnosis and level of the obstruction.

Prognosis
Surgery is rarely indicated (for suspected herniation or complications or, very occasionally, adhesional obstruction that fails to resolve).

Nausea and vomiting

This affects up to 75% of patients. It predisposes to increased bleeding, incisional hernias, aspiration pneumonia, ↓ absorption of oral medication, poor nutrition, and ↓ K^+. Causes include:
- Prolonged surgery; anaesthetic agents, e.g. etomidate, ketamine, N_2O, opioids; spinal anaesthesia; gastric dilatation from CPAP;
- Post-operative ileus; bowel obstruction; constipation; gastric reflux; peptic ulceration or bleeding; medications, including many antibiotics, NSAIDs, opiates, statins; pancreatitis; sepsis; and hyponatraemia.

Classification of antiemetics

Combining two different types of antiemetic increases efficiency.

Antidopaminergic agents
- Good against opioid nausea and vomiting, sedative, extrapyramidal side effects.
- For example, prochlorperazine 12.5mg IM, metoclopramide 10mg IV/IM/PO tds.

Antihistamines
- Sedation, tachycardias, hypotension with IV injection.
- For example, cyclizine 50mg IM/IV/PO tds.

Anticholinergics
- Active against emetic effect of opioids, sedation, confusion, dry mouth.
- For example, hyoscine (scopolamine) 0.3–0.6mg IM.

Antiserotonergics
- Lowest side effect profile of all antiemetics.
- Ondansetron 1–8mg PO/IV/IM tds, granisetron 1mg PO/IV tds.

Constipation

Failure to pass stool is common. Caused by lack of privacy, immobility, pain from wounds or anal fissures, dehydration, poor nutrition, ↓ dietary fibre, opiates, iron supplements, and spinal anaesthesia. Treat with:
- *Bulking agents*, e.g. Fybogel one sachet PO bd.
- *Stool softeners*, e.g. sodium docusate 30–60mg od PO.
- *Osmotic agents*, e.g. lactulose 5–10mL bd.
- *Stimulants*, e.g. senna one tablet bd PO, bisacodyl 5–20mg nocte PO.

Diarrhoea

Common causes in post-operative patients:
- Resolving ileus or obstruction.
- Related to underlying disease or surgery (e.g. ileal pouch or Crohn's).
- Antibiotic-related diarrhoea (send for M,C,&S).
- *Clostridium (C.) difficile* diarrhoea (send stool for *C. difficile* toxin) and pseudomembranous colitis (see 📖 p. 396).

Anastomotic leakage (see 📖 p. 420).

Neurological complications

Confusion

Confusion is common post-operatively. It is often obvious with a disoriented, uncooperative, or hallucinating patient. Frequently, it is more subtle, consisting of inactivity, quietness, slowed thinking, and labile mood, and it is only spotted by relatives or nursing staff. Actively assess whether the patient is oriented in time, person, and place. Perform a quick mini-mental state examination if you are still unsure.

Common causes of confusion

- Medication (particularly benzodiazepines, opiates, anticonvulsants).
- Stroke.
- Hypoxia, hypercapnia.
- Shock.
- Sepsis.
- Alcohol withdrawal.
- Metabolic disturbances (↓ glucose, Na^+, pH; ↑ Ca^{2+}, creatinine, urea, bilirubin).
- Post-ictal.
- Preoperative dementia.

Management

- If the patient's behaviour poses a physical danger to themselves or others, it may be necessary to sedate as first-line management. Haloperidol 2.5mg may be given up to a total of 10mg in 24h PO, IM, or IV, but if the patient remains disturbed, 2.5–5mg of midazolam should be given IV and the patient placed under close observation. ▶ Beware of sedating the hypoxic or hypotensive patient as this may trigger a cardiorespiratory arrest: confusion is a common symptom of shock and profound hypoxia.
- Assess and treat hypoxia (see 📖 p. 130) and hypotension (see 📖 p. 132).
- Reassess the drug chart: stop opiates and benzodiazepines.
- Correct abnormalities, e.g. ↓ glucose, ↓ Na.
- Alcohol withdrawal is diagnosed from a history of chronically high alcohol consumption often with raised γGT, combined with psychomotor agitation post-operatively. It can be treated with either diazepam 5–10mg tds PO/PR, haloperidol 2.5–5mg tds PO/IM/IV, or allowing the patient alcohol 1U orally.
- Perform a neurological examination to look for focal neurological deficit and consider head CT to exclude stroke.
- Reassure patient and relatives: confusion is common, almost always reversible, and it is not a sign that the patient is 'going mad'.

Stroke

Stroke is most common in vascular and cardiac surgical patients (2%), but elderly patients undergoing other major surgery are at risk.

Risk factors for stroke

- Increasing age (>80y risk of cerebrovascular accident (CVA) 5–10%).
- Diabetes.

- Previous history of stroke or transient ischaemic attack (TIA) (increases risk three-fold).
- Carotid artery atherosclerosis.
- Perioperative hypotension.
- Left-sided mural thrombus.
- Mechanical heart valve.
- Post-operative AF.

Aetiology
- *Embolic.* Carotid stenosis/atheroma, thrombus from AF.
- *Haemorrhagic.* Post-operative warfarinization.
- *Cerebral hypoperfusion.* Profound hypotension, raised intracranial pressure (ICP).
- *Hypoxia.*

Clinical features
Any deficit resolving within 24h is called a TIA. Clinical features of perioperative stroke include:
- Failure to regain consciousness once sedation has been weaned.
- Hemiplegia (middle cerebral artery or total carotid artery occlusion).
- Initial areflexia becoming hyperreflexia and rigidity after a few days.
- Aphasia, dysarthria, ataxia (gait or truncal), inadequate gag reflex.
- Visual deficits, unilateral neglect, confusion, seizures.
- Persistent, marked hypertension.
- Hypercapnia.

Diagnosis
The aim is to establish a definitive diagnosis, establish a cause to guide appropriate secondary prevention, and establish a baseline of function to help plan long-term rehabilitation or withdrawal of therapy.
- Carry out a full neurological examination (cognitive function, cranial nerves, and tone, power, reflexes, and sensation in all four limbs).
- Modern contrast head CT will show infarcts within 2h (older scanners may not pick up lesions until they are 2–3 days old. You must distinguish between haemorrhagic and ischaemic CVAs (1 in 10 are haemorrhagic). MRI is necessary to image brainstem lesions.

Initial management
- Assess the airway, breathing, and circulation.
- If the patient is unable to maintain their airway, insert a Guedel airway, bag and mask, ventilate with high flow O_2, and call an anaesthetist.
- Monitor BP, but do not attempt to correct high pressures as these are critical for adequate cerebral perfusion.
- Monitor oxygen saturations.
- Secure IV access and give colloid if indicated.
- If the patient is able to maintain their own airway and is not haemodynamically compromised, explain what has happened and reassure them.
- Perform a full neurological examination.
- Put the patient NBM if there is no gag reflex.
- Send FBC, U&E, glucose, and clotting.
- Send blood cultures if there is any history of endocarditis, pyrexia.
- Request a CT head and consider a transthoracic echo.

Haematological complications

Heparin-induced thrombocytopenia (HIT)

HIT occurs in about 5% of patients receiving heparin (5.5% of patients on bovine heparin, 1.0% with porcine heparin). It is characterized by the formation of complement-mediated heparin-dependent IgG platelet antibody. It occurs 5–10 days after initiation of heparin therapy or after the first dose of heparin in patients with previous exposure to heparin within the last 3 months.

Diagnosis
- Fall in platelet count by over 30% to <150 x 10⁹/L or by over 50%.
- *And* positive serology for HIT antibodies.
- Heparin-induced thrombocytopenia and thrombosis (HITT) occurs in about 20% of patients with HIT and is characterized by major thrombotic episodes. It has a mortality of about 30%.
- Patients may show tachyphylaxis to heparin as well as bleeding complications.

Treatment
- Discontinue all heparin therapy, including heparinized saline flushes.
- If it is at all possible, delay any surgery requiring bypass until HIT antibodies are undetectable and then follow standard heparinization, but do not use heparin in the post-operative period.
- If it is impossible to delay bypass surgery, then danaparoid and iloprost are alternatives to heparin with the major disadvantages that they cannot be reversed after bypass and require specialized assays.
- Hirudin, iloprost, danaparoid, and warfarin are alternative anticoagulants to heparin in the post-operative period.
- Discuss with haematologist.

Disseminated intravascular coagulation (DIC)

DIC may occur as a complication of sepsis, transfusion reaction, drug reaction, transplant rejection, and aortic aneurysm surgery. It is characterized by widespread activation of coagulation, resulting in the formation of intravascular fibrin, fibrin degradation products, consumption platelets, and clotting factors, and ultimately, thrombotic occlusion of vessels. Patients may present with bleeding from indwelling venous lines, wounds, and minor abrasions.

Diagnosis
There is no single diagnostic test. The following findings suggest DIC:
- Sudden fall in platelet count to <100 x 10⁹/L.
- Bleeding and/or thrombotic complications.
- ↑ APTT, PT, INR.
- ↑ fibrin degradation products.
- ↓ fibrinogen in severe DIC.

Management
The key is to treat the underlying disorder. Bleeding patients should receive FFP, platelets, blood, and cryoprecipitate as indicated by coagulation screens. Patients with thrombosis should be heparinized.

Excessive warfarinization

Warfarin inhibits carboxylation of vitamin K, inhibiting the synthesis of vitamin K dependent factors (V, VII, XI). Management depends on whether the patient is bleeding, why they are warfarinized and if urgent/emergency surgery is indicated.
- If the INR is <5.0 and the patient is not bleeding, simply omit warfarin and recheck INR daily, restarting warfarin once the INR is within range.
- If the INR is >5.0, give 10mg vitamin K PO.
- If INR is elevated and emergency reversal to normal clotting is required (e.g. for high risk surgery), IV Beriplex (mixed FII/VII/IX/X protein C/S) may be used.
- If the patient is bleeding, give FFP and up to 5mg vitamin K PO.
- If the patient has a mechanical valve, the risk of thromboembolic events when anticoagulation is reversed is <0.1% per day. Anticoagulation with heparin or warfarin should be recommenced within 1–2 weeks once any bleeding complications have resolved.

Key revision points—physiology of haemostasis
- **Vascular phase**. Vasospasm, local oedema, and haematoma.
- **Platelet phase**. Adherence of platelets activated by ADP, collagen, von Willebrand factor and mediated by IIb/IIIa, fibrinogen, 5-HT, thromboxane A2.
- **Clotting phase**:
  - **Intrinsic** (kallikrein, XII, XI, and IX).
  - **Extrinsic** (thromboplastin, VII) pathways converge on common pathway (X, thrombin, fibrinogen).

Fibrinolysis depends on plasmin, antithrombin III, proteins C and S, tissue factor pathway inhibitor.

Deep venous thrombosis and pulmonary embolism

Deep venous thrombosis (DVT) is most common in patients over 40 years of age who undergo major surgery. A post-operative increase in platelets coupled with venous endothelial trauma and stasis all contribute (Virchow's triad). If no prophylaxis is given, 30% of these patients will develop DVT and 0.1–0.2% will die from pulmonary thromboembolism (PTE).

High-risk groups (see Prophylaxis 📖 p. 72)
- Patients undergoing pelvic or hip surgery.
- Patients with malignant disease.
- Patients on the contraceptive pill (pregnancy).
- Previous history of DVT or PTE.
- Older patients. The increase in DVT is almost linear with advancing age.
- Other factors: obesity, diabetes mellitus, polycythaemia, varicose veins, cardiac and respiratory disease, thrombophilia (e.g. factor V Leiden protein C or S deficiency).

Diagnosis

Clinical
- Systemic pyrexia at 7–8 days post-operatively.
- May present with embolism (pulmonary).
- Pain, swelling of the leg, and a rise in local skin temperature.

Investigations
- DVT may be diagnosed using:
  - Duplex Doppler: less sensitive for calf DVT than thigh DVT.
  - Ascending venography: invasive, but more sensitive than duplex.
- PE may be diagnosed using:
  - CTPA (almost universally favoured now over VQ lung scans).
  - VQ lung scanning with radioactive technetium-labelled microaggregates of albumin (^{99}Tcm MAA).

Treatment

Confirm the site and the extent of the DVT by Doppler and lung scan.
- Calf vein thrombosis may be treated by compression alone.
- All other thrombi should be treated with heparin for 4–7 days (40 000U/24h), checked by bleeding times (5000–10 000U by bolus, then 1000–1500U/h IV alone), or followed by oral anticoagulation for 6–12 weeks (warfarin, checked by PT/INR).
- Lytic therapy—urokinase, streptokinase—is most effective within 24–36h of onset of DVT. This may be effective in life-threatening PE.
- Surgical thromboectomy or embolectomy is used when there is massive PTE. In bilateral ileofemoral DVT, embolism may be prevented by inserting an 'umbrella' filter into the vena cava at a level below the renal vessels.

Prevention (see 📖 p. 72).

Pulmonary embolism

Diagnosis of pulmonary embolism

PE is incorrectly diagnosed in almost 75% of patients. The differential diagnosis includes acute MI, aortic dissection, septic shock, chest infection, haemothorax, and pneumothorax. Massive PE is PE resulting in haemodynamic compromise or where >30% of the pulmonary vasculature is compromised.

Clinical features of PE

- *Symptoms*. Dyspnoea, pleuritic or dull chest pain.
- *Signs*. Tachypnoea, tachycardia, hypotension, elevated JVP.
- Risk factors for or clinical evidence of DVT.
- ECG shows RV strain pattern (S1, Q3, T3), but this is neither a specific nor a sensitive test.
- ↓ PaO_2; $PaCO_2$ may be low.
- CXR may show consolidation and effusion early on.
- Echo may show right ventricular (RV) dilatation, tricuspid regurgitation, and right atrial or RV thrombus.
- Pulmonary angiography, CT-angio, and VQ scanning are diagnostic.

Outcome

- The 30-day mortality of acute massive PE is about 50%.
- About 10% of mortality occurs within the first hour.
- Up to 80% of mortality occurs within the first 2h.
- The mortality of surgical intervention is up to 70% for patients requiring CPR or mechanical circulatory support preoperatively.
- The operative mortality of stable patients is about 30%.

Management

If the patient is haemodynamically unstable, emergency pulmonary embolectomy should be considered. In patients with large PE and no contraindications (i.e. surgery within previous 30 days), thrombolysis is the definitive management. Otherwise do the following:

- Sit the patient up and give 100% O_2.
- Patient may require intubation.
- Get IV access and give heparin 5000U bolus IV.
- Start a heparin infusion (50 000U heparin in 50mL of normal saline) at 1000–2000U/h.
- Check APTT after 6h (target APTT 70–90), adjust infusion rate accordingly, and recheck APTT after 6h.
- Once APTT is stabilized, APTT should be checked every 12–24h.
- Low molecular weight tinzaparin is licensed for use in acute PE. It has the same efficacy as unfractionated heparin without the requirement for repeated APTT checks.
- Begin warfarinization.
- Look for causes of PE.

Risk scoring

Scoring systems attempt to quantify the severity of illness so that:
- Different interventions, clinicians, or centres can be compared, adjusting for differences in case mix.
- Clinicians can predict prognosis more accurately.

Examples of risk scoring systems
- Predicting risk of dying in hospital (APACHE III).
- Quantifying morbidity (ASA score, Apgar score).
- Quantifying symptoms (NYHA angina classification).
- Predicting operative mortality (EUROscore, Parsonnet score in cardiac surgery, POSSUM).
- Predicting risk of dying on waiting list (New Zealand score in cardiac surgery).
- Predicting risk of dying for specific illnesses (Glasgow and Ranson criteria in pancreatitis).

APACHE III scoring system (Acute Physiology and Chronic Health Evaluation)

This predicts an individual's risk of dying in hospital. Twenty-seven patient variables (physiological variables such as core temperature, heart rate, BP, creatinine, age, and chronic illness variables) are entered into a programme that gives a score which can be compared against previous performance to give a risk of dying in the hospital. There are approximately another 60 hospitals worldwide where the APACHE III methodology is used to generate reports that compare their actual average ICU outcomes with those predicted by the APACHE III methodology.

EuroSCORE (European System for Cardiac Risk Evaluation)

This is a weighted additive score, based on a European sample of cardiac surgical patients. Variables such as age, renal function, and comorbidity are given points that add up to an approximate percentage of predicted perioperative mortality. Scoring systems like this are useful when consenting patients for surgery and in risk-stratifying operative outcomes so that surgeons and hospitals can be compared with each other.

POSSUM (Physiologic and Operative Severity Score for the enUmeration of Mortality and morbidity)

This is a weighted additive score. Eighteen variables are combined to produce a physiological score and an operative score, which in turn are combined to produce an estimate of the percentage risk of defined morbidity and mortality. (Variants exist for vascular, orthopaedic, and colorectal surgery.)

Critical care

Recognizing the critically ill surgical patient (see Box 2.8)

It may be obvious that a patient needs a critical care bed, e.g. the patient needing ventilation, inotropes, or dialysis. But anticipating, and maybe avoiding, this is more difficult. The first step is recognizing compensated critical illness (e.g. shock compensated by tachycardia and peripheral shutdown or respiratory failure compensated by unsustainable respiratory effort).

> **Box 2.8 Signs that should ring alarm bells**
> - **History.** 'I feel like I'm going to die.' *Timor mortis* (fear of dying) may accompany MI, hypovolaemic shock, respiratory failure. ***Never*** ignore the patient who thinks they are dying; they are often right.
> - **Nurses.** 'Mr Smith just doesn't look right.' Experienced nurses quickly recognize the patterns of critical illness; listen to them.
> - **General.** Hypothermia or hyperpyrexia, sweating.
> - **Cardiovascular.** ↓ BP, ↑↓ pulse, arrhythmias, peripheral shutdown.
> - **Respiratory.** Tachypnoea, difficulty getting full sentences out.
> - **Renal.** Oliguria <0.5mL/kg/h.
> - **Gastrointestinal.** New anorexia, nausea, and vomiting.
> - **Neurological.** Confusion, agitation or drowsiness, fits.

Immediate management

First identify and treat potentially life-threatening conditions. *Then* quantify the problem (important for referring patients to other clinicians and for establishing a baseline by which to guide treatment and monitor progress). *Finally* start looking for the underlying problem. Some of these tasks overlap. *Keep* reassessing the patient and adjust your management.
- Quickly assess airway, breathing, and circulation: ALS algorithms are printed on the inside back cover; management of shock is described on 📖 p. 100; management of haemorrhage is described on 📖 p. 102.
- Sit patient up and give high flow O_2.
- Secure IV access and take blood for FBC, U&E, amylase, glucose, LFTs, cardiac enzymes, clotting, group and save, and blood cultures.
- Take ABG: good O_2 saturations do not rule out respiratory failure and ABGs will also show acidosis and electrolyte abnormalities.
- Give 500mL gelofusine if patient not obviously fluid overloaded.
- Request a 12-lead ECG.
- Review drug, diabetic, and fluid balance charts.
- Perform a focused history and examination: ask about symptoms that have changed recently and focus your examination on that.
- Review recent bloods and X-rays and request appropriate radiology.
- If the patient needs HDU or ITU, talk to your registrar or consultant.
- A patient may need to be discharged from HDU or surgery need to be postponed: think ahead.

High dependency unit

The HDU allows a level of care between ICU and the general ward. Invasive monitoring and inotropic support are routine, but ventilation and renal support are not. Nurse:patient ratio is 1:2. Patients with single organ failure requiring basic respiratory support, including non-invasive mask ventilation with CPAP, should be admitted to HDU.

Guidelines for admission to HDU

- Need for monitored bed.
- Need for invasive monitoring.
- Need for inotropes.
- Need for CPAP or other respiratory support.
- Need for 1:2 nursing.

Intensive care unit

The ICU offers advanced ventilatory and inotropic support, renal replacement therapy, full invasive monitoring, and 1:1 nursing care.

Guidelines for admission to ITU

- Need for mechanical ventilation.
- Failure of two or more organ systems.
- Need for advanced monitoring, e.g. pulmonary artery catheter.
- Need for escalating or additional inotropes.
- Primary pathology should be reversible.
- Consultant involvement from both surgery and ITU is essential.
- Patient's stated or written preference against intensive care should be taken into account and documented.

How to use critical care

The surgical team should consider using critical care services for both elective and emergency surgical patients. Some guides follow:

- Is the elective patient in need of intensive infusional treatment prior to surgery (e.g. IV anticoagulation, IV clotting factors)? → HDU.
- Has the patient undergone major surgery with significant transfusion requirements that might lead to haemodynamic and clotting abnormalities (e.g. elective extensive pelvic surgery, aortic surgery, extensive burns surgery)? → HDU.
- Is the patient over 80, having had major abdominal, thoracic, or limb surgery? → HDU.
- Does the patient have known significant respiratory disease making intensive respiratory therapy likely? → ITU.
- Would a patient due for emergency surgery benefit from aggressive, closely monitored fluid resuscitation prior to anaesthesia? → HDU.
- Does the post-op patient need infusional inotropic support, renal replacement therapy, or invasive monitoring? → ITU/HDU.

▶ The golden rule is, 'If in doubt, ask for the advice of the critical care team—more patients can benefit than do.'

Commonly used terms in ITU

Cardiac function (see 📖 p. 620—cardiothoracic surgery).

Oxygenation and ventilation

- *Oxygenation*, the amount of oxygen in arterial blood, is described in terms of the *partial pressure of* oxygen in arterial blood (PaO_2) and the *percentage saturation of arterial haemoglobin with oxygen* (SaO_2).
- *Ventilation*, the movement of air in and out of the lungs, is described in terms of minute volume, and assessed by measuring the partial pressure of carbon dioxide in arterial blood ($PaCO_2$).
- Oxygenation is independent of minute volumes until they are very low.
- In post-operative patients, the primary cause of hypoxia is atelectasis and this must be reversed before the patient can benefit from increasing the fraction of oxygen in inspired air (FiO_2).
- *Positive end expiratory pressure* (PEEP) and CPAP treat and prevent atelectasis.
- Oxygen consumption is assessed indirectly by measuring the *percentage saturation of mixed venous haemoglobin with oxygen* (SvO_2; indirect measurement of oxygen uptake by peripheral tissues).
- Pulmonary ventilation is described in terms of four 'volumes' (*tidal volume, inspiratory reserve volume, expiratory reserve volume,* and *residual volume*) that may be combined to give four 'capacities' (*inspiratory capacity, functional residual capacity, vital capacity,* and *total lung capacity*). Tidal volume is the only measurement used on ITU.
- Loss of functional residual capacity through atelectasis, supine position, lobar consolidation and collapse, effusions, and obesity results in hypoxia. CPAP, PEEP, and physiotherapy are aimed at limiting this loss.

Invasive monitoring

Invasive monitoring is used on ITU and HDU because it provides accurate and *sensitive real-time measurements*, routes for *sampling blood*, routes for *administration of drugs*.

Arterial monitoring

Insertion technique and complications are described on 🕮 p. 196.

Indications
- Precise measurement where inotropic or mechanical support used.
- Frequent sampling of ABGs.

Contraindications
- *Absolute.* Infection at the site of insertion, distal limb ischaemia.
- *Relative.* Coagulopathy, proximal obstruction, surgical considerations.

Central venous pressure lines

Insertion technique and complications are described on 🕮 p. 198.

Indications
- Continual RA pressure (RAP) measurements in patients requiring circulatory support.
- Infusion port for some drugs that cannot be given peripherally.
- Insertion pulmonary artery catheter or transvenous pacing wires.
- Infusion port for TPN.

Contraindications
- *Absolute.* SVC syndrome, infection at the site of insertion.
- *Relative.* Coagulopathy, undrained contralateral pneumothorax, uncooperative patient. DVT of the head and neck vessels may make insertion difficult. Patients with septal defects are at risk of CVA from air emboli caused by poor technique.

Pulmonary artery catheter

Complications are as for CVP lines, additionally arrhythmias and pulmonary artery infarction or perforation. The catheter has four lumens: a proximal lumen 25cm from the tip that sits in the RA; a distal lumen connected to a pressure transducer sitting in the pulmonary artery; a balloon lumen allowing balloon inflation; a thermistor lumen.

Indications
These are indicated in patients with hypoperfusion states refractory to first- and second-line inotropic support.
- Pressure monitoring: RAP, RV pressure (RVP), PAP, pulmonary artery wedge pressure (PAWP).
- Flow monitoring: cardiac output.
- Mixed venous oxygen saturations.
- Derived parameters: systemic vascular resistance (SVR), SVR index (SVRI), pulmonary vascular resistance (PVR), PVR index (PVRI), LVSV, VO_2, DO_2.
- Temporary atrial and ventricular pacing.

Contraindications As for CV catheters (see 🕮 p. 198). Those specific to pulmonary artery catheterization include tricuspid or pulmonic valvular stenosis, RA and RV masses that may embolize, tetralogy of Fallot, severe arrhythmias, coagulopathy.

Waveforms See Fig. 2.8.

The arterial waveform

The arterial waveform has a fast upstroke and slower downstroke with a notch that represents aortic valve closure.

The CVP waveform

The waveform is composed of three upstrokes (the 'a', 'c', and 'v' waves) and two descents (the 'x' and 'y' descent). The 'a' wave—atrial systole; 'v' wave—venous return filling the RA; 'c' wave—bulging of the closed tricuspid valve cusps into the RA. The 'x' descent occurs in atrial diastole. The 'y' descent occurs in ventricular diastole.

The pulmonary artery pressure waveform

Waveform progression during correct insertion of the pulmonary artery catheter shows a sudden increase in systolic pressure as the catheter enters the RV. As the catheter enters the pulmonary artery, the diastolic pressure increases. There is a decrease in mean pressure as the catheter enters the wedge position.

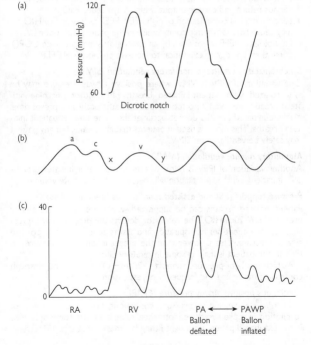

Fig. 2.8 (a) Arterial waveform. (b) Central venous pressure waveform and responses to fluid boluses. (c) Pulmonary artery pressure waveform.

Ventilation and respiratory support

Invasive methods

Intermittent positive pressure ventilation (IPPV); controlled mechanical ventilation (CMV); pressure control ventilation (PCV)

IPPV or CMV is the mode commonly used during routine surgery. Raising airway pressure forces air into the lungs via an endotracheal or tracheostomy tube. Expiration occurs when airway pressures are allowed to fall to zero. This mode is poorly tolerated by the awake patient.

Positive end-expiratory pressure (PEEP)

If, instead of allowing airway pressures to fall to zero, a small positive airways pressure is maintained throughout expiration (*positive end-expiratory pressure or PEEP*), the collapse of small airways and alveoli that occurs at the end of expiration is prevented.

- Functional residual capacity, intrapulmonary shunts, lung compliance, and PaO_2 are improved and the work of breathing is reduced.
- High levels of PEEP (>15cmH$_2$O) may be necessary to reverse established atelectasis, but increase intrathoracic pressure, reducing venous return and cardiac output, which may reduce PaO_2.
- Barotrauma is a complication of high PEEP. PEEP as low as 5cmH$_2$O may cause haemodynamic compromise in the patient with poor LV.
- Physiological PEEP is provided by an intact glottis: patients with COPD purse their lips during expiration to increase physiological PEEP.

Synchronized intermittent mandatory ventilation (SIMV)

One variation of IPPV is SIMV, where positive airway pressure may be synchronized with patient-initiated breaths. Mandatory (machine-initiated) breaths are given if no spontaneous breaths occur in a preset time. Machine-initiated breaths do not occur at the same time as patient-initiated breaths. This mode is used in patients that are awake, but any patient may safely be ventilated on SIMV.

Mandatory minute ventilation (MMV)

Another variation of IPPV is MMV where the ventilator initiates breaths only if patient-initiated ventilation falls below a preset minute volume.

Pressure support (PS) and assisted spontaneous breathing (ASB)

Patient-initiated breaths can be supported with a preset positive airway pressure of 6–20cmH$_2$O. The ventilator detects the drop in airway pressures as the patient begins inspiration and assists air inflow with a positive airway pressure. This is lower than the preset inflationary pressures in IPPV as the patient is making some inspiratory effort.

At high levels of pressure support (>20cmH$_2$O), the patient, although controlling the timing and frequency of respiration, is on IPPV.

Continuous positive airway pressure (CPAP)

In CPAP, a standing airway pressure, continuous throughout all phases of respiration, is applied via the endotracheal tube. It is more commonly used in the extubated patient via a tight fitting facemask (see 🕮 p. 131).

Non-invasive methods

Intermittent negative pressure ventilation (INPV) Virtually never used today, INPV involves placing the patient inside a tank ventilator sealed at the neck. Tank pressure is intermittently lowered, expanding the chest and lowering intrapleural pressure.

Non-invasive intermittent positive pressure ventilation (NIPPV) This is IPPV delivered by face or, more commonly, nasal mask. The patient must be cooperative in order to understand how to synchronize breaths with the ventilator. It may be used in the tiring COPD patient.

Continuous positive airway pressure (CPAP) In CPAP, a standing airway pressure, continuous throughout all phases of respiration, is applied via an entotracheal tube, tracheostomy, nasal, or, more commonly, face mask to a spontaneously breathing patient.
- This results in a kind of non-invasive PEEP, where additional alveoli are recruited with the benefits described (see 📖 p. 130).
- CPAP is a useful adjunct in the extubated patient with COPD, atelectasis, pulmonary oedema, or acute respiratory distress syndrome (ARDS).
- CPAP cannot produce ventilation by itself.

Biphasic positive pressure ventilation (BiPAP) is a solution to the problem of air trapping that can occur in patients, particularly those with COPD, on CPAP. Airway pressure is cycled at preset rates between high and low levels.

High flow (Venturi) face mask (fixed performance) The key part of the Venturi facemask is the Venturi valve which draws in an amount of air through calibrated inlets, which is mixed with O_2 flowing into the valve before entering the mask.
- More mixed air (up to 30L/min) is delivered to the mask than the patient can use: the excess escapes though holes in the mask.
- The FiO_2 is set by the choice of valve, not by the patient's breathing pattern (hence the term fixed performance).
- The maximum FiO_2 that can be delivered by a Venturi mask is about 60%. There is a minimum flow rate of O_2 for each Venturi.

Low flow (Hudson) face mask (variable performance) O_2 flows at a set rate (e.g. 2L/min) into the mask. It is diluted by air drawn into the mask, which depends on the patient's minute volumes, ranging 5–30L/min.
- The FiO_2 achieved depends primarily on the patient and the delivery system should not be used when accurate control of FiO_2 is required.
- The maximum FiO_2 that can reliably be delivered is about 30%.
- Use of a non-rebreathing mask and reservoir bag, into which high flow O_2 is drawn during expiration and then inhaled, increases FiO_2 to up to 60%: the reservoir bag must be filled with O_2 before the patient uses it.

Nasal prongs Nasal prongs deliver an FiO_2 that is determined primarily by the patient, as in a low flow mask, but they are less obtrusive, allowing the patient to expectorate and eat. They increase tracheal FiO_2 to barely more than room air levels, particularly if the patient breathes through their mouth.

Circulatory support

Principles

Improving cardiac function and end-organ perfusion involves:
• Careful fluid balance to optimize preload or 'filling' (see 📖 p. 64);
• Using vasoconstrictors and vasodilators to optimize afterload;
• Using inotropes and chronotropes to improve cardiac output (CO);
• Mechanical support in selected cases.

Inotropes

Inotropes increase inotropy (contractility)

• α-adrenergic receptor stimulation leads to ↑ SVR and PVR.
• β_1 stimulation leads to ↑ contractility, heart rate, and conduction.
• β_2 stimulation causes peripheral dilatation and bronchodilation.
• Dopamine (DA) stimulation causes coronary, renal, and mesenteric vasodilatation.

Adrenaline (epinephrine) 0.03–0.5micrograms/kg/min or bolus
Catecholamine produced by the adrenal medulla.
• *Action.* Direct agonist at α, β_1, and β_2 receptors.
• *Pharmacodynamics.* Instant onset, half-life 2min. Metabolized by MAO.
• *Indications.* Cardiac arrest (asystole, ventricular fibrillation (VF), electromechanical delay (EMD)); anaphylaxis; low CO states; bronchospasm.

Dopamine 3–10micrograms/kg/min
A catecholamine precursor to noradrenaline (NA) and adrenaline.
• *Action.* α, β_1, β_2, and DA_1 agonist, and release of stored neuronal NA. At the lower doses, β and DA effects (increased heart rate (HR), contractility) predominate. At >10micrograms/kg/min, α effects predominate (↑ SVR, dysrhythmias).
• *Pharmacodynamics.* Fast onset, slow offset. Metabolized by monoamine oxidase (MAO).
• *Indications.* Low CO states; renal insufficiency.

Milrinone 0.3–0.8micrograms/kg/min
Bipyridine derivative that inhibits phosphodiesterase.
• *Action.* Potent inotropic and vasodilator effects.
• *Pharmacodynamics.* Half-life is 4h. Metabolism is hepatic.
• *Indication.* Low CO state in the setting of ↑ SVR.

Vasopressors

Vasopressors cause vasoconstriction

• α_2-adrenergic stimulation increases SVR and PVR.
• α_1-adrenergic stimulation ↑ contractility without ↑ HR.

Noradrenaline (norepinephrine) 0.03–1.0micrograms/kg/min

Catecholamine produced by the adrenal medulla.
- *Action.* Direct α agonist: potent vasoconstriction + β_1 effect = ↑ BP.
- *Pharmacodynamics.* Immediate onset; half-life 2min.
- *Indication.* Hypotension because of low SVR in good to high CO states.

Chronotropes

> **Chronotropes increase heart rate**
> - β_1 stimulation leads to ↑ contractility, HR, and conduction.
> - Muscarinic cholinergic activity is predominantly parasympathetic.

Atropine (0.3–1mg IV bolus)

Atropine is a belladonna alkaloid.
- *Action.* A competitive antagonist at muscarinic cholinergic receptors, reducing parasympathetic tone to 'reveal' underlying sympathetic tone.
- *Pharmacodynamics.* Almost instant onset. When given IV, offset is 15–30min. When given IM, SC, or PO, 4h. Renal elimination.
- *Indication.* Bradydysrhythmias, reduction of oral secretions.

Isoprenaline (0.01–0.3micrograms/kg/min)

Synthetic catecholamine.
- *Action.* Direct β_1 (↑ contractility, conductivity, and HR) and β_2 ↑ (vasodilatation and bronchodilatation) effect. No α activity.
- *Pharmacodynamics.* Plasma half-life 2min. Hepatic metabolism by MAO, 40% conjugated, 60% excreted unchanged.
- *Indication.* Bradycardia unresponsive to atropine.

Mechanical support

Intra-aortic balloon counterpulsation

Mechanism

The intra-aortic balloon pump (IABP) is a polyethylene balloon filled with helium, ranging from 2 to 50cm^3 in size, that sits in the descending aorta just distal to the left subclavian artery. The balloon inflates in early diastole, improving coronary perfusion, and deflates just before systole, reducing afterload. The myocardial oxygen supply:demand ratio is improved and CO may be increased by up to 40%.

Indications

Weaning from cardiopulmonary bypass, refractory ischaemia, cardiogenic shock.

Contraindications
- Aortic regurgitation (AR) (balloon inflation during diastole will worsen AR).
- Aortic dissection.

Ventricular assist devices (VADs) These are pumps that are anastomosed to the great vessels or cardiac chambers to support failing right, left, or both ventricles.

Renal support

The main aims of treatment of renal failure are:
• Maintain renal perfusion.
• Optimize fluid balance.
• Provide adequate enteral support.
• Correct hyperkalaemia and acidosis.
• Identify and treat sepsis.
• Target therapy to underlying pathology.
• Provide renal replacement therapy.

Haemodialysis and haemofiltration

Indications for renal replacement therapy
• Refractory hyperkalemia (see 🕮 p. 111).
• Refractory acidosis.
• Pulmonary oedema.
• Drug toxicity.
• Progressive uraemia or uraemia associated with pericarditis, encephalopathy, seizures, or coagulopathy.

There are two main techniques of renal replacement therapy used on cardiac ICUs: haemodialysis and haemofiltration. In both techniques, access to the circulation is required and blood passes through an extracorporeal circuit that includes either a dialyser or a haemofilter.
• In haemodialysis, blood flows along one side of a *semipermeable* membrane as a solution of *crystalloids is pumped* against the other side of the membrane, against the direction of blood flow.
• In haemofiltration, *blood under pressure* passes down one side of a *highly permeable* membrane on the other side of which is a static crystalloid solution.
• In haemodialysis, removal of solutes depends on diffusion: molecules move from high to low concentration and smaller molecules move faster so the amount of solute removed depends on its concentration in the dialysis fluid and on the size of the molecule.
• In haemofiltration, removal of solutes with a molecular weight up to 20 000 depends on convective flow as in glomerular filtration: all molecules are removed at a similar rate and virtually all ions are removed.
• In haemodialysis, large molecules are not efficiently removed.
• In haemofiltration, large molecules are so effectively removed that drugs such as heparin, insulin, and vancomycin may need to be replaced and reduction in circulating inflammation mediators and pyrogens leads to a reduction in pyrexia and systemic inflammation.
• In haemodialysis, controlled amounts of sodium and water are removed by creation of a transmembrane pressure gradient.
• In haemofiltration, large amounts of salt and water are removed and must be replaced by an infusion of an appropriate amount of physiologic crystalloid into the distal port of the haemofilter.

Types of haemofiltration

Haemofiltration has become an increasingly popular form of renal replacement therapy for acute renal failure post-operatively, even though it is several times more expensive than dialysis. This is because the continuous nature of the process avoids the big swings in fluid balance and electrolytes that characterize dialysis. There are several variants.

Continuous arteriovenous haemofiltration (CAVH) This is the original and simplest form of filtration. The femoral artery and vein are cannulated and blood passes through the haemofilter under arterial pressure alone. It is therefore less appropriate for patients with low CO states. Prolonged arterial cannulation carries complications (see 📖 p. 197).

Continuous arteriovenous haemodialysis with filtration Because clearance rates are as low as 10mL/h with CAVH, a dialysis circuit is added to the equipment, improving clearance rates at considerable cost.

Continuous venovenous haemofiltration (CVVH) An occlusive pump is incorporated into the circuit to drive blood so that venous cannulation is all that is required. This also allows control of blood flow and filtration rate. Clearance of up to 100mL/min can be achieved. This is the most commonly used system in ICUs.

Continuous venovenous haemodialysis with filtration Some systems add haemodialysis to the CVVH circuit for additional fine control.

Management of the haemofiltered patient

A double lumen catheter (Vascath) is inserted into a central vein. The blood pump is set at 125mL/min and the haemofiltration rate to 25mL/min. The replacement fluid pump is programmed to balance the inflow and outflow of fluid to achieve a preset rate of fluid loss. The circuit is heparinized with an infusion of 200–1600U/h. Lactate is the commonest replacement anion, but in lactic acidosis, a lactate-free replacement solution must be employed. Mg^{2+}, Ca^{2+}, PO_4, and HCO_3 are replaced. Hypotension is common when commencing haemofiltration.

Enteral support

(See also 📖 p. 66.) Neglecting the patient's nutritional needs increases morbidity and mortality.

Routine management

- Patients may be started on oral intake directly after most forms of surgery unless contraindicated. There is good evidence of reduced pulmonary, septic, and anastomotic complications in patients fed early.
- Patients with a history of dyspepsia or peptic ulceration should be commenced electively on an IV proton pump inhibitor (PPI).
- Analgesia should be downscaled from IV and oral opiates to non-opiate analgesia such as paracetamol 1g qds PO/PR as soon as possible to avoid ileus, constipation, anorexia, nausea, and vomiting.
- Avoid NSAID analgesia in patients at risk of peptic ulceration.
- Give regular IV antiemetics to treat persistent nausea and vomiting.

Enteral nutrition

This is nutrition using the GI tract. It is superior to, safer, and cheaper than TPN.

Routes/methods for supplemented enteral nutrition

- Sip feeds.
- Fine bore NG tube (NGT) with use of infusion pump.
- Nasojejunal tube (needs radiographic imaging).
- Percutaneous endoscopic gastrostomy (PEG) and jejunostomy.
- Open surgical gastrostomy or jejunostomy.

> ### Examples of enteral feeds
> - Standard feeds—Osmolite®, Nutrison® standard.
> - Fibre enriched—Jevity®, Nutrison® Multi-Fibre.
> - High energy—Nutrison® Energy, Ensure® Plus.

Enteral tube feeds come in sterile, ready to hang 500mL and 1000mL packs. Standard feeds are nutritionally complete and provide 1kcal/mL. They are based on whole protein. Fibre-enriched feeds also provide 1kcal/mL. They contain soy polysaccharides that are soluble, but remain undigested passing to the colon where they are fermented by bacteria to produce short chain fatty acids, promoting absorption of sodium and water and reducing diarrhoea. They are also probiotic. High energy feeds provide 1.5kcal/mlL and are used in patients requiring reduced fluid input.

- Renal failure patients require high energy, low volume, and electrolyte feeds. Nepro® provides 2kcal/mL and high protein content.
- Drugs can be given by the NGT being used for enteral feeding. Liquid preparations designed for oral administration should ideally be used as crushed tablets may block the tube. The feed should be stopped and the NGT flushed with saline before and after administration of drugs.
- The therapeutic effect of warfarin is reduced by the vitamin K content in feeds; it is frequently necessary to increase the dose of warfarin.

- Phenytoin interacts with enteral feeds, which should be stopped for 2h before and after phenytoin administration.

Indications for supplementary enteral feeding
- Inadequate oral intake due to anorexia, practical difficulties with feeding, being on ITU/HDU, drug-induced nausea, poor oral health or dentition.
- Hypercatabolism exceeding normal intake (e.g. chronic major sepsis, malignancy, trauma, burns).
- Gut intact, but absorption impaired excessive losses; chronic diarrhoea, high output stoma or fistula (usually low residue or elemental feeds to maximize absorption).

Complications of supplementary enteral feeding
- *Complications of feeding tube.* Malposition, blockage (wound infection around jejunostomy tubes).
- *Complications of administration.* Pulmonary aspiration, regurgitations, diarrhoea, bloating, nausea, cramps.
- *Complications of contents.* Vitamin and trace mineral deficiencies, electrolyte imbalances, drug interactions.

Diarrhoea is the most common complication. If feed-related, reducing the osmotic load is effective (using half-strength feed or slowing the infusion). Omeprazole, Lomotil®, and erythromycin may be tried. It is mandatory to exclude other causes of diarrhoea such as subacute obstruction and infectious causes (particularly *Clostridium difficile*).

Total and peripheral parenteral nutrition (TPN, PPN)

TPN consists of specially formulated feed given IV. Because TPN solutions have high osmolality, they cause thrombophlebitis if infused into peripheral veins. They are given via central lines (subclavian or internal jugular) which may be tunnelled for long-term use. PPN uses heparin, in-line filtration, buffering, fine bore cannulas, and reduced osmolality feeds to avoid thrombophlebitis.

Indications
- Failure of bowel to absorb food, e.g. radiation damage, severe acute enteritis, or malabsorption syndromes.
- Failure of adequate length of bowel for absorption (short bowel syndrome due to Crohn's disease or after massive intestinal resection).
- GI tract not accessible for enteral route, e.g. acute severe pancreatitis, oesophagogastric surgery, or disease where tube feeding not possible.
- Failure of enteral feeding to accomplish nutritional targets (rare).

Complications
- Complications of CV catheters (see ☐ p. 199).
- Late complications: sepsis, migration, erosion, DVT, occlusion.
- Metabolic complications: ↑↓ glucose, K^+, Na^+, ↑ Ca^{2+}, ↓ PO_4, ↓ Zn, Mg, folate.

Sepsis, SIRS, MODS, and ALI

Systemic inflammatory response syndrome (SIRS) is a pro-inflammatory state that does not include a documented source of infection. It may lead to multiple organ dysfunction syndrome (MODS).

Definitions

SIRS
- Any two or more of the four following signs:
  - Tachycardia >90 beats/min.
  - Tachypnoea >20 breaths/min.
  - Pyrexia >38°C (or hypothermia <36°C).
  - White blood count >12 × 10⁹/L (or <4 × 10⁹/L).
- *Without* identifiable bacteraemia or need for organ support *and* in the setting of a known cause of endothelial inflammation such as:
  - Suspected infection.
  - Pancreatitis.
  - Ischaemia.
  - Multiple trauma and tissue injury.
  - Haemorrhagic shock.
  - Immune-mediated organ injury.

Sepsis
Systemic response to infection manifested by two or more of:
- Tachycardia >90 beats/min.
- Tachypnoea >20 breaths/min.
- Pyrexia >38°C (or hypothermia <36°C).
- White blood count >12 × 10⁹/L (or <4 × 10⁹/L).

Multiple organ failure Presence of altered organ function in an acutely ill patient such that homeostasis cannot be maintained without intervention.

Acute lung injury (ALI)
- Acute onset.
- PaO_2/FiO_2 <300.
- Bilateral infiltrates on CXR.
- PAWP <18mmHg or no clinical evidence of raised left atrial pressure.

Acute/adult respiratory distress syndrome (ARDS) As for ALI, except PaO_2/FiO_2 <200.

Pathophysiology

The pathophysiology involves systems involved in inflammation, immunity, ischaemia, and homeostasis, including complement, clotting and cytokine cascades, cell-mediated immunity, and humoral immunity.
- Metabolic acidosis is a frequent accompaniment to SIRS and it is derived principally from lactate.
- SIRS may affect all organ systems and may lead to MODS.

- Cell signalling molecules involved include interleukins IL-1, IL-5, and IL-6; chemokines; tumour necrosis factor (TNF).
- Theories explaining why SIRS develops include:
  - Immunologically mediated inflammation.
  - ↑ intestinal permeability and colonization with Gram −ve anaerobes that produce endotoxins that migrate across the mucosa to drive the inflammatory and immune response.
  - 'Second hit' hypothesis.

Acute lung injury (ALI)

Thirty per cent of patients with SIRS develop ALI. It is the pulmonary manifestation of the global physiological insult (rarely occurs in isolation). ARDS is one end of the continuum of ALI. Management of ALI is supportive, including prone ventilation and aggressive diuresis or early ultrafiltration.

Investigations

These are aimed at excluding differential diagnoses such as overwhelming sepsis, cardiogenic shock, hypovolaemic shock, and hypersensitivity reactions as well as identifying an underlying cause.
- U&E, LFTs, serum amylase, lactate and cardiac enzymes.
- FBC, APTT, PT, fibrinogen, D-dimers.
- Cultures of blood, urine, sputum, stool.
- ABGs.
- Pulmonary artery catheter measurements of cardiac function and mixed venous oxygen saturations.
- Cytokine assays can be used as markers of severity.

Management

- Volume resuscitation:
  - Aims to achieve normovolaemia: increases CO and oxygen delivery without large increase in oxygen consumption.
  - Hypervolaemia appropriate in selected cases.
  - Albumin probably beneficial in selected cases.
  - Pulmonary artery catheter may guide management.
- Maintenance of oxygen delivery:
  - Airway protection and ventilatory support usually necessary.
  - Inotropic support of cardiac function has important role.
  - Vasoactive drugs selected so that BP is not maintained at the expense of splanchnic vasoconstriction and hypoperfusion.
- Organ support:
  - In addition to cardiovascular and respiratory support, these patients frequently need renal, hepatic, and enteral support.
  - Attempts to reduce translocation, e.g. introduction of competing bacteria (e.g. lactobacillus of yoghurt), early enteral nutrition, particularly with the use of immunostimulating enteral diets.

Prognosis Mortality ranges from 25% to100%, depending on the number and type of organ failures involved, age, and pre-existing comorbidity.

Surgical pathology

Cellular injury

Causative agents

Cellular injury is caused by:
- Trauma.
- Thermal injury.
- Chemicals, including drugs.
- Infectious organisms.
- Ionizing radiation.

Mechanisms of injury

These causative agents cause cell damage via a number of mechanisms.
- *Mechanical disruption*. Trauma, freezing, osmotic imbalance.
- *Failure of membrane integrity*. Failure of ion pumps, cytolysis, trauma.
- *Blockage of metabolic pathways*. Cellular respiration (e.g. cyanide), protein synthesis (e.g. streptomycin), DNA damage or loss (e.g. X-rays).
- *Deficiency of essential metabolites*. Oxygen (ischaemia), glucose (diabetic ketoacidosis), hormones (↓ trophic hormones results in apoptosis).
- *Free radicals*. Toxins (e.g. carbon tetrachloride), ischaemia-reperfusion injury, intracellular killing of bacteria.

Necrosis

Necrosis is death of tissue or cells.

Coagulative necrosis
This is the most common form of necrosis and occurs in all organs. Cells retain their shape as cell proteins coagulate and metabolic activity stops. Digestion by macrophages may cause the tissue to become soft. Histologically, there is progressive loss of staining. The presence of necrotic material normally provokes an inflammatory response.

Colliquative necrosis
This occurs in the brain because of the lack of tissue architecture provided by substantial surrounding stroma.

Caseous necrosis
Dead tissue lacks any structure and is characterized by a white, soft, or liquid 'cheesy' appearance. This is common in TB.

Gangrene
Necrosis with dessication or putrefaction (see p. 158).

Fibrinoid necrosis
In malignant hypertension, necrosis of smooth muscle vessel walls allows seepage of plasma into the media and deposition of fibrin.

Fat necrosis
- *Direct trauma*. Release of extracellular fat produces an inflammatory response, fibrosis and eventually, in some cases, a palpable mass.
- *Acute pancreatitis*. Fat is digested by pancreatic lipase to produce fatty acids which precipitate with calcium in the process of saponification.

Apoptosis (programmed cell death) is the cell-mediated, controlled elimination of individual cells.

Apoptosis

Apoptosis is a physiological process requiring energy. It is the normal means of maintaining the size of an organ in the face of continuing cell turnover or a reduction in size during atrophy. It is mediated by endogenous endonucleases. The cell shrinks and fragments into apoptotic bodies. Examples include:

- *Physiological.* Epithelium of GI tract, bone marrow, clonal selection in immune system, targets of cytotoxic T cells.
- *Pathological.* After exposure to ionizing radiation, chemotherapy, smooth muscle cells around atherosclerotic plaque, viral hepatitis.

Inflammation

Inflammation is the local physiological response to tissue injury. It can be acute or chronic.

Acute inflammation

This is the initial tissue reaction to a wide range of agents: *accumulation of neutrophil polymorphs in the extracellular space* is diagnostic. It lasts hours to days and is usually described with the suffix '-itis'.

Causes
- Physical and chemical, e.g. mechanical trauma, X-rays, acid, alkali.
- Infection: bacteria, viruses, parasites, fungi, or protozoa.
- Ischaemia.
- Hypersensitivity.

Macroscopic appearance
Calor, rubor, tumor, dolor, and functio laesa (heat, redness, swelling, pain, and impaired function). Special macroscopic appearances include:
- *Serous.* Inflammation + abundant fluid-rich exudates, e.g. peritonitis.
- *Catarrhal.* Inflammation + mucus hypersecretion, e.g. common cold.
- *Haemorrhagic.* Inflammation + vascular injury, e.g. pancreatitis.
- *Suppurative.* Inflammation + pus produced to form abscess or empyema.
- *Fibrinous.* Exudates contain fibrin which forms coating, e.g. pericarditis.
- *Membranous.* Coating of fibrin and epithelial cells, e.g. laryngitis.
- *Pseudomembranous.* Superficial mucosal ulceration with slough, e.g. pseudomembranous colitis secondary to *C. difficile* (see 📖 p. 396).
- *Necrotizing (gangrenous).* Inflammation + tissue necrosis (see 📖 p. 158).

Microscopic changes
Mediated by *endogenous chemicals* released by cells (histamine, prostaglandins, leukotrienes, serotonin, and lymphokines) and plasma factors (complement, kinin, coagulation, and fibrinolytic cascades). Changes are:
- Changes in vessel calibre and flow.
  - Immediate and transient smooth muscle vasoconstriction.
  - Vasodilation (active hyperaemia) lasting 15min to hours.
  - Capillaries, then arterioles dilate to increase blood flow.
- Increased vascular permeability and fluid exudates.
  - Capillary hydrostatic pressure is increased.
  - Endothelial cells contract, creating gaps.
  - Plasma proteins escape into extracellular space.
  - Increase in colloid osmotic pressure draws more fluid.
- Formation of cellular exudates.
  - Accumulation of neutrophil polymorphs in extracellular space.
  - Begins with margination of neutrophils (flow next to vessel walls).
  - Neutrophils then adhere to vessel walls: mechanism unknown.
  - Migrate by amoeboid movement through gaps between cells.

- Neutrophil polymorphs phagocytose debris and kill microbes intracellularly using oxygen-dependent (hydrogen peroxide and hydroxyl radicals) and -independent (lysozymes) means.

Sequelae of acute inflammation

- *Resolution*. Restoration of tissue to normal; likely if minimal tissue damage, rapid destruction of causal agent, rapid removal of exudates by good vascular drainage, and organ with restorative capacity, e.g. liver.
- *Suppuration*. Formation of pus (see 📖 p. 144).
- *Organization*. Replacement by granulation tissue.
- *Chronic inflammation*.

Chronic inflammation

This is an inflammation where *lymphocytes, plasma cells, and macrophages* predominate, granulation tissue often accompanies.

Causes

- Resistance of infective agent to phagocytosis (TB, viral infections).
- Foreign body (endogenous, e.g. urate or exogenous, e.g. asbestos).
- Autoimmune (e.g. contact hypersensitivity, RA, organ-specific).
- Primary granulomatous disease (e.g. Crohn's, sarcoidosis).
- Unkown aetiology (e.g. ulcerative colitis).

Macroscopic appearances

The commonest appearances are:

- Chronic ulcer, e.g. peptic ulcer;
- Chronic abscess cavity, e.g. empyema;
- Thickening of wall of hollow viscus, e.g. Crohn's disease;
- Granulomatous inflammation, e.g. TB;
- Fibrosis, e.g. chronic cholecystitis.

Microscopic changes

Lymphocytes, plasma cells, and macrophages (see 📖 p. 145) predominate; neutrophil polymorphs are scarce, eosinophil polymorphs are present. Fluid exudate is not prominent.

Granuloma

This is different to granulation tissue (see 📖 p. 147).

A **granuloma** is an aggregate of epithelioid histiocytes.

Causes

- *Specific infections*.
  - Endogenous. necrotic bone or fat, keratin, urate.
  - Exogenous. Talc, silicone, asbestos, sutures.
- *Drugs*. Sulphonamides, allopurinol.
- *Unknown*. Crohn's, sarcoidosis, Wegener's granulomatosis.

Wound healing

Classification of wounds
- **Clean.** Non-traumatic wounds with no break in surgical technique, no septic focus, and no viscus opened (e.g. hernia repair).
- **Clean contaminated.** Non-traumatic wounds with contaminated entry into a viscus, but with minimal spillage (e.g. elective cholecystectomy).
- **Contaminated.** Clean, traumatic wounds or significant spillage from a viscus or acute inflammation (e.g. emergency appendectomy).
- **Dirty.** Includes traumatic wounds from a dirty source or when significant bacterial contamination or release of pus is encountered.

General principles of healing
Tissue healing in any organ follows some basic principles:
- Cells may be *labile* (good capacity to regenerate, e.g. surface epithelial cells), stable (capacity to regenerate slowly, e.g. hepatocytes), or permanent (no capacity to regenerate, e.g. nerve and striated muscle cells).
- Tissue architecture is important: complex arrangements cannot be reconstructed if destroyed, e.g. renal glomeruli.
- *Complete restitution* occurs when part of a labile population of cells is damaged, e.g. a minor skin abrasion.

Key revision points—the four stages of wound healing
When specialized tissue is destroyed, it cannot be replaced and a stereotyped response called **repair** then follows in four stages:
- **Haemostasis** (immediate). In response to exposed collagen, platelets aggregate at the wound and degranulate, releasing inflammatory mediators. Clotting and complement cascades activated. Thrombus formation and reactive vasospasm achieve haemostasis.
- **Inflammation** (0–3 days). Vasodilation and increased capillary permeability allow inflammatory cells to enter wound and cause swelling. Neutrophils amplify inflammatory response by release of cytokines, reduce infection by bacterial killing, and debride damaged tissue. Macrophages follow and secrete cytokines, growth factors, and collagenases. They phagocytose bacteria and dead tissue and orchestrate fibroblast migration, proliferation, and collagen production.
- **Proliferation** (3 days–3 weeks). Fibroblasts migrate into the wound and synthesize collagen. Specialized myofibroblasts containing actin cause wound contraction. Angiogenesis is stimulated by hypoxia and cytokines and granulation tissue forms.
- **Remodelling** (3 weeks–1y). Reorientation and maturation of collagen fibres increases wound strength.

- *Granulation* tissue is the combination of capillary loops and myofibroblasts. This is unrelated to a granuloma (see 📖 p. 145).
- *Organization* is the process where specialized tissues are repaired by formation of mature connective tissue, e.g. pneumonia or infarcts.
- *Wound contraction* mediated by myofibroblasts; can reduce the tissue defect by up to 80%, but can lead to problems, e.g. burns contractures.
- *Collagen* is secreted at the same time to form a scar.

Factors affecting wound healing

- Impaired arterial supply or venous drainage (global or local).
- Excessive movement, local distension, or distal obstruction.
- Infection, malignancy, foreign body, necrotic tissue, smoking.
- *Malnutrition.* Obesity, recent weight loss, nutrient deficiency.
- *Immunosuppressive.* Cancer, steroids, immunosuppressants, HIV.
- *Anticancer therapies.* Radiotherapy and chemotherapy.
- *Metabolic.* Diabetes, jaundice, uraemia, musculoskeletal diseases, age.

Wound healing in specific tissues

Skin: first intention healing

This takes place where there is close apposition of clean wound edges.
- Thrombosis in cut blood vessels prevents haematoma formation.
- Coagulated blood forms a surface scab which keeps the wound clean.
- Fibrin precipitates to form a weak framework between the two edges.
- Capillaries proliferate to bridge the gap.
- Fibroblasts secrete collagen into the fibrin network.
- Basal epidermal cells bridge the gap and are eventually resorbed.
- The elastic network in the dermis cannot be replaced.

Skin: second intention healing

This takes place in wounds where skin edges cannot be cleanly apposed.
- There is phagocytosis to remove debris.
- Granulation tissue to fill in defects.
- Epithelial regeneration covers the surface.

Gastrointestinal tract

- *Erosion* is loss of part of the thickness of the mucosa.
  - Adjacent epithelial cells proliferate to regenerate the mucosa.
  - Healing may take place this way in a matter of hours.
- *Ulceration* is loss of the full thickness of the mucosa.
  - Mucosa is replaced from the margins.
  - The muscularis propria cannot be regenerated: it is replaced by scar.
  - Damaged blood vessels bleed, fibrin covers the raw surfaces.
  - Macrophages migrate in and phagocytose dead tissue.
  - Granulation tissue is produced in the base.
  - If the cause persists, the ulcer becomes chronic.
  - Fibrous scar tissue may result in contractions.

Ulcers

An **ulcer** is a breach in an epithelial surface.

Classification
Venous, arterial, diabetic, neuropathic, malignant, traumatic.

Features to note on examination
- *Site.* Neck, groin, and axilla (TB); legs and feet (vascular); anywhere (malignant).
- *Surface.* Usually depressed. Elevated in malignancy, vascular granulations.
- *Size.* Measure the ulcer. Is it large by comparison to the length of history?
- *Shape.* Oval, circular, serpiginous, straight edges.
- *Edge.* Eroded (actively spreading), shelved (healing), punched out (syphilitic), rolled or everted (malignant).
- *Base.* Fixed to underlying structures? Mobile? Indurated? Penetrating?
- *Discharge.* Purulent (infection), watery (TB), bleeding (granulation or malignancy).
- *Pain.* Usually occurs during the extension phase of non-specific ulcers. In diabetic patients, ulcers are relatively painless.
- *Number.* Widespread locally (local infection such as cellulitis), widespread generally (constitutional upset).
- *Progress.* Short history (pyogenic), chronic (vascular or trophic, e.g. post-phlebitic syndrome, decubitus ulceration of paraplegia).
- *Lymph nodes.* In the region of an ulcer may indicate secondary infection or malignant change.

Natural history
- *Extension.* There is discharge, thickened base, inflamed margin. Slough and exudates cover the surface.
- *Transition.* Slough separates and the base becomes clean. The discharge becomes scanty, the margins less inflamed.
- *Repair.* Granulation becomes fibrous tissue and forms a scar after re-epithelialization.

Investigations
History, biopsy and histology, serology, as indicated by presentation.

Chronic leg ulcers
Their aetiology is diverse, but can usually be diagnosed clinically.

Venous ulcers
Part of post-phlebitic limb syndrome where there may be a history of past DVT. The ulcer is associated with oedema, *lipodermatosclerosis* (woody thickening of soft tissues around the calf), and venous congestion with secondary calf perforators and varicose veins. The ulcer is usually over the medial malleolus, but can be large, involving the whole of the gaiter region.

- If pulses are absent in the foot, there may be an arterial element which can be excluded by measurement of the ankle to brachial pressure index (ABPI).
- If any doubt persists, a vascular referral for arterial reconstruction should be considered, but four-layer bandaging must be avoided when there is arterial insufficiency.

Arterial ulcers
These are often multiple and occur distally over and between the toes or at pressure points such as heels or malleoli. They may occur elsewhere on the leg, usually when there is an associated diabetic or venous element. There is usually a history of arterial disease, particularly peripheral vascular disease with claudication.

- Unlike venous ulcers where bacterial colonization is common, the presence of organisms suggests infection, particularly when there is moisture around the ulcers: wet gangrene (caused by staphylococci and streptococci, not clostridia, see later) may ensue with cellulitis.
- If the leg is kept dry, infection is minimized and a line of demarcation may aid in decision-making for the level of amputation.
- Arterial reconstruction should be considered before this stage.

Diabetic ulcers
These commonly occur in conjunction with arterial disease. They represent large- and small-vessel disease with an impaired ability to heal and increased susceptibility to infection. Ulcers may occur in the arterial distribution, particularly at pressure points, and involve deep tissue infections (such as plantar abscesses) and osteomyelitis. The associated diabetic neuropathy with *Charcot's joints* presents with deformed feet and joints, which are susceptible to ulceration.

- Management involves good diabetic and ulcer care, which includes orthotist help with shoes and gait.
- Surgery aims to avoid major amputation, but requires debridement of necrotic tissue, drainage of abscesses, and excision of dead tissue, often involving bone as 'ray' excisions of toes.

Other causes
Include pressure, vasculitic, lymphatic, infective, and artefactual causes. Leg ulcer clinics have emphasized the value of a team approach.

Cysts, sinuses, and fistulas

Cysts

A **cyst** is a collection of fluid in a sac lined by endothelium or epithelium which usually secretes the fluid.
- **True cysts** are lined by endo- or epithelium.
- **False cysts** are the result of exudation or degeneration, e.g. pseudocyst of pancreas, cystic degeneration in a tumour.

Classification
Congenital
- *Sequestration dermoid*. Due to displacement of epithelium along embryonic fissures during closure, e.g. skin. Sites include outer and inner borders of orbit, midline of the body, anterior triangle of neck (brachial cyst), (cf. implantation dermoid due to skin implantation from injury).
- *Tubulo-dermoid/tubulo-embryonic*. Abnormal budding of tubular structures, e.g. enteric cysts, post-anal dermoid, thyroglossal cyst.
- *Dilatation of vestigial remnants*. For example, urachal, vitellointestinal, paradental and branchial cleft cysts, hydatid of Morgagni, Rathke's pouch.

Acquired
- *Retention cysts*. Due to the blocking of a glandular or excretory duct, e.g. sebaceous cyst (sweat gland); ranula (salivary gland); and cysts of the pancreas, gall bladder, parotid, breast, epididymis, Bartholin's glands, hydronephrosis, hydrosalpinx.
- *Distension cysts*. Due to the distension of closed cavities as a result of exudation or secretion, e.g. thyroid or ovarian cysts; hygroma (lymphatic cysts), hydrocoele, ganglia, bursas (false cysts).
- *Cystic tumours*. For example, cystadenoma, cystadenocarcinoma of ovary.
- *Parasitic cysts*. For example, hydatid cysts (*Taenia echinococcus*).
- *Pseudocysts*. Due to necrosis of haemorrhage with liquefaction and encapsulation, e.g. necrotic tumours, cerebral softening, or coalescence of inflammatory fluid collections, e.g. pseudocyst of pancreas.

Clinical features
Subcutaneous/superficial
Smooth, spherical, soft, and fluctuant when palpated in two planes with the fingers at right angles to each other. If tense contents, may produce pain in the cyst or surrounding tissue. If the fluid is clear, the swelling will transilluminate. Ultrasound and aspiration of contents are methods of determining whether a given swelling is cystic and may differentiate a cyst from a lipoma. May compress surrounding tissues. May produce pain if complications supervene. They are also subject to infection, torsion if on a pedicle, haemorrhage, and calcification.

Treatment
- *Excision.* Only if symptomatic, cosmetic, or concern over diagnosis.
- *Marsupialization* (deroofing and suture of the lining to skin). If chronic or infected.
- *Drainage* (deep site). If symptomatic or complicated. Not if concern over malignancy.

Sinuses/fistulas

- A **sinus** is a blind epithelial track, lined by granulation tissue which extends from a free surface into the tissues, e.g. pilonidal sinus.
- A **fistula** is an abnormal communication between two epithelial surfaces. It is lined by granulation tissue and colonized by bacteria, e.g. fistula-in-ano, pancreaticocutaneous, colovesical, vesicovaginal.

Causes
- Specific disease, e.g. Crohn's.
- Abscess formation and spontaneous drainage, e.g. diverticular abscess discharging into vagina with fistula formation.
- Penetrating wounds.
- Iatrogenic (e.g. anastomotic leak discharging via wound).
- Neoplastic.

Persistence of a fistula is due to the following
- Presence of foreign material, e.g. suture/bone in a sinus.
- Distal obstruction of the viscus of origin.
- Continuing active sepsis, e.g. TB, actinomycosis.
- Epithelialization of the track.
- Chronic inflammation, e.g. Crohn's.
- Malignancy in the track.

Investigation
Establish the extent by sinography/fistulogram. MRI scan is often helpful.

Treatment
Principles of sinus treatment:
- Ensure adequate drainage, laying it open and remove granulations.
- Remove septic material, foreign bodies.
- Biopsy sinus wall if concern over underlying diagnosis.
- Loose packs may be used to help drainage.

Principles of fistula treatment:
- Treat any sepsis, fluid imbalances, and poor nutrition if associated.
- Ensure good drainage to prevent fistula extension.
- Identify the anatomy, use examination under anaesthetic (EUA) or imaging if required.
- Biopsy the fistula if concern over underlying diagnosis.
- Definitive treatment requires:
  - Excision of the organ of origin or closure of the site of origin.
  - Removal of chronic fistula track and surrounding inflamed tissue.
  - Closure of 'recipient' organ if internal or drainage of external site if to skin.

Atherosclerosis

Atherosclerosis is a degenerative disease of large and medium-sized arteries characterized by lipid deposition and fibrosis.

Aetiology

Reversible risk factors include smoking, hypercholesterolaemia, obesity, and hypertension. Irreversible risk factors include diabetes, male sex, age, and family history.

Pathological features

- There are three stages of atheromatous lesion; *fatty streaks* are linear lesions on the artery lumen, composed of lipid-filled macrophages, and which progress to *fibrolipid plaques* and finally, *complex lesions*.
- In sites predisposed to atherosclerosis (sites of vessel bifurcation, turbulent flow, post-stenotic areas, areas denuded of endothelial cells), lipid-laden macrophages enter the vessel wall via gaps between endothelial cells.
- A fibrolipid plaque contains a mixture of macrophages and smooth muscle cells which migrate into the plaque, capped by a layer of fibrous tissue.
- Growth factors, particularly platelet-derived growth factor (PDGF), stimulate the proliferation of intimal smooth muscle cells and the synthesis of collagen, elastin, and mucopolysaccharide.
- Lipid accumulates within the plaque extracellularly and in the myocytes, ultimately producing foam cells.
- Cell death eventually ensues with the release of intracellular lipids, calcification, and a chronic inflammatory reaction.
- High levels of circulating LDL-cholesterol are thought to lead to atherosclerosis by damaging endothelium, both directly by increasing membrane viscosity and indirectly through free radical formation, and by inducing secretion of PDGF.
- In larger vessels such as the aorta, atherosclerotic plaques may release atheroemboli and mural thrombus or impinge on the vessel media, causing tissue atrophy resulting in aneurysm formation or dissection.
- *Acute MI* is caused by three processes in coronary vessels: progressive atherosclerosis, disruption of unstable plaque with acute thrombosis, and acute haemorrhage into the intima around the plaque.

Thromboembolic disease

Thrombus

A **thrombus** is a solid mass of blood constituents formed within the vascular system.

The formation, structure, and appearance of thrombus and clot are completely different. Clinical features of thrombus—see 📖 p. 120.

Aetiology

Described by Virchow, the three types of risk factors for thrombus are called Virchow's triad (see Box 3.1). Not all three are needed: any one of them may result in thrombus formation in arteries or veins. Arterial thrombus is most commonly associated with *atheroma*, venous thrombus with *stasis*.

Box 3.1 Virchow's triad

- **Disruption in the blood vessel endothelium.**
  - Atheromatous plaque, e.g. acute MI.
  - Thrombophlebitis, e.g. DVT.
  - Trauma, e.g. from pressure, surgery, fractures, previous thrombus.
- **Disruption in the pattern of blood flow.**
  - Stasis, e.g. immobilization, surgery, low CO states.
  - Turbulence, e.g. post-stenotic, atherosclerotic plaques.
- **Changes in blood constituents.**
  - Age.
  - Smoking.
  - Malignancy.
  - DIC, HITT.
  - Pregnancy, oral contraceptive pill.

Thrombus formation

Wherever thrombus forms, the principal mechanisms are similar.
- Initial trigger is one or more of Virchow's triad.
- Fibrin deposition on vessel wall and formation of platelet layer.
- Red cells trapped in fibrin meshwork on top of platelet layer.
- Mass projects into lumen, causing turbulent blood flow.
- Thrombus grows in direction of blood flow: propagation.
- In veins, alternating patterns of white platelets and red blood cells may be seen: *lines of Zahn.*
- *Thrombophlebitis* is inflammation of veins secondary to thrombus.
- *Phlebothrombosis* is thrombus formation secondary to phlebitis.
- *Phlegmasia alba dolens* (white painful leg) occurs after slow thrombosis formation in the ileofemoral veins and is a chronic condition.
- *Phlegmasia cerulean dolens* (blue painful leg) is due to acute massive ileofemoral venous thrombosis and can result in shock and gangrene.
- *Thrombophlebitis migrans* are transient thromboses in previously healthy veins anywhere in the body, suggesting visceral cancer.

Embolism

An **embolism** is a mobile mass of material in the vascular system capable of blocking its lumen.

Types of embolism

The aetiology is very different, depending on the cause of embolism. The clinical effects depend on the territory supplied by the vessel that is blocked. Emboli can be divided into:

- Systemic emboli (see 🕮 p. 642) (cause stroke, end-organ ischaemia, MI);
- PE (see 🕮 p. 120).

Both types of embolism can be further classified by the substance involved:

- *Thrombus.* Most emboli are derived from thrombi.
- *Gas.* Injection or entraining of air, decompression sickness.
- *Fat.* Long bone fractures, severe burns, extensive soft tissue trauma.
- *Amniotic fluid.* ↑ Intrauterine pressure forces fluid into uterine veins and into systemic circulation.
- *Septic emboli.* Vegetations from heart valves.
- *Atheromatous plaque.* Peripheral vascular disease, iatrogenic.
- *Tumour.* Common route of metastasis.
- *Foreign bodies.* IV drug users, medically inserted catheters.

Clot

A **clot** is a solid collection of blood cells within a fibrin network.

Clot forms in vessels after death or outside the body as part of the response to trauma. Activation of the clotting cascade (see 🕮 p. 119) results in formation of fibrin from fibrinogen, resulting in the formation of fibrin meshwork that enmeshes cells in a solid, elastic clot.

Ischaemia and infarction

Ischaemia is tissue effect due to insufficient oxygen delivery.
Infarction is tissue death due to insufficient oxygen delivery.

Oxygen supply-demand mismatch is caused by:

- Vascular narrowing (atherosclerosis, thrombus, embolus, spasm).
- Global hypoperfusion (shock, cardiopulmonary bypass).
- Hypoxaemia (anaemia, hypoxia).
- Vascular compression (ventricular distension, venous occlusion).
- Increased oxygen demand (exercise, pregnancy, hyperthyroidism).

Pathological features

The shape of the infarct depends on the territory and perfusion of the occluded vessel.

- *Seconds.* Change from aerobic to anaerobic metabolism.
- *Minutes.* ↓ Contractility of muscle, cell and mitochondria swell.

- *Hours.* Myocyte death, coagulation necrosis, muscle pale, oedematous.
- *Days.* Inflammatory exudates with polymorphonuclear leucocytes, then fibroblast infiltration beginning scar formation; macroscopically, the infarcted area appears yellow and rubbery with haemorrhagic border.
- *Weeks.* Neovascularization and margins.
- *Months.* Scar maturation—tough, white, contracted area.

Gangrene and capillary ischaemia

Gangrene is ischaemic tissue necrosis with dessication (**dry gangrene**) or putrefaction (**wet gangrene**).

Gangrene

Aetiology

- *Thrombosis,* e.g. appendiceal artery secondary to inflammation.
- *Embolus,* e.g. atherosclerotic emboli in peripheral vascular disease.
- *Extrinsic compression,* e.g. fracture, organ torsion, tourniquet.

Clinical appearances

Dry gangrene

The affected limb, digit, or organ is black because of breakdown of haemoglobin, dry, and shrivelled. Dry gangrene shows little or no tendency to spread. A zone of demarcation appears between the dead and viable tissue and separation begins to take place by aseptic ulceration in a few days.

Wet gangrene

Veins as well as arteries are blocked. Pain is initially severe, but lessens as the patient becomes more septic. There is always infection (putrefaction). The skin and superficial tissues become blistered. There is a broad zone of ulceration which separates it from normal tissue. Proximal spread is a feature, leading to septicaemia and death.

Gas gangrene

Gangrene complicated by infection with gas-producing anaerobic bacteria, e.g. *Clostridium perfringens.* Gases elaborated from putrefaction lead to surgical emphysema and crepitus (see 📖 p. 175).

Principles of treatment

- *Systemic treatment.*
  - Aggressive fluid resuscitation is often necessary.
  - Pain relief (IV morphine 5–10mg).
  - IV antibiotics—broad-spectrum (e.g. benzylpenicillin, metronidazole, piperacillin/tazobactam, or according to microbiological advice).
- *Conservative treatment.* Only possible for non-vital organs affected by dry gangrene (e.g. toes/forefoot). Aim is to let the affected areas mummify and spontaneously separate.
- *Surgical salvage procedures.* Conservative excision possibly combined with reconstruction or restoration of blood supply (e.g. foot amputation and bypass surgery for distal lower limb gangrene).
- *Radical surgical excision.* Only possible where affected organ is completely resectable (e.g. limbs, perineal tissues)—excision must be radical in spreading or gas gangrene. Ensure all pus is released, all affected tissue (not just the necrosed area) is excised back to bleeding healthy tissue. Often requires 'relook' surgery to ensure adequate excision of infected tissue.

- *Palliative care*. Consider for unresectable gangrene (e.g. retroperitoneal gangrene, very extensive intestinal gangrene) or for elderly sick patients where surgery is inappropriate.

Capillary ischaemia

This is ischaemia mediated by injury to capillaries.

- *Frostbite*. Exposure to cold with freezing results in fixed capillary contraction, ischaemia, and infarction.
- *Trenchfoot*. Exposure to cold without freezing results in capillary contraction followed by fixed dilation.
- DIC (see p. 116).
- Cryoglobulinaemia, sickle cell, parasites.

Tumours

Definitions
- **Metaplasia**. Reversible transformation of one type of terminally differentiated cell into another fully differentiated cell type.
- **Dysplasia**. Potentially premalignant condition characterized by increased cell growth, atypical morphology, and altered differentiation.
- **Neoplasia**. Autonomous abnormal growth of cells which persists after the initiating stimulus has been removed.
- A **neoplasm** is a lesion resulting from neoplasia.

Metaplasia
This represents an adaptive response of a tissue to environmental stress. It is mediated by changes in expression of genes involved in cellular differentiation. *It does not progress to malignancy*: if the environmental changes persist, dysplasia may result and progress to malignancy. For example:
- Change from ciliated to squamous cells in the respiratory epithelium of the trachea and bronchi in smokers;
- Change from squamous to columnar cells in the oesophageal epithelium of patients with gastro-oesophageal reflux disease (Barrett's) (see 📖 p. 280).

Dysplasia
Potentially premalignant condition. May be a response to chronic inflammation or exposure to carcinogens. Early forms may be reversible: severe dysplasia has a high risk of progression to malignancy, for example:
- Dysplasia arising in colonic epithelium due to chronic ulcerative colitis.
- Squamous dysplasia in the bronchi of smokers (sputum cytology).

Classification of tumours
Use this classification to give a differential diagnosis for any neoplasm.
- *Tissue of origin*. Organ and tissue type (see Table 3.1).
- *Behaviour*. Benign or malignant.
- *Primary or secondary*.

Benign tumours
- Slow growing, usually encapsulated, do not metastasize, do not recur if completely excised, rarely endanger life. Effects are due to size and site.
- *Histology*: well differentiated, low mitotic rate, resemble tissue of origin.

Malignant tumours
- These expand and infiltrate locally, encapsulation is rare, metastasize to other organs via blood, lymphatics or body spaces, endanger life if untreated.
- *Histology*: varying degrees of differentiation from tissue of origin, pleomorphic (variable cell shapes), high mitotic rate.

Table 3.1 Structural classification

Tissue of origin	Tumour type
Epithelium	**Benign**: papilloma, adenoma (glandular epithelium)
	Malignant: carcinoma (adenocarcinoma, squamous cell carcinoma indicate cell types)
Connective tissue	**Benign**: fibroma (fibrous tissue), lipoma (fat), chondroma (cartilage), osteoma (bone), leiomyoma (smooth muscle), rhabdomyoma (striated muscle)
	Malignant: sarcoma, e.g. fibrosarcoma, osteosarcoma, etc. (if well differentiated); spindle cell sarcoma, etc. (if poorly differentiated)
Neural tissue	These arise from nerve cells, nerve sheaths, and supporting tissues, e.g. astrocytoma, medulloblastoma, neurilemmoma, neuroma, etc.
Haemopoietic	The leukaemias, Hodgkin's disease, multiple myeloma, lymphosarcoma, reticulosarcoma
Melanocytes	Melanoma
Mixed origins	E.g. fibroadenoma, nephroblastoma, teratoma (all three germ layers), choriocarcinoma
Developmental blastomas	E.g. neuroblastoma (adrenal medulla), nephroblastoma (kidney), retinoblastoma (eye)

Invasion

Invasion is the most important single criterion for malignancy and is also responsible for clinical signs and prognosis as well as dictating surgical management. Factors that enable tumours to invade tissues include:

• Increased cellular motility.
• Loss of contact inhibition of migration and growth.
• Secretion of proteolytic enzymes, such as collagenase, which weakens normal connective tissue bonds.
• Decreased cellular adhesion.

Metastasis

Metastasis is a consequence of these invasive properties: it is the process by which malignant tumours spread from their site of origin (primary tumour) to form secondary tumours at distant sites. Carcinomatosis denotes extensive metastatic disease. The routes of metastasis are:

• *Haematogenous*. Via the bloodstream.
  • Five tumours—breast, bronchus, kidney, thyroid, prostate—classically metastasize via haematogenous spread to bone.
  • Lung, liver, and brain are common sites for secondaries.
• *Lymphatic*. To local, regional, and systemic nodes.
• *Transcoelomic*. Across pleural, pericardial, and peritoneal cavities.
• *Implantation*. During surgery or along biopsy tracks.

Carcinogenesis

Carcinogenesis is the process that results in malignant neoplasm formation. Usually more than one carcinogen is necessary to produce a tumour, a process which may occur in several steps—**multistep hypothesis**.

- *Initiators* produce a permanent change in the cells, but do not themselves cause cancer, e.g. ionizing radiation: this change may be in the form of gene mutation.
- *Promoters* stimulate clonal proliferation of initiated cells, e.g. dietary factors and hormones: they are not mutagenic.
- *Latency* is the time between exposure to carcinogen and clinical recognition of tumour due to:
  - Time taken for clonal proliferation to produce a significant cell mass.
  - Time taken for exposure to multiple necessary carcinogens.
- *Persistence* is when clonal proliferation no longer requires the presence of initiators or promoters and the tumour cells exhibit autonomous growth.

See Table 3.2 for a list of common risk factors for cancer.

Tumour growth

Tumour doubling time depends on cell *cycle time, growth function*, and *cell loss fraction*. In tumours such as leukaemias, the doubling time remains remarkably constant: the cell mass increases proportionally with time. This is *exponential growth*. In solid tumours, doubling time slows as size increases. This is referred to as *Gompertzian growth*.

Genetic abnormalities in tumours

Two genetic mechanisms of carcinogenesis are proposed:
- *Oncogenes*. Enhanced expression of stimulatory dominant genes.
- *Tumour suppressor genes*. Inactivation of recessive inhibitory genes.

Oncogenes

At least 60 oncogenes have been identified. They can be classified according to the function of the gene product (e.g. growth factors, cell signalling agents). The proteins produced (oncoproteins) can be produced in abnormal quantities or be abnormally active forms and cause:
- Independence from extrinsic growth factors.
- Production of tumours in immunotolerant animals.
- Production of proteases to assist in invasion of normal tissues.
- Reduced cell cohesiveness assisting metastasis.
- Growth to higher cell densities and abnormal cellular orientation.

Examples include *BRCA1, p53, k-ras, APC, DCC*.

Table 3.2 Common risk factors for cancer

Known carcinogen	Type of cancer
Chemicals	
Polyaromatic hydrocarbons	Lung cancer (smoking), skin cancers
Aromatic amines	Bladder cancer (rubber and dye workers)
Alkylating agents	Leukaemia
Viruses	
HIV	Kaposi's sarcoma, lymphoma
Epstein–Barr virus	Burkitt's lymphoma, nasopharyngeal cancer
Human papillomavirus	Squamous papilloma (wart), cervical cancer
Hepatitis B virus	Liver cell carcinoma
Radiation	
UV light (UVB>UVA)	Malignant melanoma, basal cell carcinoma
Ionizing radiation	Particularly breast, bone, thyroid, marrow
Biological agents	
Hormones, e.g. oestrogens	Breast and endometrial cancer
Mycotoxins, e.g. aflatoxins	Liver cell carcinoma
Parasites, e.g. schistosoma	Bladder cancer
Miscellaneous	
Asbestos	Mesothelioma and lung cancer
Nickel	Nasal and lung cancer
Host factors	**Type of cancer**
Race	
Caucasians	Malignant melanoma, stomach cancer
Diet	
High dietary fat	Breast, colorectal cancer
Alcohol	Breast cancer
Gender, inherited risks	
Female sex	Breast cancer
Familial polyposis coli	Colorectal cancer
Multiple endocrine neoplasia	Phaeo, parathyroid, medullary cancer thyroid
BRCA1–17q21	Breast, ovarian and prostate cancer
Premalignant lesions and conditions	
Adenomatous rectal polyp	Colorectal adenocarcinoma
Mammary ductal hyperplasia	Breast carcinoma
Ulcerative colitis	Colorectal adenocarcinoma
Transplacental exposure	
Diethylstiboesterol	Vaginal adenocarcinoma

Screening

Screening is testing any population for a disease.

The aim is reduction in morbidity and mortality from screened diseases.

Requirements for successful screening
- Screening *test* must be:
  - Sensitive (see 📖 p. 7).
  - Specific (see 📖 p. 7).
  - Safe.
  - Inexpensive.
  - Acceptable.
- The *population* screened must be:
  - Easily identified and contactable.
  - Compliant.
- The *disease* screened must be:
  - Detectable in a treatable, premalignant form or earlier stage.
  - Preventable or more amenable to successful or curative treatment.
  - A sufficient burden on the population to justify cost of screening.
  - Chronic or of suitable evolution for sporadic testing to detect it.

Disadvantages of screening
- Cost (time and resources).
- The benefit may be small.
- False positive tests may be physically or psychologically detrimental.

Examples of screening programmes
Abdominal aortic aneurysm (4000 deaths/y)
The UK multicentre aneurysm screening study of 68 000 men showed screening halves aneurysm-related deaths by reducing risk of rupture. The conclusion was that aneurysm screening should be offered in the UK. The MASS study showed a benefit where other studies failed because:
- It was adequately powered (see 📖 p. 8).
- Screening compliance was higher:
  - GP-based ultrasound had a better compliance than specialist clinics.
  - Participants unlikely to attend were excluded from the study.

Breast cancer (14 000 deaths/y)
A meta-analysis of thirteen breast cancer screening trials concluded that screening mammography significantly reduced breast cancer mortality in women aged 50–74. A BMJ analysis concluded that:
- For every 1000 women screened over 10y, around 200 (depending on age) are recalled because of an abnormal result and of these:
  - Around 60 will have at least one biopsy.
  - About 15 will have invasive cancer and 5 will have ductal carcinoma *in situ* (DCIS).

- About 0.5, 2, 3, and 2 fewer deaths from breast cancer occur over 10y per 1000 women aged 40, 50, 60, and 70y, respectively, who choose to be screened.
- Ten per cent of invasive carcinoma is not radiologically detectable.
- Risk of a false positive screen is approximately 25% over 10y.
- Studies suggest up to a 30% reduction in mortality from screen-detected early breast cancer.
- Features looked for on screening mammography include: spiculated calcification, microcalcification.

What is offered?
- Since 1988, population-based screening offered.
- Starts age 50 and continues to age 70 (covers peak ages of incidence of new diagnoses and excludes low risk younger women—prevents 'psychological morbidity of screening the well').
- Seventy per cent of women offered it accept screening (lowest take-up in lower socio-economic groups and those difficult to contact, e.g. rapidly changing addresses or no fixed address).
- Two-view (lateral and oblique) mammography of both breasts.
- Suspicious or malignant-looking lesions invited for clinical assessment by standard triple assessment.

Cervical cancer (1500 deaths/y)
Since the mid-1980s, incidence of and mortality from cervical cancer in women under 70 in England and Wales has fallen. Screening is thought to be the most likely explanation. A BMJ analysis concluded that:
- In the NHS cervical screening programme, 1000 women need to be screened for 35 years to prevent one death:
  - 150 have an abnormal result and 75 need repeat for inadequate test.
  - 80 undergo biopsy.
  - 55 have an abnormal biopsy result.
  - 2 have carcinoma, the rest have dysplasia.
- At least one woman dies within the 35y despite being screened.

Prostate cancer (9000 deaths/y)
A third of men over 50y have evidence of prostate cancer at post-mortem, but less than 1% of these have clinically active disease. Screening is controversial because:
- Prostate-specific antigen (PSA), rectal examination, and transrectal ultrasound have low specificity and sensitivity alone or in combination.
- Treatment of prostate cancer is controversial (see 📖 p. 374).
- No randomized trial has shown a survival benefit in screened populations: screening may cause more harm than good.
- Screening can be carried out on request despite the evidence above.

Colorectal cancer (16 000 deaths/y)
The lifetime risk of colorectal cancer is about 1 in 20. A nationwide screening programme is likely, following current pilot centres:
- Several possible screening tests exist:
  - Faecal occult blood (low sensitivity, 90% specificity)—requires colonoscopy for positive results (false positives common).

- Colonoscopy (sensitivity and specificity near 100%).
- Flexible sigmoidoscopy (sensitivity 80%, specificity near 100%).
- Colorectal cancer is suited to screening:
  - It has a detectable premalignant phase.
  - It is detectable at an earlier and potentially highly treatable stage.
  - Screening has been shown to be cost-effective and acceptable.

Grading and staging

- **Staging** is the process of assessing the extent of local and systemic spread of a malignant tumour or the identification of features which are risk factors for spread.
- **Grading** is the process of assessing the degree of differentiation of a malignant tumour.

Key facts

The objectives of staging and grading a tumour are:
- To plan appropriate (treatment) for the individual patient.
- To give an estimate of the prognosis.
- To compare similar cases when assessing outcomes or designing clinical trials.

Staging and grading methods

Staging

The commonest system is the internationally agreed TNM classification (see Table 3.3). It is not appropriate for leukaemia, lymphomas, or myeloma. A four-stage classification (I, II, III, IV) is also often used and is compatible with TNM. Specific staging systems also exist for some tumour sites (e.g. Duke's stage in colorectal cancer, see 📖 p. 400).

Staging may be:
- *Radiological* (often performed preoperatively): indicated by the prefix 'r' before the letter (e.g. rT3, rM1). If different radiological modalities are used, separate prefixes can be used, e.g. 'u' for ultrasound (uT2). Radiological staging is used to plan treatment (e.g. neoadjuvant therapy, selection for surgery, planning of surgery).
- *Pathological* (performed on surgical specimens): indicated by the prefix 'p' before the letter (e.g. pT3, pN2, pM1). If preoperative radiotherapy is used, the prefix 'y' is used to denote that the pathological stage may have been modified by this (e.g. ypT2). Pathological staging is used to plan adjuvant treatment (chemotherapy or radiotherapy) and for informing prognosis.

An example of lung cancer staging is:
- Stage I (T1N0, T2N0), 85% 5y survival with surgery.
- Stage II (T1N1, T2N1, T3N0), 60% 5y survival with surgery.
- Stage IIIa (T3N1 or any N2), 20% 5y survival with surgery.
- Stage IIIb (any T4, any N3), <20% 5y survival, no benefit with surgery.
- Stage IV (M1), <10% 5y survival, no benefit with surgery.

Other pathological features may be included with the TNM system for some tumours, for example:
- Presence of extratumoural vascular invasion V0 or V1.
- Presence of extratumoural lymphatic invasion Ly0 or Ly1.
- Presence of viable tumour cells at or within 1mm of the surgical margin of excision R0, R1 (microscopic), R2 (macroscopic).

Table 3.3 Basic form of TNM classification*

Classification	Interpretation
Primary tumour (T)	
TX	Primary tumour cannot be evaluated
T0	No evidence of primary tumour
Tis	Tumour *in situ*
T1, T2, T3, T4	Size and extent of primary tumour
Regional lymph nodes (N)	
NX	Regional lymph nodes cannot be evaluated
N0	No regional lymph node involvement
N1, N2, N3	Number and location of involved lymph nodes
Distant metastasis (M)	
MX	Distant metastasis cannot be evaluated
M0	No distant metastasis
M1	Distant metastasis

* Additional codes used with the TNM: pul, pulmonary; hep, hepatic; V, vascular; Ly, lymphatic vessels; R, radial margin. Prefixes used with the TNM: u, ultrasound; r, radiological; p, pathological.

Histological grading

Gives a guide to the behaviour of a cancer by describing the degree of differentiation of the tumour (e.g. breast cancer).

- Grade 1, represents the least malignant tumours.
- Grade 2, 25–50% of the cells are undifferentiated.
- Grade 3, 50–75% of the cells are undifferentiated.
- Grade 4, >75% of the cells are undifferentiated.

Other methods of describing tumours

- Depth of invasion (e.g. Breslow thickness in malignant melanoma).
- Tumour type (e.g. small cell versus non-small cell lung cancer).

Tumour markers

Key facts
- Tumour markers (see Table 3.4) are complex molecules, often proteins that can be detected by a variety of techniques, including chemical, immunological, or bioactivity testing.
- Most are molecules normally produced by normal cells in small amounts, but which may be produced in increased amounts by tumour cells due to changes in cellular function (e.g. increased production, increased gene expression, decreased degradation, increased release).

Testing
Testing is most commonly *in vitro* via serum measurements or testing tissue specimens. Common uses include:
- Screening (detection of subclinical disease).
- Diagnosis (including differentiation of tumour origin in metastatic disease).
- Monitoring response to treatment.
- Monitoring for development of recurrence.

Non-tumour related elevations in tumour marker levels (reducing the specificity of these tests for tumours) may occur due to:
- Increased production/release due to inflammation, infection, trauma, or surgery.
- Decreased removal/destruction due to renal or liver disease.

Abbreviations for some tumour markers
- AFP (alpha-fetoprotein).
- β-HCG (beta-human chorionic gonadotrophin).
- PAP (placental alkaline phosphatase).
- CEA (carcinoembryonic antigen).
- LDH (lactic dehydrogenase).
- PSA (prostate-specific antigen).

Table 3.4 Commonly used tumour markers

Marker	Useful in	Notes/use
AFP	Hepatoma; teratoma (75% of cases); pancreatic carcinoma (some patients)	Elevated in liver disease, e.g. hepatitis, cirrhosis, and pregnancy
β-HCG	Choriocarcinoma (almost all cases); testicular tumours/teratoma (75%); other germ cell tumours	Measured both in blood and urine
PAP	Seminoma; ovarian adenocarcinoma	
CEA	Colonic adenocarcinoma; ovarian adenocarcinoma; advanced breast cancer; pancreatic cancer	Not useful for diagnosis or screening. Used to monitor response to treatment and identify relapse in tumours showing raised CEA at diagnosis. May be elevated in pancreatitis, ulcerative colitis, gastritis, and heavy smokers
CA 19–9	Pancreatic cancer (80%); advanced colorectal cancer (75%)	A polysialated antigen (Lewis blood group antigen). Ratio of CA 19–9:CEA most sensitive for pancreatic cancer diagnosis
LDH	Lymphoma	
Thyroglobulin	Thyroid cancer	Used to monitor and identify relapse after treatment
Calcitonin	Medullary carcinoma of the thyroid	Used to monitor and identify relapse after treatment
PSA	Prostate cancer	May be measured in serum and tissue by immunohistochemistry. Serum level closely relates to disease status
Alkaline phosphatase	Osteosarcoma	Also raised in bony metastases, osteitis, Paget's disease

Surgical microbiology

Key facts

- Three-quarters of nosocomial infection occur in surgical patients who account for 40% of hospital inpatients.
- Risk factors for wound infection include the type of surgery, patient age, malnutrition, immunosuppression, obesity, lack of appropriate antibiotic prophylaxis, foreign bodies, and residual malignancy or necrotic tissue.

Nosocomial infections are acquired in hospital.
Community acquired infections are acquired outside hospital.

Sources of surgical infection

Three-quarters of nosocomial infections occur in surgical patients (see Table 3.5) who account for 40% of hospital inpatients. Sources of infection include:

- Patient's own body flora:
  - Failure of correct aseptic technique.
  - Contaminated surgery (see 🕮 p. 146).
- Indirect contact:
  - Contact from hands of doctors, nursing staff, patients, visitors.
  - Contaminated surfaces, e.g. door handles, cups.
- Direct inoculation:
  - Surgeon or environmental flora through failure of aseptic technique.
  - Contaminated instruments or dressings.
  - Colonization of indwelling drains, catheters, intravenous lines.
- Airborne contamination:
  - Skin and clothing of staff, patients, and visitors.
  - Air flow in operating theatre or ward.
- Haematogenous spread:
  - Intravenous and intra-arterial lines.
  - Contaminated infusions.
  - Sepsis at other anatomical sites.
- Food and waterborne.
- Faecal-oral.
- Insect borne.

Risk factors for wound infection

- General:
  - Age.
  - Malnutrition, obesity, malnutrition.
  - Immunosuppression, including steroid therapy, chemotherapy.
  - Endocrine and metabolic disorders, e.g. diabetes, jaundice, uraemia.
  - Hypoxia and anaemia.
- Local:
  - Type of surgery (see Table 3.5), lengthy procedures.
  - Necrotic tissue.
  - Residual local malignancy.
  - Foreign bodies, including prosthetic implants.
  - Ischaemia, haematoma.

Table 3.5 Expected wound infection rates after surgical procedures

Type of surgery	Rate of post-operative infection (%)
Clean (no viscus opened), e.g. hernia repair	<2
Clean contaminated (viscus opened minimal spillage), e.g. cholecystectomy	<10
Contaminated (open viscus with spillage or inflammatory disease), e.g. simple appendicectomy	15–20
Dirty (pus or perforation or incision through abscess), e.g. perforated appendicectomy	>40

- Microbiology:
  - Lack of antibiotic prophylaxis.
  - Type and virulence of organism, size of inoculate.

Modes of occupational infections of health workers

- Direct percutaneous inoculation of infected blood (e.g. needle-stick injury, scalpel wounds).
- Entry of infection through minute skin abrasions after contact with spilled infectious bodily fluids (e.g. blood, saliva, semen, urine, faeces).
- Entry of infection via mucosal surfaces after exposure to contaminated infectious bodily fluids (e.g. eye splashes in theatre, faecal-oral route).
- Transfer of infection by fomites (e.g. via contaminated equipment—prions transferred by neurosurgical equipment).

Procedures designed to minimize transmission

See also 📖 p. 174 for HIV and hepatitis.
- Identify infected (infectious) patients by serology.
- Identify potentially infected (infectious) patients by risk factors (e.g. IV drug users at risk from hepatitis B carriage).
- Specific procedures for the care of infected (infectious) patients (e.g. barrier nursing for *C. difficile* diarrhoea).
- Careful disposal of disposable items related to patient care.
- Specific treatment and sterilization of non-disposable equipment.
- Additional/specific precautions for theatre staff:
  - Make all procedures 'safe' procedures by having the highest standards of safety and care using instruments and sharps: remember ALL patients may be infected/infectious.
  - Wearing of plastic aprons in procedures with expected soiling with urine/faeces/ascites.
  - Wearing of two pairs of gloves to reduce the risk of skin exposure when gloves tear.
  - Wearing of re-enforced gloves for procedures with a high risk of penetrating injury (e.g. fragmented fractures).
  - Wearing of glasses, goggles, or visors for eye protection.
  - Handle all sharps using a transfer container: never pass them hand to hand.
  - Don't allow unnecessary blood or fluid spillage.

Surgically important organisms

Normal body flora

These are usually involved in infections in surgical patients and include:

Staphylococci

- Normal flora of skin, oropharynx, and nasopharynx.
- *S. aureus* is an important pathogen in many surgical infections.
- *S. aureus* is the only staphylococcus that can coagulate plasma.
- 'Coagulase negative' effectively means non *S. aureus* staph, e.g. *S. epidermis*: they are usually dismissed as contaminants, but they are an increasingly common cause of line and prosthesis infections, particularly in immunocompromised patients.
- *Antibiotic sensitivities:* cephalosporins especially cefuroxime, gentamicin, fusidic acid, vancomycin, rifampicin, teicoplanin.
- *Antiseptic sensitivities:* chlorhexidine, povidone-iodine.
- Methicillin-resistant *S. aureus (MRSA)* is resistant to all cephalosporins; vancomycin, teicoplanin, fusidic acid should be reserved to treat this.

Streptococci

- Normal flora of skin, oropharynx, and nasopharynx.
- 'α-haemolytic' streptococci haemolyse blood agar, e.g. *S. pyogenes*.
- 'β-haemolytic' streptococci also haemolyse erythrocytes, e.g. *S. viridens*.
- Pneumococci and enterococci (below) are subtypes of streptococci.
- *S. pyogenes* has been called 'the most important human pathogen': it causes 'strep throat', a range of skin infections, septicaemia, necrotizing fasciitis, toxic shock syndrome, and valvular disease in rheumatic fever.
- *Antibiotic sensitivities:* penicillin, erythromycin, cephalosporins, clindamycin, fusidic acid, mupirocin.
- *Antiseptic sensitivities:* chlorhexidine, povidone-iodine.

Enterococci

- Normal flora of large intestine.
- These are an increasingly important cause of nosocomial infections.
- Involved in wound infections, intra-abdominal sepsis, urinary tract infections, intravascular line infections, and dialysis-related infections.
- *Antibiotic sensitivities:* enterococci are intrinsically resistant to many antibiotics, including all cephalosporins, and must usually be treated by a combination drug regime, e.g. ampicillin plus glycoside.
- Vancomycin-resistant *enterococcus (VRE)* is resistant to all cephalosporins and vancomycin, and sometimes teicoplanin.

'The Gram-negative rods'

- Normal flora of large intestine.
- Gram-negative bacilli (also known as *coliforms*) include *Escherichia coli*, *Salmonella*, *Klebsiella*, *Enterobacter*, and *Proteus*.
- *Pseudomonas* and *Actinobacter* are non-coliform Gram-negatives.
- *Antibiotic sensitivities:* most are intrinsically resistant to penicillin and there is increasing resistance to amoxicillin and ampicillin; cephalosporins are the commonest first-line treatment for non-resistant forms or 'extended range' penicillins (e.g. piperacillin/

tazobactam), aminoglycosides (e.g. gentamicin, streptomycin, amikacin, tobramycin), alone or in combination with cephalosporins, offer good bactericidal action.

Anaerobes
- Normal flora of skin, oropharynx, large bowel, terminal ileum, and genitourinary tract.
- Include *Bacteroides* and clostridia (bowel).
- *C. difficile* causes pseudomembranous colitis (see 🕮 p. 396).
- Cause anaerobic infections, including cellulitis, gas gangrene, empyemas, and colonize diabetic foot ulcers.
- Act usually with aerobes to produce 'synergistic' necrotizing infections of skin, fascia, and muscle spontaneously or after trauma or surgery.
- *Antibiotic sensitivities:* metronidazole is only active against anaerobes and resistance is rare; most anaerobes are also sensitive to penicillins, cephalosporins, clindamycin, erythromycin, and co-trimoxazole.

Specific infections

Gas gangrene
Gas gangrene is caused by *Clostridium perfringens*, a Gram-positive bacillus, found in soil or faeces. Injury may be trivial. More common in immuno-compromised patients. There is exudate and gas in the tissues; skeletal muscle is affected. Oedema, spreading gangrene, and systemic signs follow. Aggressive debridement and fasciotomies are required, with resuscitation, organ support, and penicillin (2g 4-hourly IV) and metronidazole.

Synergistic spreading gangrene (Meleney's or Fournier's gangrene)
Also known as *necrotizing fasciitis*. The organisms involved are not clostridial, but rather aerobes and synergistic microaerophilic/anaerobes. Patients may be immunocompromised. The initial wound might have been minor or an uneventful operation. Severe wound pain and gas in the tissues (crepitus) may be seen: the extent of subdermal gangrene may not be apparent. Systemic support and antibiotics are required, with excision of involved tissues.

Tetanus
This is a rare infection in the UK, but is common in many parts of the world, with a mortality rate of about 60%. The causal organism, *Clostridium tetani*, produces a powerful exotoxin which is neurotoxic. It enters the spinal cord via peripheral nerves where it blocks inhibitory spinal reflexes. It is found widely: infection often follows a trivial puncture wound. Treatment is benzylpenicillin, 1g every 6h IV, metronidazole, and human anti-tetanus immunoglobulin 30U/kg IM. If a wound is present, it is excised and left open to heal by secondary intention. Immunization with 10-yearly boosters is protective.

Soft tissue infections

Cellulitis is the presence of actively dividing infectious bacteria within the skin tissues.

Abscess is a liquid collection of pus lined by granulation tissue and fibrosis (if chronic).

Lymphangitis is the presence of actively dividing infectious bacteria in the lymphatic vessels of an area of the body.

Fasciitis is inflammation of connective tissue that may be infective.

Myositis is infection or inflammation of muscle tissue.

Cellulitis

Pathological features

- Skin entry by pathogenic bacteria (scratch, ulcer, hair follicle).
- Usually Gram +ve cocci (e.g. *Streptococcus pyogenes, S. aureus*).
- Usually heals by resolution if treated promptly.
- Spread may result in *lymphangitis*, suppuration results in a *furuncle* (skin gland), *carbuncle* (upper dermis), or an *abscess* (deep skin tissue).

Clinical features

- Skin widely involved: warm, red (usually blanches with pressure), swollen (often pitting), and exquisitely painful.
- Crepitus indicates the development of gas-forming tissue necrosis which may be an emergency (see 📖 p. 175).

Treatment

- IV antibiotics: benzylpenicillin (1g qds) and flucloxacillin (500mg qds).
- Always assess with microscopy and culture, if possible.

Abscess

Pathological features

- Contain polymorphonuclear neutrophils (PMNs)/macrophages, lymphocytes (live and dead), bacteria (dead and viable), and liquefied tissue products.
- May rupture ('pointing'), discharge into another organ (forming a fistula eventually), or open onto another epithelial surface (sinus) (see 📖 p. 151).
- Incomplete treatment due to resistant organisms (mycobacteria) or poor treatment may lead to chronic abscesses.
- Complete elimination of the organisms in a chronic abscess without drainage can lead to a 'sterile abscess' ('anti-bioma').

Typical causes

- Suppuration of tissue infection (e.g. renal abscess from pyelonephritis).
- Contained infected collections (e.g. subphrenic abscesses).
- Haematogenous spread during bacteraemias (e.g. cerebral abscesses).

Diagnosis

- Deep abscesses are characterized by swing fever, rigors, high WCC, and high CRP. Untreated, they lead to catabolism, weight loss, and a falling serum albumin. Ultrasound, CT, MRI, or isotope studies may be necessary to confirm the diagnosis.

Treatment

- Drain the pus, e.g. incision and drainage (perianal abscess), CT-guided drain (renal abscess), closed surgical drainage (chest empyema), or surgical drainage and debridement (intra-abdominal abscess).
- IV antibiotics (may require course of several weeks, indicating PICC line insertion).

Fasciitis

Suspect when pain, oedema, and skin necrosis appear within 24–48h of injury or operation.

Signs

The skin may be normal, oedematous, or mottled. There may be spiking fever, hypotension, mental confusion.

Treatment

- IV fluids; extensive excision may be indicated.
- Antibiotics on the basis of Gram stain.
- Dress incisions with moist gauze impregnated with dilute aqueous antiseptics. Change these frequently under general anaesthetic.

Myositis

The bacterial infection has penetrated and destroyed muscle bundles.

Cause

Usually *Clostridium perfringens*, a Gram-positive, anaerobic, spore-forming rod.

Management

- Recognize the condition: there is oedema and serosanguinous exudate; exposed muscle is swollen and ranges from salmon pink to
- deep green/black in appearance. Crepitation may be present. There is a 'sickly sweet' smell.
- Excise dead tissue until healthy, contractile, bleeding muscle is encountered.
- Carry out Gram staining immediately. Streptococcal myositis rarely needs amputation, clostridial may.
- Replace extracellular fluid (ECF) deficit. Transfuse if needed.
- High-dose penicillin (IM or IV, 0.6–1.2g every 2h). May need antianaerobic therapy.
- Excision of all infected tissue may necessitate full thickness excision of abdominal wall with prosthetic mesh replacement. Amputations are performed by guillotine technique and the wounds packed open.
- There is no proven advantage to hydrogen peroxide dressings or the use of hyperbaric oxygen, but passive immunization in proven clostridial gangrene has been suggested, using a variety of bacterially derived products.

Osteomyelitis Covered on 📖 pp. 558–62.

Blood-borne viruses and surgery

Viral hepatitis

- Commonest liver disease in the world.
- May cause acute liver failure or chronic active hepatitis.

Hepatitis A

Formerly known as infectious hepatitis. This is the most common form of jaundice in children and young adults.

- Spread is by the faecal-oral route; the incubation period is 1 month.
- The antibody to the virus is anti-HAV.
- There is no vaccine and health care workers do not have to be tested.

Hepatitis B

- Double-shelled DNA virus: 565 new cases in UK in 2000. Ten per cent of adults fail to clear the virus after infection. Up to 5% people worldwide are carriers.
- Infection is largely blood-borne and is transmitted by blood transfusion, inoculation, sharing syringes (drug addicts), sexual intercourse during menstruation (with an infected partner), and anal intercourse.
- *Transmission from a contaminated sharps injury is 30%.*
- *Antigens appear in the serum*: HBsAg, the surface antigen; HBcAg, the hepatitis core antigen; HBeAg, the 'e' antigen; the Dane particle; double-stranded DNA; and DNA polymerase activity.
- Antibodies formed against these antigens (*anti-HBs, anti-HBe*) can be detected in the peripheral blood:
  - *HBsAg +ve.* Failure to clear infection, residual infectivity.
  - *HBsAb +ve.* Protection marker from immunization or infection.
  - *HBeAg +ve.* Close correlation of infectivity.
- Hospital staff are routinely offered vaccination for hepatitis B:
  - Infectious carriers may not perform exposure-prone procedures.
  - Vaccination against hepatitis B is not compulsory. The alternatives are frequent testing to check infectivity or limited clinical practice.
  - The NHS Injury Benefits Scheme provides some benefits where hepatitis B has been occupationally acquired.
- *Treatment.* Any health care worker who remains HBeAg +ve may undergo antiviral therapy under supervision by a hepatologist including:
  - Immunomodulation with interferon.
  - Viral suppression with nucleoside analogues.

Hepatitis C

RNA virus which causes cirrhosis of the liver and primary liver cancer. There is no vaccination. Detected in 1 in 150 screened blood donations: 0.4% of the UK population are chronically infected. *Transmission from a contaminated sharps injury is 2–3%.* Surgeons must be tested for hepatitis C and may not carry out exposure-prone procedures if hepatitis C +ve.

Human immunodeficiency virus (HIV)

Double-stranded RNA retrovirus transmitted by passage of infected body fluids from one person to another by several methods: anal and vaginal sexual intercourse, peripartum, sharps, and infected blood products.

- HIV infection results in widespread immunological dysfunction, manifested by a fall in CD4 +ve lymphocytes, monocytes, and antigen-presenting cells (APCs).
- There is usually a 3-month asymptomatic, but infective viraemia.
- During this period, ELISA tests for HIV antibodies are negative.
- At seroconversion, an acute illness can occur.
- This is followed by generalized lymphadenopathy.
- Acquired immunodeficiency syndrome (AIDS) develops in 5–10y.
- Median survival with untreated AIDS is 2y, treated is >20y.

High risk populations (2004 WHO statistics)
- Prevalence in adult population of southern Africa is 15–30%.
- Prevalence in adult population of sub-Saharan Africa is 5–15%.
- Prevalence in homosexual men at London genitourinary clinics is 10%.
- Prevalence of HIV in injecting drug users in UK is about 1%.

High risk procedures
The UK General Medical Council (GMC) has made it clear that surgeons are obliged, if required, to operate on patients with AIDS or HIV infection. Always use universal precautions. High risk procedures include:
- Any invasive procedure in HIV +ve patients.
- Invasive procedures in at-risk populations (see above).
- Biopsies for the diagnosis of opportunistic infection or suspected HIV.
- Procedures to deal with malignancies, e.g. Kaposi's sarcoma, B-cell and non-Hodgkin's lymphoma, squamous oral carcinoma.

Precautions and post-exposure prophylaxis (PEP)
- The HIV risk from an HIV contaminated hollow needle is 0.3%.
- The risk from splashes on broken skin or mucous membranes is 0.1%.
- *PEP* ▶ Go to occupational health or A&E out of hours. PEP reduces the risk of seroconversion by over 80% if started within 1h of exposure; PEP is continued for 4 weeks. Side effects include diarrhoea and vomiting.

Universal precautions
These are designed to protect workers from exposure to diseases spread by blood and body fluids. ▶ *All* patients are assumed to be infectious for blood-borne diseases, including HIV.
- They apply to blood; amniotic, synovial, pleural, peritoneal and pericardial fluid; semen, vaginal secretions; and CSF.
- They do not apply to faeces, sputum, urine, vomit, or saliva.
- Universal precautions include:
  - Use of protective clothing, e.g. gloves, gowns, masks, eye-guards.
  - Removing hazards from work place, e.g. sharps bins, ventilation.
  - Work practice, e.g. hand washing, handling of sharps, transport of soiled goods, reducing unnecessary procedures.
  - Single use disposable injection equipment.
  - Hospital policy for all sharps injuries: squeeze, wash, and report.

Bleeding and coagulation

Blood products and transfusion reactions are described on 📖 pp. 96–9.

Haemostasis

This is the physiological process by which bleeding is controlled. It has four components:

- *Vessel wall response*, primarily vasoconstriction due to smooth muscle contraction, is the first response.
- *Platelet activity* results in formation of a platelet plug.
  - Platelets *adhere* to exposed endothelial collagen, a process which required von Willebrand factor (VWF) (factor VIII).
  - Release of adenosine diphosphate (ADP), arachidonic acid, prostaglandin, and thromboxane A2 promotes *platelet aggregation*.
  - Aggregated platelets react with thrombin and fibrin, forming a *plug*.
  - *Aspirin* irreversibly inhibits the cyclooxygenase-mediated formation of prostaglandin, lasting for the life of the platelet (7–10 days); *clopidogrel* irreversibly inhibits ADP-mediated aggregation (7–10 days).
- The *coagulation cascade* converts prothrombin to thrombin to produce a fibrin clot: two interacting pathways are involved.
  - The *intrinsic pathway* involves only normal blood components and starts when factor XII (Hageman factor) is activated by binding to a damaged vessel, resulting in the sequential activation of factors XI, IX, VIII, and X.
  - The *extrinsic pathway* requires thromboplastin (a tissue phospholipid) which forms a complex with calcium and factor VII, which activates factor X.
  - Both these pathways converge at the activation of factor X, which converts *prothrombin to thrombin*: thrombin converts soluble *fibrinogen to fibrin* to produce a stable clot.
  - All of the soluble factors are manufactured by the liver except factor VIII (made by endothelium).
  - *Warfarin* inhibits the manufacture of vitamin K-dependent clotting factors (prothrombin, VII, IX, and X): taking 3–4 days to have effect.
- The *fibrinolytic system* terminates thrombus propagation to maintain circulating blood in a fluid state; it depends on four proteins.
  - *Plasmin*, a serine protease which is produced by the action of thrombin on plasminogen and attacks unstable bonds between fibrin molecules to generate fibrin degradation products.
  - *Antithrombin III* which deactivates thrombin, XIIa, IXa, and Xa.
  - *Proteins C and S* which prevent thrombin generation by binding factors Va and VIIIa. *Tissue factor pathway inhibitor*, produced by platelets, inhibits factors Xa and VIIa.
  - *Heparin* potentiates antithrombin III with immediate effect; protamine binds heparin, reversing its effect almost immediately.

Disorders of haemostasis

These can be thought of in terms of the four components below:

- *Vessel wall abnormalities*, e.g. Henoch–Schönlein purpura, Cushing's syndrome, steroid use, vitamin C deficiency (scurvy).

- *Platelet abnormalities.*
  - *Thrombocytopaenia* ($<100 \times 10^9/L^3$) caused by reduced production (bone marrow failure, radiotherapy, chemotherapy, infiltrative disease, e.g. neoplasia, leukaemia); faulty maturation (e.g. folate and B12 deficiency); abnormal distribution (splenomegaly); increased destruction (autoimmune disorders, drugs, DIC, haemorrhage); dilutional thrombocytopaenia in massive banked blood transfusion.
  - *Abnormal function*, e.g. von Willebrand's disease, uraemia, idiopathic causes, drug effects, especially aspirin and clopidogrel.
- *Coagulation abnormalities.*
  - *Congenital*, e.g. haemophilia A (↓ factor VIII), haemophilia B or Christmas disease (↓ factor IX), von Willebrand's disease (↓ VWF).
  - *Acquired*, e.g. DIC (see 📖 p. 118); ↓ vitamin K (which is produced by gut flora) secondary to poor nutrition, antibiotic therapy, obstructive jaundice; liver disease; exogenous anticoagulants.

Preoperative evaluation of haemostasis

NICE guidelines
- Routine testing not recommended unless patient is ASA 3 as a result of renal disease.
- For at-risk patients undergoing 'major +' cardiac or neurosurgery, testing may be considered.

History and examination
- Ask about bleeding problems, e.g. menorrhagia, bruising, family history of bleeding, and medication (specifically aspirin, clopidogrel, and warfarin which should all be stopped 5 days before elective surgery) (see 📖 p. 72).
- Look for petechiae and purpura, jaundice, and hepatosplenomegaly.

Laboratory investigation
- *Platelet count.* Normally $200–400 \times 10^9/L$; $70 \times 10^9/L$ is needed for surgical haemostasis, $<20 \times 10^9/L$ results in spontaneous bleeding.
- *Blood film.* Estimate of platelet count and indicates morphology.
- *Bleeding time.* Useful as normal bleeding time indicates normal platelets, normal function, and normal vascular response to injury, but uncommonly used as a screening test.
- *Prothrombin time (PT).* Reflects the extrinsic pathway (I, II, V, VII, X).
- *Partial thromboplastin time (PTT).* Reflects the intrinsic pathway (all factors except VII).
- Individual clotting factor assays.
- *Thrombin time (TT).* Rate of conversion from fibrin to fibrinogen.
- *Fibrin degradation products.* These are released by the action of plasmin and are raised in DIC.

Principles of management
- Indications for FFP, platelets, and anti-fibrinolytics are listed on 📖 p. 96.
- IV heparin may be reversed with protamine and/or FFP.
- Warfarin may be reversed over 12–24h with 1mg vitamin K SC or acutely with FFP.

Anaemia and polycythaemia

Anaemia

This is a reduction in haemoglobin concentration below normal (approximately 13–16g/dL in men, 11.5–15g/dL in females). It is classified as follows:

- *Decreased red cell production.*
  - Haematinic deficiency (↓ Fe, B12 folic acid).
  - Bone marrow failure (congenital, chemotherapy, radiotherapy, infiltrative disease).
- *Abnormal red cell maturation.*
  - Myelodysplasia.
  - Sideroblastic anaemia.
- *Increased red cell destruction* (haemolytic anaemias).
  - Inherited (e.g. sickle cell, thalassaemia).
  - Acquired (e.g. autoimmune, DIC—see 🕮 p. 118).
- *Chronic disease* (common cause of anaemia in surgical patients).
  - Renal failure (↓ production of erythropoietin).
  - Endocrine, liver disease.

Iron deficiency anaemia

Commonest cause of anaemia in surgical patients. Causes include:
- Menstruation (in 15% of females).
- GI losses (peptic ulcer, oesophagitis, gastric carcinoma, colorectal carcinoma).
- Reduced iron uptake (poor diet, coeliac disease, malabsorption).

Sickle cell anaemia

Single base substitution gene defect causing an amino acid substitution in haemoglobin, making HbS instead of HbA. Deoxygenated HbS polymerizes and causes red blood cells to sickle, resulting in occlusion of small blood vessels and infarction. Common in black Africans. Homozygotes have high levels of HbS and are prone to crises. Heterozygotes ('sickle trait') are only symptomatic in hypoxic conditions, e.g. unpressurized aircraft, limb ischaemia.

- Most patients are diagnosed: screening for sickle cell is widespread.
- The patient typically has an Hb of 6–8g/dL, reticulocytes 10–20%.
- There are three types of sickle cell 'crisis':
  - *Thrombotic crises.* Precipitate by cold, dehydration, infection, ischaemia, may mimic acute abdomen or pneumonia, priapism;
  - *Aplastic crises.* Due to parvoviruses and require urgent transfusion;
  - *Sequestration crises.* Spleen and liver enlarge rapidly from trapped erythrocytes, resulting in right upper quadrant (RUQ) pain, ↑ INR, ↑ LFT, ↓↓ Hb.
- Treatment involves removing causes and decreasing percentage of HbS.
  - Keep warm and well hydrated, if necessary with IV fluids.
  - Give O_2.

- Give opiate analgesia.
- Empirical antibiotics if any evidence of sepsis.
- If Hb <6g/L, give blood; if Hb >9g/dL, exchange transfusion.
- Exchange transfusion to maintain HbA >60% before cardiac surgery.

Thalassaemia

Thalassaemias are genetic diseases of Hb synthesis, resulting in underproduction of one chain which results in destruction of red cells while they are still in the bone marrow. α-thalassaemia leads to ↓ α chain production with unbalanced β chain production and β-thalassaemia leads to ↓ β chain production. Common in the Mediterranean to Far East.
- Severity correlates with the genetic deficit.
- Death may result by 1y of age without transfusion.
- Symptoms of iron overload after 10y: endocrine failure, liver disease, and cardiac toxicity.
- Death at 20–30y due to cardiac siderosis.

Preoperative screening of anaemia: NICE guidelines
- FBC 'should be considered' for all surgery in adults >60y of age.
- FBC is recommended for 'intermediate' surgery (e.g. primary repair of inguinal hernia, varicose vein surgery) in adults >60y of age.
- FBC is recommended in any adult undergoing major surgery.
- Sickle cell screening is recommended in any patient of African descent undergoing a general anaesthetic: *consent* should be obtained.

Preoperative evaluation of anaemia

↓ *Mean cell volume (MCV) or microcytic anaemia*
- Iron deficiency (blood loss, dietary): ↓ serum ferritin and iron, ↑ total iron binding capacity (TIBC).
- Thalassaemia (↑ serum iron and ferritin, ↓ TIBC).
- Hyperthyroidism.

↑ *MCV or macrocytic anaemia*
- B12 or folate deficiency (dietary, pernicious anaemia, anti-folate drugs).
- Alcohol.
- Liver disease.
- Myelodysplasia and bone marrow infiltration.
- Hypothyroidism.

Normal MCV or normocytic anaemia
Anaemia of chronic disease, renal failure, bone marrow failure, haemolysis, pregnancy, dilutional.

Management of anaemia
- Elective patients should be investigated and treated appropriately.
- Blood transfusion (see 📖 p. 96) is indicated in patients with Hb <8g/dL undergoing emergency or elective surgery.
- Evidence suggests that maintaining Hb 7–9g/dL has a better outcome than maintaining Hb 10–12g/dL, except in patients with unstable angina.

Polycythaemia
- *Relative* (↓ plasma volume. Dehydration from alcohol or diuretics).
- *Absolute* (↑ red cell mass).
  - *Primary* (polycythaemia rubra vera).
  - *Secondary* (altitude, smoking, COPD, tumours, e.g. fibroids).
- Treat underlying cause; consider venesection.

Chapter 4

Practical procedures

Endotracheal intubation

Key facts

Indicated in cardiac arrest, serious head injury, certain acute respiratory and trauma settings, and prior to many surgical operations.

- ▶ Effective bag-and-mask ventilation is better than ineffective attempts at endotracheal intubation in the arrest setting.
- ▶ Except in a dire emergency, this procedure should not be performed without expert supervision.

Equipment

- Empty 10mL syringe.
- Endotracheal tube (ET; size 8–9 for females and 9–11 for males).
- Laryngoscope.
- Ribbon to secure tube, lubricating jelly.
- Connection tubing, Ambubag, and O_2 (cylinder or wall connection).
- Working wall suction, tubing, and Yankauer.

Preparation

- Move bed forward so that you can stand behind patient's head and raise it so that you are working a comfortable height. Put on gloves.
- *Elective setting.* Pre-oxygenate the patient; attach pulse oximeter to patient, connect Ambubag to 100% O_2, use effective bag-and-mask ventilation for 2–3min to achieve O_2 saturations >95%.
- *Emergency setting.* Suction mouth (aspiration is major risk, bag-and-mask ventilation with Ambubag, and 100% O_2).
- Check laryngoscope light works and blade opens and ET tube cuff inflates and deflates with 10mL syringe.
- Remove any dentures and suction again any saliva and secretions.
- Extend the neck.
- Insert the laryngoscope, pushing the tongue to the left.
- Advance the scope anterior to the epiglottis and pull gently, but firmly, upwards to expose the vocal cords.
- Insert the lubricated ET tube between the cords into the trachea.
- Confirm correct positioning of the tube by observing chest movements and listening over lung bases and stomach.
- Progressively inflate the cuff and attach ventilation equipment.
- Confirm correct cuff inflation by listening for whistling or bubbling in the larynx suggesting air leak and secure the tube in place with ribbon.
- ▶ Patients not in cardiac arrest or who maintain a gag reflex will need anaesthetizing prior to oropharyngeal intubation, i.e. administration of inducing agent plus muscle relaxant: this should be done only under supervision of a trained anaesthetist.
- ▶ The best setting to learn intubation is preoperatively in the anaesthetic room of a theatre with good supervision in controlled conditions.

Tips and pitfalls

- *Oesophageal intubation.* Potentially fatal if not recognized. Always check for bilateral breath sounds, chest movement, absence of stomach sounds, pulse oximetry, blood gas, and capnography, if available. Bag-

and-mask ventilation is the safest and most effective way to oxygenate a patient if you are not experienced at endotracheal intubation.
- *Cannot visualize vocal cords.* Ask for 'cricoid pressure'—firm downwards pressure from an assistant over the cricoid can help bring cords into view. Some patients are 'difficult intubations' just because of their particular anatomy and build; the safest way to maintain their airway is to avoid repeat attempts at intubation, resume bag-and-mask ventilation, and wait for senior help.
- *Inadequate cuff pressure.* Too little and airway not protected from aspiration, too much and pressure injury can result in erosion or stenosis. The balloon should feel as firm as your fingertip.

Key revision points—anatomy of the lower pharynx and larynx (Fig. 4.1)

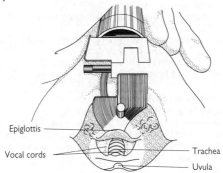

Epiglottis

Vocal cords

Trachea

Uvula

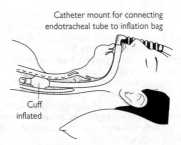

Catheter mount for connecting endotracheal tube to inflation bag

Cuff inflated

Fig. 4.1 (a) Diagram of the larynx as seen at intubation. (b) Correct position of inflated endotracheal tube cuff.

Cardioversion

Key facts
- Synchronized direct current (DC) cardioversion is the treatment of choice for tachyarrhythmias compromising cardiac output (CO), such as AF and supraventricular tachycardia (SVT) and for AF refractory to chemical cardioversion.

Checklist for elective DC cardioversion
- Is it indicated? Is the patient still in AF?
- Is it safe (see 📖 p. 189)?
  - Either AF has lasted <24h; or
  - The patient must have had at least 6 weeks of formal anticoagulation; or
  - The patient must have a TOE excluding intracardiac thrombus.
- Is the patient ready?
  - The potassium should be 4.5–5.0 (otherwise, repeat AF likely).
  - The INR, if anticoagulated, should be >2.0.
  - The patient should have a valid consent form.
- The patient should be starved for 6h.

DC cardioversion for AF and SVT
Patient should be anaesthetized: some anaesthesiologists prefer not to intubate, managing the airway with a bag and mask. You can either use adhesive external defibrillator pads which remain fixed to the patient until the procedure is completed or handheld paddles and gel pads. As soon as the anaesthesiologist is happy:
- Expose chest.
- Place pads on chest in position shown in Fig. 4.2: the aim is to direct as much of the current as possible through the heart.
- Place three ECG electrodes on the patient as shown and connect to the defibrillator so that an ECG trace is visible.
- Switch defibrillator on and turn dial on to appropriate power setting (100J, 200J, 360J).
- ▶ *Press the 'SYNC' button and ensure that each R wave is accented on the ECG: failure to do this can mean that a DC shock is delivered while the myocardium is repolarizing, resulting in VF. Check that the 'SYNC' button is on before every shock for AF.*
- If you are using handheld paddles, hold them firmly on the gel pads.
- Perform a visual sweep to check that no one is in contact with the patient at the same time as saying clearly, 'Charging. Stand clear'.
- Press the 'CHARGE' button.
- Press the 'SHOCK' button when the machine is charged.
- If the shock has been delivered successfully, the patient's muscles will contract violently: anyone in contact with the patient risks experiencing an electric shock.
- Check the rhythm.
- If still AF, press the 'CHARGE' button and repeat the sequence.

Complications of DC cardioversion
- Complications of general anaesthesia (see 📖 p. 218).
- Systemic embolization (see 📖 pp. 155, 642.)
- Failure to cardiovert.
- Burns from incorrect application of gel pads.
- Muscle pain from involuntary contraction.
- Arrhythmias, including asystole and ventricular fibrillation (VF).

Common pitfalls
Failure to deliver a shock
Check that the defibrillator is switched on and adequately charged. Check that the correct power setting has been selected. Change the machine.

Failure to cardiovert
Check the latest available serum K^+ was 4.5–5.0. Check that the correct power setting has been selected. Replace gel pads with fresh ones. Reposition the patient on their side and the pads as shown and try two further shocks at 200J (see Fig. 4.2). Don't start at too low a power setting: each shock leaves the myocardium less sensitive to further shocks. There is some evidence that 360J as the first power setting results in less myocardial damage and a better conversion rate than multiple shocks at lower power settings.

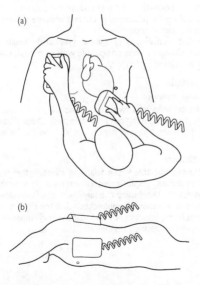

Fig. 4.2 Using defibrillators. (a) Correct positioning for defibrillation and cardioversion. (b) Alternative positioning for synchronized DC cardioversion.

Defibrillation

Key facts
- Defibrillation is the treatment of choice for VF and pulseless VT.
- *Biphasic defibrillators* cycle current direction every 10ms: the same amount of current (roughly 12amp and 1500V) is delivered, but with less energy (200J compared to 360J in older monophasic models), reducing the risk of burns and myocardial damage.

External defibrillation for VF and pulseless VT
Do not delay defibrillation for manoeuvres such as intubation, massage, or administration of drugs.
- Expose chest.
- Place gel pads on chest in position shown in Fig. 4.2: the aim is to direct as much of the current as possible through the heart.
- Switch defibrillator on and turn dial on to appropriate power setting (200J for external defibrillation).
- Press 'CHARGE' button.
- If you are using handheld paddles instead of adhesive external defibrillator pads, place them firmly on gel electrodes and hold.
- Perform a visual sweep to check that no one is in contact with the patient at the same time as saying clearly, 'Charging. Stand clear'.
- Press the red/orange 'SHOCK' button on the paddles.
- If the shock has been delivered successfully, the patient's muscles will contract violently: personnel in contact with the patient may experience an electric shock.
- Check the rhythm: if VF, charge again and repeat the sequence.
- If the rhythm changes to one compatible with an output, check the pulse before proceeding further.

Common pitfalls
Failure to deliver a shock
Check that the defibrillator is switched on and adequately charged. Check that the correct power setting has been selected. Check that the 'SYNC' button is *off* if you are trying to defibrillate VF. Change the machine and paddles.

Failure to defibrillate
Exclude causes of intractable VF, i.e. failure to effect rhythm changes compatible with an output despite repeated attempts. In internal defibrillation, decompress the heart using massage (with the flows down if you're on cardiopulmonary bypass). Double-check that the rhythm is not in fact asystole. Epinephrine, lidocaine, or amiodarone may improve chances of converting VF and maintaining rhythm.

Venepuncture

Key facts

This is a mandatory skill to learn for all doctors, but many patients will have 'difficult' veins and regular practice is needed.

Indications

Obtaining venous blood samples for laboratory analysis, venesection.

Equipment

- Tourniquet.
- 23G or 21G needle, vacutainer holder.
- Syringe (appropriate size: 10–20mL).
- Alcohol swabs.
- Appropriate laboratory sample tubes.
- Cotton wool ball and tape.
- Pillow if the vein looks difficult.

Most hospitals now have vacuum tube systems as an alternative to the 'needle and syringe' approach for obtaining blood samples.

Preparation

Apply tourniquet above the elbow and inspect the arm for suitable engorged veins. Place arm on a pillow, especially if you may be a while.

Method

- Clean the skin thoroughly with alcohol at the site of access.
- Tether the skin distal to the site with the thumb of your left hand.
- Pass the needle obliquely through the skin at a point approximately 2mm distal to the point of planned entry to the vein.
- Advance the needle slowly until a 'give' is felt as the vein is entered and a 'flashback' is seen in the needle: push vacutainer onto holder.
- Aspirate the desired amount of blood while holding the barrel of the syringe firmly.
- Release the tourniquet *before* gently withdrawing needle and syringe.
- Apply pressure to the site to arrest any bleeding. Do not assume the patient can help with this, e.g. stroke patients.

Tips and pitfalls

- *Poor veins.* If the patient is cold and the samples non-urgent, place the arm in warm water as this may aid venodilation. Veins on the dorsum of the hand may be the only ones readily available; try using a smaller or butterfly needle to obtain samples. Aspirate gently using a syringe on a butterfly needle, not a vacutainer as this may collapse veins.
- *Obese patients.* Try the dorsum of the hand or the radial aspect of the wrist, access may be easier here.
- *Failed attempts.* Repeated failed attempts will distress the patient and demoralize the doctor! Ask someone to help. If the samples are extremely urgent, a femoral stab may be the best option for obtaining blood samples, e.g. during cardiac arrest.

- *IV cannulae.* If blood samples and IV access are needed, obtain samples through the cannula—simple and saves the patient another needle, although be careful to draw blood slowly as haemolysis is more common via a cannula.
- *Sample bottles and request forms.* Ensure these are labelled correctly and the appropriate tests are ordered. If in doubt about a particular investigation, seek advice from a senior or the laboratory.
- *Blood cultures.* Ensure that the skin is swabbed thoroughly. Do not touch the skin again unless sterile gloves are worn. Once the sample is taken, change the needle before transferring the sample to the appropriate culture bottle. Document whether the patient was on antibiotics at the time of the sample and ensure the sample is not placed in the fridge during transfer to the lab.

Key revision points—venous drainage of the upper limb

- Superficial venous system.
  - **Cephalic vein.** Commences from the lateral end of the dorsal venous network overlying the **anatomical snuffbox**, ascending the lateral and anterolateral aspect of the arm to the **deltopectoral groove**, piercing the clavipectoral fascia to join the **axillary vein**.
  - **Basilic vein.** Commences from medial end of the dorsal venous network, ascending along medial and anteromedial aspect of forearm, piercing the deep fascia to join the **venae comitantes of the brachial artery** which eventually join the **axillary vein**.
  - **Median cubital vein.** Connects these two veins in the cubital fossa.
- Deep system: venae comitantes of ulnar, radial, and brachial artery, which flow into the axillary vein.
- Most common sites for **phlebotomy** and cannulation are:
  - Dorsal venous network.
  - Median cubital vein.
- Cephalic vein in the forearm.

Intravenous cannulation

Key facts

A similar skill to that of simple venepuncture, but needs plenty of practice to become competent. If having difficulty, observe a few experts in action; an ideal setting is in the anaesthetic room of theatres.

Indications

Venous access for administration of IV fluids, blood, or IV drugs.

Equipment

- Tourniquet.
- Cannula (20G or 18G) (see Table 4.1).
- Adhesive dressing/tape.
- Alcohol swabs.
- 5mL syringe containing 0.9% saline or heparinized saline.
- IV fluid bag with giving set, if necessary.

Preparation

Apply tourniquet above or below the elbow and inspect the arm for suitable engorged veins.

Method

- Clean the skin thoroughly at the site of access; put on sterile gloves.
- Identify a suitable vein.
- Tether the skin distal to the proposed site of puncture.
- Pass the cannula obliquely through the skin at a point approximately 2mm distal to the point you wish to enter the vein.
- Advance the cannula smoothly until the vein is entered: a 'give' will be felt and a 'flashback' seen in the hub of the cannula.
- Hold the hub of the needle with one hand and advance the cannula into the vein, while maintaining skin fixation until the cannula is well into the vein.
- Remove the tourniquet and press on the vein proximal to the cannula as the needle is removed. Apply the screw cap to the end of the cannula.

Table 4.1 Size and function of different cannulae

Colour	Size	Flow (mL/min)	Use
Blue	22G	31	Small veins, paediatrics
Pink	20G	55	Slow infusions
Green	18G	90	IV fluids, drugs, transfusions
White	17G	135	
Grey	16G	170	Rapid IV fluids, emergencies
Brown	14G	265	

- Secure the cannula in place with a dressing.
- If the cannula is not going to be used immediately, flush with heparinized saline.

Tips and pitfalls

- *Poor veins, obese patients, and failed attempts.* See 'Venepuncture' section (see 📖 p. 192).
- *Agitated or fitting patients.* Try not to place the cannula over a joint as these tend to become easily dislodged or 'tissued'.
- *Secure the cannula.* Cannulae are all too easily dislodged because of poor fixation to the skin. Use of two cannula dressings (one placed above and one below) and a bandage is often needed.
- *Hairy arm.* Shaving the skin at the planned cannula site seems tedious, but will allow the cannula to be secured adequately.
- *Non-dominant hand.* Placing the cannula in the non-dominant hand, if possible, will allow the patient a little bit more freedom and may prevent the cannula becoming dislodged easily.
- *Fragile veins.* Tends to be a problem in elderly or debilitated patients. Try using a smaller cannula; the dorsum of the hand is often ideal site.
- *Poor peripheral access.* In some patients with multiple collapsed or damaged veins, alternative cannula sites may have to be considered, e.g. feet. If peripheral cannulation becomes impossible, a central line will have to be considered.
- *Blood transfusion.* If blood is being given IV, then an 18G or 16G cannula will be needed.

Complete failure to cannulate

- Is a cannula necessary?
  - Can IV medication or fluids be omitted until elective central/long line insertion is possible?
  - Can medication or fluids be given orally or via NGT?
  - Discuss with microbiology if antibiotics are involved: changing route of administration often requires appropriate changes in antibiotic.
  - Fluid and insulin regimes can be modified to be given subcutaneously if desperate.
  - Many painkillers and antiemetics can be given PR or IM.
- Ask another member of your team to try: sometimes a 'fresh' pair of hands is all that is needed.
- If no one in your team can site the cannula, ask the on-call anaesthetist if they can help, but remember they are *not* a cannulation service and do not ask them until you have asked every member of your team unless it is an emergency!
- If peripheral access is impossible or required for a long time (e.g. IV antibiotic regimes for infected prostheses), consider:
  - Elective PICC line insertion (long-term line inserted electively by specialist nurse into the basilic vein);
  - Elective central line insertion: this should be done in an anaesthetic room rather than on ward and during daytime hours (📖 p. 198).
  - Femoral line insertion (less ideal as this site is more prone to line sepsis).

Arterial puncture and lines

Key facts

Arterial puncture is needed to sample ABGs; if serial measurements are required or continuous monitoring of arterial blood pressure is needed, then an arterial line should be sited (see 📖 p. 128).

Equipment

- Arterial puncture only requires a 22G needle on the green 5mL blood gas syringe, an alcohol swab, and cotton wool.
- Arterial line insertion equipment generally comes prepacked in sterile kits, but if unavailable, you will need:
  - Two 20G arterial cannulas with guidewire.
  - Connectors, transducer, and three-way tap.
  - 2mL 1% lidocaine.
  - 5mL syringe and blue needle.
  - 10mL saline.
  - Skin prep, sterile gloves, small drape.
  - Gauze swabs.

Preparation

- Explain the procedure to the patient if appropriate.
- It is good practice to perform Allen's test (see below) to demonstrate that the ulnar arterial supply to the hand arcades is intact.
- For radial artery cannula insertion, place the forearm on a pillow so that the wrist is dorsiflexed; for femoral artery insertion, abduct and flex the hip slightly.

Landmarks

- *Radial artery*. Lies between tendon of flexor carpi radialis and head of radius.
- *Femoral artery*. Lies midway between the anterior superior iliac spine and the symphysis pubis.

Technique

- Prepare and check equipment and prep skin; put on sterile gloves.
- Infiltrate local anaesthetic in the skin, but avoid distorting the anatomy.
- Palpate pulse between two fingers for 2–3cm.
- Pass cannula at 45° into skin.
- Once the cannula is *in situ*, aspirate and flush via the three-way tap.

Transfixion technique (see Fig. 4.3)

The cannula is passed through both artery walls, the needle completely withdrawn, and the cannula then withdrawn slowly until flashback occurs, at which point it is advanced into the artery.

Partial transfixion technique

The cannula is advanced until flashback stops and the needle withdrawn while holding the cannula steady which is then advanced into the artery.

Artery not transfixed
The cannula is advanced carefully in 0.5mm increments until flashback is seen, at which point the catheter is slid off the needle in the artery.

Guidewire
A guidewire is useful where it is possible to get flashback, but difficult to advance the catheter up the artery.

Complications

Ischaemia, thrombosis, bleeding, damage to radial and median nerve. Inadvertent intra-arterial injection of drugs.

Allen's test

Allen's test demonstrates a patent palmar collateral circulation: the patient clenches his fist to exclude blood from palm and the doctor firmly compresses both ulnar and radial pulses while patient opens his palm, which should be blanched. The doctor releases the ulnar compression whilst still occluding the radial pulse: the palm becomes pink in <5s if there is good collateral supply from the ulnar artery (see 📖 p. 647). About 3% of people do not have a collateral palmar supply and hand ischaemia is a real risk if the radial artery is cannulated.

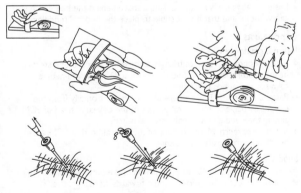

Fig. 4.3 Transfixion technique of arterial cannula insertion.

Insertion of central venous catheter

Key facts

Indications are listed on 📖 p. 128. Cannulae can be single or multi-lumen, sheaths (for insertion of pulmonary artery (PA) catheters and pacing wires), tunnelled, or long lines.

Equipment

- Appropriate central venous (CV) catheter.
- Ultrasound probe and condom if ultrasound is to be utilized.
- Enough three-way taps for all individual lumens.
- 10mL 1% lidocaine.
- 10mL syringe.
- Blue needle and a green needle.
- 20mL saline.
- 2 or 3/0 silk on a large handheld needle.
- 11-blade scalpel.
- Skin prep, sterile drape, sterile gloves, and gown.
- Gauze swabs, dressing.

Preparation

- Explain the procedure to the patient if appropriate.
- Ask a nurse to be present.
- Patient's ECG and pulse oximetry should be continually monitored.
- Ensure that there is adequate light, a space behind the bed which you can work in, and that it is possible to place the bed in Trendelenberg.

Landmarks

Internal jugular vein

- *Central approach.* Apex of triangle formed by clavicular and sternal heads of sternocleidomastoid (SCM) muscle, aiming the needle towards the opposite nipple.
- *Posterior approach.* Point where line drawn horizontally from the cricoid cartilage to the lateral border of the clavicular head of SCM, aiming the needle towards the sternal notch.
- *Anterior approach.* Medial border of the sternal head of SCM, aiming needle towards ipsilateral needle.

Subclavian vein

Advance the needle at 45° to the junction of the outer and middle third of the clavicle 1–2cm, then direct needle towards sternal groove.

Technique

There are numerous techniques: only one is described below.
- Prep the patient, gown, and glove.
- Drape so that all landmarks are exposed.
- Palpate the carotid pulse.
- Infiltrate local anaesthetic around the planned puncture site.
- Spend 2–3min laying out the equipment in the order of use, secure three-way taps to central line, and turn to closed position.
- Ask the nurse to place the bed in 10–20° of Trendelenberg.

- Ballot the internal jugular vein.
- Using aseptic technique and a 20G catheter on a 10mL syringe, enter the skin at 45° as described in 'Landmarks' section (see 📖 p. 196).
- On aspirating venous blood, remove the syringe and needle, but leave the catheter *in situ*: check that the puncture is venous, not arterial, by attaching manometry tubing, letting it fill with blood, and holding it up—level should fall if venous.
- Pass the guidewire down the catheter, keeping hold of it at all times.
- Once an adequate length of wire is in place, remove the catheter over the wire, and apply pressure to the vein.
- Make a 3mm nick in the skin over the wire with a scalpel.
- Pass the dilators over the wire through the skin, but not into the vein.
- Remove the dilators, apply pressure, and pass the CV cannula over the wire into the vein up to an appropriate length.
- The wire normally protrudes through the brown (proximal) lumen of a triple lumen line which should therefore be left open.
- Aspirate, flush, and close all lumens and suture the catheter to the skin.
- Check that there is a satisfactory pressure trace if a transducer is used.
- Chest X-ray (CXR) to identify pneumothorax.

Complications
Immediate
Damage to nearby structures (carotid artery puncture, pneumothorax, haemothorax, chylothorax, brachial plexus injury, arrhythmias), air embolism, loss of guidewire into right side of heart, haematoma.

Late
Sepsis, thromboembolism, arteriovenous (AV) fistula formation.

Key revision points—anatomy of the internal jugular vein
- In the upper neck, the internal jugular vein may be cannulated as it lies within the carotid sheath. The important relations here are:
  - Sheath is just anterior to the anterior border of SCM.
  - Carotid artery is anteromedial.
  - Vagus nerve lies between the two.
- In the lower neck, the internal jugular vein may be cannulated as it lies behind the SCM. The important relations are:
  - Vein lies 45° lateral and 45° inferior to the junction of the sternal and clavicular heads of the SCM.
  - The pleural lies inferomedial.
  - The subclavian artery lies lateral.
- The internal jugular drains into the brachiocephalic vein; on the right, this is shorter and drains more vertically into the superior vena cava (SVC), making the internal jugular vein cannulae easier to pass into the SVC.

Chest drain insertion

Key facts

There are three main options for most patients with pleural effusions or pneumothoraces that need intervention:

- *Needle thoracentesis*. Used for first-time treatment of simple effusions or pneumothoraces with low likelihood of recurrence.
- *Pigtail thoracostomy*. A 16G tube inserted using modified Seldinger technique; good for simple pneumothorax or effusion.
- *Chest tube*. Large bore tube inserted, either blunt (recommended) or using trocar to treat tension pneumothorax, recurrent pneumothorax, haemothorax, or empyema. Indications are listed below.

Indications (British Thoracic Society guidelines)

- Pneumothorax.
  - In any ventilated patient.
  - Tension pneumothorax after initial needle relief.
  - Persistent or recurrent pneumothorax after simple aspiration.
  - Large secondary spontaneous pneumothorax in patients over 50y.
- Malignant pleural effusion.
- Empyema and complicated parapneumonic pleural effusion.
- Traumatic haemopneumothorax.
- Post-operative, e.g. thoracotomy, oesophagectomy, cardiac surgery.

Equipment

- 28G intercostal drain.
- Underwater seal containing water to up to mark.
- Connection tubing.
- Line clamp.
- Roberts or other instrument for blunt dissection.
- 20mL 1% lidocaine.
- 10mL syringe.
- Blue needle and a green needle.
- 20mL saline.
- 2 or 3/0 silk on a large handheld needle.
- 11-blade scalpel.
- Skin prep, sterile drape, gloves and gown, gauze swabs.

Preparation

- Explain the procedure to the patient if appropriate; recheck side on X-ray and sign consent form.
- Ensure continual monitoring of pulse oximetry.
- Position the patient at 45° with the arm abducted.

Technique

- Usual insertion site is the *5th intercostal space in the mid-axillary line*.
- It may extend anteriorly to the anterior axillary line.
- Prep and drape the skin, gown, and glove.
- Infiltrate site for tube insertion with local anaesthetic, ensuring anaesthesia at all layers down to and including parietal pleura and the periosteum of the ribs posterior to the line of the incision.

- A 2cm transverse skin incision is made and the intercostal space (see Fig. 4.4) is dissected bluntly.
- Place purse string suture and suture to secure drain now.
- Firmly and carefully pass a blunt-ended clamp over the lower rib through the pleura (you will feel a pop as the tissue gives) and spread to widen the hole.
- Place a finger into the pleural space to ensure there are no adhesions.
- Pass a chest tube *without a trocar* into the pleural space, guiding it superiorly for a pneumothorax and basally for a haemothorax.
- Secure drain with at least one strong suture and connect immediately to an underwater seal and place on −20mmH$_2$O suction.

Tips and pitfalls

- *Misplacement.* Subcutaneous (more common in obese patients), intraparenchymal; always check for an air leak on coughing and a swing to confirm that the chest tube is in the pleural space, particularly if no effusion draining.
- *Trauma to other structures (diaphragm, spleen, liver, heart, aorta, lung parenchyma, intercostal arteries).* Entry sites too low (common mistake, remember you are much less likely to cause damage if you are too high than if you are too low), too posterior or trocar used instead of blunt dissection. Stay on the top of the lower rib to avoid injuring the intercostal artery and causing a haemothorax.
- *Surgical emphysema.* Implies there is massive air leak not being drained effectively by the chest tube. Is the tube blocked, kinked, pulled out so that holes are communicating with skin, in too far so that it is wedged in fissure, in the subcutaneous tissue rather than the pleura?
- *Wound infection, empyema.*
- *Pain.*

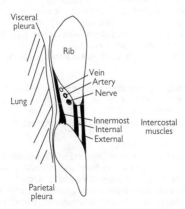

Fig. 4.4 Anatomy of the intercostal space.

Management of chest drains

Technique of insertion is described on 🕮 p. 200. This section describes the types of chest drainage systems available and basic protocols for managing chest drains.

Types of drainage system

Underwater seal

Underwater seal drains used to consist of three bottles connected by tubing, the third bottle providing suction control determined by the depth the connection tube penetrated below the water level in the bottle. Now most hospital wards have reliable high volume, low pressure wall suction, which means that simple, lightweight, single underwater seal bottles can be used instead of the cumbersome three-bottle systems. The system has to be kept upright.

• Underwater seals are suitable for any condition requiring chest drainage.
• They can be used with or without suction.
• Suction is usually –2–5kPa.

Heimlich valves

The Heimlich valve is a one-way flutter valve within rigid tubing. It can be connected to a standard chest drain. The system allows air and fluid out of the chest cavity, but prevents both from entering. The system has to be open to air, which makes collecting liquid effluent more difficult.

Heimlich valves are usually considered in patients with a permanent air leak for whom surgery is not appropriate and for whom the main goal of therapy is discharge to home or palliative care.

Portex bag

• The Portex bag was designed as an ambulatory chest drainage system. It consists of a Heimlich valve within a drainage bag which has a capacity of about 1500mL and can be emptied intermittently. This drainage system cannot be connected to suction.
• These drains are indicated in patients with chronic pleural collections, in whom surgery is not appropriate.
• As the systems are airtight, an air leak is a contraindication.

Suction

Almost all conditions can be safely managed by an underwater seal system without suction, but suction helps to reinflate the acutely collapsed lung and improves drainage of fluid. There is a huge range in surgeons' preferences for suction protocols: the points below represent commonly used protocols.

• 1kPa = 7.5mmHg = 10cmH$_2$O.
• Suction should be high volume, low pressure: approximately 2–3kPa.
• Blocked suction tubing or a blocked filter at the wall is the equivalent of clamping the drain; have a low threshold for suspecting either.
• Most patients with chest drains should be on suction; the exceptions to this are patients with pneumonectomies who are not placed on suction.

- Ventilated patients cannot generate their own negative intrapleural pressures and therefore all chest drains in these patients, with the exception of post-pneumonectomy drains, should be placed on suction.
- It is usually safe for a patient with an underwater seal on wall suction to mobilize off suction for brief periods.
- Discontinue suction in extubated patients after 24–48h when the lung is fully inflated on CXR and there is no air leak (the drain does not bubble when the patient coughs).
- Suction is unlikely to secure expansion in the lung that has been collapsed chronically; it is most effective in the immediate post-operative period.

Clamping drains

More patients have died as a result of clamped drains than unclamped drains. The practice of clamping chest drains during transfer is a dangerous one. It reveals a failure to understand how a modern underwater seal drain works as well as reflecting outmoded practice that dates back to the time of TB when drain bottles contained caustic sterilizing fluid that could drain back into the patient if lifted above the level of the chest during transfer. The only indications for clamping a chest drain are below.

Post-pneumonectomy

The post-pneumonectomy chest drain is usually clamped for an hour at a time and unclamped briefly to allow blood to drain. Leaving the drain unclamped risks causing mediastinal shift towards the pneumonectomy side and cardiovascular compromise. The drain is usually removed on day 1 post-operatively.

Massive haemothorax or effusion

If more than 1500mL of fluid is drained immediately on insertion of a chest tube and/or the patient appears haemodynamically compromised as a result of drainage, it is appropriate to clamp the drain for a brief period. In massive haemothorax, the effect is to attempt to tamponade the bleed, buying a little time to organize surgical exploration. In a massive effusion, this allows time for the lung to expand without re-expansion pulmonary oedema and to reduce mediastinal shift caused by rapid drainage.

Decision making in long-term drains

Occasionally, a surgeon may decide to see if a patient with a chronic effusion or air leak can manage without a drain by clamping the drain. Tension pneumothorax may result from doing this in a patient with an air leak. Such patients must be observed frequently for any sign of respiratory or haemodynamic compromise, surgical emphysema, or radiological evidence of lung collapse, and if any of the above occur, the drain must be unclamped and placed on underwater seal. If the patient tolerates the clamp for 24h, it is usually possible to remove the drain.

Pericardiocentesis

Key facts

- Occasionally used, usually by cardiologists under fluoroscopic guidance, to relieve acute pericardial tamponade.
- There is almost no indication, outside emergencies in an under-equipped setting, to perform this procedure blindly without fluoroscopic or echo guidance.
- In an emergency due to trauma where tamponade is due to active bleeding, clots will prevent effective needle aspiration and a thoracotomy, sternotomy, or subxiphoid incision, depending on the circumstances, should be performed.

Equipment

- Pericardiocentesis needle or catheter.
- 10mL 1% lidocaine.
- 10mL syringe.
- 18G catheter.
- 20mL saline.
- 2 or 3/0 silk on a large handheld needle.
- 11-blade scalpel.
- Skin prep.
- Sterile drape.
- Sterile gloves and gown.
- Gauze swabs.

Preparation

- Explain the procedure to the patient where appropriate.
- Ensure patient has continual ECG monitoring.

Landmarks

One half centimetre below and to the left of the xiphoid, aiming at 45° to skin, pointing at left shoulder or nipple.

Technique (see Fig. 4.5)

- Prep and drape the skin, gown, and glove.
- Infiltrate 5mL 1% subcutaneous lidocaine and make a nick in the skin.
- To begin, identify the needle entry site 0.5cm immediately to the left of the xiphoid tip.
- Insert the catheter, applying continuous aspiration in the direction described above.
- After needle entry into the skin and SC tissue, watch the ECG monitor (or echo/fluoroscopic screening monitor if available) as the needle is slowly advanced; if there are ectopics or changes in the ST segments, stop and withdraw the needle a few mm.
- When in contact with the pericardium, advance the needle a few cm into the pericardial space.
- If ST segment elevation is present, this indicates contact with the myocardium and the needle should be withdrawn slightly into the pericardial space where no ST segment elevation should be seen.

- When in the pericardial space, withdraw needle from catheter and aspirate fluid.
- If the tamponade is successfully reduced, right atrial pressures should be decreased, cardiac output should increase and pulsus paradoxus should disappear.
- Echocardiography, normally transoesophageal, is required to show reduction in the size of the collection and improvement in the signs of tamponade such as compression of right atrium and ventricle.
- Clotted blood cannot be evacuated in this way; a patient with tamponade from a haemopericardium needs emergency surgical evacuation, usually via a sternotomy if trauma is suspected.

Complications
- Cardiac puncture.
- Laceration of a coronary artery.
- Air emboli.
- Cardiac arrhythmias.
- Haemothorax.
- Pneumothorax.
- Infection.

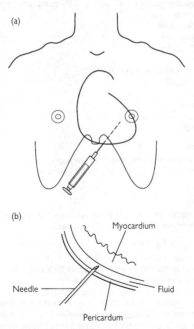

Fig. 4.5 Technique of pericardiocentesis. (a) Landmarks for needle. (b) Pericardiocentesis.

Cricothyroidotomy

Indications
Emergency need for a surgical airway
- Major maxillofacial injury.
- Oral burns.
- Fractured larynx.
- Need for tracheal toilet in the extubated patient.

Needle cricothyroidotomy
- Patient peri-arrest.
- Use the landmarks described below.
- Omit local anaesthetic infiltration, cut-down, and dissection.
- Pass a 12G (brown or larger) needle directly though the cricoid membrane.
- Oxygenate using jet insufflation until a formal airway can be established.

Equipment
- Minitracheostomy, size 6.0 ET tube or 12G cannula in emergencies.
- Artery forceps.
- 10mL 1% lidocaine.
- 10mL syringe.
- Blue needle and a green needle.
- 20mL saline.
- 2 or 3/0 silk on a large handheld needle.
- 11-blade scalpel.
- Skin prep.
- Sterile drape.
- Sterile gloves and gown.
- Gauze swabs.

Preparation
- Explain procedure to the patient where appropriate.
- The trauma patient's C-spine should be immobilized in the neutral position.

Landmarks
The cricoid membrane is a small diamond-shaped membrane, palpable just below the prominence of the thyroid cartilage.

Technique (see Fig. 4.6)
- Prep and drape, put on sterile gloves.
- If the patient is conscious and maintaining their own airway, infiltrate local anaesthetic using aseptic technique.
- Stabilize the thyroid cartilage with the left hand.
- With your right hand, make a 2cm transverse incision (smaller for minitracheostomy) through the skin overlying the cricothyroid membrane and then straight through the cricothyroid membrane.
- Now turn the scalpel blade 90° within the airway so that it acts as a temporary retractor.

- Place an artery forceps through the incision and open it, remove the scalpel, and insert a size 6.0 ET tube.
- Suction the tube, secure, and connect to a source of oxygen.
- Some minitracheostomy kits use the Seldinger technique; aspirating air freely is a sign that the needle is in the trachea and that a guidewire can be gently passed down the lumen.

Complications
- Bleeding.
- Loss of airway.
- Recurrent laryngeal nerve injury.
- Vocal cord injury.

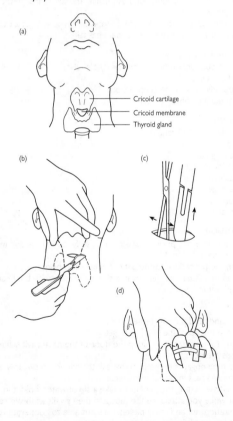

Fig. 4.6 Technique of cricothyroidotomy. (a) Structures involved. (b) Incision. (c) Keeping cricothyroidotomy patent. (d) Inserting mini-thyroidostomy.

Nasogastric tube insertion

Key facts

- Nasogastric tubes (NGT) are used to decompress the stomach and to administer enteral feeding and drugs in patients that cannot manage oral intake. Enteral feeding is covered on ⬜ p. 136.
- Inadvertent placement of an NGT into the bronchial tree can cause aspiration pneumonia or even respiratory arrest if it is then used to administer feeds or other fluids; placement must always be systematically checked (see ⬜ p. 209) on a CXR prior to use.
- Never replace an NGT in an oesophagectomy patient without discussing it with a senior; you risk pushing the tube through the fresh anastomosis.
- It is worth learning how to place these; usually you will get a call when the person who normally places them has failed.

Indications

- Intestinal obstruction (wide bore or Ryle's tube).
- Paralytic ileus.
- Perioperative gastric decompression.
- Enteral feeding (fine bore tube).

Equipment

- NGT (sizes 10–12 French).
- Gloves.
- Lubricating gel.
- Lignocaine throat spray.
- NG collection bag.
- Litmus paper.
- Stethoscope.
- Sticky tape.

Preparation

- Chill NGT in fridge prior to passing. This stiffens the tube and makes it easier to pass.
- Explain the procedure to the patient where appropriate.
- Position the patient, preferably in a sitting position, with the head tilted slightly forward.

Method

- Wash hands and put on sterile gloves.
- Lubricate the tip of the NGT with gel.
- Pass the tube horizontally along the floor of the nasal cavity, aiming towards the occiput.
- As the tube engages in the pharynx, ask the patient to swallow and the tube should pass into the oesophagus.
- Some advise getting the patient to take a sip of water, hold it in their mount while you introduce the tube and then swallow; this introduces an aspiration risk and many patients are not able to cooperate to this extent because of pain, nausea, confusion, etc.

- Advance the tube approximately 40–60cm.
- *Check the position of the tube* as follows:
  - Aspirating gastric contents which will turn blue litmus red; *and*
  - Insufflate 20mL air down the tube; if in stomach, should produce bubbling which can be heard on auscultation over the stomach; *and*
  - All feeding tubes must be X-rayed prior to use to exclude inadvertent bronchial intubation; you must be able to follow the NGT all the way down to the fundus of the stomach on the CXR. Always double-check you cannot see the tube in the bronchial tree or pleura. This is the only true confirmation that NGT is in stomach.
- Tape tube securely to nostril and attach end to bag/suction.

Tips and pitfalls

- *Patient has problems swallowing.* Ask the patient to swallow sips of water as the tube is passed.
- *Constant coiling in the mouth.* Tube may be soft; cool in the fridge.
- *Resistance to passing.* There may be an anatomical reason for this, e.g. oesophageal stricture. The tube may need to be passed under X–ray control.
- *Tube migration.* Just because the tube was in the correct position yesterday does not mean it is today; patients pull at these, work them out of the oesophagus with their tongue into a coil at the back of the throat. If called to assess, always look at the back of the pharynx ('Open your mouth and say *Ah*') and get a CXR.
- *Aspiration of tube feeds.* In the hypoxic or obtunded patient on NGT feeds, think of aspiration. Stop the feeds. Sit the patient up and give O_2. Assess the tube position. If you suspect aspiration (tube feeds visible in mouth, coughing up feeds, tube in bronchus on CXR), call for senior help; the patient may need a bronchoscopy and/or intubation.

Urethral catheterization

Key facts
- Foley catheters are useful to monitor urine output hourly (renal failure, fluid balance) and in immobile patients.
- Catheterization of female patients is usually performed by nursing staff; it is useful to learn the technique as you will be asked to try if they fail!

Indications
- Perioperative monitoring of urinary output.
- Acute urinary retention.
- Chronic urinary retention.
- Aid to abdominal or pelvic surgery.
- Incontinence.

Male catheterization
Equipment
- Foley catheter (size 12–20G, 14G most commonly used).
- Dressing/catheter pack containing drapes.
- Cleansing solution, sterile gloves (two pairs).
- Lidocaine gel.
- Gauze swabs, drainage bag and/or universal specimen pot for midstream urine (MSU).

Preparation
- Consent the patient, explaining the procedure.
- Lay patient supine.
- Expose the genital area and cover with a sterile drape with a hole in it.

Method
- Clean hands and put on sterile gloves.
- Pick up the glans penis with your non-dominant 'dirty' hand through the hole in the drape; the other hand will be your 'clean' hand.
- Holding a swab soaked in sterile saline with your clean hand, retract the foreskin and clean the urethral orifice and glans thoroughly so your gloved fingers only touch the swab, not the glans penis.
- Without letting go of the penis, discard the swab and pick up the sterile lidocaine gel with your clean hand and inject into the urethra.
- Still holding the penis in a vertical position, introduce the catheter with the clean hand and advance gently for approximately 10cm.
- Lower the penis to lie horizontally and advance the catheter fully (through the prostatic urethra) up to the hilt.
- Inflate the balloon now in the bladder via the smaller catheter channel with the 10mL sterile water; some catheters have an integral bulb of air which, when squeezed, inflates the balloon.
- ▶ *NEVER inflate the balloon until the catheter is fully inserted as this risks inflating the balloon within the prostatic urethra, causing urethral rupture; ideally you should see urine before inflating the balloon.*
- Attach a catheter bag firmly to the catheter.
- ▶ *Replace the foreskin to avoid paraphimosis.*

Tips and pitfalls
- *Difficulty identifying urethral orifice.* Sometimes orifice is located in the glans penis. If just difficulty retracting foreskin, use plenty of gel.
- *No urine immediately.*
  - The bladder has just been emptied; insert a 2mL syringe into the end of the catheter and aspirate any residual urine.
  - The catheter tip may be blocked with lidocaine gel; try gently instilling 15–20mL of sterile water and gently aspirating.
- *Still no urine.* The patient may be anuric or a false passage may have been created; palpate to see if the bladder is empty or if you can feel the catheter balloon (which should not normally be palpable).
  - Treat anuria appropriately (see 📖 p. 112).
  - Consult a senior colleague if a false passage may have been created.
- *Inability to insert.* Try a smaller catheter or a silastic (firmer). If unsuccessful, ask a senior for help; suprapubic catheterization may be needed (see 📖 p. 212).
- *Decompression of grossly distended bladder.* Rapid decompression of a distended bladder (e.g. from chronic retention) may result in mucosal haemorrhage. Empty the bladder by 250–500mL every 30min until empty. Then monitor urine output closely as a brisk diuresis and dehydration may follow.
- *Bypassing catheter.* Usually due to catheter blockage. Check urine output, flush the catheter, and observe. If urine is flowing down the catheter and bypassing it, the catheter may be too small; try a slightly larger size.
- *Catheter stops draining.* The catheter may be kinked or blocked. Flush as above; if unsuccessful, try inserting a new catheter. Is the patient oliguric or anuric? Treat appropriately (see 📖 p. 64).

Female catheterization
▶ *In many hospitals, males are not allowed to catheterize awake females. Check before doing do and request a female chaperone.*

Equipment As for male catheterization.

Preparation Lie patient on back with knees bent. Ask the patient to place heels together and allow knees to fall apart as far as possible.

Method
A similar technique is employed here to male catheterization, but note the following:
- Separate the labia minora with the left hand and ensure the whole genital area is adequately cleaned using the right hand.
- Identify the external urethral orifice. If this proves difficult in obese patients, an assistant may help by retracting the dependent fat from the pubic area.
- Lubricate the tip of the catheter with sterile water or lidocaine gel and pass gently into the urethra.

Tips and pitfalls
- *Difficulty identifying urethral orifice.* After warning the patient, place an index finger in the vagina to elevate the anterior vulva. Guide the catheter along the finger into the urethra.

Suprapubic catheterization

Indications
Urinary retention with failed or contraindicated urethral catheterization.

Cautions
- Do not perform suprapubic catheterization on a patient with known bladder tumour or previous bladder surgery; seek expert advice.
- Ensure by clinical examination (and if available, ultrasound bladder scanning) that the bladder is full and distended.

Equipment
- Dressing pack.
- Gloves.
- Cleansing solution.
- Two 10mL syringes.
- 25G and 21G needle.
- 10mL 1% lidocaine.
- Prepacked suprapubic catheter set (usually containing catheter, trocar, and scalpel).
- 1/0 silk suture.
- Catheter bag.

Preparation
- Explain the procedure and consent the patient.
- Lie patient supine and expose abdomen.
- Confirm clinically an enlarged, tense bladder.
- Identify catheterization site, 3–4cm (two finger breadths) above the symphysis pubis (see Fig. 4.7).

Method
- Clean the skin thoroughly around the site and apply drapes.
- Inject lignocaine into skin and subcutaneous tissues, injecting and aspirating in turn *until urine is withdrawn*.
- Two systems for introducing a suprapubic catheter are available.

'Nottingham' introducer (uses trocar)
- Make a 5mm incision at the identified site.
- Advance the catheter, with trocar in place, through the incision and subcutaneous tissues. A 'give' will be felt as the bladder is entered.
- Withdraw the trocar and ensure that there is free flow of urine from the catheter.
- Inflate the catheter balloon and suture the flange of the catheter to the skin.
- Attach a catheter bag.

Bonnano (modified Seldinger technique)
- Make a 5mm nick in the skin.
- Take the introducer needle and advance it, aspirating until urine is withdrawn.

- Remove the syringe and pass the guidewire down the needle into the bladder, then remove the needle, holding the guidewire in place.
- Pass the dilator firmly over the wire into the bladder.
- Remove the dilator and pass the catheter into the bladder, securing it as above.

Tips and pitfalls

- *Bypassing urine.* With some types of catheter and trocar, urine may initially bypass the catheter. This will cease with full advancement of the catheter and decompression of the bladder.
- *No urine or faeculent matter in catheter.* Obtain help; you may have entered the peritoneum or bowel.

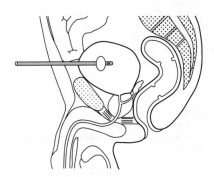

Fig. 4.7 Site of typical suprapubic catheter insertion.

Paracentesis abdominis

Key facts
This is a useful technique in some patients for the diagnosis and management of ascites, often in a patient with malignancy.

Indications
- Diagnostic evaluation of ascites.
- Therapeutic drainage of ascites.

Equipment
- Dressing pack.
- Gloves.
- Cleansing solution.
- 10mL syringe and 21G and 25G needles.
- 10mL 1% lidocaine.
- 60mL syringe with 16G aspiration needle for diagnostic 'tap'.
- Bonano catheter or paracentesis catheter, three-way tap, and collecting bag for therapeutic drainage.
- Specimen container if appropriate.
- Dressing.

Preparation
- Explain the procedure and consent the patient.
- Position the patient supine and expose the abdomen.
- Percuss out and identify the position of ascites.
- Identify a suitable tap site; the right lower quadrant is the commonest with the patient turned semilateral to ensure the ascites fills this area (see Fig. 4.8).

Method
- Prepare the skin at the appropriate site and place sterile drapes.
- Infiltrate local anaesthetic into skin and subcutaneous tissues down to the peritoneum. Aspirate as the needle is advanced to avoid accidental vessel puncture.

Diagnostic tap
- Introduce the aspiration needle through the skin and subcutaneous tissues while aspirating. A 'give' should be felt and fluid freely aspirated as the peritoneal cavity is entered.
- Withdraw 15–20mL of fluid for a diagnostic evaluation.
- Remove the aspiration needle carefully and apply an occlusive dressing.

Therapeutic drainage
- Introduce catheter into abdominal wall until a 'give' is felt. Trial aspirate with a syringe to ensure ascites returned.
- Slide catheter over the needle into the peritoneal cavity. Stop if resistance is encountered.
- Allow up to 1000mL of ascites slowly over 1–2h.

Tips and pitfalls

- *Unable to aspirate adequate quantity of fluid.* The ascites may be loculated. Drainage under ultrasound guidance may be helpful.
- *Blood or faeculent material.* Continual staining of the ascitic fluid with fresh blood or any staining with faeculent material may indicate puncture of a vessel or viscus. This is potentially serious; inform a senior colleague.
- *Peritoneal catheter.* Some patients who require repeated ascitic taps might benefit from placement of a temporary intraperitoneal catheter to allow daily drainage of ascites for symptomatic relief. There is a risk of peritonitis with these devices and only a short period of use is usually recommended, e.g. 2–3 days.

The volume of ascites drained should be closely monitored along with the patient's serum albumin and overall fluid balance. A maximum drainage of 2L/day is usually advised.

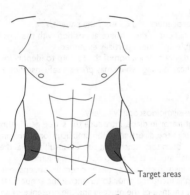

Target areas

Fig. 4.8 Target areas for ascitic tap at the level of the umbilicus, 3–4cm lateral to the mid-inguinal line.

Rigid sigmoidoscopy

Key facts
This is a useful skill to learn. It is usually performed in the outpatient department as part of the investigation of lower GI complaints, but may have to be performed on the ward, e.g. acute admissions with rectal bleeding.

Indications
- Investigation of anorectal symptoms.
- Visualization of the rectum.

Equipment
- Rigid sigmoidoscope with obturator and light source.
- Lubricating jelly.
- Gloves.
- Gauze swabs.

Preparation
- Explain the procedure and consent the patient.
- Position the patient in the left lateral position with the hips flexed as fully as possible and knees partially extended.
- Carry out a digital examination of the rectum to identify low-placed lesions or faecal loading, which may prevent safe insertion or obscure a useful view.

Method
- Lubricate the sigmoidoscope with jelly.
- With the obturator in place, introduce the scope gently through the anal sphincter in the direction of the umbilicus for approximately 5cm.
- Remove the obturator; attach light source, insufflator, and eyepiece.
- Introduce small amounts of air to open up the lumen.
- Advance the instrument slowly under direct vision, ensuring that a patent lumen is identified prior to advancing the scope further.
- Note the appearance of the mucosa and the presence of any mucosal lesions. The level of any lesion should also be noted using the marked scale on the outer casing of the sigmoidoscope.
- If the patient experiences significant discomfort, do not persist.
- Withdraw the scope slowly, again under direct vision.
- Clean the area around the patient's anus.

Tips and pitfalls
- *Biopsy.* Unless experienced in the skill, do not attempt biopsy of lesions. Note and document their position and inform a senior colleague.
- *Unable to see the upper rectum.* Remember that the rectum has a sacral curvature, often pronounced in women; *GENTLY* use the tip of the scope as a 'lever' to push the anterior wall of the rectum forward to open to lumen. If this isn't easy and painless, don't persist; it may represent pathology.

- *Rectosigmoid junction.* Negotiation of the rectosigmoid junction can be difficult. The best view that can be hoped for is to see the last sigmoid fold above the junction. Do not attempt to pass the scope into the distal sigmoid; this is the role of flexible sigmoidoscopy.

Key revision points—anatomy of the rectum

- The rectum is said to start at the level of S2, but a distance of 15cm from the anorectal junction is used to define pathology which is termed 'rectal'.
- The rectum has two main angles.
  - The first is the **acute anorectal angle** which slopes posteriorly and is formed in part by the pull of the sling of levator ani.
  - The second is the **sacral curvature** which runs throughout the rectum, sloping progressively anteriorly up to the level of the rectosigmoid junction.
- Three 'lateral valves' are commonly described, but are only the mucosal folds of the rectum equivalent to the colonic folds.
- The peritoneal-lined 'pouch of Douglas' (or rectovesical pouch in males) extends a variable distance down the anterior wall of the rectum. Its contents (e.g. sigmoid colon) may be easily palpable, particularly in elderly females.
- The upper third is covered by peritoneum anterolaterally, the middle third just anteriorly, and the lower third is entirely extraperitoneal.
- The rectum has a complete outer longitudinal muscle coat (thus diverticular disease does not occur in the rectum).
- The rectum and associated mesorectal fat, blood vessels, and lymph nodes are enclosed and separated from the 'true' pelvic organs by a fascial sheet—the mesorectum.

Local anaesthesia

Local anaesthesia is used in a variety of settings and is easy to deliver. It is essential to become familiar with the different agents, their relative merits, and potential dangers.

Indications

- Minor procedures requiring anaesthesia, e.g. insertion of a chest drain, CV access, suprapubic catheterization, etc.
- Excision of skin or subcutaneous lesions.
- Infiltration of surgical wounds post-operatively.

Cautions

- *Allergy.* Do not use local anaesthesia if there is a history of allergy to local anaesthetic.
- *Infection at site of infiltration.* Injection may spread infection. The effect of the local anaesthetic will be diminished (due to an acidic environment) and injection may be more painful.
- *Increased risk of toxicity.* Heart block, low cardiac output, epilepsy, myasthenia gravis, hepatic impairment, porphyria, β-blocker, or cimetidine therapy.
- *Epinephrine.* Causes vasoconstriction, reducing bleeding locally and prolonging anaesthetic effect. It should not be used for injections into fingers, toes, ears, or penis (all supplied by end arteries) or where skin flaps are involved to reduce the chance of flap necrosis.

Agents The two most commonly used agents are lidocaine and bupivacaine. Other agents, e.g. prilocaine, are less commonly used.

Lidocaine (previously known as lignocaine)
Used for local infiltration for minor procedures.
- *Concentrations.* 0.5%, 1%, and 2%. Plain solutions (with no added adrenaline) or solutions containing adrenaline.
- *Duration of action.* Rapid onset (2–3min), lasts 30–90min.
- *Maximum dose.*
  - *Plain solutions.* 3mg/kg, 20mL 1% or 10mL 2% for 70kg adult.
  - *Solutions with adrenaline.* 7mg/kg as systemic absorption is much slower, 50mL 1% or 25mL 2% for 70kg adult.

Bupivacaine
Useful in some prolonged procedures, wound infiltration, and regional blocks as it has a longer duration of action than lidocaine.
- *Concentrations.* 0.25–0.75% plain solutions or with adrenaline.
- *Duration of action.* Slower onset than lidocaine; effects last 3–8h.
- *Maximum dose.* 3mg/kg for an adult, 2mg/kg for a child.

Equipment
- Syringe.
- Needles 21G–25G.
- Alcohol swabs.

Preparation

- Identify site of infiltration and check for any sign of infection or obvious subcutaneous blood vessels.
- Calculate maximum dose of anaesthetic for each individual patient.
- Draw up anaesthetic and check details of drug and dose.

Method

- Clean area with alcohol swabs.
- Inject anaesthetic slowly with a fine needle to area required, aspirating before each delivery to prevent accidental IV injection.
- Injecting local anaesthetic in a fan-shaped area subcutaneously from a single injection is often more comfortable for the patient.
- *Field block.* Injecting anaesthetic into the tissues surrounding the area which is to be anaesthetized (e.g. a cutaneous lesion) will often produce a field block, including the area itself.

Toxicity

This is caused by an overdose of local anaesthetic with systemic absorption or by accidental IV injection.

Symptoms and signs

- *Neurological.* Drowsiness, confusion, slurred speech, light-headedness, tinnitus, numbness of tongue or mouth, convulsions, and coma.
- *Cardiovascular.* Early tachycardia and hypertension, late bradycardia, hypotension, cardiac arrhythmias, and cardiac arrest may ensue.
- These features usually will occur at a peak of 10–25min after subcutaneous injection, but occur immediately with IV injection.

Treatment

- Stop procedure.
- Maintain the patient's airway and provide oxygen.
- Ensure IV access.
- Perform an ECG.
- *Convulsions.* Diazepam 5–10mg IV, slowly.
- *Hypotension.* Raise end of bed and initiate IV fluids.
- *Bradycardia.* Usually resolves, atropine is rarely needed.

Tips and pitfalls

- ▶ *You are more likely to achieve good anaesthetic block with a large volume of less concentrated local than a small volume of more concentrated local anaesthetic; generally use 1%, rather than 2%.*
- Allow 2–3min for the local to take effect; spend this time setting up your instruments and draping the patient.
- *Accidental IV injection.* See toxicity section above.
- *Inadequate analgesia.* Infiltrate more anaesthetic up to the patient's maximum calculated dose. If the patient is still not tolerating the procedure, alternative anaesthetic methods may have to be considered, e.g. regional anaesthesia (note maximum local anaesthetic dose), sedation, or general anaesthetic.
- The smaller the needle and the more slowly you inject initially, the less painful it is for the patient.

Intercostal nerve block

This may be a useful skill to learn, although it is usually performed by anaesthetists.

Indications
- Pain due to fractured ribs.
- Post-thoracotomy pain relief.

Equipment
- Dressing pack.
- Skin antiseptic.
- Gloves.
- 20mL syringe and needle.
- 20mL of local anaesthetic, e.g. bupivacaine.

Preparation
The patient is positioned as for pleural aspiration (see 'Pleural aspiration', 📖 p. 635) and the site of infiltration is identified.
- *Broken ribs.* Medial to the site of fracture on the posterior aspect of the chest wall.
- *Post-thoracotomy.* Medial to the posterior edge of the scar on the posterior chest wall.

Method
- Ensure that the skin is prepared thoroughly with antiseptic. Drapes are placed appropriately.
- Insert the needle and syringe containing anaesthetic through the skin, inferior to the rib (unlike pleural aspiration) associated with the nerve to be blocked.
- Aspirate the syringe to ensure that the needle has not entered a blood vessel or the pleural space. If no blood or air is withdrawn, the site is infiltrated with 4–5mL of anaesthetic.
- This is repeated at various sites.
- Obtain a CXR to ensure a pneumothorax has not complicated the procedure.

Note
- *Multiple blocks.* Ensure that the patient does not receive a toxic dose of local anaesthetic.
- *Air or blood is aspirated.* Withdraw the needle slowly, get a CXR.

Mechanism of action of local anaesthetics
Local anaesthetic works by blocking Na channels in the nerve membrane, preventing propagation of the action potential. Small, non-myelinated pain fibres are blocked first. Large, myelinated fibres that conduct impulses from pressure senses are the last to be blocked.

Head and neck surgery

Thyroglossal cyst, sinus, and fistula

Key facts
- Thyroglossal cyst is a fluid-filled sac resulting from incomplete closure of the thyroglossal duct.
- Thyroglossal sinus results from persistence of the whole duct.
- Incidence <1%; ♂:♀ 1:1.

Anatomy (see Fig. 5.1)
The thyroglossal duct arises embryologically between the first and second pharyngeal pouches. It runs as a hollow tube from the foramen caecum on the dorsal surface of the tongue, becoming a solid cord of cells migrating through the tongue and into the midline of the neck. The tract usually passes in front of the hyoid bone and then loops up behind it before descending in the midline of the neck where the cells divide to form the two lobes of the thyroid gland either side of the midline. The duct normally atrophies in the sixth week of gestation.

Clinical features
- Usually presents in children or young adults.
- Ninety per cent present as a painless midline cyst.
- Ten per cent appear on one side of the midline, usually the left.
- Seventy-five per cent appear in front of the hyoid bone and the majority of the rest at any point to the root of the neck.
- The cyst elevates on protruding tongue if attached to hyoid or if attached to isthmus of thyroid elevates on swallowing.
- Five per cent become infected presenting as a painful, red neck swelling.
- Fifteen per cent have a fistula to the skin (due to infection or incomplete excision).
- Papillary carcinoma of the thyroglossal ductal cells is rare. Treatment is by excision.

Diagnosis and investigations
- Ultrasound-scan is investigation of choice.
- CT scan will often reveal a well circumscribed cyst related to the midline of the hyoid bone.
- Fine needle aspiration may reveal a cloudy infected fluid or a straw-coloured fluid.

Treatment
Infected thyroglossal cyst
- Majority respond to antibiotics.
- Surgical drainage if abscess formed or failure to respond to antibiotics.
- Elective excision of the cyst once acute infection has resolved.

Surgery
- Excision is recommended for most cysts.
- Remove through a transverse midline incision in a skin crease.

- Divide the platysma muscle and excise the cyst using sharp and blunt dissection.
- On the deep surface, it is attached to the hyoid bone; excise approximately 1cm of the bone in midline, removing any underlying thyroglossal duct epithelium. This is Sistrunk's procedure.
- Close the wound in layers with a suction drain.
- If there is a fistula or sinus in the neck, excise it through a transverse elliptical incision. Again use blunt dissection and remove the middle part of the hyoid bone ('Sistrunk procedure').

Complications These are usually very few. Remove the drain the next day and discharge the patient.

The important structures that must be considered when operating on the thyroid gland include:
- Recurrent laryngeal nerve.
- Superior laryngeal nerve.
- Parathyroid glands.
- Trachea.
- Common carotid artery.
- Internal jugular vein (not depicted).

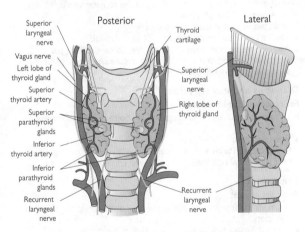

Fig. 5.1 The anatomy of the region of the thyroid gland. Reproduced with permission from Longmore, M. et al. (2007). *Oxford Handbook of Clinical Medicine*, 7th edn. Oxford University Press, Oxford.

Branchial cyst, sinus, and fistula

Key facts
- Disputed aetiology. Theories include:
  - Cystic degeneration of epithelial derivatives of the first, second, or third branchial clefts.
  - Cystic degeneration of epithelial elements in a cervical lymph node.
- A branchial fistula is a tract running from the neck skin through to the posterior pillar of the fauces; these are very rare.
- A branchial sinus occurs when the lower part of this tract remains open on to the neck skin surface.
- A branchial abscess is an infected branchial cyst.

Clinical features
- Presents as a neck lump, usually painless.
- They typically present in early adulthood.
- Sixty to seventy per cent are anterior to the upper third of the sternomastoid muscle with the posterior border lying beneath the sternomastoid. Other sites include:
  - Parotid gland.
  - Anterior to the lower two-thirds of the sternomastoid.
  - Anterior to the pharynx.
  - In the posterior triangle of the neck.
- Two-thirds occur on the left side; 2% are bilateral.
- May present with an acute branchial cyst abscess causing pain, increased swelling, and occasionally, pressure symptoms (difficulty swallowing or breathing).

Diagnosis and investigation
For branchial cyst or abscess
- Ultrasound scan is first investigation of choice. CT/MRI for complex cases.
- Fine needle aspiration biopsy:
  - *Abscesses.* Purulent fluid is obtained that may culture organisms.
  - *Cysts.* Straw-coloured fluid containing cholesterol crystals.

Treatment
Branchial abscess
- Drain via a transverse incision in the neck at the point of maximum convexity.
- Suture a Yeates type drain.
- Give antibiotics and make no attempt to remove the cyst until the infection has resolved completely.

Branchial cyst
- Most cysts are excised to achieve a diagnosis and prevent symptoms or complications.
- Place a transverse incision over the cyst, preferably in a transverse skin crease, long enough to match the size of the cyst.

- Divide the platysma and the deep fascia over the anterior border of the sternomastoid and retract the muscle posteriorly.
- Remove the cyst, usually by blunt/sharp dissection.
- Use suction drainage and close the wound in layers.
- If the cystic lesion is in the parotid gland and cannot be distinguished from any other parotid lesion, extend a preauricular incision into the neck as for a superficial parotidectomy.

Branchial fistula
- Excise a sinus of fistula through a horizontal elliptical incision around the neck opening.
- Blunt and sharp dissection of sinus tract as far as possible.
- If the upper end of the tract cannot be reached, make a further transverse incision at a higher level ('stepladder' incisions).
- Sometimes the tract runs between the internal and external carotid arteries and sometimes up to the pharyngeal wall in the region of the middle constrictor.
- Close the wounds in layers with suction drainage.

Complications

A branchial cyst at any site often lies near important nerves. Previous infections causing fibrosis will increase the risk of damaging them. The following nerves are at risk:
- Hypoglossal nerve (tongue deviates to affected side on protrusion).
- Mandibular branch of the facial nerve (movement of lower lip).
- Great auricular nerve (numb ear).
- Accessory nerve (paralysis of trapezius: weakness of arm abduction, asymmetry, and chronic pain).

Salivary calculi

Key facts

- Salivary gland calculi occur most commonly within the submandibular ductal tree (80%), 20% in the parotid.
- Composed of calcium phosphate and carbonate; may be related to sialadenitis (inflammation of a salivary gland).
- Most common in adults.
- No proven relationship with other calculi, e.g. renal.

Clinical features

- Pain and swelling of the affected gland on eating and drinking.
- If there is partial obstruction of the duct, the swelling can last minutes to several hours.
- Complete obstruction leads to persistent swelling and infection.
- The patient may also experience colicky pain in the duct when eating.

Points in the examination of the submandibular gland

- Examine the gland from behind and feel the swelling by running the finger backwards under the jaw. If you cannot feel a lump, ask the patient to suck a sour sweet and re-examine them
- Examine the duct orifice from the front. Ask the patient to open their mouth wide and point their tongue upwards. The ducts lie near the midline at the root of the tongue. Are they red? Is there pus? Can you see an impacted stone?
- Examine the gland bimanually from the front. Wear gloves and place the finger of one hand over the gland. The index of the other hand is placed in the mucosal surface of the mandible and the gland palpated between the two.

Diagnosis and investigations

- Radiographs of the submandibular gland, parotid gland, and ducts are helpful. Twenty per cent of submandibular and 80% of parotid calculi are radiolucent.
  - Lower occlusal X-ray of the teeth will show a stone in the distal portion of submandibular duct.
  - A lateral oblique X-ray or orthopantomogram (OPT) of the mandible will show a calculus in the submandibular gland.
- Submandibular duct radiography (sialography) is technically difficult and rarely done.
- Parotid sialography may show a filling defect. Sialectasis is often seen. May provide therapeutic benefit due to flushing out of debris in the ductal tree.
- Ultrasound scanning of parotid and submandibular glands is often the choice of investigation by head and neck radiologists.

Treatment

- Stones in the intra-oral part of the ducts can be removed under local anaesthesia. Steady the stone with a Babcock's forceps and incise directly over it. Remove the stone; leave the duct marsupialized.
- Stones within the submandibular gland require removal of the gland itself.
- Removal of a calculus from the parotid gland is a rare operation. Most calculi are at the distal end of parotid duct (as it does an 'S' bend through buccinator muscle) and can be released by intra-oral incision of parotid duct papilla.
- Most parotid gland obstructive/inflammatory disease is treated conservatively with sialogogues and intermittent massage of the gland towards the duct. Duct dilation using lacrimal probes is useful as most strictures/obstruction occur at the 'S' portion noted above.

Key revision points—anatomy and physiology of salivary glands

- Salivary glands produce: saliva-containing water; electrolytes (especially K^+ and HCO_3^-); varying amounts of mucus and enzymes.
- The parotid is a pure serous gland. It responds to salivary stimuli, e.g. food in mouth, smell. There is little resting flow. The submandibular is mixed with serous and mucous acini, responds to salivary stimuli, and has a resting flow, which contributes along with sublingual and minor glands to maintain mouth moisture.
- Saliva functions to lubricate, aid mastication, aid taste, suppress oral bacteria, initiate starch digestion.
- Submandibular duct is palpable in the floor of the mouth and enters mouth from gland on the sublingual papilla near the midline.
- Parotid duct is palpable over the anterior border of masseter and enters the mouth on the medial wall of the cheek after passing through buccinator muscle via an 'S' bend.
- The facial nerve trunk lies between the deep and superficial parts of the parotid gland and divides into five branches (pes anseris) within the superficial portion.

Acute parotitis

Key facts
- Parotitis is inflammation of the parotid gland. Causes include:
  - Acute or chronic obstruction (now commonest cause).
  - Bacterial (ascending parotitis), less common.
  - Viral infection, e.g. paramyxovirus (mumps), HIV.
  - Inflammatory disorders, e.g. Sjögren's syndrome, sarcoidosis.
  - Any cause of inflammation of lymph nodes within the parotid gland.
- Most patients develop this condition as an acute episode of a chronic obstructive sialadenitis.

Clinical features
- Obstructive parotitis occurs more commonly in adults.
- Presents as an acutely painful preauricular swelling.
- There is often a history of recurrent, intermittent swelling of the gland.
- The gland is usually tender on palpation.
- The patient may be toxic with fever and raised WCC, and pus may exude from the opening of the parotid duct opposite the crown of the second upper molar tooth.
- Elderly, debilitated, dehydrated patients with poor oral hygiene or who are on anticholinergic drugs are at greatest risk.

Diagnosis and investigations
- Plain X-rays to determine whether radio-opaque calculi are present in the duct or gland.
- Ultrasound or CT scanning may help differentiate between stones, inflammation, and tumour.
- If pus is present, take a bacteriology swab and send it to the lab. The commonest infecting organism is *Staphylococcus aureus*.

Treatment
Acute parotitis
- Most patients respond to antibiotics:
  - Give amoxicillin 500mg tds, IV if necessary.
  - Rehydrate dehydrated and debilitated patients.
  - Good oral nursing care with chlorhexadine mouth rinses.
- Review patients by clinical examination after the infection has subsided to make sure that the obstruction was not due to a parotid tumour.
- If a parotid abscess develops, it should be drained surgically:
  - Make an incision over the abscess under general anaesthetic where it appears to be pointing, parallel to the branches of the facial nerve to avoid damaging them.
  - Open the abscess with sinus forceps and place a Yeates drain in the wound.

Recurrent parotitis
- Teach patients with recurrent parotitis to massage the gland in order to express saliva from the duct.
- Dilatation of the duct with lacrimal probes can assist drainage.

- Remove radio-opaque calculi, if possible.
- Advise the patient to keep an emergency supply of antibiotics at home.
- If recurrent parotitis persists for months or years, a total parotidectomy is curative.

Salivary gland tumours

Key facts Salivary gland tumours are rare, accounting for 0.4% of all malignant tumours; 80% arise in the parotid gland.

Clinical features Most patients present with a slow-growing lump in the affected gland. Pain, paraesthesia (e.g. lingual nerve in submandibular gland), facial palsy (parotid gland) imply malignancy. Salivary tumours of minor glands in upper aerodigestive tract (UADT) present as a lump. Fifty per cent of these are malignant.

Clinicopathological features

Pleomorphic adenoma

- Eighty per cent of benign parotid tumours.
- ♂:♀ 1:1.
- Peak incidence 30–50y.
- Composed of epithelial and mesothelial cells that form a mucous matrix, often with chondromatous components.
- The tumour grows slowly and has no true capsule so that strands of tumour cells protrude into normal surrounding tissue. Local extension may be widespread with recurrence if excision is incomplete.
- Malignant change (adenocarcinoma) occurs in 20% after 10y and is seen in asymptomatic deep lobe parotid tumours.

Warthin's tumour (adenolymphoma)

- Usually affects men >50y; 10% are bilateral.
- Benign and presents as a slow-growing soft swelling.
- Successfully treated by wide local excision.

Malignant tumours

Mucoepidermoid tumour

- Low grade malignancy, though variable behaviour.
- Most grow slowly, invading locally and eventually metastasizing to neck lymph nodes, lung, and skin.

Adenoid cystic carcinoma

- A slow growing malignant tumour with indolent behaviour.
- Perineural invasion propensity and facial palsy common with extension through stylomastoid foramen. Lung metastasis common.
- Often regarded as incurable, but individuals can lead a normal life over 20–30y before succumbing.
- Treatment is extensive wide local excision, with nerve/organ preservation where possible. Post-operative radiotherapy has a role. Radiotherapy also has a role in controlling lung symptoms if they arise.

Acinic cell carcinoma

♀ > ♂; slow-growing, but may metastasize unexpectedly. Surgery is the treatment of choice.

Squamous cell carcinoma, adenocarcinomas, and undifferentiated carcinomas

- Generally high grade malignant tumours.

- Often rapid local invasion into extraparotid tissues and infratemporal fossa, leading to pain and trismus.
- There may be skin fixation or ulceration with facial nerve palsy and invasion of the external auditory canal; incurable; palliative radiotherapy.

Diagnosis and investigations
- Clinical examination is still of great importance in assessing extent.
- CT scanning may help differentiate between stones, inflammation, and tumour.
- MRI scanning offers the most sensitive investigation for assessment of local invasion and involvement of surrounding structures.
- PET CT is useful for assessing metastases.

Treatment
Benign parotid tumours
- Excise the parotid gland superficial to the facial nerve (superficial parotidectomy). Deep lobe tumours should have a facial nerve-sparing total parotidectomy.
- Enucleation is inadequate and often leads to local recurrence that is difficult to manage.

Benign tumours in other salivary glands
Excision of the entire gland (e.g. simple submandibulectomy).

Malignant tumours
- Radical local excision (to sacrifice or preserve the facial nerve in parotid tumours is controversial).
- May be accompanied by neck dissection, especially in parotid tumours.

Complications of parotid surgery
- Facial nerve injury (risk varies according to procedure: lowest in primary surgery for benign tumours < redo surgery < surgery for malignancy). Seventy-five per cent neurapraxia with complete or extensive recovery of function; 25% neurolysis with little or no recovery (may be treated by nerve interposition grafting).
- Frey's syndrome:
  - Late complication of surgery in up to 25% of patients.
  - Facial flushing and sweating of the skin innervated by the auriculotemporal nerve when the patient salivates.
  - Caused in this case by division of the parasympathetic secretomotor fibres that innervate the parotid gland: they may regenerate erratically to control cutaneous secretomotor functions.
  - Subcutaneous botox injection is useful.

Prognosis
- Recurrence of benign tumours. May develop 20y after surgery, especially in the patient where enucleation, rather than superficial parotidectomy has been performed.
- Five-year survival rate for all malignancies approximately 60%.

Head and neck cancer

Key facts
- Head and neck cancer refers to cancer of UADT; 90% are squamous cell carcinomas (SCC).
- UK incidence 8–15 in 100 000 and rising. Wide geographical variation, e.g. Indian subcontinent: 40% of all cancers.
- ♂:♀, 2:1, female incidence rising.
- Predisposing factors:
  - *Carcinogens*. Tobacco, alcohol, betel nut chewing;
  - *Infection*. Hyperplastic candidiasis, human papilloma virus (HPV) 16;
  - *Extrinsic factors*. UV light in lip cancer;
  - *Intrinsic factors*. Diet poor in fruit, vegetables, and fish oils, immunodeficiency/suppression.

Clinical features
- Peak incidence 40+y (increasing incidence in younger patients).
- Persistent oral ulcer with induration, bleeding, often painful.
- Persistent oral swelling, e.g. large tonsil, unexplained loose teeth.
- Unexplained earache: common in tongue, oropharyngeal tumours.
- Dysphagia, odynophagia occur in oro/hypopharyngeal cancer.
- Hoarseness lasting >3 weeks.
- Persistent unilateral serosanguineous nasal discharge.
- Unresolved head or neck swellings of >3 weeks.
- Examination of the neck is mandatory and should include all levels of neck lymph nodes. Bilateral nodal spread common.
- Six per cent of patients have a synchronous SCC present in the aerodigestive tract (mouth, larynx, lungs, oesophagus).

Diagnosis, investigations, staging, assessment
- Fibre optic nasendoscopy to examine nasopharynx, base of tongue, hypopharynx, larynx.
- Fine needle cytology for neck mass.
- *Imaging*. CT of head and neck and chest with MRI in selected cases. PET CT for unknown primary tumours, metastatic disease assessment.
- Haematology, biochemistry, ECG, lung function tests as patients usually have high comorbidities.
- *Examination under anaesthetic (EUA)*. Measure tumour size, biopsy. Panendoscopy to exclude synchronous tumours of UADT.
- Extraction of any diseased teeth, especially if in possible radiotherapy treatment field to prevent osteoradionecrosis.
- All patients should be seen by dietician, speech and language therapist, clinical nurse specialist, and restorative dentist.

- In TNM system, T1–4 stage is complex and depends on anatomical site; N1–3 stage applies to all sites.

Treatment
- Surgery, radiotherapy ± chemotherapy, or combination of all and may be done with curative intent or palliation.

- Function and quality of life are important outcomes. Gastrostomy/ NGT feeding often required during treatment.

Treatment of primary tumour
- Approximately equal cure rate for T1, T2 tumours with surgery or primary radiotherapy. Surgery is usually offered for oral cancer, sometimes for T1 larynx (laser surgery). Radiotherapy ± chemotherapy have better functional outcome in pharyngeal, posterior one-third tongue cancers.
- Larger T3, T4 tumours involving bone/cartilage are best managed surgically, e.g. laryngectomy, and often require adjuvant radiotherapy.

Treatment of the neck
- N0 necks may have occult nodal metastases, depending on tumour site, e.g. >50% for pharynx, and should have either a selective neck dissection or radiotherapy.
- Single node disease (N1) should have either a neck dissection or radical radiotherapy.
- Bulky nodal disease (N2, N3) should have a comprehensive neck dissection followed by radiotherapy or vice versa.

Neck dissections
These are either comprehensive or selective. Selective dissection removes groups of nodes likely to have occult metastases. Comprehensive includes radical neck dissection (removal of all five levels of lymph nodes, accessory nerve, internal jugular vein, and sternomastoid muscle) and modified or functional neck dissection:
- Type 1 preserves the accessory nerve.
- Type 2 preserves the accessory nerve and internal jugular vein.
- Type 3 preserves the accessory nerve, internal jugular vein, and sternomastoid muscle.

Reconstruction of surgical defect
- Good functional outcome (speech, eating, swallowing) is aim of reconstruction of surgical defect in the UADT.
- Options include:
  - Primary closure, e.g. small tongue tumour.
  - Local flap, e.g. nasolabial to floor of mouth.
  - Regional flap, e.g. pectoralis major to retromolar region.
  - Free microvascular transfer flaps offer great versatility, e.g. radial forearm for lining, fibula for bone, anterior thigh for bulk.
  - Prosthesis, e.g. obturator for palatal defect.

Prognosis
- Crude overall 5y survival is 30–40% and of those deaths, 50% die from other causes, usually tobacco-related.
- HPV 16 positive cancers appear to have better outcome.

Facial trauma

Key facts
- Eighty-five per cent of facial injuries are from assault, often with alcohol/drugs involved; the remaining from falls, sports, road accidents, industrial injuries.
- Ten to twenty per cent have associated head injury, 2% cervical spine injury.
- Fracture incidence: nose > zygoma > mandible > maxilla. Panfacial fractures indicate high energy impact or multiple blows.

Emergency situations in facial injuries
As part of 1° and 2° survey, pay special attention to:
- *Airway*. Severely displaced fractures, tissue swelling (which may get worse), blood, dislodged teeth can compromise airway, especially with associated head injury; intubate if in doubt.
- *Bleeding*. Profuse bleeding can occur in midface fractures or deep tongue wounds, requiring early theatre for suturing, nasal packing/ fracture stabilization. Swallowed blood is often vomited.
- *Retrobulbar bleed*. May follow even minor injury. Orbital swelling can mask it. Cardinal signs are pain, proptosis, and falling visual acuity. Treatment is lateral canthotomy under LA, then theatre for orbital drainage via infra-orbital incision to open ocular muscle cone; 90min window before blindness sets in.

Key clinical examination points
- Examine the eye even if it means opening swollen eyelids: check visual acuity. Any diplopia indicates orbital fat/muscle entrapment in orbital complex fracture. Orbital blow-out fracture may have enophthalmos.
- Dental occlusion (bite): ask patient if bite feels normal. If not, then a fracture is likely. Manually check continuity of mandible. Fractures in teeth-bearing segment are compound fractures. In maxilla, grasp upper incisor teeth and any movement suggests maxillary fracture.
- Mental nerve or infra-orbital nerve paraesthesia indicates mandibular or orbital floor/zygoma fracture, respectively.
- Look for deformity, e.g. nose deviation, flattened cheek, forehead hollow.

Investigations
- *Imaging*. Plain X-rays, OPT, and PA skull for fractured mandible; occipitomental 30°, 45° views for zygoma fracture. For complex fractures, CT with 3D reconstruction. Coronal CT/MRI is useful in orbital complex injuries.
- Clinical photographs as a record which may be used in court.
- Other tests, e.g. ECG, Hb, U&Es for falls in the elderly.

Treatment
- Head injuries, soft tissue lacerations, and direct trauma to the eye take precedence.

- Fractures involving the teeth are compound and antibiotics are required, e.g. amoxicillin or erythromycin if allergic to penicillin.
- Timing: mandibular fractures involving tooth-bearing segments and any soft tissue lacerations should be treated within 24h. Uncomplicated fractures of orbit/malar/frontal bone/nose/maxilla are best treated when facial swelling has settled. Optimum time is 5–10 days.
- All patients with orbital/malar/maxilla fractures must not blow their nose for 10 days to prevent surgical emphysema of soft tissues.
- Undisplaced fractures may be treated conservatively. Advise soft diet if tooth-bearing fragments involved.
- The aim of active treatment is to restore function and correct any deformity, e.g. diplopia from orbital complex fracture; decompression of any nerves involved in fracture line (infra-orbital, inferior dental, frontal nerves); restoration of dental occlusion to correct bite (mandibular/maxillary fractures); correct deformity (fractured nose/ zygoma).
- Fractures may be treated by closed reduction, e.g. intermaxillary fixation with wires or open reduction using mini-fracture plates. Surgical access to fractures may be intra-oral, incisions around the eye for orbit, submandibular for mandible, bicoronal to frontal bone.
- Patients who have had an unprovoked assault may experience post-traumatic stress disorder and benefit from referral to clinical psychologist.

Neck space infections

Key facts

- Ninety per cent of neck space infections are of dental origin, especially lower molar teeth.
- Ten per cent are from tonsils and infected epidermoid, branchial, and thyroglossal cysts.
- Their importance is risk of airway obstruction, septicaemia, and mediastinitis; mortality risk from overwhelming sepsis.

Anatomy

The investing layer of cervical fascia is attached to mastoid, superior nuchal line, lower border of mandible, hyoid and descends to the clavicle. It splits to enclose sternomastoid and trapezius muscles and thus forms a structural collar to the neck. Medially lie the pharynx, larynx, trachea, and upper oesophagus which is in direct continuity with the mediastinum. As it splits to enclose parotid gland, a deep layer is formed attached to base of skull, merging with the upper end of the carotid sheath and pharyngobasilar fascia posteriorly. It also splits to enclose the submandibular gland with deep layer attached to mylohyoid line. As a result, a number of important anatomical compartments or potential spaces exist (see Fig. 5.2).

- *Sublingual.* Floor of mouth above mylohyoid.
- *Submental.* Anterior upper neck below mylohyoid.
- *Submandibular.* Below mylohyoid around submandibular gland.
- *Parapharyngeal.* Deep to parotid, lateral to pharynx.
- *Pterygoid.* Pterygomaxillary fissure.

These are all interconnected and continue inferiorly down the neck following outside the tough carotid sheath into the mediastinum. Related are buccal and submasseteric spaces that are not connected.

Clinical features

- Infection may present as a localized fluctuant swelling or it may present as a spreading cellulitis with a brawny, hard, tender, hot, erythematous mass. Often it is a mixture of both. Necrotizing faciitis is rare and has high mortality.
- There is usually a history of toothache, sore throat, previous neck swelling, e.g. branchial cyst.
- Cardinal signs of severity include: fever, trismus, hot potato speech, dysphagia, stridor, tachycardia, and respiratory rate increase.
- Bilateral sublingual/submental/submandibular swelling (Ludwig's angina) is particularly aggressive.

Investigations

- Temperature, HR, BP, respiratory rate.
- WCC.
- *Imaging.* OPT if dental cause expected. Ultrasound scan can localize any deep space collection. CT, including chest, is useful in severe cases.

Treatment

- Admit if systemically unwell or any cardinal signs of severity as above.
- *IV antibiotics*. Co-amoxiclav or clindamycin if allergic to penicillin.
- Contact anaesthetist as may need fibre optic intubation.
- Theatre before sunset if systemic sepsis.

Surgical management

- Remove cause of infection, e.g. extract offending teeth, incise quinsy of tonsil.
- Incise and drain at dependent point any localized abscess.
- Send pus sample for culture and sensitivity.

Exploration of neck spaces

Use a submandibular incision, incise platysma and cervical fascia. Using Hilton's method, find lower border of mandible, then explore medially; this is the submandibular space; go anteriorly to open up sublingual space. To open parapharyngeal space and pterygoid space, push forceps up medial ramus of mandible and open forceps. If there is swelling extending to root of neck, make a second incision above clavicle and medial to sternomastoid. Suture in a corrugated type drain.

If intubation difficult or airway compromised, e.g. unrelieved trismus on induction, do a tracheostomy. The swelling often gets worse before it gets better. You may need to re-explore the neck. Book ITU bed in severe cases.

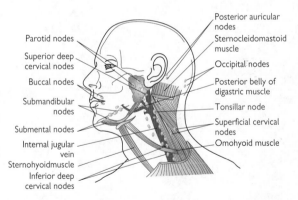

Fig. 5.2 The distribution of lymph nodes in the neck. Reproduced with permission from Longmore, M. *et al.* (2007). *Oxford Handbook of Clinical Medicine*, 7th edn. Oxford University Press, Oxford.

Breast and endocrine surgery

Breast cancer

Key facts
- Total of 35 000 new cases per year; 1 in 9 lifetime risk for women.
- Commonest in Western Europe; least common in Japan and Africa.
- Incidence increases with age.
- One per cent occurs in men.
- Five per cent related to identifiable genetic abnormality (BRAC1, BRAC2, ataxia–telangectasia genes.)
- Sixty per cent present as symptomatic disease; 40% during screening.

Pathological features
Eighty per cent ductal adenocarcinoma; 20% lobular, mucinous tubular or medullary adenocarcinoma. Most carcinomas believed to originate as *in situ* carcinoma before becoming invasive; 70% express oestrogen or progesterone receptors.

Clinical features
Breast lump
- Commonest presenting symptom.
- Usually painless (unless inflammatory carcinoma).
- Hard and gritty feeling.
- May be immobile (held within breast tissue), tethered (attached to surrounding breast tissue or skin), or fixed (attached to chest wall).
- Ill-defined; irregular with poorly defined edges.

Nipple abnormalities
- Nipple may be the prime site of disease (Bowen's disease), presenting as an eczema-like change.
- Nipples may be affected by an underlying cancer:
  - Destroyed.
  - Inverted.
  - Deviated.
  - Associated bloody discharge.

Skin changes
- Carcinoma beneath skin causes dimpling, puckering, or colour changes.
- Late presentation may be with skin ulceration or fungation of the carcinoma through the skin.
- Lymphoedema of the skin (*peau d'orange*) suggests local lymph node involvement *or locally advanced cancer*.
- Extensive inflammatory changes of the skin are associated with inflammatory carcinoma (aggressive form).

Systemic features
- Systemic features include weight loss, anorexia, bone pain, jaundice, malignant pleural, pericardial effusions, and anaemia.

Diagnosis and investigation

Diagnostic tests

- All breast lumps or suspected carcinomas are investigated with triple assessment.
- Clinical examination (as above).
- Radiological assessment:
  - *Mammography usual*, particularly over age 35y.
  - *Ultrasound scan* used to assess the presence of involved lymph nodes; sometimes used under age 35 because increased tissue density reduces sensitivity and specificity of mammography.
  - *MRI* used in lobular carcinoma to assess the extent of the disease, multifocality, and the opposite breast.
- *Younger women with dense breast tissue*. For screening purpose in patients with strong family history.

Tissue diagnosis

- Core biopsy or fine needle aspiration cytology (FNAC) of the breast lesion ± axillary nodes.
- Core biopsy also finds oestrogen receptor status, differentiates between invasive carcinomas and *in situ* carcinoma (ductal carcinoma *in situ*, DCIS).

Staging investigations

Systemic staging is usually reserved for patients following surgical treatment with a tumour who are at risk of systemic disease.

- Staging CT scan (chest, abdomen, and pelvis).
- Liver ultrasound.
- Chest X-ray.
- Bone scan.
- LFTs, serum calcium.
- Specific investigations for organ-specific suspected metastases.

Treatment Surgical treatment is described on p. 242.

Medical treatment

In non-metastatic disease, medical therapy is adjuvant to reduce the risk of systemic relapse, usually after primary surgery. It is occasionally used as a treatment of choice of elderly or those unfit/inappropriate for surgery.

- *Endocrine therapy*.
  - Used in (o)estrogen receptor (ER) +ve patients.
  - Anti-oestrogens like tamoxifen or aromatase inhibitors (letrozole).
  - Post-menopausal patients—letrozole (caution osteoporosis).
  - Premenopausal patients—tamoxifen.
  - Herceptin—given in Her-2 receptor +ve patients.
- *Chemotherapy* (e.g. anthracyclines, cyclophosphamide, 5-FU, methotrexate). Offered to patients with high risk features (+ve nodes, poor grade, young patients).

In metastatic disease, medical therapy is palliative to increase survival time and includes:

- *Endocrine therapy*. As above.
- *Chemotherapy* (e.g. anthracyclines, taxanes, herceptin).
- *Radiotherapy*. To reduce pain of bony metastases or symptoms from cerebral or liver disease.

Surgical treatment of breast cancer

Surgery is the mainstay of non-metastatic disease. Options for treatment of the primary tumour are as follows.

Wide local excision

- To ensure clear margins.
- Commonest procedure.
- Breast-conserving, provided breast is adequate size and tumour location appropriate (not central/retro-areolar).
- Usually combined with local radiotherapy to residual breast to reduce risk of local recurrence.

Simple mastectomy

- Best local treatment and cosmetic result for large tumours (especially in small breast), central location, late presentation with complications such as ulceration.
- Also used for multifocal tumours or where there is evidence of widespread *in situ* changes.
- Adjuvant breast radiotherapy is very rarely necessary.
- Performed with reconstruction at the same time or later stage including:
  - Latissimus dorsi flap;
  - TRAM flap;
  - Prosthesis (see 📖 p. 618).

Surgical management of regional lymph nodes

Axillary node sampling

- Minimum of four nodes should be retrieved.
- Avoids complete disruption to axillary lymph drainage, reducing risk of lymphoedema.
- Is inadequate for treatment of the axilla. If nodes are +ve, they require adjuvant radiotherapy to axilla or *axillary node clearance*.

Axillary node clearance

- Optimizes diagnosis and treatment of axilla.
- Increases risk of lymphoedema greatly.

Sentinel node biopsy

- One or two nodes primarily draining tumour identified by radioactive tracer or dye injected around tumour and node(s).
- Identify positive nodes, then require a full axillary clearance.
- Avoids major axillary surgery where not necessary.

Surgery for metastatic disease

Surgery in metastatic disease is limited to procedures for symptomatic control of local disease (e.g. mastectomy to remove fungating tumour).

Ductal carcinoma *in situ* (DCIS)

- Precancerous condition.
- Ten to fifty per cent develop invasive ductal cancers.

- Mammograms show microcalcification.
- Pathologically graded to low grade, intermediate grade, and high grade.
- DCIS is treated with wide local excision with clear margin.
- Mastectomy needed in larger breast lesions or multifocal disease.
- High grade DCIS treated by post-operative radiotherapy after wide local excision.
- Axillary surgery is not needed as there is no potential for lymph node metastasis.

Breast cancer screening

Aims

- To identify asymptomatic (hopefully early) invasive breast cancer.
- To identify asymptomatic carcinoma *in situ*.
- Features looked for on screening mammography include: spiculated calcification; microcalcification.

What is offered?

- Since 1988, population-based screening has been offered.
- Arranged regionally with centrally activated postal invitation.
- *Starts age 50 and continues to age 70 (cover peak ages of incidence of new diagnoses and excludes low risk younger women—'prevents psychological morbidity of screening the well'); plans to extend screening age group from 47–74y.*
- Two view (lateral and oblique) mammography of both breasts.
- Suspicious or malignant-looking lesions invited for clinical assessment by standard triple assessment.

Results

- Seventy per cent of women offered it will accept screening (lowest take-up in socio-economic groups and those difficult to contact, e.g. rapidly changing addresses or no fixed address).
- Ten per cent of invasive carcinoma is not radiologically detectable (false negative rate).
- Risk of a false positive screening is approximately 25% over 10y of screening.
- For every 1000 women screened over 10y, around 200 are recalled because of an abnormal result.
  - Sixty (6%) will have at least one biopsy.
  - Fifteen (1.5%) will have invasive cancer.
  - Five (0.5%) will have DCIS.
- Absolute reduction in cancer deaths due to screening over 10y are:
  - 0.5 per 1000 at age 40.
  - 2 per 1000 at age 50.
  - 3 per 1000 at age 60.
  - 2 per 1000 at age 70.
- Studies suggest up to a 30% reduction in mortality from screen-detected early breast cancer.

Benign breast disease

Most benign breast conditions arise from pathology related to abnormalities of the normal development and involution of the breast (ANDI). Other benign diseases are related to infection or trauma.

Fibroadenoma

Benign overgrowth of one lobule of the breast. Usually isolated, may be multiple or giant, especially in Afro-Caribbeans. Commonest under age 30, but may occur at any age up to menopause.
- *Features.* Painless, mobile, discrete lump.
- *Diagnosis.* Ultrasound usually conclusive.
- *Treatment.* Excision if concern over diagnosis, cosmesis, or symptoms.

Cysts

Almost always benign, filled with green-yellow fluid. Often associated with fibrocystic disease (below).
- *Features.* Round, symmetrical lump(s); may be discrete or multiple. Occasionally painful.
- *Diagnosis.* Aspiration—typical fluid returned; residual mass or recurrent cysts—mammography to exclude associated tumour.
- *Treatment.* Repeated aspiration; hormone manipulation occasionally useful for multiple recurrent cysts.

Fibrocystic disease

Combination of localized fibrosis, inflammation, cyst formation, and hormone-driven breast pain. Occurs almost exclusively between menarche and menopause (15–55y).
- *Features.* Cyclical pain and swelling, 'lumpy' breasts, multiple breast cysts.
- *Diagnosis.* Lumps usually require triple assessment (even once a diagnosis of fibrocystic disease is made—any woman *may* develop a carcinoma).
- *Treatment.* Reassurance, anti-inflammatories, hormone or 'cellular' manipulation (e.g. γ-linoleic acid/evening primrose oil, combined oral contraceptive (COC) pill, cyst aspiration).

Breast infections

Lactational mastitis

Due to acute staphylococcal infection of mammary ducts. May degenerate into an acute lactational abscess. Treat with oral antibiotics and (repeated) aspiration if abscess occurs. No need to stop lactating.

Recurrent mastitis/mammary duct ectasia

Due to dilated, scarred, chronically inflamed subareolar mammary ducts. Associated with smoking. Present with recurrent yellow-green nipple discharge or recurrent breast abscesses. Infection is usually mixed anaerobic based. Treatment with metronidazole and drainage of acute abscesses. Surgery is rarely necessary.

Traumatic fat necrosis

Post-traumatic disorder of breast tissue caused by the organization of acute traumatic injury by:

- Fibrosis.
- Organized local haematoma.
- Occasionally calcification.

Presents with new, painless or painful breast lump, often poorly defined. History of trauma is often absent.

Diagnosis may be difficult even on triple assessment. Failure to resolve or doubt about diagnosis after assessment is an indication for excision biopsy.

Acute breast pain

Causes and features

Breast origin

- *Breast abscess.* Acute severe, localized pain in the breast, associated with swelling, redness, and sometimes purulent nipple discharge. Most common in breastfeeding women. May be due to chronic mastitis/mammary duct ectasia (see 📖 p. 246)—occasionally recurrent.
- *Mastitis.* Recurrent intermittent breast pain with swelling, tenderness, seropurulent nipple discharge. Most common in smokers; associated with mammary duct ectasia (see 📖 p. 246).
- *Fibrocystic disease* (see 📖 p. 246). Usually recurrent or chronic breast pain, but may be acute isolated episode. Often multifocal and associated with tender vague swelling or 'lumpiness'.

Non-breast origin

- *Musculoskeletal.* Often onset after exercise, coughing, or straining, but not always. No associated breast symptoms. Pain usually sharp and precipitated by movement or breathing. Often tender deep to breast tissue and over other chest wall areas (e.g. costochondral junctions in costochondritis (Tietze's disease)). May be due to pleural disease (post-pneumonic, post-pulmonary embolism, viral pleurodynia (Bornholm's disease)).
- *Visceral.* May be due to atypical angina or acute coronary syndrome.
- *Skin pathology.* Such as infected sebaceous cysts, cellulitis, skin abscess.

Emergency management

Establish a diagnosis

- Good inspection and careful history taking is usually all that is required.
- Imaging is rarely necessary and is often painful if the pathology is primary breast. Mammography should be avoided due to the breast compression required. Breast ultrasound may help, particularly in the diagnosis of breast abscess.
- Consider specialist referral or opinion if PE, cardiac ischaemia, or pneumonia suspected. CXR is simple, but often unhelpful.

Early treatment

- Give adequate analgesia. NSAIDs (diclofenac (Voltarol®) 50mg PO or 100mg PR) are effective in most causes. Opiates may be necessary.
- Breast abscesses may be effectively aspirated for relief of pressure symptoms under local anaesthetic. Formal incision and drainage is often avoided, especially in lactational abscesses.

Definitive management

- *Breast abscess.* If lactational, oral antibiotics (including flucloxacillin 500mg tds) and aspirational drainage (often repeated several times on a daily or alternate day basis). If associated with chronic mastitis, oral antibiotics (to include metronidazole 400mg PO tds or co-amoxiclav 750mg tds PO).
- *Fibrocystic disease.* NSAIDS (e.g. ibuprofen 400mg prn), γ-linoleic acid, danazol, occasionally tamoxifen.

Goitre

Key facts

- *Goitre* refers to an enlarged thyroid gland (from the Latin *guttur*, meaning throat).
- For clinical practice, 'enlargement' is taken to mean a thyroid gland that is easily visible or palpable with the neck in neutral position.

Pathological features

- Goitres result from follicular cell hyperplasia at one or multiple sites within the thyroid gland.
- The mechanism is multifactorial—genetic, environmental, dietary, endocrine, and other factors.

On the basis of clinical and pathological features, goitre can be subclassified as follows.
- *Epidemiology.*
  - Endemic.
  - Sporadic.
  - Familial.
- *Morphology.*
  - Diffuse.
  - Nodular.
    — Multinodular.
    — Solitary nodules.
- *Thyroid function status.*
  - Toxic.
  - Non-toxic.
- *Location.*
  - Cervical.
  - Retrosternal.
  - Intrathoracic.

Clinical features

Sporadic nodular goitre

- Commonest surgical presentation of thyroid disease.
- Generally asymptomatic and usually present with a neck mass or compressive symptoms.
- Present as a small, diffuse, or nodular goitre and is generally euthyroid.

Compressive symptoms

- More likely to occur in patients with a retrosternal extension (at the thoracic inlet, the bony structures create a limited space that cannot expand).
- Growth of the goitre may cause:
  - Dyspnoea (worse when lying flat) due to tracheal displacement.
  - Dysphagia due to oesophageal compression.
  - Voice changes due to recurrent laryngeal nerve (RLN) pressure.

- Distended neck veins, facial plethora, swelling, and stridor due to superior vena caval compression (worse with arms raised above the head—'Pemberton's sign').

Cosmesis May or may not be a significant problem—varies widely.

Hyperthyroidism or hypothyroidism
- The vast majority of patients with goitre will be euthyroid.
- May be apparent clinically or biochemically (hyper = ↑ free T$_4$, ↓ TSH; hypo = ↓ free T$_4$, ↑ TSH).

Diagnosis and investigations
- *Thyroid function tests* ((TFTs) for TSH and free T$_4$). Usually normal, especially outside endemic areas.
- *CXR.* Look for tracheal deviation and a retrosternal shadow.
- *Thoracic CT.* Used to define the anatomy in patients with large intrathoracic extension.
- *Preoperative laryngoscopy.* To assess the possibility of pre-existing RLN palsy.

Treatment
Surgical treatment
- Indications include:
  - Relief of local compressive symptoms.
  - Cosmetic deformity.
  - Prevention of progressive thyroid enlargement.
- Thyroid lobectomy is feasible if there is asymmetric enlargement with only the one lobe creating the obstructive symptoms. This avoids the need for long-term thyroxine replacement (important mainly in areas where medical facilities are limited).
- Total thyroidectomy offers immediate improvement of obstructive symptoms, minimal morbidity in experienced hands, less risk of recurrent symptoms, particularly in large or retrosternal goitres.

Medical treatment
- Oral levothyroxine (₁T$_4$). Used to reduce the size of goitres in patients with iodine deficiency or subclinical hypothyroidism (i.e. when a raised TSH stimulates the enlargement of the thyroid gland).
- Radioactive iodine (^{131}I). Induces a gradual destruction of thyroid tissue, with a decrease in goitre volume up to 50% in 2y. Large (or repeated) doses of ^{131}I are needed. Used for non-toxic goitres (more in Europe than UK or USA).
- The risks of radioactive iodine are:
  - Radiation thyroiditis (acute thyroid swelling can potentially be dangerous in patients with large substernal goitres).
  - Temporary thyrotoxicosis (due to rapid release of preformed hormones from the destroyed follicles).
  - Late hypothyroidism due to over-destruction of the gland.

Thyrotoxicosis

Key facts
- Hyperthyroidism occurs in 27 in 1000 women and 3 in 1000 men in the UK.
- Graves' disease is the most common cause of hyperthyroidism.

Causes and pathological features
- TSH-secreting pituitary adenoma.
- Autoimmune stimulation (Graves' disease) (Fig. 6.1).
  - Thyroid-stimulating antibodies (IgG) bind to TSH receptors and stimulate the thyroid cells to produce and secrete excessive amounts of thyroid hormones.
  - Thyroid gland hypertrophies and becomes diffusely enlarged.
  - The autoimmune process leads to mucopolysaccharide infiltration of the extra-ocular muscles and may lead to exophthalmos.
- T_3, T_4 secreting site in the thyroid.
  - Nodule in a multinodular goitre ('Plummer's syndrome').
  - Adenoma or (very rarely) carcinoma.
- Thyroiditis (large amount of preformed hormones are released after the destruction of follicles, with transient thyrotoxicosis).
- Exogenous intake of thyroid hormones (factitious thyrotoxicosis).

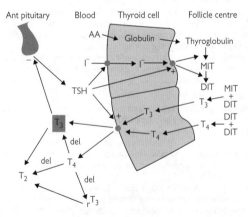

Fig. 6.1 Physiology of thyroid hormone secretion. AA, amino acids; del, deiodination (especially of liver and kidney); DIT, di-iodotyrosine; MIT, mono-iodotyrosine; TSH, thyroid-stimulating hormone.

Clinical features (any cause)

- Weight loss, heat intolerance, sweating (due to stimulated metabolism and heat production).
- Tremor, nervousness, irritability, emotional disturbance, tiredness, and lethargy (due to CNS overactivity).
- Cardiac features are caused by beta-adrenergic sympathetic activity: Palpitations, tachycardia, and arrhythmias.
- Eye signs can be:
  - Minimal/mild (soft tissue oedema, chemosis).
  - Very prominent (severe exophthalmos, corneal ulcers, diplopia).
  - Ophthalmopathy is usually bilateral, but may only involve one eye.
- Pretibial myxoedema, thyroid acropachy, vitiligo, and alopecia are rare.

Thyroid storm (thyrotoxic crisis)

- Rare presentation of extreme signs of thyrotoxicosis and severe metabolic disturbances.
- Precipitated by non-thyroid surgery, major trauma, infection, imaging studies with iodinated contrast medium in patients with unrecognized thyrotoxicosis.
- Features are insomnia, anorexia, vomiting, diarrhoea, marked sweating, fever, marked tachycardia.
- Early clinical diagnosis of the condition and immediate treatment decrease the risk of fatal outcome.

Diagnosis and investigations

- TFTs. ↓ TSH level, ↑ free T_4, and free T_3 (in all causes, but pituitary).
- Positive serology for thyroid autoantibodies.
- Radioactive iodine scan (or technetium scan). Helpful in distinguishing the diagnosis of Graves' disease, thyroiditis, toxic nodule (unilateral uptake with negative scan on the contralateral side), or toxic multinodular goitre.

Treatment

Medical treatment

- Antithyroid drugs block hormone synthesis:
  - Carbimazole 20mg bd, then reducing dose (especially in UK).
  - Propylthiouracil 200mg bd (especially in USA): blocks the peripheral conversion of T_4 to T_3.
- Beta-blockers (propranolol 40–120mg/day) are used to control tachycardia and tremor.
- Radioactive iodine (^{131}I; see 📖 p. 251 for risks). Contraindicated in severe eye disease (could worsen after ^{131}I treatment), young women (risk of teratogenicity in pregnancy), patients who are main carers of small children.

Surgical treatment

- *Total thyroidectomy* (for Graves' disease). Indicated in patients who are not candidates for ^{131}I therapy. It is the treatment of choice in those with eye disease and patients where control of symptoms has been difficult on medication. Slightly higher risk of RLN injury and hypoparathyroidism (due to increased vascularity of the gland and the local fibrosis).
- *Thyroid lobectomy*. For isolated nodules or adenomas.

Thyroid tumours—types and features

Key facts

- Solitary thyroid nodule is the most common thyroid disorder.
- Ultrasound studies show that up to 50% of patients have thyroid nodules by the age of 50.
- Although thyroid nodules are common, malignant nodules are rare (incidence of 4 in 100 000 individuals per year).

Pathological features

- *Colloid nodule.*
  - The most commonly encountered solitary thyroid nodule.
  - Ultrasound examination may reveal numerous other small nodules as part of a multinodular gland.
  - Nodules are formed mainly of collagenous material interspersed with benign thyroid cells with little or no malignant potential.
- *Follicular adenoma.*
  - Benign tumour that grows in a glandular or follicular pattern.
  - Tends to develop slowly with a pseudocapsule of compressed normal thyroid tissue.
- *Papillary carcinoma.*
  - Most common malignant neoplasm of the thyroid.
  - Malignant cells show typical cytological features (nuclear 'grooves', intranuclear inclusions, or 'optically clear nuclei'—'Orphan Annie cells').
  - Spread tends to be via lymphatics to local lymph nodes.
- *Follicular carcinomas.* Malignant tumours divided into two histologically distinct groups.
  - *Minimally invasive.* Usually small, encapsulated neoplasms that show invasion only into the tumour capsule; vascular and lymphatic invasion is normally absent; associated with an excellent prognosis.
  - *Widely invasive.* Invasion through the capsule into the surrounding thyroid tissue; they can replace the entire thyroid, invade local structures, and display haematogenous metastases.
- *Medullary thyroid cancer.* Rare, derived from calcitonin-secreting C-cells of the thyroid.
  - *Sporadic.* Single, unilateral, and presenting in isolated patients with a neck mass and often cervical lymphadenopathy.
  - *Familial.* Either as part of the multiple endocrine neoplasia (MEN) type 2 (see 📖 p. 262) or non-MEN familial tumours when cancers may be multiple and multifocal, arising in a background of diffuse C-cell hyperplasia.
- *Anaplastic thyroid cancer.* Very rare and extremely aggressive tumour, characteristically occurring in older women.
- *Thyroid lymphoma.*
  - Tumour of mucosa-associated lymphoid tissue (MALToma).
  - Classified as diffuse B-cell non-Hodgkin's lymphomas.
  - Rarely associated with longstanding Hashimoto's thyroiditis.

Clinical features

Most thyroid nodules are asymptomatic, presenting as a chance finding by the patient or during a routine general examination. Clinical assessment should include an assessment of risk factors related to malignancy (see Table 6.1).

Table 6.1 Clinical features

Sex	Thyroid nodules—females > males. A solitary nodule in a man is more likely to represent a cancer.
Age	Nodules in children and old patients are more likely to represent a cancer.
Family history	MEN2A and MEN2B (medullary Ca).
Geographic	
Previous neck irradiation	
Solitary versus multiple nodules	
Nodule characteristics	Firm/hard or fixed nodules are more likely to be a cancer. Rapid increase in size of a previously static longstanding nodule is worrying (particularly in an elderly patient).
Local lymphadenopathy	
Voice changes	RLN palsy is a sign of invasive cancer.

Retrosternal extension should be assessed.

Differential diagnosis of neck swellings (see Table 6.2)

Table 6.2 Differential diagnosis

Congenital conditions	Thyroglossal tract abnormalities Branchial cyst Cystic hygroma Cervical rib
Tumours	Thyroid Salivary glands Chemodectoma (carotid body tumour) Sarcoma Lipoma, fibroma
Lymph nodes	Primary malignancy (lymphomas, leukaemias) Secondary malignancy (skin, nasopharynx, mouth, oesophagus, thyroid, breast, or occult) Inflammatory conditions (tonsillitis, dental, mononucleosis, toxoplasma, HIV, cat scratch fever)
Diverticulae	Oesophagus
Traumatic	Sternocleidomastoid 'tumour'

Thyroid tumours—diagnosis and treatment

Diagnosis and investigation

- TFTs (free T_4, TSH levels).
- Thyroid autoantibodies.
- *Fine needle aspiration biopsy* (FNAB). Mandatory for all thyroid nodules. An 18G needle is used to obtain a sample for cytological analysis. The results are presented on a 5-point scale.
  - Thy1, non-diagnostic sample (though this may be expected if the nodule contains cystic fluid).
  - Thy2, benign colloid nodule.
  - Thy3, follicular lesion (i.e. either an adenoma or a carcinoma, the distinction being possible only after excision biopsy and histological analysis).
  - Thy4, suspicious, but not diagnostic of papillary cancer.
  - Thy5, diagnostic for thyroid cancer.
- *Neck ultrasound.* Sometimes used to assess the size and characteristics of a nodule and to determine whether the nodule is solitary or part of multinodular goitre.

Treatment

Surgical treatment

- Thyroid lobectomy, including the isthmus and pyramidal lobe (if present), is the minimum operation for thyroid tumours. It is curative for colloid nodule (alleviating pressure symptoms), enables full histological diagnosis in suspicious (Thy3) follicular lesions, whilst being considered curative for minimal papillary cancers (<1cm) and for minimally invasive follicular cancers.
- Total thyroidectomy at initial operation is indicated for cytologically proven cancers. Completion total thyroidectomy (following thyroid lobectomy) is deemed necessary for papillary thyroid cancers larger than 2cm in diameter or histologically proven widely invasive follicular cancer after initial lobectomy.
- Total thyroidectomy plus cervical nodal dissection. A modified (selective) functional neck dissection is performed in patients presenting with palpable lymphadenopathy and in patients with medullary thyroid cancer.

Medical treatment for patients with thyroid cancer

- T_3 substitution (levothyronine, 20 micrograms tds) is used in the immediate post-operative period in patients due to undergo ^{131}I-whole body scan. The shorter half-life of T_3 means it can be stopped for only 2 weeks to allow a rise in TSH that would favour uptake of ^{131}I in any remaining thyroid cells.
- ^{131}I is administered to patients with thyroid cancer following total thyroidectomy. The ^{131}I is extremely effective in killing any residual thyroid cells or metastatic cells that may be present.

- T_4 replacement in slightly higher doses (thyroxine, 100–200 micrograms od) is used to maintain a suppressed TSH. This has been shown to decrease the possibility of contralateral disease in patients undergoing lobectomy for thyroid cancer and to reduce the risk of local recurrence or metastatic disease in patients who underwent total thyroidectomy.
- Recombinant human TSH (rhTSH) has recently become available as a means of inducing ^{131}I uptake without having to stop thyroid hormone replacement therapy (therefore avoiding the distressing symptoms of hypothyroidism in the weeks before and after the ^{131}I scan).

Key revision points—anatomy of the thyroid gland

- The thyroid consists of two lateral lobes that make up 90% of the gland substance and a central midline isthmus with a small pyramidal lobe.
- Each lobe contains lobules that comprise follicles containing colloid and lined by thyroid epithelial cells with parafollicular C (calcitonin-secreting) cells.
- The **arterial supply** is from superior thyroid arteries (2) from the external carotid (related to the external laryngeal nerves in their course), and the inferior thyroid arteries (2) from the subclavian artery (related to the recurrent laryngeal nerves).
- Four parathyroid glands are usually found posteromedial to the mid-upper and inferior poles of the lateral lobes.

Post-thyroid surgery emergencies

Neck bleeding

May occur immediately (in recovery) or late (on the ward, sometimes due to infection).

- *Symptoms.* Usually due to the pressure of a haematoma on neck structures: dyspnoea, pain, sensation of neck swelling.
- *Signs.* Stridor, neck swelling, bleeding from wound, cyanosis (if high pressure compression of neck).

Resuscitation

- If the patient is at all unwell, *call for senior help*—acute bleeding can be rapidly life-threatening.
- If possible, establish large calibre IV access. Give crystalloid fluid up to 1000mL if tachycardic or hypotensive.
- Give high flow O_2 (8L/min via non-rebreathing mask).
- Consider opening the wound immediately. If the patient is cyanosed or unconscious, cardiorespiratory arrest may be imminent and loss of blood from opening the wound will be trivial in comparison.

Early treatment Returning to theatre to deal with the cause is the definitive treatment and the patient may be transferred while resuscitation and emergency treatment are continuing.

Acute bilateral recurrent laryngeal nerve injury

- Extremely rare; due to surgical technique.
- Causes acute paralysis (and therefore adduction) of both vocal cords, leading to acute airway obstruction.
- Usually noticed immediately after extubation.
- *Signs.* Acute severe stridor, falling O_2 saturations, and cyanosis.

Resuscitation

- Usually conducted by the anaesthetist.
- Reintubation or, if not possible, immediate cricothyroidotomy.
- Usually recovers as the nerve injuries are rarely both complete.

Acute thyrotoxic crisis

- Rare due to improved medical pre-conditioning of patients prior to surgery for thyrotoxic conditions.
- May occur due to handling of the gland.
- Has features similar to those of acute severe thyrotoxicosis (see 📖 p. 252).
- *Features.* Sweating, fever, tachycardia (may include tachydysrrhythmias such as AF or atrial flutter), hypertension.

Resuscitation

- Ensure the patient has large calibre IV access. Crystalloid may be required if there is marked vasodilatation with hypotension, but tachycardia may not represent fluid depletion.
- Give high flow O_2 (8L/min via non-rebreathing mask).

- Catheterize and monitor urine output.
- Severely ill patients may need transfer to critical care due to the need for control of adrenal amine release and the cardiac effects of excessive thyroid hormones.

Primary hyperparathyroidism

Key facts
- Primary hyperparathyroidism (PHPT) is a common endocrine disease.
- Prevalence is highest among post-menopausal women, with 1 in 500 possibly being affected.
- Most patients are identified by an incidental finding of raised serum calcium during investigations for another condition.

Pathological features
- Eighty-five per cent have a single parathyroid adenoma. Most of these tumours are small, less than 1g (normal glands are 30–50mg).
- Ten to fifteen per cent have multigland hyperplasia, either as a sporadic disease or in association with familial disease (e.g. MEN syndromes, see 📖 p. 262).
- Parathyroid cancer is rare, representing less than 1% of patients.

Clinical features
- Classical symptoms are described as:
  - *Moans.* Psychological/psychiatric symptoms (lethargy, depressed mood).
  - *Groans.* Non-specific GI symptoms (abdominal pain, constipation).
  - *Bones.* Aches/pains localized in large joints.
  - *Stones.* Calcium-based renal stones.
- Polyuria, polydipsia, and nocturia are also common features.
- More than half of patients report no specific symptoms and accept most of the symptoms as part of 'generally getting older'.
- *Hypercalcaemic crisis* can occur in patients with PHPT exposed to severe dehydration (e.g. diarrhoea/vomiting). In severe cases, patients can present in coma.

Diagnosis and investigations
- ↑ Corrected serum calcium is highly suggestive if unexplained, but not diagnostic.
- ↑ Serum parathyroid hormone concentration (PTH) in the presence of hypercalcaemia confirms the diagnosis (e.g. bone metastases (breast, renal, thyroid carcinoma) have a low (i.e. inhibited) PTH concentration).
- High resolution neck ultrasound may identify tumours.
- Sestamibi (radioisotope) scanning used to localize adenomas (accurate in 50%) and allows a focused approach (minimally invasive parathyroidectomy).

Treatment
Surgical treatment
- Bilateral neck exploration, visualization of all four parathyroid glands with excision of the enlarged one(s), has, for many years, been the standard treatment. It remains the treatment for those with negative localization scans.

- When imaging studies identify reliably the position of the adenoma, patients can undergo *minimally invasive parathyroidectomy* (MIP). This is a focused neck exploration through a lateral cervical scar, aiming to remove the adenoma visualized on scanning and not to explore the other parathyroid glands.

Medical treatment
- Hypercalcaemic crisis needs aggressive rehydration.
- Establish large calibre IV access. Give 1L in first hour, further 4–6L in first 24h.
- Monitor urine output and CVP until normalized.
- Furosemide can be added to increase urinary excretion of calcium once rehydration is adequate.
- Bisphosphonates (e.g. IV pamidronate) should be avoided in PHPT when parathyroidectomy is anticipated since they impair the ability to maintain normocalcaemia after the excision of an overactive parathyroid adenoma.

Multiple endocrine neoplasia

Key facts
- Familial endocrine diseases constitute a group of rare conditions.
- Familial syndromes are autosomal dominant diseases involving tumours of several endocrine glands in a synchronous or metachronous pattern.

Clinicopathological features
Multiple endocrine neoplasia type I (MEN-1)
A syndrome of the '3Ps'.
- *Parathyroid* gland tumours. By age 40, 95% of patients have hypercalcaemia which is the commonest manifestation.
- *Pancreatic* islet cell tumours.
  - Prevalence of 30–75%.
  - Usually multicentric, slow-growing.
  - Secrete multiple polypeptides (insulin and gastrin commonest).
  - Gastrinoma leads to Zollinger–Ellison syndrome (recurrent and multiple peptic ulcers, severe reflux oesophagitis, and diarrhoea).
  - Rarer tumours are VIPoma, glucagonoma, somatostatinoma.
- Anterior *pituitary* tumours.
  - Detected in 15–40%.
  - Commonest is prolactinoma.
  - Rarer are GH- (causes acromegaly) or ACTH- (causes Cushing's disease) secreting tumours.

Carcinoid tumours (thymus, lungs, foregut), adrenal tumours, lipomas, and pinealomas have also been reported to appear in MEN-1 patients.

MEN-1 gene, *Chr11*, encodes a nuclear protein, *menin* (role unclear).

Multiple endocrine neoplasia type II (MEN-2) Has two forms.

MEN-2A Syndrome with the following features.
- Medullary thyroid carcinoma (MTC).
  - Originates in the calcitonin-secreting parafollicular C-cells (derivatives of the neuroectodermal tube);
  - Commonly multicentric and bilateral and appear on a background of C-cell hyperplasia;
  - Presents as unilateral or bilateral thyroid nodules with/without associated cervical lymphadenopathy;
  - Associated secretion of other (some unidentified) peptides can lead to severe diarrhoea.
- Phaeochromocytoma (in 50% of patients; see p. 268 for features).
- Primary hyperparathyroidism (15% of patients).

MEN-2B Syndrome with the following features.
- MTC.
- Phaeochromocytoma.
- 'Marfanoid-specific body habitus' (tall, slender, high arched palate, and long extremities), 90% of patients.

MEN-2B is associated with mucosal neuromas and intestinal ganglioneuromatosis and characteristic facial appearance.

MEN-2 gene, *Chr10*, encodes a cell surface glycoprotein member of receptor tyrosine kinases (RET proto-oncogene). Point mutations in specific parts of the RET gene lead to specific clinical syndromes (genotype–phenotype correlation). Because of near complete penetrance, all gene carriers are likely to be affected.

Familial MTC A syndrome of isolated familial with MTC.

Diagnosis and investigations
MEN-1
- Biochemical screening from second decade in known families (serum calcium, PTH, prolactin, and insulin growth factor-1 (IGF-1) for pituitary lesions, and serum glucose, insulin, gastrin, and chromogranin for pancreatic tumours).
- Genetic screening can be used for offspring of known index cases. Because 10% of *menin* mutations are *de novo*, siblings of an index case are not necessarily at risk.

MEN-2
- Genetic screening for point mutations of the *RET* gene has 100% accuracy for identifying carriers (before biochemical abnormalities).
- Affected children are offered total thyroidectomy at an age related to the individual risk of each mutation (as early as 3y old for some aggressive mutations).
- Biochemical screening with 24h urine excretion of catecholamines and metanephrines and serum calcium and PTH are measured annually.

Treatment
Surgical treatment
MEN-1
- Parathyroidectomy.
- Pancreatic tumours. Enucleation of individual tumours in the head of the pancreas and distal pancreatectomy for tumours in the tail/body.
- Hypophysectomy and external beam irradiation are considered for pituitary tumours.

MEN-2
- Total thyroidectomy (TT) indicated in patients identified by genetic screening. Symptomatic patients need TT and cervical nodal dissection for the lymph nodes on the involved side.
- Laparoscopic adrenalectomy for phaeochromocytoma.
- Parathyroidectomy for MTC in patients belonging to families in which hyperparathyroidism is frequently associated.

Medical treatment

MEN-1 Prolactinomas can be treated with dopamine agonists (bromo-criptine/cabergoline).

Cushing's syndrome

Key facts

A syndrome of excess levels of plasma cortisol and associated clinical features.

Causes
- Commonest cause is iatrogenic administration of steroids.
- Primary adrenal disease (50% of patients).
  - Unilateral. Cortical adenoma or cortical carcinoma.
  - Bilateral. ACTH-independent macronodular adrenal hyperplasia or pigmented nodular adrenal cortical disease.
- Secondary adrenal disease.
  - ACTH-secreting pituitary adenoma (Cushing's disease, 25%).
  - Ectopic ACTH secretion (25%) from other malignant tumours (e.g. small cell lung carcinoma).

Clinical features

- Weight gain. Obesity is predominantly truncal with a protuberant abdomen and a 'buffalo hump'.
- Muscle weakness, especially thigh and upper arms (add to the overall appearance, likened to a 'lemon on sticks').
- Menstrual irregularities, headache, and backache are common presenting symptoms.
- Psychological changes are commonly overlooked: lethargy/depression, paranoid ideas, hallucinations, and a tendency to suicide.
- Plethora, acne, striae, and multiple bruising are common, as is hirsutism.
- Hypertension, osteoporosis, and impaired glucose tolerance/diabetes.

All these symptoms and signs are non-specific and not exclusively related to Cushing syndrome.

Diagnosis and investigations

Diagnosis is by proving cortisol excess and then by establishing the cause.
- *Loss of normal circadian rhythm of cortisol secretion.* Samples taken at 9 a.m. and midnight demonstrate a loss of the normal morning peak and night nadir.
- *Persistent increase in cortisol levels.* 24h urine cortisol levels are elevated, but false positive results can appear in obese patients, athletes, and patients suffering stress.
- *Overnight dexamethasone test.* After administration of 1mg dexamethasone in the evening, the morning cortisol is inhibited in normal patients, but not in Cushing's syndrome. It is a very valuable outpatient screening test.
- *Low dose dexamethasone test.* Administration of 0.5mg dexamethasone qds for 48h fails to inhibit plasma cortisol and urine cortisol and metabolites.
- *ACTH levels* are inhibited in primary adrenal disease (see above) and are increased in patients with pituitary adenomas and ectopic secretion.

- *High dose dexamethasone test.* Administration of 2mg dexamethasone qds for 48h inhibits ACTH secretion from pituitary tumours and leads to a drop in cortisol levels in such patients. The test is negative in primary adrenal disease and in ectopic ACTH secretion.
- *Imaging.*
  - Abdominal CT or MRI scanning demonstrates whether there is a solitary adrenal tumour (with an atrophic contralateral gland) or whether both adrenals are enlarged. Cancer should be strongly suspected in tumours greater than 7cm.
  - Pituitary MRI usually demonstrates tumours over 10mm; small microadenomas may need confirmation by measuring ACTH concentrations in the inferior petrosal sinuses (to demonstrate laterality of the tumour).

Treatment

Surgical treatment

- Unilateral adrenalectomy (may be laparoscopic). For patients with primary adrenal disease.
- Bilateral adrenalectomy. For patients with pituitary ACTH-secreting adenomas who failed pituitary surgery or gamma-knife treatment. It is also needed for the very rare patients with ACTH-independent bilateral adrenal hyperplasia.

Medical treatment

- Metyrapone and ketoconazole can be used preoperatively to decrease cortisol synthesis, but their efficacy is limited.
- Cortisol replacement after unilateral or bilateral adrenalectomy is vital.
  - Patients with solitary adrenal tumours have the contralateral adrenal gland atrophied and it may take up to 1y for a return to normal function. Start on 50–100mg IV tds hydrocortisone post-operatively. Maintenance dose is usually prednisolone orally long-term.
  - Patients should be informed about the possibility of an Addisonian crisis triggered by any illness that could impair their ability to continue medication (e.g. severe diarrhoea/vomiting episodes). They should wear a bracelet and carry a card with details of their condition.
- Mineralocorticoid replacement (fludrocortisone 0.1mg) is also necessary after bilateral adrenalectomy.

Conn's syndrome

Key facts

- Syndrome of hypertension, severe hypokalaemia, and aldosterone hypersecretion with suppression of plasma renin activity.
- Originally described in 1954 by Dr Jerome Conn; caused by a benign adrenocortical tumour.

Causes and pathological features

- Aldosterone-producing adenomas are usually solitary tumours involving only one adrenal gland. Most adenomas are small (<2cm in diameter). Aldosterone-producing adenomas (APA) account for about 50–75% of cases of primary hyperaldosteronism (PAL).
- Other causes are idiopathic bilateral adrenal hyperplasia (25–30% of cases) and familial hyperaldosteronism (very rare cases).
  - *Type I familial hyperaldosteronism.* Autonomous aldosterone hypersecretion that is suppressible by dexamethasone (mutation in the ACTH-responsive regulatory portion of the *11b-hydroxylase* gene).
  - *Type II familial hyperaldosteronism.* Autosomal dominant autonomous aldosterone hypersecretion that is *not* suppressible by dexamethasone.

Clinical features

PAL is characterized by:

- *Hypertension.* Moderate to severe and indistinguishable from other forms of hypertension (up to 10% of new diagnoses of hypertension);
- *Hypokalaemia.* Signs include muscle weakness, cramping, intermittent paralysis, headaches, polydipsia, polyuria, and nocturia.

Diagnosis and investigations

- Serum and urinary K^+ levels. PAL suspected if serum K^+ <3mmol/L and urinary K^+ excretion >40mmol/L per day. (Spironolactone or ACE inhibitors should be stopped prior to testing and any K^+ deficit corrected.)
- Ratio of plasma aldosterone concentration to plasma renin activity, PAC/PRA (i.e. aldosterone/renin ratio, ARR).
  - Aldosterone is elevated in all cases (normal 2.2–15ng/dL).
  - In PAL, plasma renin activity is suppressed.
  - PAC:PRA ratio of >50 is diagnostic for PAL.
  - False positive due to beta-blockers, clonidine, NSAIDS, renal impairment, and the contraceptive pill.
  - False negative due to diuretics, ACE inhibitors, renovascular hypertension, malignant hypertension, calcium blockers, and very low Na^+ diets.
- Aldosterone suppression test.
  - Inability to suppress aldosterone with a high Na^+ diet.
  - Oral Na^+ (9g/day for 3 days) and 0.5mg of fludrocortisone are given and a 24h urine sample obtained.

- Na+ values >200mEq with aldosterone levels >12micrograms/L are diagnostic.
- Normokalaemia should be ensured prior to testing as the test may precipitate hypokalaemia. The test is positive in only 3 of 10 patients with Conn's syndrome.
- Posture test.
  - ↑ PAC after standing for 4h in bilateral adrenal hyperplasia.
  - ↓ PAC after standing for 4h in unilateral disease (i.e. adrenocortical adenoma, Conn's syndrome).
  - APAs are unresponsive to angiotensin, but still follow the circadian rhythm of ACTH/cortisol.
- Adrenal imaging.
  - CT scan. To localize the cause.
  - If a solitary unilateral macroadenoma (>1cm), no other localization studies are necessary and treatment is unilateral adrenalectomy.
- Adrenal venous sampling (AVS) is useful when CT localization has failed.

Patients in whom localization is not achieved may have bilateral adrenal hyperplasia and should be treated medically.

Treatment

Surgical treatment

Laparoscopic adrenalectomy for aldosterone-secreting adenomas. Hypokalaemia should be corrected before the operation by the use of spironolactone, oral potassium, or both. Normalization of BP after treatment with spironolactone is a good predictor of the successful treatment of hypertension after unilateral adrenalectomy.

Medical treatment

Spironolactone can control hypertension and correct K+ levels in the preparation for surgical treatment.

Phaeochromocytoma

Key facts
- Rare—incidence of 2–8 cases per million population/year.
- Many cases probably remain undiagnosed.

Clinicopathological features
- Said to follow the '10% rule':
  - 10% are multifocal.
  - 10% are bilateral.
  - 10% are extra-adrenal.
  - 10% are malignant.
  - 10% occur in children.
- Originate from the neural crest tissue that forms the adrenal medulla, sympathetic chain, and visceral autonomic tissue.
- Most common active products are catecholamines (adrenaline, dopamine, and noradrenaline), but vasopression, somatostatin, ACTH, and oxytocin may also be secreted.
- Excess catecholamine secretion leads to characteristic episodes ('attacks') of:
  - Headache.
  - Sweating.
  - Palpitations.
  - Paroxysmal hypertension, tachydysrrhythmias, and a feeling of 'impending doom or death' may also occur.
- Attacks can be triggered by activities causing mechanical pressure on the tumour (e.g. physical exercise, defecation, intercourse), by ingestion of alcohol, labour, general anaesthesia, and surgical procedures.
- Only 50% of patients have persistent hypertension. The other 50% have normal BP or are hypotensive between the acute episodes.

Diagnosis and investigations
Consider the diagnosis in patients with characteristic paroxysmal episodes, those with unusually labile or intermitted hypertension, those with a family history of phaeochromocytoma or related conditions (see MEN syndromes), and in hypertensive children.
- 24h urine collection and assessment for vanillylmandelic acid (VMA) and noradrenaline is most accurate for diagnosis (97% sensitive).
- Clonidine suppression test (failure of urine levels to fall after clonidine dose) confirms the diagnosis where urine levels are borderline.
- Provocative testing (e.g. stimulation with bolus IV glucagon) is rarely necessary and not without risk.

Localizing studies
- Thoraco-abdominal CT or MRI scanning. First-line test, especially for adrenal and sympathetic chain tumours.
- MIBG (meta-iodo-benzyl-guanidine) scanning localizes extra-adrenal sites not seen on CT or MRI.

Treatment

Medical treatment

- It is imperative to control BP prior to contemplating any surgical intervention.
- Alpha-blockade (e.g. phenoxybenzamine 10mg bd/tds up to the maximum dose tolerated) until hypertension controlled.
- Beta-blockade (e.g. propranolol) can be added *after* hypertension controlled to control the beta-adrenergic effects (tachycardia).
- Alternative treatments with doxazosin (alpha-/beta-blocker) or calcium channel blockers have been described, but are not widely used.

Surgical treatment

- The principle of surgery is complete resection of the tumour (with clear negative margins if suspected of malignancy).
- Laparoscopic adrenalectomy is the treatment of choice for smaller adrenal tumours (<8cm); open adrenalectomy for larger tumours.
- Local or radical excision is appropriate for extra-adrenal tumours.

Key revision points—anatomy of the adrenal gland

- Two main regions—cortex (steroid producing) and medulla (catecholamine-producing).
- Three cortical zones.
  - Glomerulosa (outer)—mineralocorticoids (aldosterone).
  - Fasciculata (middle)—glucocorticoids (cortisol).
  - Reticularis (inner)—sex hormones (andosterone).
- Blood supply.
  - Arterial supply is triple—mainly suprarenal artery, some from renal artery and inferior phrenic artery.
  - Venous drainage—usually single vein to the vena cava (right suprarenal vein is very short).
- Innervation.
  - Autonomic—sympathetic from greater splanchnic nerve (T12), parasympathetic from vagus (X) via coeliac plexus.
  - Somatic—from pudendal nerve (S2, 3, 4) to supply external urethral sphincter.

Upper gastrointestinal surgery

Upper gastrointestinal endoscopy

There are four types of endoscopy looking at the upper gastrointestinal (GI) and pancreaticobiliary tracts.

Gastroscopy

Correctly termed oesophago-gastro-duodenoscopy (OGD). Allows direct visualization of pathology, small channel biopsies to be taken, and minor interventions (e.g. injection).

Indications

- Investigation of dysphagia.
- Investigation of dyspepsia, reflux disease, upper abdominal pain.
- Investigation of acute or chronic upper GI bleeding.
- Investigation of iron deficiency anaemia (with colonoscopy).
- Therapeutic interventions for upper GI pathology:
  - Balloon dilatation of benign strictures.
  - Endoluminal stenting of malignant strictures.
  - Injection, coagulation, or banding of bleeding sources, including ulcers, varices, tumours, and vascular malformations.
  - Resection of early neoplastic lesions in stomach and oesophagus (endoscopic mucosal resection (EMR)).

Preparation and procedure

- Patient should be starved for 4h (except in emergency indications).
- IV access may be used.
- Always performed with local anaesthetic throat spray (lidocaine).
- Often performed with IV sedation (e.g. midazolam 3mg).

Risks and complications

- *Perforation* (usually of the oesophagus). Median risk approximately 1 in 3000; highest in elderly, with oesophageal pathology, during therapeutic interventions.
- *Bleeding.* Commonest after biopsies or therapeutic procedures.
- *Respiratory depression and arrest.* Related to overmedication with sedative; commonest in frail, low body weight, elderly patients.

Endoscopic ultrasound (EUS)

Utilizes a video endoscope with an ultrasound scanner in its tip.

Indications

- Staging of oesophageal, gastric, or pancreatic cancers.
- Investigation of pancreatic cysts/tumours.
- Investigation of possible distal common bile duct stones/sludge.
- Guided biopsy of pancreatic, peri-oesophageal, or perigastric masses/lymph nodes.
- Guided drainage of pancreatic (pseudo)cysts.
- Guided coeliac plexus blockade.

Endoscopic retrograde cholangiopancreatography (ERCP)
Indications
- Investigation of possible biliary disease (common bile duct stones, biliary strictures, biliary tumours, biliary injuries, intrahepatic biliary disease) only where non-interventional imaging (e.g. magnetic resonance cholangiopancreatogram (MRCP), CT cholangiography) is not possible.
- Investigation of pancreatic disease (pancreatic duct strictures, pancreatic duct abnormalities).
- Therapeutic interventions for pancreatico-biliary disease:
  - Stenting for common bile duct stones, strictures, and tumours, post-operative bile leak.
  - Sphincterotomy for the extraction of biliary stones.

Preparation and procedure
- Patient should be starved for 4h (except in emergency indications).
- IV access required.
- Always performed with local anaesthetic throat spray (lidocaine).
- Always performed with IV sedation (e.g. midazolam 5mg) and occasionally, analgesia (pethidine 50mg, fentanyl).
- Performed under X-ray screening guidance, often in X-ray department.
- May be performed under GA.
- LFTs and INR needed prior to procedure.

Risks and complications
- *Perforation* (of the oesophagus or of the duodenum). Median risk approximately 1 in 1000; highest in elderly, with pathology, during therapeutic interventions, especially sphincterotomy.
- *Bleeding.* Commonest after biopsies or therapeutic procedures, especially sphincterotomy; usually controlled by balloon pressure, may require open surgery.
- *Post-ERCP pancreatitis.*
- *Post-ERCP cholangitis.* Particularly in jaundiced patient in whom procedure has been unsuccessful.
- *Respiratory depression and arrest.* Related to overmedication with sedative; commonest in frail, low body weight, elderly patients.

Ileoscopy
Often termed 'push endoscopy'. Performed with long length thin calibre endoscope, aiming to intubate past the duodenojejunal junction and visualize the first loops of the upper small bowel.

Indications
- Investigation of undiagnosed upper GI bleeding (possibly due to proximal small bowel pathology).
- Investigation of abdominal pain.
- Investigation of upper small bowel Crohn's disease.

Preparation and procedure As for gastroscopy.

Risks and complications As for gastroscopy.

Oesophageal motility disorders

Key facts A spectrum of diseases involving failure of coordination or contraction of the oesophagus and its related muscular structures.

Pathological features In some cases, degeneration of the inner and outer myenteric plexuses can be demonstrated, but often no structural abnormality is seen.

Clinical features

Achalasia
- Peak ages of incidence in young adulthood (idiopathic) and old age (mostly degenerational).
- Slowly progressive dysphagia. Initially worse for fluids than solids.
- Frequent regurgitation of undigested food common late in the disease.
- Secondary recurrent respiratory infections due to aspiration.

Diffuse oesophageal spasm
- Commonest in young adults; ♂ > ♀.
- Characterized by acute pain along the length of the oesophagus induced by ingestion, especially of hot or cold substances (odynophagia).

Diagnosis and investigations

Achalasia
- *Video barium swallow.* A characteristic failure of relaxation of the lower oesophagus with a smooth outline 'rat's tail' or 'bird beak'.
- *Oesophageal manometry.* Hypertonic lower oesophageal high pressure zone with failure of relaxation normally induced by swallowing; in chronic cases, the proximal oesophagus may be adynamic.
- *Oesophagoscopy.* To exclude benign and malignant strictures.

Diffuse oesophageal spasm
- *Video barium swallow.* 'Corkscrew' appearance of the oesophagus caused by discoordinated diffuse contractions.
- *Oesophageal manometry.* Diffuse hypertonicity and failure of relaxation; little or no evidence of coordinated progressive peristalsis during episodes, but normal peristalsis when asymptomatic.
- *Oesophagoscopy.* Required to exclude underlying associated malignancy.

Treatment

Achalasia
- *Endoscopically guided controlled balloon dilatation* (fixed pressure). Successful in up to 80% of patients; low complication rates (perforation); may need multiple procedures over time.
- *Botulinum toxin injections.* Success in some patients failing dilatation.

- *Surgical myotomy (Heller's cardiomyotomy).* Usually performed laparoscopically with division of the lower oesophageal circular muscle fibres; highly successful in resistant cases; mostly applicable to young patients. Specific complications include reflux, obstruction of gastro-oesophageal junction, oesophageal perforation.

Diffuse oesophageal spasm

- Oral calcium channel blockers or relaxants, e.g. benzodiazepines.
- Long-acting nitric oxide donors (smooth muscle relaxant).
- Widespread oesophageal pneumatic dilatations (often repeated).
- Long surgical open myotomy, rarely undertaken.

Key revision points—anatomy and physiology of the oesophagus

- Upper two-thirds. Stratified squamous epithelial-lined (develops squamous carcinoma), striated skeletal muscle, lymphatic drainage to neck and mediastinal nodes, somatic innervation of sensation (e.g. moderately accurate location of level of pathology).
- Lower third. Transition to columnar epithelium (develops adenocarcinoma), transition to smooth muscle, lymphatic drainage to gastric and para-aortic nodes, visceral innervation (poor localization of pathology).
- Gastro-oesophageal junction is site of portosystemic anastomosis (between left gastric and (hemi)azygous veins)—may develop gastric or oesophageal varices.
- Upper oesophageal sphincter (UOS) = cricopharyngeus.
- Lower oesophageal sphincter (LOS) = functional zone of high pressure above the gastro-oesophageal junction. Relaxants include alcohol.
- Swallowing requires intact and coordinated innervation from vagus (UOS, oesophagus, LOS) and intramural myenteric plexus.

Pharyngeal pouch

Key facts

- An acquired 'pulsion' diverticulum arising in the relatively fibrous tissue between the inferior constrictor and cricopharyngeus muscle—'Killian's dehiscence'.
- Arises primarily as a result of failure of appropriate coordinated relaxation of the cricopharyngeus, causing increased pressure on the tissues directly above during swallowing.
- Typically occurs in the elderly.
- Associated with lower cranial nerve dysfunction (e.g. motor neuron disease, previous CVA).

Pathological features

- Acquired diverticulum (fibrous tissue and serosa without muscle fibres in most of the wall).
- Tends to lie to one side of the midline due to the cervical spine directly behind.

Clinical features

- Upper cervical dysphagia.
- Intermittent 'lump' appearing to the side of the neck on swallowing.
- Regurgitation of food—undigested.
- Nocturnal aspiration—'waking up coughing'.

Diagnosis and investigations

- Diagnosis may be made on observed swallowing with a transient neck swelling appearing.
- Video barium swallow will show filling of pouch.

▶ Gastroscopy should be avoided unless there is a question of associated pathology since the pouch is easily missed and easily damaged or perforated by inadvertent intubation.

Treatment

Endoscopic stapled pharyngoplasty—side-to-side stapling of pouch to the upper oesophagus, which also divides the cricopharyngeus muscle.

Hiatus hernia

Key facts

The presence of part or all of the stomach within the thoracic cavity, usually by protrusion through the oesophageal hiatus in the diaphragm (see Fig. 7.1).

- Very common; ♀ > ♂; majority are asymptomatic.
- May or may not be associated with gastro-oesophageal reflux disease (GORD).
- Predisposing factors include obesity, previous surgery.

Clinico-pathological features

Sliding hernia

- Results from axial displacement of upper stomach through the oesophageal hiatus, usually with stretching of the phrenico-oesophageal membrane.
- By far, the commonest form; may result in GORD.

Rolling (para-oesophageal) hernia

Results from the displacement of part or all of the fundus and body of the stomach through a defect in the phrenico-oesophageal membrane such that it comes to lie alongside the normal oesophagus.

- Much less common.
- Symptoms include hiccough, 'pressure' in the chest, odynophagia.
- May result in volvulus or become incarcerated and cause obstruction.

Diagnosis and investigations

- *Upper GI endoscopy* (OGD). To exclude oesophageal mucosal pathology
- *Video barium swallow.* Usually identifies the type and extent.
- *CT scanning of the thorax.* Investigation of choice in acute presentations.

Treatment

Medical (mainly for GORD symptoms)

- *Reduce acid production.* Stop smoking, lose weight, reduce alcohol consumption.
- *Counteract acid secretion.* Proton pump inhibitors (PPIs), symptomatic relief with antacids, mucosal protectants.
- *Promote oesophageal and gastric emptying.* Promotilants, e.g. metoclopramide.

Surgical

Rarely required. Indicated for:

- Persistent symptoms despite maximal medical therapy;
- Established complications of rolling hernia such as volvulus or obstruction.

Elective procedure of choice is laparoscopic (or occasionally open) reduction of the hernia and fixation (gastropexy), usually with plication of the oesophageal opening (cural plication), occasionally with a fundoplication (e.g. Nissen's operation) if GORD symptoms predominate. Acute presentations may rarely require a partial gastrectomy.

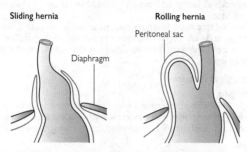

Fig. 7.1 Hiatus hernia—sliding and rolling. Reproduced with permission from Longmore, M. et al. (2007). *Oxford Handbook of Clinical Medicine*, 7th edn. Oxford University Press, Oxford.

Gastro-oesophageal reflux disease

Key facts

- Pathologically excessive entry of gastric contents into the oesophagus.
- Reflux occurs in 'normals' up to 5% of the time.
- Commonest in middle-aged adults.
- Usually due to gastric acid, but also due to bile reflux.
- Contributory factors include:
  - *Reduced tone in the lower oesophageal sphincter.* Idiopathic, alcohol, drugs, previous surgery, secondary to existing peptic stricture.
  - *Increased intragastric pressure.* Coughing, delayed gastric emptying, large meal.

Pathological features

Oesophagitis

- Results in inflammatory changes in the squamous-lined oesophagus.
- Varies in severity from minor mucosal erythema and erosions to extensive circumferential ulceration and stricturing (graded I to IV).

Stricture

- Chronic fibrosis and epithelial destruction may result in stricturing.
- Eventually shortening and narrowing of the lower oesophagus.
- May lead to fixation and susceptibility to further reflux.

Oesophageal metaplasia ('Barrett's oesophagus')

- May develop as a result of gastro-oesophageal reflux; possibly more commonly in biliary reflux.
- Normal *squamous epithelium* is replaced by *columnar epithelium (metaplasia)*.
- *Dysplasia* and premalignant change may occur in the columnar epithelium.

Clinical features

- Dyspepsia may be the only feature; may radiate to back and left of neck.
- True reflux may occur with acid in the pharynx.
- Commonly worse at night, after large meals, and when recumbent.
- Dysphagia may occur if there is associated ulceration or a stricture.

Diagnosis and investigations

Under the age of 45 Symptoms are relatively common and can be treated empirically. Investigation is only required if symptoms fail to respond to treatment.

Over the age of 45 Reflux can be confirmed by 24h continuous pH monitoring. Peaks of pH change must correspond to symptoms. OGD should be performed in all new cases over the age of 45 to exclude oesophageal malignancy.

Treatment

Medical

- *Reduce acid reflux.* ↓ Smoking, ↓ weight, ↓ alcohol consumption.
- *Counteract acid secretion.* PPI (e.g. omeprazole 20mg od), symptomatic relief with antacids (e.g. Gaviscon® 10mL PO od).
- ↑ *Gastric and oesophageal emptying.* Promotilants, e.g. metoclopramide 10mg tds PO.

Surgical

Procedure of choice is laparoscopic fundoplication, *'Nissen's operation'* (wrapping fundus of the stomach around the intra-abdominal oesophagus to augment high pressure zone).

Rarely required. Indicated for:
- Persistent symptoms despite maximal medical therapy.
- Large volume reflux with risk of aspiration pneumonia.
- Complications of reflux, including stricture and severe ulceration.

Uncertain role in the prevention of progressive dysplasia in Barrett's oesophageal metaplasia in the absence of symptoms.

Oesophageal tumours

Key facts and pathological features
There are several types of oesophageal tumours.

Adenocarcinoma
- Rapidly increasing incidence in western world; ♂:♀, 5:1.
- Commonest in Western Europe.
- Associated with dietary nitrosamines, GORD, and Barrett's metaplasia.
- Most commonly occurs in the lower third of the oesophagus.

Squamous carcinoma
- Incidence slightly reducing in western world. Commonest in Japan, northern China, and South Africa; ♂:♀, 3:1.
- Associated with smoking, alcohol intake, diet poor in fresh fruit and vegetables, chronic achalasia, chronic caustic strictures.
- May occur anywhere in the oesophagus.

Rhabdomyo(sarco)ma Malignant tumour of skeletal muscle wall of the oesophagus; very rare.

Lipoma and gastrointestinal stromal tumours (GIST, see 📖 p. 292) Rare.

Clinical features
- *Dysphagia.* Any new symptoms of dysphagia, especially over the age of 45, should be assumed to be due to tumour until proven otherwise.
- *Haematemesis.* Rarely the presenting symptom.
- *Incidental/screening.* Occasionally identified as a result of follow-up/screening for *Barrett's metaplasia*, achalasia, or reflux disease. Presence of high grade dysplasia in Barrett's is associated with the presence of an occult adenocarcinoma in 30%.
- *Features of disseminated disease.* Cervical lymphadenopathy, hepatomegaly due to metastases, epigastric mass due to para-aortic lymphadenopathy.
- *Symptoms of local invasion.* Dysphonia in recurrent laryngeal nerve palsy, cough and haemoptysis in tracheal invasion, neck swelling in superior vena cava (SVC) obstruction, Horner's syndrome in sympathetic chain invasion.

Diagnosis and investigations
- Diagnosis usually by flexible oesophagoscopy and biopsy.
- Barium swallow only indicated for failed intubation or suspected post-cricoid carcinoma (often missed by endoscopy).

Staging investigations
- *Local staging.* Endoluminal ultrasound scan to assess depth of invasion.
- *Regional staging.* CT scanning to evaluate local invasion, locoregional lymphadenopathy, liver disease; laparoscopy to assess for peritoneal disease in junctional tumours.
- *Disseminated disease.* PET scanning may be used to exclude occult disseminated disease in patients otherwise considered for potentially curative treatment.

Treatment

Palliative

Most patients present with incurable disease and require palliation.

- Dysphagia can be treated by endoluminal self-expanding metal stenting (SEMS), external beam radiotherapy; surgery is very rarely indicated for palliation.
- Metastases. Systemic chemotherapy if symptomatic.

Potentially curative

- *Squamous carcinoma.* Radical external beam chemoradiotherapy or neoadjuvant chemotherapy followed by surgery (radical resection).
- *Adenocarcinoma (large).* Neoadjuvant chemotherapy followed by surgery (radical resection).
- *Adenocarcinoma (small) or high grade dysplasia in Barrett's.* Surgical resection/EMR/ablation.

Peptic ulcer disease

Key facts

- Peptic ulceration develops when a breakdown in the mucosal defence of the stomach or duodenum leads to a mucosal breach.
- May be acute and transient (e.g. stress ulceration after surgery, in acutely unwell ITU patients).
- If the repair system fails to deal with the breakdown of the mucosa, it may become chronic.
- The term 'peptic' refers to ulcers in columnar mucosa in the lower oesophagus, stomach, duodenum, or small bowel, usually due to the action of acid.

Classification

Peptic ulcers can be broadly classified into:

- Gastric ulcers (type I, body and fundal).
- Duodenal and gastric ulcers (type II, prepyloric).
- Atypical ulceration.

Gastric ulceration

- ♂:♀, 3:1; peak age of incidence 50y.
- Associated with *Helicobacter (H.) pylori* in 45% of cases and with high alcohol intake, smoking, NSAID use, normal or low acid secretion.

Duodenal and type II gastric ulceration

- ♂:♀, 5:1; peak age of incidence 25–30y.
- Associated with *H. pylori* in 85% of cases and with high acid secretion, smoking, NSAID use.

Atypical ulceration

- Usually due to either atypical sites of gastric acid secretion (e.g. ectopic gastric mucosa in a Meckel's diverticulum) or abnormally high levels of acid secretion (e.g. *Zollinger–Ellison syndrome*; see 🕮 p. 285).
- Associated with ulceration that fails to respond to maximal medical therapy, multiple ulcers, ulcers in abnormal locations (e.g. distal duodenum or small bowel).

Clinical features

- Nausea and epigastric pain.
- Duodenal ulceration typified by hunger pains with central back pain *relieved by food*; pain is often cyclical and occurs in the early hours of the morning.
- Gastric ulceration typified by *pain precipitated by food* with associated weight loss and anorexia; pain less cyclical.
- Vomiting and upper abdominal distension suggest gastric outlet obstruction.

Diagnosis and investigations

- *Gastroscopy.* Commonest diagnostic test.
- *Barium meal.* May be used if gastroscopy contraindicated.

- *Urease testing.* To assess for presence of *H. pylori* can be performed on antral biopsies from gastroscopy or as a CO_2 breath test.
- *Fasting serum gastrin levels.* If hypergastrinaemia suspected.

Complications

- Acute upper GI bleeding (see 📖 p. 294).
- Iron deficiency anaemia due to chronic low level bleeding.
- Perforation (see 📖 p. 296).
- Gastric outlet obstruction due to chronic scarring at or around the pylorus.

Treatment

Medical

- Advice to reduce alcohol intake, stop smoking, avoidance of NSAIDs.
- PPIs (e.g. omeprazole 20mg PO od, lansoprazole) or H_2 blockers (e.g. ranitidine 150mg PO bd, cimetidine 400mg PO bd) if intolerant to PPI.
- Topical antacids (e.g. Gaviscon®, sucralfate, colloidal bismuth), especially for acute ulceration post-operatively or in ITU patients.
- *H. pylori* eradication therapy (usually triple therapy of metronidazole, PPI, and clarithromycin).

Surgical

Rarely necessary with the very highly effective acid-reducing drugs and eradication therapy. Indications include the following.

- Gastric outlet obstruction not responsive or suitable for endoscopic dilatation. Usual procedure is pyloroplasty (with or without highly selective vagotomy) or type II partial gastrectomy (Bilroth II or polya).
- Failure to respond to maximal medical treatment with severe symptoms or due to habitual recidivism. Procedure is type I partial gastrectomy for type I gastric ulcer or type II partial gastrectomy for duodenal ulcer.
- Emergency indications include:
  - Perforation (see 📖 p. 296);
  - Bleeding (see 📖 p. 294).

Zollinger–Ellison syndrome

- Due to hypergastrinaemia causing extensive, persistent, or typical ulceration.
- Commonest cause is benign secretory gastrinoma (usually intrapancreatic); occasionally cause is malignant gastrinoma (associated with MEN syndromes).
- Diagnosed by raised serum gastrin level, tumour located by CT scanning, angiography, selective pancreatic venous cannulation at surgery.
- Treatment. Resection of pancreatic tissue containing tumour.

Gastric tumours

May arise from the tissues of the mucosa (adenocarcinoma), connective tissue of the stomach wall (previously known as leiomyoma or leiomyosarcoma, but part of the spectrum of disease called gastrointestinal stromal tumours (GISTs); see 📖 p. 292), the neuroendocrine tissue (carcinoid tumours; see 📖 p. 292), or the lymphoid tissue (lymphomas).

Key facts

Adenocarcinoma; commonest age of incidence >50y; ♂:♀, 3:1. Predisposing factors include:
- Diet rich in nitrosamines (smoked or fresh fish, pickled fruit);
- Chronic atrophic gastritis;
- Blood group A;
- Chronic gastric ulceration related to *H. pylori*.

Clinical features

Symptoms
- Dyspepsia (any new onset of dyspepsia over the age of 45 should be considered to be due to adenocarcinoma until proven otherwise).
- Weight loss, anorexia, and lethargy.
- Anaemia (iron deficiency due to chronic blood loss).
- Occasionally presents as acute upper GI bleeding (see 📖 p. 294).
- Dysphagia uncommon unless involving the proximal fundus and gastro-oesophageal junction.

Signs
- Weight loss.
- Palpable epigastric mass.
- Palpable supraclavicular lymph node (Troisier's sign) suggests disseminated disease.

Diagnosis and investigation
- Diagnosis usually by gastroscopy (barium meal may be required if gastroscopy contraindicated).
- Staging (see Table 7.1) investigations include:
  - Thoraco-abdominal CT scan to assess for distant metastases and local lymphadenopathy.
  - Endoluminal ultrasound to assess for local disease.
  - Laparoscopy (for patients considered for potential resection) to exclude small volume peritoneal metastases.

Treatment

Unfortunately, in the UK, the majority of tumours are metastatic or unresectable due to local extension and so not suitable for consideration of surgical treatment for cure. The majority of treatment is directed at symptoms and palliation. When a tumour is considered potentially curable, the treatment offered is based on the extent of disease at staging.

Table 7.1 TNM staging of gastric cancers

T (tumour)	N (nodes)	M (metastases)
Tis, *in situ* within mucosa	N0, no lymph nodes	P (peritoneal metastases)
T1, confined to submucosa	N1, involved nodes within 3cm of primary	P0, no peritoneal metastases
T2, confined to muscle wall	N2, involved nodes more than 3cm from primary	P1/2/3, peritoneal metastases in increasing extent
T3, involvement of serosal surface		H (hepatic metastases)
T4, involvement of other organs		H0, no hepatic metastases
		H1/2/3, hepatic metastases in increasing extent

Early gastric cancer (T1 or 2, N0/1, P0, H0)
- Suitable for attempted curative resection if patient medically fit enough.
- Surgery. Radical gastrectomy usually preceded by neoadjuvant chemotherapy in patients fit.
- Patients now frequently offered preoperative and post-operative chemotherapy.
- Local resection or ablation has an uncertain place in treatment.

Advanced gastric cancer (T3 or more or any of N2/P1+/H1+)
- Patients will be offered pre- and post-operative chemotherapy.
- Surgical intervention unlikely to be curative.
- May be undertaken for palliative treatment.
- Local ablation for symptom control occasionally possible.
- Palliative chemotherapy occasionally effective for disseminated disease.

> **Key revision points—anatomy and physiology of the stomach**
> - The fundus is predominantly a storage zone with few active cells.
> - The body contains mostly chief cells (secrete pepsinogen; stimulated by gastrin and local ACh release) and oxyntic cells (secrete H^+; stimulated by gastrin, histamine, and ACh; inhibited by H^+, secretin, and GIP).
> - The antrum contains G cells (secrete gastrin; stimulated by ACh from vagus, stretch; inhibited by VIP, secretin, H^+).
> - The pyloric sphincter is a functional sphincter of circular muscle.
> - Arterial supply is profuse (gastric ischaemia is rare) via coeliac axis—left gastric, splenic, and common hepatic arteries.
> - Lymphatic drainage follows arteries and is profuse (significant lymph node metastases are usually fatal).

Chronic intestinal ischaemia

Caused by chronic reduction in blood supply to the intestine without acute threat to the viability of the bowel.

Key facts

Chronic intestinal ischaemia is uncommon. Usually presents with vague symptoms and diagnosis is often prolonged. Causes include:

- Progressive atherosclerosis affecting the visceral vessels; usually requires more than one vessel to be affected (e.g. superior mesenteric artery occlusion and coeliac artery stenosis).
- Obliterative small vessel disease (e.g. thromboangiitis obliterans, systemic sclerosis, severe diabetic vasculopathy).

Clinical features

Symptoms

- Commonest symptom is *mesenteric angina*, chronic central abdominal pain brought on by eating; associated with nausea and vomiting.
- May present with weight loss, general anorexia, and malnutrition.
- Often associated with other features of extensive vascular disease such as renal impairment, coronary disease, claudication.

Signs

Weight loss, central abdominal tenderness.

Diagnosis and investigations

- Usually diagnosed by imaging of the visceral arteries in combination with clinical symptoms. Methods of imaging visceral vessels include:
  - CT angiogram.
  - MR angiogram.
  - Transfemoral digital subtraction angiogram/aortogram.
- Other investigations should include:
  - Assessment of renal function.
  - Assessment of coronary circulation.
  - Exclusion of aneurysmal disease.
- Small vessel disease may require autoimmune screen.

Complications

- Acute intestinal ischaemia is less common due to the development of collaterals although, if undiagnosed, loss of all visceral vessels results in eventual pan-intestinal infarction.
- Chronic ischaemic strictures due to focally severe ischaemia.

Treatment

Medical

- Stop smoking.
- Control of hypertension; treatment of any hyperlipidaemia.
- Aspirin 75mg od to prevent thromboembolic events.
- Control diabetes if present.
- Treatment of autoimmune disease if present.

Interventional

Commonest treatment for large vessel stenosis is radiologically guided stenting. Risks converting stenosis to acute occlusion with the risk of precipitating emergency surgery. Not possible if the stenosis is at the aortic ostium of the vessel affected.

Surgical

- Rarely indicated. Commonest procedure is external iliac to ileocolic artery side-to-side bypass.
- Overall prognosis is poor as the underlying disease process is often widespread and progressive.

Key revision points—anatomy and physiology of the small intestine

- Duodenum is a secretory and digestive organ; described in four parts (second part admits the common bile and pancreatic ducts via the ampulla of Vater on the medial wall).
- Jejunum is a secretory and digestive organ. Typical features include: thick, red-purple wall; prominent plicae circulares; single arterial arcades with long mesenteric vessels.
- Ileum is predominantly an absorptive organ. Typical features include: thin blue-purple wall; prominent lymphoid aggregates; multilayered mesenteric arterial arcades.
- Terminal ileum is a specialized area of ileum, particularly concerned with absorption of bile salts, vitamin B12/IF complex.

Surgery for morbid obesity

Key facts

- Approximately 25% of UK adult population are classified as obese, a body mass index (BMI) of greater than 30kg/m^2.
- Admissions to hospital due to obesity-related disease have increased eightfold in the last 10y.
- Obese patients are exposed to an increased risk of chronic diseases, particularly type 2 diabetes, hypertension, hyperlipidaemia, and arthritis.
- Increased risk of some forms of cancer (colon and endometrial).

Clinical features

Symptoms

- The symptoms of obesity are generally related to the underlying condition that develops in association with it.
- Commonly, patients find their physical capacity is reduced and they become short of breath more easily on exertion

Signs

- Examination of obese patients can be challenging as their size can reduce the ability to elicit clinical signs.
- Assess for signs of respiratory disease, dyspnoea at rest.
- Investigation of possible biliary disease (common bile duct stones, biliary strictures, biliary tumours, biliary injuries, intrahepatic biliary disease).
- Investigation of pancreatic disease (pancreatic duct strictures, pancreatic duct abnormalities).
- Therapeutic interventions for pancreatico-biliary disease:
  - Stenting for common bile duct stones, strictures, tumours.
  - Sphincterotomy for the extraction of biliary stones.

Diagnosis and investigations

Exclude underlying endocrine disorders—Cushing's disease, hypothyroidism, polycystic ovarian syndrome.

Treatment

Medical

- Diabetic control. Oral hypoglycaemics and insulin, if necessary.
- Medication for anti-hypertensive and cardiovascular disease.
- Psychological and dietetic support for weight loss programme.
- Anti-obesity medication. Orlistat (reduces fat absorption) is the commonest.

Surgical

- Should only be considered after non-surgical treatments have failed and patient has been through a preoperative assessment to ensure they are able to make the necessary post-operative dietary and lifestyle changes.
- Procedures have either a restrictive or malabsorptive effect.

- Adjustable gastric banding is the commonest restrictive operation (the band is placed around the cardia of the stomach and restricts the volume of food, but not liquid, that can be ingested at one time).
- Gastric bypass involves a restrictive element (division of the stomach to create a small remnant) and a malabsorptive element (division and re-anastomosis of small bowel to reduce its ability to absorb food).
- These procedures are most commonly performed laparoscopically.

Small bowel tumours

Key facts

The small bowel is a rare location for tumours. Tumours may arise from:
- *Mucosa* small bowel—adenocarcinoma (<5% of all GI malignancies).
- *Neuroendocrine tissue*, e.g. carcinoid tumours.
- *Connective tissue* of the bowel wall, e.g. GIST, lipoma.
- *Lymphoid tissue* (lymphoma).

Adenocarcinoma of small bowel
- Forty per cent of all small bowel tumours.
- Commonest in the duodenojejunal junction and proximal jejunum; least common in the mid- and distal ileum.
- Associations:
  - Familial adenomatous polyposis (third commonest location of adenocarcinoma after colorectum and duodenum).
  - Peutz–Jegher's syndrome.
  - Crohn's disease.
  - Untreated longstanding coeliac disease.

Carcinoid tumours
- Twenty-five per cent of all small bowel tumours.
- Commonest in the distal small bowel; may arise in the appendix or Meckel's diverticulum.
- Majority are benign (non-metastatic).
- May produce enteric hormones (e.g. 5-HT, kallikrein, substance P); hormone effects only occur when the primary is able to secrete hormones into the systemic circulation or when hepatitic metastases secrete into the caval circulation (*carcinoid syndrome*; see 📖 p. 293).

GIST (gastrointestinal stromal tumours)
- Ten per cent of small bowel tumours.
- Arise from the mesenchymal tissues of the bowel wall and mesentery (smooth muscle cells, fibroblasts, lipocytes).
- Previously called variously leiomyo(sarc)oma, lipo(sarco)ma.
- Tumours of myenteric plexus tissues are a variant called GANT (gastrointestinal autonomic nerve tumours).

Primary lymphoma
- Twenty per cent of small bowel tumours.
- Arise from the lymphoid tissue of the small bowel wall.
- Almost always non-Hodgkin's; commonest are B-cell lymphomas arising from the mucosa-associated lymphoid tissue (MALTomas).

Clinical features
- *Adenocarcinoma of small bowel.* Often presents late with metastases; may present with small bowel obstruction, recurrent abdominal pain, or recurrent/occult GI bleeding.
- *Carcinoid tumours.* Commonest presentation is incidental finding after appendicectomy or Meckel's diverticulectomy.

- *Carcinoid syndrome.* Rare (typified by flushing, tachycardia, colicky abdominal pain, diarrhoea, wheezing).
- *GIST.* Often present with slow-growing abdominal mass, vague abdominal pain; may present with occult GI bleeding due to tumour ulceration.
- *Primary lymphoma.* Presents with malaise, abdominal pain, diarrhoea; may present with acute perforation or small bowel obstruction.

Diagnosis and investigations

Common diagnostic tests for all are:
- *CT chest and abdomen.* Identifies primary tumour, assesses extent of involvement of other tissues, assesses possible metastatic disease.
- *CT angiography.* For assessment of particularly vascular tumours or GISTs lying close to major visceral vessels to establish resectability.
- *Small bowel contrast study.* Rarely required for identification of primary tumours.
- *Ileoscopy.* May demonstrate proximal lesions presenting with occult, recurrent upper GI bleeding.

Complications

- *Bleeding.* Common with adenocarcinoma and some GISTs.
- *Obstruction.* Especially adenocarcinoma, GISTs, GANTs, and lymphoma.
- *Perforation.* Commonest with lymphoma, especially shortly after starting chemotherapy (due to bowel wall replacement by tumour); also occurs with adenocarcinoma.
- *Malabsorption.* Often with lymphoma if widespread.

Treatment

Surgery

- Primary surgical resection with macroscopic clearance of tumour for adenocarcinoma, carcinoid, GISTs, GANTs.
  - Potentially curative for non-metastatic disease.
  - Palliative to prevent complications if disease is metastatic.
- Surgical resection may be indicated for primary lymphoma prior to chemotherapy if there is a high risk of perforation of primary.
- Surgical resection of metastases is uncommon.

Medical

- *Chemotherapy.* Lymphoma and metastatic adenocarcinoma.
- *Hepatic abalation/embolization.* Used to treat carcinoid metastases to treat symptoms of carcinoid syndrome.
- *Imatinib (Glivec®)* (anti-CD113). Treatment for GISTs that are positive for c-Kit.

Acute haematemesis

Key facts

See Table 7.2 for predicting mortality of acute upper GI bleeding.
- Incidence 1 in 1000 adults per year in UK.
- Twenty per cent require intervention because of ongoing bleeding or rebleeding.
- Haematemesis is vomiting of blood, usually due to bleeding proximal to the duodenojejunal junction.
- Melaena is the passage of altered blood (dark purple, pitch black, or 'tarry', usually due to bleeding below the gastro-oesophageal junction.

Causes and features

- *Peptic (gastric or duodenal) ulceration* (benign, 50%). Fresh red blood with clots, occasionally mixed with food.
- *Oesophageal varices.* Copious dark red venous blood with little mixing with food; features of portal hypertension (e.g. caput medusa).
- *Oesophageal ulceration.* Small volumes of bright red blood/streaks typical.
- *Oesophageal trauma* ('Mallory–Weiss tear'). Small volumes of fresh bright blood preceded by violent or prolonged vomiting or retching.
- Vascular malformations/lesions (e.g. 'Dieu la Foy').
- Gastric carcinoma, leiomyoma.
- *Aortoenteric fistula.* Copious bright red blood (often rapidly fatal).

Associated or predisposing conditions

- Agents affecting mucosal health—NSAIDs, steroids, alcohol, major trauma, or massive burns.
- Agents worsening risk of bleeding—anticoagulants.

Emergency management

Resuscitation

- Establish large calibre IV access; give crystalloid fluid up to 1000mL if tachycardic or hypotensive. Only use O −ve blood if the patient is *in extremis*; otherwise wait for cross-matched blood if transfusion needed.
- Catheterize and place on a fluid balance chart if hypotensive.
- Send blood for FBC (Hb, WCC), U&E (Na, K), LFTs (albumin), cross-match (at least 3U if haematemesis large), clotting.
- Always consider alerting HDU/ITU if very unwell.
- Monitor pulse rate, BP, and urine output (urinary catheter).
- Insertion of a Sengstaken–Blakemore gastro-oesophageal tube may be a life-saving resuscitation manoeuvre.

Establish a diagnosis

- Urgent OGD is the investigation of choice (at least within 24h).
  - May require ongoing resuscitation with anaesthetist present.
  - Allows diagnosis and biopsy if appropriate.
  - May allow therapeutic interventions including adrenaline injection, heater probe coagulation, banding of varices, clipping vessel.

- Angiography.
  - Occasionally suitable for active bleeding due to invasive intervention done in radiology department.
  - May allow selective embolization in some patients with recurrent bleeding.

Early treatment
- Give IV PPI (e.g. omeprazole 40mg IV); stop all NSAIDs.
- Blood transfusion if large volume haematemesis or drop in Hb.
- Ensure the appropriate surgical team knows of the patient in case surgical intervention is required.
- Known or suspected liver disease—consider FFP to correct clotting.
- Surgery may be required if:
  - Massive haemorrhage requiring ongoing resuscitation.
  - Failed initial endoscopic treatment with ongoing bleeding.
  - Rebleeding not suitable for repeated endoscopic treatment.

Definitive management

Varices (see 📖 p. 322)
- Endoscopy coagulation or banding/interventional radiology/surgery.
- IV vasopressin or analogues.

Gastric/duodenal ulcer
- Endoscopic coagulation or injection; may be repeated if suitable ulcer.
- Surgery for failed primary management or rebleeding that is unsuitable for attempted repeat endoscopic treatment.
- Surgical options—local excision of gastric ulcer or partial gastrectomy; under-running of duodenal ulcer.
- *H. pylori* eradication (triple therapy).

Gastric carcinoma
- Endoscopic treatment often not effective.
- Partial or subtotal gastrectomy (often palliative, rarely curative).

Oesophageal trauma Oral antacids.

Aortoenteric fistula Surgery if the patient survives beyond diagnosis.

Table 7.2 Rockall score for predicting mortality of acute upper GI bleeding*

	Rockall score		
	0	1	2
Age (y)	<60	60–79	>80
Shock	None	HR >100bpm	Systolic BP <100mmHg
Comorbidities	None		Cardiac	Hepatorenal disease Carcinoma

* Percentage mortality for scores: 0, <1%; 1, 3%; 2, 6%; 3, 11%; 4, 25%; 5, 40%; 6, >80%.

Acute upper GI perforation

Causes and features

- Duodenal ulceration.
- Gastric ulceration (usually anterior prepyloric; less commonly anterior body).
- Gastric carcinoma.
- Traumatic, e.g. fish bone perforation.
- Ischaemic (usually secondary to gastric volvulus).

Symptoms

- Acute onset upper abdominal pain. Severe, constant, worse with breathing and moving; may radiate to back or shoulders.
- Prodrome of upper abdominal pain (in benign or malignant ulceration).
- Copious vomiting and upper abdominal distension suggest volvulus.
- Prodrome of weight loss, dyspepsia, and anorexia suggests carcinoma.

Signs

- Generalized peritonism common ('board-like' generalized rigidity with marked guarding and tenderness).
- Localized upper abdominal peritonism may occur, especially with previous surgery where adhesions may act to contain the contamination.
- Mild fever, pallor, tachycardia, and hypotension (often profound due to autonomic reaction); typically respond quickly to modest fluid resuscitation.

Emergency management

Resuscitation

- Establish large calibre IV access; give crystalloid fluid up to 1000mL if tachycardic or hypotensive.
- Catheterize and place on a fluid balance chart.
- Send blood for FBC (Hb, WCC), U&E (Na, K), LFTs (albumin), group and save, clotting.

Establish a diagnosis

- Erect CXR (looking for free gas). If the CXR is non-diagnostic, a lateral decubitus abdominal film can be performed, although a CT is more common.
- CT scan if diagnosis unclear on CXR; may demonstrate presence of gastric carcinoma.

Early treatment

- Once the diagnosis of perforation is confirmed on clinical or radiological grounds, the treatment is surgical unless:
  - The patient declines.
  - The patient is considered unlikely to survive and supportive care is deemed more appropriate.
- Conservative management. IV PPI, limited oral intake, active physiotherapy—has a very limited role in management; it offers an outcome similar to that of surgery only in cases where the perforation

has sealed at the time of presentation, there is no haemodynamic instability, and there are no signs of peritonism.

Definitive management

Duodenal ulcer
- Sutured closure with omental patch.
- Empirical oral triple therapy for *H. pylori*.
- Definitive surgery (partial gastrectomy, vagotomy, and drainage procedure) should only be performed for recurrent perforation, failed fully compliant medical therapy, recidivist non-compliant patient.

Gastric ulcer
- Sutured closure with omental patch if prepyloric.
- Local excision and sutured closure if body.

Gastric carcinoma Partial gastrectomy (usually palliative).

Traumatic Sutured closure.

Volvulus with ischaemia Usually subtotal gastrectomy.

Acute appendicitis

Causes and features

▶ Commonest cause of urgent abdominal surgery and the common provisional diagnosis of all emergency surgical admissions in the UK.
- Can affect any age, but uncommon under the age of 4 and over the age of 80. Peak age of incidence is early teens to early twenties. Three types:
  - *Mucosal.* Mildest form usually diagnosed by pathology reporting.
  - *Phlegmonous.* Typified by slow onset and relatively slow progression.
  - *Necrotic.* Often due to acute bacterial infection with ischaemic necrosis; leads to perforation unless treated by surgery.

Differential diagnosis
- Children.
  - Non-specific abdominal pain, including 'mesenteric adenitis'.
  - Meckel's diverticulitis.
  - Ovarian cyst/menstrual symptoms (peri-menarchal girls).
- Adults.
  - *Terminal ileal pathology.* Crohn's, Meckel's diverticulitis, gastroenteritis.
  - *Retroperitoneal pathology.* Pancreatitis, renal colic.
  - *Ovarian pathology.* Ectopic pregnancy, cyst, infection, menstrual pain.
- Older adults.
  - *Ileocaecal pathology.* Caecal diverticulitis, caecal tumours.
  - *Colonic pathology.* Sigmoid diverticulitis.
  - *Ovarian pathology.* Cysts, infection, tumours.

Clinical features
- *Symptoms.*
  - Malaise, anorexia, and fever.
  - Diarrhoea common and may be mistaken for acute (gastro) enteritis.
  - Abdominal pain starts centrally and localizes to the right iliac fossa (RIF).
  - Abdominal pain caused by coughing and moving.
- *Signs.*
  - Fever, tachycardia.
  - Abdominal tenderness. Peritonism suggests perforation (local or generalized). Often maximal over *'McBurney's point'* (see opposite), but only if appendix is in conventional anatomical position.
  - Palpation of left iliac fossa (LIF) causes pain worse in RIF (*Rovsing's sign*).
- Investigations may be normal and none are diagnostic or exclusive (see 📖 p. 299).

Complications
- Perforation (localized or generalized).
- RIF 'appendix' mass (usually appendicitis with densely adherent caecum and omentum, forming a 'mass').
- RIF abscess (usually 2° to perforated retrocaecal appendicitis).
- Pelvic abscess (usually 2° to perforated pelvic appendicitis).

Emergency management

Resuscitation

- Establish IV access.
- Catheterize and place on a fluid balance chart only if ↓ BP or septic.
- Request FBC (Hb, WCC), U&E (Na, K), CRP (usually ↑ WCC, CRP).

Establish a diagnosis

- The diagnosis is a clinical one in all but exceptional cases and investigations are usually unnecessary.
- CT is appropriate in adults, especially over the age of 65 or if the diagnosis is unclear since the differential diagnosis is much wider and appendicitis relatively less likely above this age.
- CT is the best investigation in suspected appendix mass or abscess.
- Ultrasound scan (pelvic) is indicated in young women of childbearing age if ovarian pathology is suspected.
- Laparoscopy is a useful surgical diagnostic manoeuvre, allowing diagnosis of pelvic pathology, e.g. pelvic inflammatory disease (PID) without a major abdominal incision.

Early treatment Avoid giving IV antibiotics without a clear diagnosis.

Definitive management

▶ Acute appendicitis

- Open or laparoscopic appendicectomy.
- IV antibiotics on induction; continued antibiotics only indicated for perforation.

Appendix mass or appendix abscess

- IV antibiotics (e.g. cefuroxime 750mg tds + metronidazole 500mg tds).
- If symptoms settle, delayed (interval) appendicectomy after 6 weeks.
- If symptoms fail to settle, may need acute appendicectomy.
- Appendix abscess may be amenable to CT-guided drainage.

Key revision points—anatomy of appendicectomy

- Commonly **retrocaecal,** but may be pelvic, retroileal, or retrocolic.
- *Taenia coli of caecum converge at base of appendix* and aid location, especially in difficult locations.
- Small mesentery with sole blood supply from **appendicular artery** (a terminal branch ileocolic) which may thrombose causing gangrene.
- Principles of **appendicectomy** are as follows:
  - **Muscle splitting gridiron** incision centred at **McBurney's point.**
  - **Lapararoscopic approach** increasingly popular.
  - Appendix is carefully located and delivered into the wound.
  - The mesentery of the appendix is divided and ligated.
  - The appendix is clamped and tied at the base and excised.
  - Some surgeons invaginate the stump using a purse-string in the wall of the caecum round the base of the appendix.

Acute peritonitis

Defined as acute inflammation in the peritoneal cavity.

Causes

May be primary (rare) or secondary (common).

- Primary peritonitis. Typically streptococcal with probable portal of entry via bloodstream rather than intra-abdominal organs.
- Commonest causes of secondary peritonitis are:
  - *Acute perforated appendicitis* (see 📖 p. 298)—commonest cause of peritonitis especially in under 45s.
  - *Acute perforated diverticular disease* (see 📖 p. 404)—commonest cause in elderly.
  - *Upper GI perforation* (see 📖 p. 296).
  - Perforated tumours (colonic or gastric).
  - Perforated ischaemic bowel, e.g. due to adhesions.
  - Acute pancreatitis (usually inflammatory rather than infective).
  - Peritoneal dialysis-related—often atypical or cutaneous organisms gaining entry via contaminated dialysate bags or catheter.
  - Post-surgical intervention, e.g. anastomotic leak, enteric injury.

Clinical features

There are features common to all causes. Additional features suggestive of an underlying cause should also be sought, particularly in the history.

Symptoms

- Anorexia and fever.
- Severe generalized abdominal pain radiating to shoulders and back.
- Abdominal pain worse with movement, coughing, sneezing.

Signs

- Fever, tachycardia.
- Generalized abdominal tenderness with guarding and rigidity.
- Differential maximal tenderness *may* indicate the possible underlying cause.
- Gentle palpation may allow identification of an underlying mass.

Emergency management

Resuscitation

- Establish large calibre IV access.
- Catheterize and place on a fluid balance chart.
- Send blood for FBC (Hb, WCC), U&E (Na, K), CRP, amylase, group and save.
- ABGs if shocked or ischaemic bowel/pancreatitis suspected.

Establish a diagnosis

Most causes of acute peritonitis require surgery to correct them, but surgery is contraindicated in most cases of acute pancreatitis.

Diagnostic investigations are indicated if the patient would otherwise be a candidate for surgical intervention.

- Blood investigations may show neutrophilia, ↑ CRP.
- Raised amylase may suggest pancreatitis.
- Abdominal CT scanning is the investigation of choice for diagnosis. It should reliably exclude acute pancreatitis and often locate the probable source of the pathology.
- Laparoscopy is occasionally useful in patients where a formal laparotomy should be avoided if possible.

Early treatment
IV antibiotics are appropriate without a clear diagnosis, especially if surgery is likely (e.g. metronidazole 500mg IV tds + cefuroxime 750mg IV tds).

Definitive management

Acute appendicitis See 📖 p. 298.

Upper GI perforation See 📖 p. 296.
Perforated diverticular disease
- IV antibiotics (e.g. cefuroxime 750mg tds + metronidazole 500mg tds).
- Surgical treatment involves resection of the affected segment. Depending on the length of time from perforation, extent of the contamination, and extent of inflammation in the affected segment, the bowel may be anastomosed (primary anastomosis) or the proximal end brought out on to the abdominal wall as an end colostomy ('Hartmann's type' resection).

Perforated tumour
Surgical resection is required even if palliative. Ends of bowel may be re-anastomosed or exteriorized as stomas, depending on the circumstances (degree of contamination, underlying pathology).

Primary peritonitis or continuous ambulatory peritoneal dialysis (CAPD)-related peritonitis
- A diligent and systematic search is necessary to ensure there is no occult source of perforation as a cause.
- Primary treatment is extensive lavage of all quadrants and treatment with appropriate antibiotics (guided by culture results from peritoneal fluid).

Acute abdominal pain

Acute abdominal pain is the commonest emergency presentation to hospitals in the UK. It is often a daunting challenge to the admitting team because of the huge differential diagnosis possible, and the wide range of tests available to try and establish a diagnosis. Be methodical and remember some simple rules.

- Take a proper history and examination; do not work to the diagnosis given to you by the referring doctor.
- Resuscitate the patient properly and give adequate analgesia; this often helps to clarify the diagnosis. There is *no* reason to withhold analgesia prior to 'senior' clinical examination.
- Try to clarify if you think the patient has signs of peritonitis (localized or generalized); this will narrow the differential and may require surgery as part of the diagnostic work-up.

Causes

Causes approximate to the fact that pathology of underlying structures in each region tend to give rise to abdominal pain maximal in that region (see Box 7.1). Although a good guide, it is wise to remember that viscera are often mobile and pain often radiates to adjacent sections of the abdomen.

Clinical features

Each condition has its own clinical features, but here are some rules to follow.

Symptoms and signs

- Constant pain, gradual in onset, but progressive worsening suggests an underlying inflammatory cause.
- Intermittent pain that is poorly localized suggests colic arising from a visceral structure.
- Central and lower abdominal pain in children (under the age of 12) is self-limiting (non-specific) in 70%, from benign gynaecological causes in 25% (girls), and only pathological in 10–20%.
- Severe pain out of proportion to the clinical signs suggests ischaemic bowel until proven otherwise.
- Pain in the loin or back arises from (at least partially) retroperitoneal structures; consider the pancreas, renal tract, and abdominal aorta.

Emergency management

Resuscitation

- Establish IV access.
- Catheterize and place on a fluid balance chart only if hypotensive.
- Give adequate analgesia. If renal pathology is suspected, diclofenac (Voltarol®) 100mg PR is very effective (avoid in asthma and renal disease). If intra-abdominal pathology is suspected, 5–10mg morphine IV is reasonable. Morphine IV *never* hides established clinical signs; it often helps to clarify the diagnosis by its anxiolytic effect on patients.
- Send blood for FBC (Hb, WCC), U&E (Na, K), amylase, LFTs, CRP, group and save.

Box 7.1 Causes of acute abdominal pain arranged according to abdominal region

Right hypochondriac	*Epigastric*	*Left hypochondriac*
• Right lower lobe pneumonia/ embolism • Cholecystitis • Biliary colic • Hepatitis	• Pancreatitis • Gastritis • Peptic ulcer • Myocardial infarction	• Left lower lobe pneumonia/ embolism • Large bowel obstruction
Right lumbar	*Umbilical*	*Left lumbar*
• Renal colic • Appendicitis	• Intestinal obstruction • Intestinal ischaemia • Aortic aneurysm • Gastroenteritis • Crohn's disease	• Renal colic • Large bowel obstruction
Right iliac	*Hypogastric*	*Left iliac*
• Appendicitis • Crohn's disease • Right tubo-ovarian pathology	• Cystitis • Urinary retention • Dysmenorrhoea • Endometriosis	• Sigmoid diverticulitis • Left tubo-ovarian pathology

Establish a diagnosis

The time frame for the diagnosis of acute abdominal pain varies according to the presentation. It is not uncommon for 12–24h of 'masterful inactivity' to be used to allow the diagnosis to be clarified. Young patients with central and mild RIF pain are typical of this sort of management. Do not assume this is normal. Some causes of acute abdominal pain require diagnosis and management immediately upon admission or within 6–8h or less. Try to be thoughtful in diagnostic tests; many may be requested, but usually only one or two are really useful.

- Blood investigations are very rarely diagnostic. Serum amylase more than 3x normal maximum is very highly suggestive of acute pancreatitis.
- Plain abdominal radiographs are very rarely diagnostic.
- Always request a plain erect chest radiograph; it is the first-line test of choice for free abdominal air.
- Upper abdominal ultrasound is an excellent investigation for suspected hepatobiliary pathology.
- Pelvic ultrasound (transabdominal or transvaginal) is a good test for suspected tubo-ovarian disease.
- CT scanning may well be indicated and is a good 'general survey' of the abdomen, but exposes the patient to significant radiation and should not be routinely requested.

Early treatment
- IV antibiotics are inappropriate without a clear diagnosis; they will suppress, but may not adequately treat, developing infection.
- Until a definitive management plan is established, concentrate on fluid balance, analgesia, and monitoring vital signs.

Gynaecological causes of lower abdominal pain

Gynaecological pathologies are a common cause of lower abdominal pain, not only in women of childbearing age, but they can also affect post-menopausal women.

Causes

- Complications of menstruation. Retrograde menstruation, mid-cycle ovulation pain ('Mittelschmerz').
- Ovarian cyst. Acute swelling, rupture, torsion.
- Tubo-ovarian infection, including PID, abscess.
- Ectopic pregnancy, including rupture.

Clinicopathological features

Complications of menstruation

- Commonest during development of regular periods.
- Typically cyclical pains, often sharp and sudden in onset.
- May have marked tenderness bordering on peritonitis.
- Normal blood investigations; self-limiting.

Ovarian cyst complications

- Commonest in mid-childbearing years.
- May have severe pain with few clinical signs.
- Normal blood investigations.

Tubo-ovarian infection

- Commonly caused by *Escherichia coli*, *Bacteroides fragilis*, *Streptococcus* sp.
- Associated with cervical disease or instrumentation.
- Sexually-transmitted infections can cause tubo-ovarian sepsis, which may be more chronic and recurrent (*Neisseria gonorrhoeae*, *Chlamydia trachomatis*).
- Associated with multiple sexual partners and unprotected intercourse.
- Pyrexia, mild tachycardia, occasional purulent vaginal discharge.
- Often affects both sides causing bilateral pain and tenderness.

Ectopic pregnancy

- May occur at any age.
- Commonest site is the Fallopian tube (ampulla, tube, or isthmus).
- Associated with previous tubal disease or surgery.
- Menstrual irregularity or a 'late' period is common, but not uniform.
- May give rise to symptoms whilst enlarging with unilateral pelvic pain.
- Symptoms increase with complications (bleeding into site of pregnancy, free rupture with bleeding into pelvis and peritoneal cavity).
- Typified by lower abdominal pain without fever.
- Hypotension with tachycardia suggests active intra-abdominal bleeding, but is fortunately rare at presentation.

Emergency management

Resuscitation

- Establish large calibre IV access if an ectopic pregnancy is suspected.
- Catheterize and place on a fluid balance chart only if hypotensive.
- Give adequate analgesia (5–10mg morphine IV is reasonable).
- Send blood for FBC (Hb, WCC), U&E (Na, K), CRP, group and save.

Establish a diagnosis

- Urine β-HCG (and serum β-HCG where urine test is positive since this is more reliable). *All women of childbearing age should be assumed to be pregnant until proven otherwise.* Pregnancy testing may be negative in ectopic pregnancy if the fetus is already dead by the time of presentation.
- High vaginal swabs should be taken if tubo-ovarian sepsis is suspected.
- Pelvic ultrasound (transabdominal or transvaginal) is the diagnostic investigation of choice unless the patient is acutely unstable. It has a high sensitivity and good specificity.
- Laparoscopy is a very common diagnostic investigation. It allows a firm diagnosis of most gynaecological pathology and may be therapeutic (e.g. pelvic lavage, cyst treatment).

Early treatment

- IV antibiotics for a clear diagnosis of pelvic infection.
- If ruptured or bleeding ectopic pregnancy is seriously considered, make sure the surgical and gynaecological teams are aware. Direct transfer to theatre may be necessary.

Definitive management

- *Complications of menstruation.* Conservative management—pelvic lavage if laparoscopy is performed.
- *Ovarian cyst complications.* Ovarian preservation if below the age of menopause; cystectomy or drainage where possible.
- *Tubo-ovarian infection.* Cephradine 500mg tds PO and metronidazole 400mg PO tds for non-sexually transmitted infections; metronidazole 400mg PO for chlamydia; IV penicillin for neisserial infections.
- *Ectopic pregnancy.* Conservation or reconstruction of the affected tube/ovary wherever possible. If not salvageable, unilateral salpingo-oophrectomy.

Intra-abdominal abscess

Key facts

Intra-abdominal sepsis can present as an intra-abdominal abscess if the sepsis is contained by tissues or anatomy. Common locations are:
- Alongside the organ of origin (e.g. paracolic in diverticulitis, parapancreatic after infected pancreatitis).
- Pelvic (especially after pelvic sepsis such as appendicitis or after generalized peritoneal infection).
- Subphrenic (e.g. after upper GI perforation).

Causes

- Sigmoid diverticulitis (see 📖 p. 404).
- Acute appendicitis (see 📖 p. 298).
- Severe acute cholecystitis (see 📖 p. 316).
- Upper GI perforation (see 📖 p. 296).
- Post-anastomotic leakage (see 📖 p. 420).
- Infected acute pancreatitis (see 📖 p. 332).
- Post-trauma.

Clinical features

Depending on the source, the preceding pathology may have specific clinical features, but the development of an abscess gives rise to certain common features independent of the origin.

Symptoms
- Malaise, anorexia.
- Localized abdominal pain—constant.

Signs
- Swinging fever, typically peaks in excess of 38.5°C occurring twice a day.
- Tachycardia tends to follow the temperature.
- Localized abdominal tenderness with a possible mass if abscess in an accessible position (e.g. paracolic).

Emergency management

Resuscitation
- Establish large calibre IV access if the patient is unwell.
- Catheterize and place on a fluid balance chart only if hypotensive.
- Give adequate analgesia (e.g. 5–10mg morphine IV).
- Send blood for FBC (Hb, WCC), U&E (Na, K), CRP, group and save.

Establish a diagnosis
- Helical CT scanning is the diagnostic investigation of choice.
- Pelvic ultrasound (transabdominal or transvaginal) is occasionally useful if a pelvic abscess is suspected and CT scanning is to be avoided due to age.

Early treatment IV antibiotics are appropriate if the patient is septic and should be given according to the most likely underlying diagnosis and organisms.

Definitive management

- Radiologically guided drainage by ultrasound or CT scanning wherever possible. Limitations include retroperitoneal or intermesenteric abscesses with dangerous access or complex multiloculated abscesses.
- Open surgical drainage usually only indicated if:
  - Radiological drainage not possible or safe.
  - Radiological drainage fails to deal with the clinical symptoms or abscess recurs.
  - Surgical treatment is required for the primary underlying pathology.

Liver, pancreatic, and biliary surgery

Jaundice—causes and diagnosis

Key facts
Jaundice is clinically apparent at serum bilirubin levels above 40mmol.

Key revision points—physiology of bile
- Unconjugated bilirubin formed mainly in spleen by the breakdown of haemoglobin.
- It is insoluble and is transported in the plasma bound to albumin.
- Taken up by the liver by active transport, it is converted in the hepatocytes into conjugated bilirubin (water-soluble).
- It is excreted into the bile canaliculi and via the main bile ducts into the duodenum.
- Ten per cent of the unconjugated bilirubin is reduced to urobilinogen by small intestinal bacteria, reabsorbed in the terminal ileum, and then excreted in the urine (enterohepatic circulation).
- Ninety per cent is converted by colonic bacteria to stercobilinogen which is excreted in faeces.

Causes and features
Pre-hepatic jaundice (haemolytic)
- Congenital abnormalities of red cell structure or content (e.g. hereditary spherocytosis, sickle cell disease).
- Autoimmune haemolytic anaemia.
- Transfusion reactions.
- Drug toxicity.

Hepatic jaundice (hepatocellular)
- *Hepatic unconjugated hyperbilirubinaemia.*
  - Gilbert's syndrome. Deficiency or abnormalities of unconjugated bilirubin uptake system.
  - Crigler–Najjar syndrome. Abnormality of conjugation process enzymes.
- *Hepatic conjugated hyperbilirubinaemia.*
  - Infection. Viral (e.g. hepatitis A, B, C, EBV, CMV); bacterial (e.g. liver abscess, leptospirosis); parasitic (e.g. amoebic).
  - Drugs, e.g. paracetamol overdose, antipsychotics, antibiotics.
  - Non-infective hepatitis, e.g. chronic active hepatitis, alcohol-related.

Post-hepatic jaundice (obstructive)
- *Intraluminal abnormalities of bile ducts.*
  - Gallstones.
  - Blood clot.
  - Parasites (e.g. flukes).
- *Mural abnormalities of bile ducts.*
  - Cholangiocarcinoma.
  - Congenital atresia.
  - Sclerosing cholangitis.

- Biliary cirrhosis (primary (autoimmune) or secondary to sepsis).
- Traumatic/post-surgical stricture.
- *Extrinsic compression of bile ducts.*
  - Pancreatitis.
  - Tumours, e.g. head of pancreas, ampulla of Vater.
  - Lymphadenopathy of porta hepatis nodes.

Diagnosis and investigations

History
Common aspects overlooked in the clinical history of jaundiced patients.
- Family history of blood disorders.
- Recent foreign travel and work (exposure to infective agents).
- Recent drugs or changes in medications.
- Recent surgery or anaesthesia.
- History of gallstones.
- Alcohol intake, cholangitis (pain, fever, rigors), and carcinoma, especially the head of the pancreas.

Basic tests
- Reticulocytosis, abnormal blood film (haemolysis).
- ↑ Prothrombin time.
- 'Hepatitis screen' (viral titres for hepatitis A, B, C, CMV, EBV).
- Immunology (anti-smooth muscle antibodies (chronic active hepatitis) and anti-mitochondrial antibodies (primary biliary cirrhosis)).
- LFTs (see Table 8.1).

Advanced tests
- Ultrasound scan (liver, gall bladder, bile ducts, and pancreas).
  - Excludes the presence of extrahepatic obstruction (dilated common bile duct).
  - May locate cause and site of obstruction.
  - Examines hepatic parenchyma in possible hepatitis.
- Magnetic resonance cholangiopancreatography (MRCP) for suspected extrahepatic obstruction with no cause seen on ultrasound.
- Liver biopsy (ultrasound-guided) for suspected hepatitis.

Table 8.1 Liver function tests in jaundice

	Haemolytic	Hepatocellular	Obstructive
Unconjugated bilirubin	Increased	Increased	Normal
Alkaline phosphatase	Normal	Normal	Much increased
γ glutamyl transferase	Normal	Increased	Much increased
Transaminases	Normal	Increased	Normal
Lactate dehydrogenase	Normal	Increased	Normal

Jaundice—management

Complications of jaundice

- *Renal failure* (hepatorenal syndrome). Caused by a combination of infection, dehydration, and a direct effect of high levels of bilirubin and other toxic products of metabolism on the kidney; mortality is highest when the patient is over 65 with an elevated blood urea.
- *Biliary infection* (cholangitis). Commonest in obstructive jaundice or with previously damaged biliary tree; commonly due to Gram –ve bacteria (e.g. *Escherichia coli, Pseudomonas*).
- *Deranged coagulation.* Due to decreased synthesis of vitamin K dependent clotting factors (III, VII, IX, X) and impaired platelet function.
- *Relative immunosuppression.* Predisposes to systemic infections (e.g. chest infection) and reduces wound healing due to combinations of jaundice, infection, and reduced proteosynthesis.

Acute presentation—general treatment

Fluid balance
- *Correct dehydration.* Give up to 1000mL IV crystalloid if there is no pre-exisisting liver disease; sodium input should be carefully monitored in pre-exisisting liver disease—ask for senior advice.
- Monitor hourly urine output—urethral catheter.
- *Treat infection.* Take blood cultures if the patient is pyrexial. Give IV antibiotics according to local protocol (e.g. cefuroxime 750mg IV tds, IV gentamicin, PO or IV ciprofloxacin (500mg IV)); treatment of bile duct obstruction may be required urgently (e.g. radiologically-guided drainage, ERCP, or rarely, surgery); consider prophylactic antibiotics.
- *Check clotting times* (APTT, PT). Give vitamin K 10mg IV stat if PT is prolonged.
- *Ensure adequate nutrition.* Ensure the patient has a dietetic review; enteral feeding is optimum, but may require a fine bore NGT or, very occasionally, a surgical gastrostomy or jejunostomy.
- Preoperative biliary decompression has not been proven to reduce post-operative complications.

Acute presentation—specific treatments

- *Endoscopic procedures* (ERCP).
  - Sphincterotomy. Used for common bile duct stone extraction, treatment of ampullary strictures due to tumours or inflammation.
  - Stent insertion (plastic or expanding metal). Used for bile duct stones that cannot be removed easily, post-operative or benign strictures, malignant strictures, external compression of bile duct.
- *Percutaneous transhepatic cholangiogram* (PTC). Used for stent insertion (often in combination with ERCP), temporary external drainage of obstructed biliary system.
- *Surgical drainage* (e.g. choledochoduodenostomy). Very rarely used if other interventions failed due to very high morbidity and mortality.

Elective presentation—specific treatments

- Haemolytic jaundice.
  - Steroids for autoimmune case.
  - Splenectomy (laparoscopic). Rarely used for hereditary causes and failed medical treatment.
- Obstructive jaundice.
  - ERCP and PTC may be used as above for stones, strictures, compression.
  - Surgical drainage (e.g. choledochoduodenostomy or cholecystojejunostomy) used for failed interventional treatments.
  - Surgical resection, e.g. Whipple's pancreaticoduodenectomy. Used for very selected cases where pancreatic or distal bile duct tumours are benign or malignant, but potentially curable on staging; staging of potentially suitable patients may include endoscopic ultrasound, CT scan, ERCP or MRCP, visceral arteriography, laparoscopy.
- Hepatocellular jaundice.
  - Remove causative agent and support liver function.
  - Consider transplantation in specific circumstances.
- Selective arteriography of the hepatic, coeliac, and superior mesenteric arteries gives information about anatomical variants, vessel invasion, tumour operability.

Prognosis in acute jaundice

Adverse risk factors include:

- Age >65y.
- Elevated plasma urea.
- Elevated plasma bilirubin (>200g/L).
- Uncontrolled sepsis and multiple organ dysfunction (typically acute tubular necrosis).
- Underlying malignant disease.

Gall bladder stones

Key facts Present in 10% of people >50y in the UK.

Pathological features

Bile has three major constituents:
- Bile salts (primary—cholic and chenodeoxycholic acids; secondary—deoxycholic and lithocholic acids).
- Phospholipids (90% lecithin).
- Cholesterol.

Bile containing excess cholesterol relative to bile salts and lecithin predisposes to gallstone formation.

Types of gallstones
- Pure cholesterol (10%). Often solitary, large (>2.5cm), round.
- Pure pigment (bile salts 10%). Pigment stones are of two types:
  - Black (associated with haemolytic disease).
  - Brown (associated with chronic cholangitis and biliary parasites).
- Mixed (80%). Most common; usually multiple.

Predisposing conditions
- Increasing age.
- Female (pregnancy and use of the oral contraceptive).
- Obesity.
- Multiparity.
- Chronic haemolytic disorders (only for pigment stones).
- Long-term parenteral nutrition (alteration of bile constituents).
- Previous surgery (e.g. vagotomy or resection of the terminal ileum) or disease involving the distal small bowel (e.g. Crohn's disease)—alteration of bile constituents.

Clinical features (common presentations)

Biliary colic Intermittent severe epigastric and right upper quadrant pain; usually associated with nausea and vomiting. Resolves after few hours; tenderness over gall bladder during acute episodes.

Acute cholecystitis
Severe continuous right upper quadrant pain; often radiates to right flank and back associated with anorexia and pyrexia. Tenderness over gall bladder during inspiration (Murphy's sign).
  Complications of acute cholecystitis include:
- Formation of an empyema or abscess of the gall bladder (rare). Indicated by high swinging fever and severe localized pain;
- Perforation with biliary peritonitis (very rare).
- Cholecystoenteric fistula formation (may lead to a gallstone entering and obstructing the distal ileum ('gallstone ileus'; see p. 302);
- Jaundice due to compression of the adjacent common bile duct by pressure ('Mirizzi syndrome').

Chronic cholecystitis Repeated episode of infection causes thickening and fibrosis of gall bladder.

Mucocele Stone in neck of gall bladder; bile is absorbed, but mucus secretion continues, producing a large, tense globular mass in right upper quadrant.

Empyema Abscess of gall bladder.

Diagnosis and investigations

- FBC, U&E, LFTs, blood culture, serum amylase—in acute presentations
- *Abdominal X-ray*. Only 10% of calculi are radio-opaque.
- *Oral cholecystogram* (Graham–Cole test). Rarely used.
- *Ultrasound*. Procedure of choice; identifies stones, determines wall thickness, and assesses ductal dilatation.
- *Hepatobiliary iminodiacetic acid (HIDA) scan*. Useful when ultrasound findings are equivocal.

Surgical treatment

Cholecystectomy

Majority done laparoscopically; often done as a day case. This is the treatment of choice for all patients fit for GA. Indicated for:

- Patients with symptoms deemed to be due to gall bladder stones.
- Asymptomatic patients with gall bladder stones at risk of complications (diabetics, porcelain gall bladder (15–20% associated with carcinoma), history of pancreatitis, long-term immunosuppressed).

Risks of laparoscopic cholecystectomy

- Conversion to open operation, 5–10%.
- Bile duct injury, <1%.
- Bleeding, 2%.
- Bile leak, 1%.

Non-surgical treatments

Percutaneous drainage of gall bladder

- Done under ultrasound or CT guidance.
- Used for empyema of the gall bladder in patients unsuitable for emergency cholecystectomy.
- After resolution of the infection, the calculi may be removed percutaneously.

Dissolution therapy

- Rarely used. Requires a functioning gall bladder, small stones.
- Problems—requires prolonged treatment, <70% response, high rate of recurrence of stones, side effects of medication (diarrhoea, pruritus).

Extracorporeal shock wave lithotripsy Hardly ever used; risk of visceral injury and high risk of stone recurrence.

Common bile duct stones

Key facts
- Types of stones as per gall bladder stones (see 📖 p. 316).
- Common bile duct (CBD) stones present in 10% of patients with gallstones.
- Most pass from the gall bladder into the CBD (secondary duct stones).
- Rarely form within the CBD (primary duct stones); almost always associated with partial duct obstruction.

Clinicopathological features

Asymptomatic Usually found incidentally on ultrasound for gall bladder stones.

Obstructive jaundice
- Usually due to CBD stone causing obstruction; rarely due to stone-induced CBD stricture.
- Anorexia, nausea, itching.
- Dark urine and pale stools.
- Epigastric pain and fever more common with CBD stones than other cause; due to associated low grade bile infection.
- A palpable, distended gall bladder is rare with CBD stones.

> **Courvoisier's law**
> 'If in the presence of jaundice, the gall bladder is palpable, then the cause of the jaundice is unlikely to be due to stone.'
>   This is due to the fact that CBD stones originate in the gall bladder which is usually scarred and fibrotic, preventing distension.

Ascending cholangitis Constant severe right upper quadrant pain, obstructive jaundice, and high swinging fever ('Charcot's triad').

Acute pancreatitis Sixty per cent of acute pancreatitis in adults in the UK is due to gallstones (see 📖 p. 316).

Diagnosis and investigations
Basic tests
FBC (↑ WCC in cholangitis and pancreatitis), U&E, creatinine, LFTs (↑ conjugated bilirubin and alkaline phosphatase), serum amylase (↑ in pancreatitis), clotting studies.

Advanced tests
Ultrasound (transabdominal)
- Best first-line investigation.
- Accuracy low for distal CBD stones, in acute presentations, obesity, with extensive overlying bowel gas.

MRCP
- Investigation of choice for inconclusive ultrasound result.
- Non-invasive, avoids radiation exposure, highly accurate.

ERCP
- Used diagnostically for patients unable to tolerate MRCP (claustrophobia).
- Mainly reserved for therapeutic interventions:
  - Endoscopic sphincterotomy (ES) and stone extraction or destruction (lithotrypsy).
  - Stent insertion for unextractable stones.
- Risks of ERCP (↑ with ES):
  - Haemorrhage.
  - Acute pancreatitis.
  - Ascending infection.
  - Perforation (usually retroduodenal, may cause peritonitis).

PTC
- Used for failure of ERCP as therapeutic procedure (often in combination with ERCP).
- Risks include sepsis, tube movement, leakage around the tube, and dehydration.

Treatment
Principles of treatment of CBD stones are as follows.

Emergency treatment of CBD stones
- Indicated in unresolving gallstone pancreatitis, unresolving ascending cholangitis.
- Usually ERCP with stone extraction or stent insertion.
- Occasionally PTC required.

Elective treatment of CBD stones
- Indicated for:
  - All patients having had complications (pancreatitis, cholangitis, obstructive jaundice).
  - All patients with gall bladder stones due for cholecystectomy.
- Usually by ERCP or combined ERCP/PTC.
- Common bile duct exploration required at time of cholecystectomy (laparoscopic or open) if ERCP/PTC fail or impossible or as surgeon's preference. Open CBD exploration may require a T-tube to be left in the CBD.

Treatment of persistent CBD stones after cholecystectomy
- Rarely necessary with more accurate preoperative diagnosis and more effective preoperative treatments.
- Stones can be extracted via a T-tube track if present (6 weeks after surgery with radiologically guided basket extraction).
- Post-operative ERCP is rarely required.

Chronic pancreatitis

Key facts

- Characterized by recurrent or persistent abdominal pain arising from the pancreas.
- Often associated with exocrine or endocrine pancreatic insufficiency.
- Characterized by irreversible destruction and fibrosis of pancreatic parenchyma.
- May arise following one or more episodes of acute pancreatitis or may be a chronic progressive process *de novo*.

Pathological features

- The process may affect the whole or part of the gland (focal).
- The head tends to be the most severely involved part in chronic alcohol disease.
- Features of acute pancreatitis may occur—oedema, acute inflammatory infiltrate, focal necrosis, intraparenchymal haemorrhage.
- Chronic inflammatory changes cause progressive disorganization of the pancreas:
  - Glandular atrophy and duct ectasia.
  - Microcalcification and intraductal stone formation with cystic changes secondary to duct occlusion.

Causes and clinical features

Causes

- Recurrent acute pancreatitis of any cause, especially alcohol.
- Secondary to pancreatic ductal obstruction:
  - Pancreatic head cysts, tumours.
  - Pancreatic duct strictures—post-surgery, ERCP, parasitic infestation.
  - Congenital pancreatic abnormalities (pancreas divisum, annular pancreas).
  - Cystic fibrosis.
- Associated with autoimmune diseases (primary biliary cirrhosis, primary sclerosing cholangitis).
- Congenital idiopathic chronic pancreatitis.

Features of chronic inflammation

- Recurrent or chronic abdominal pain:
  - Typically epigastric, radiating to the back and requiring opiates.
  - Worse with food, alcohol.

Features of exocrine failure

- Anorexia and weight loss (due to protein malabsorption).
- Steatorrhoea (due to fat malabsorption); soft, greasy, foul-smelling stools that typically float on water.

Features of endocrine failure Insulin-dependent diabetes mellitus (due to loss of β islet cells).

Diagnosis and investigations

Basic tests
- Plain abdominal X-ray may show pancreatic calcification.
- Abdominal ultrasound may show cystic change and duct dilatation within the pancreas.

Advanced tests
- *Pancreatic CT scan.*
  - May identify a cause, e.g. anatomical variants, tumours, cysts.
  - May show extent of disease. Pancreatic atrophy, disorganization of pancreatic ducts, altered acinar pattern with fibrosis, calcification, and cystic change.
- *MRI scan.* May show the same changes as CT.
- *ERCP.* Demonstrates irregularity of the pancreatic duct strictures, calculi, dilated segments ('chain of lakes'), and changes in first and second order branches and cyst formation; a secondary effect from involvement of the head is stricture of the bile duct, leading to an 'obstructive' pattern of LFTs.

Treatment
- *Prevention of cause/progressive damage.*
  - Stop alcohol, deal with gallstones, treat autoimmune disease.
  - Encourage a diet rich in antioxidants (vitamins A, C, E, selenium).
- *Control symptoms/complications.*
  - Dietary modifications. Adequate carbohydrates and protein, reduced fat.
  - Pancreatic exocrine enzyme supplements (e.g. Creon®).
  - Analgesia. May require opiates (e.g. MST) or coeliac plexus block.
  - Control of diabetes mellitus often requires insulin; control is often difficult due to variable pancreatic function.

Surgical treatment Indications include the following.
- Treatment of reversible cause (anatomical abnormalities, tumours, cysts, ductal strictures and stones). Operations used include those to remove causes and those to drain an obstructed pancreatic duct:
  - Pancreaticoduodenectomy (Whipple procedure).
  - Partial pancreatectomy of the head (Frey procedure) or tail (distal pancreatectomy).
  - Pancreaticojejunostomy (Peustow or Duval procedure).
- Treatment of severe intractable pain or multiple relapses. Operations are usually to resect affected portion:
  - Partial pancreatectomy of the head (Frey procedure) or tail (distal pancreatectomy).
  - Total pancreatectomy.
- Complications (pseudocyst, obstruction, fistula, infections, portal hypertension).

Resectional surgery is associated with increasing risk of exocrine and endocrine pancreatic failure and high risk of complications. All surgery is associated with a risk of symptom recurrence due to recurrent or progressive disease.

Portal hypertension

Key facts Normal portal vein pressure is 5–10mmHg. Portal hypertension (PH) develops when the portal pressure is greater than 12mmHg.

Causes and pathological features

Causes

- *Prehepatic.* Congenital portal vein atresia or portal vein thrombosis due to neonatal umbilical sepsis, phlebitis of the portal vein from abdominal infection (e.g. acute appendicitis or diverticulitis), trauma, or a thrombosed portocaval shunt.
- *Hepatic.* Cirrhosis (e.g. alcoholic most frequently in the UK), chronic active hepatitis, and parasitic diseases (e.g. schistosomiasis).
- *Post-hepatic.* Budd–Chiari syndrome (hepatic vein thrombosis), constrictive pericarditis, or tricuspid valve incompetence (rare).

Features and complications

- Decreased or reversed portal blood flow to the liver promotes the development of portosystemic anastomosis between the portal system and systemic circulation:
  - Left gastric vein into the oesophageal veins at the gastro-oesophageal junction—oesophageal and gastric varices.
  - Superior rectal into inferior rectal veins at the lower rectum—rectal varices.
  - Obliterated umbilical vein into the epigastric veins—'caput medusae'.
- Oesophageal or gastric varices may bleed torrentially.
- Liver cell dysfunction/liver failure occurs in hepatic and post-hepatic causes.
- Ascites. In part due to portal hypertension, but may be due to associated liver dysfunction.
- Splenomegaly (hypersplenism may result).
- The Child–Pugh classification is used to assess the severity of portal hypertension (see Table 8.2).

Diagnosis and investigations

Many investigations may be used at different times in PH.

- FBC, U&Es, LFTs, and clotting.
- Screening tests for causes of cirrhosis (see 📖 p. 324).
- CT and ultrasound scan to assess liver morphology, diagnose PH, and assess cause.
- Transabdominal Doppler ultrasound to assess blood flow in the portal vein and hepatic artery.
- Gastroscopy in acute variceal bleeding (see 📖 p. 272).

Treatment

Cause

- Anticoagulation for Budd–Chiari syndrome.
- Treatment for hepatic causes.

Table 8.2 The Child–Pugh classification of portal hypertension

	1 point	2 points	3 points
Bilirubin (µmol/L)	<34	34–51	>51
Albumin (g/L)	>35	28–35	<28
PT (s)	<3	3–10	>10
Ascites	None	Moderate	Moderate–severe
Encephalopathy	None	Moderate	Moderate–severe

Grade A: 5–6 points; Grade B: 7–9 points; Grade C: 10–15 points.

Chronic complications
- *Oesphago-gastric varices.*
  - Beta-blockers (e.g. propranolol or nadolol) reduce portal venous pressure.
  - Repeated injection sclerotherapy or variceal ligation.
  - Elective portosystemic shunts (e.g. splenorenal anastomosis).
  - Liver transplant may be considered for treatment if associated with severe liver disease.
- *Rectal varices.* Injection sclerotherapy.
- *Symptomatic splenomegaly or hypersplenism.* Splenectomy (laparoscopic or open).
- *Ascites.* Oral spironolactone; in cases of tense ascites, paracentesis may be required with IV albumin replacement.

Acute complications Bleeding oesophago-gastric varices.

Key revision points—anatomy of portal circulation
- The hepatic portal circulation carries blood from the GI tract (from the distal oesophagus to the anorectal junction) to the liver.
- Portosystemic anastomoses occur in 'junctional' areas of venous drainage.
  - Left gastric veins (portal) and oesophageal veins (hemi/azygous veins) at the gastro-oesophageal junction.
  - Superior rectal veins (portal) and inferior rectal veins (pudendal veins) in the lower rectum.
  - Pancreatic and duodenal veins (portal) and retroperitoneal (hemi/azygous) veins in the upper retroperitoneum.
  - Umbilical vein (portal) into the epigastric veins at the umbilicus.
- Portal venous blood drains into liver venous sinusoids and hence into the hepatic veins.

Cirrhosis of the liver

Key facts
- Commonest cause of liver failure in the UK.
- Commonest cause is alcohol-related.

Causes
- *Congenital.*
  - Haemochromatosis.
  - Wilson's disease.
  - Other metabolic disorders (e.g. α1-anti-trypsin deficiency).
- *Acquired.*
  - Alcohol intake.
  - Chronic hepatitis (autoimmune, infective types B, C, and D, drug-induced).
  - Primary biliary cirrhosis.
  - Secondary biliary cirrhosis (gallstones, strictures, cholangitis).
  - Hepatic vein obstruction, e.g. Budd–Chiari syndrome.
  - Idiopathic.

Pathological features
Cirrhosis is characterized by fibrosis of the liver parenchyma, nodular regeneration, and hepatocellular necrosis.
- Micronodular form. Small and uniform nodules (<4mm in diameter), separated by thin fibrous septa uniformly throughout the liver.
- Macronodular form. Larger nodules separated by wider scars and irregularly distributed throughout the liver.
- Mixed.

Clinical features
- One-third of cirrhosis patients are compensated, i.e. do not produce any clinical symptoms, and are incidentally discovered during a medical examination, at operation, or at autopsy.
- Two-thirds are decompensated, i.e. have features of liver cell dysfunction or complications.

Features fall into three broad groups.

Portal hypertension See p. 322.
Hepatocellular failure
- Jaundice.
- Spider naevi.
- Ascites.
- Hypoalbuminaemia.
- Clotting disorders.
- Encephalopathy.
- Gynaecomastia and testicular atrophy.
- Hepatorenal syndrome (renal failure in the setting of hepatic failure due to renal vasoconstriction of unknown aetiology).

Malignant change
- Hepatatocellular carcinoma (particularly chronic hepatitis B infection).
- Often indicated by sudden rapid decrease in hepatocellular function.

Diagnosis and investigation
Diagnosis of cause
- Metabolic screen (e.g. serum copper).
- Hepatitis screen (A, B, C, D, E; EBV, CMV).
- Autoimmune screen (anti-mitochondrial antibodies, anti-smooth muscle antibodies).
- Abdominal ultrasound and CT may show type of cirrhosis, intra- or extra-hepatic biliary dilatation, extrahepatic obstructive causes.
- Liver biopsy to confirm diagnosis and establish type, activity, evolution, and cause.

Investigation of severity or complications
- LFTs (transaminases, γGT, albumin, bilirubin).
- Clotting studies (PT).
- Transabdominal ultrasound or CT scan (splenomegaly and ascites).

Treatment
Removal of the cause/prevent progression
- Abstinence from alcohol.
- Interferon α. Chronic hepatitis B, response rate <50%.
- Combination therapy (interferon α and ribavirin for 6 months. Moderate to severe hepatitis C.
- Immunosuppression for autoimmune causes.

Treatment of complications
- PH (see 📖 p. 322).
- *Encephalopathy*. Treatment aims to lower the amount of nitrogen absorbed from the gut.
  - Administration of oral lactulose.
  - Oral, non-absorbable antibiotics.
  - Careful IV fluid replacement to prevent sodium overload.
  - Diet of high carbohydrate, low salt, moderate protein.
- *Ascites*. Oral spironolactone; in cases of tense ascites, paracentesis may be required with IV albumin replacement.
- *Decompensated hepatocellular failure*. Consider liver transplant.

Pancreatic cancer

Key facts
- Fourth commonest solid organ cancer in the UK.
- Incidence is increasing rapidly.
- Eighty per cent of cases occur between the sixth and seventh decades.
- Risk factors include cigarette smoking, increasing age, high fat diet, diabetes mellitus, excessive alcoholism, and chronic pancreatitis.
- Occupational hazards, e.g. exposure to naphthylene and benzidine.
- There may be hereditary factors involved as 1 in 20 patients with pancreatic cancer have a family history of pancreatic cancer.

Pathological features
- Ninety per cent ductal adenocarcinoma.
- Seven per cent mucinous cystic neoplasms (mucinous cystadenoma/cystadenocarcinoma), serous cystadenoma, and papillary cystic tumour.
- Three per cent islet cell tumours.

Clinical features
Carcinoma of the head of pancreas (65%)
- Obstructive jaundice (90%). Due to compression or invasion of the CBD. Gall bladder is typically palpable.
- Pain (70%). Epigastric or left upper quadrant, often vague and radiates to the back.
- Hepatomegaly. Due to metastases.
- Anorexia, nausea and vomiting, fatigue, malaise, dyspepsia, and pruritus.
- Acute pancreatitis. Occasionally the first presenting feature.
- Thrombophlebitis migrans (10%). Presents as emboli; splenic vein thrombosis may lead to splenomegaly in 10% of patients.

Carcinoma of the body (25%) and tail (10%)
- Usually asymptomatic in the early stages.
- Weight loss and back pain (60%).
- Epigastric mass.
- Jaundice suggests spread to hepatic hilar lymph nodes or metastases.
- Thrombophlebitis migrans (7%).
- Diabetes mellitus (15%).

Diagnosis and investigations
- FBC, LFTs, blood sugar.
- Elevated serum CA 19–9 (sensitivity 90%; specificity 70% for diagnosis). Level correlates with the tumour volume.
- Transabdominal ultrasound scan (sensitivity 70%; 30% in lesions <2cm).
- Doppler ultrasound images blood flow in the portal vein and superior mesenteric vessels.
- Helical CT scan of pancreas with dual phase IV contrast assesses size of the primary lesion, vascular invasion, and distant metastasis.

- FNAC. Usually CT or ultrasound-guided (specificity 99%; sensitivity 50–70%).
- EUS more accurate than CT in detecting pancreatic lesions <3cm in diameter and peripancreatic lymph node involvement.
- PET may help differentiate neoplastic from non-neoplastic lesions and may be used to exclude extra-pancreatic spread that would preclude surgical resection.
- ERCP is 85% accurate; can provide cytology as well as achieving biliary drainage via insertion of a stent.
- Selective angiography or CT angiography used to assess resectability based on encasement of the major vessels.
- Laparoscopy used to rule out peritoneal disease and liver metastasis <2cm prior to offering surgical resection.

Treatment
Palliative treatment
The majority of tumours (95%) are not suitable for surgical resection due to presence of metastases, local invasion, involved lymph glands, age, or comorbidity of patient.

Relief of jaundice
Obstructive jaundice is associated with pruritus, coagulopathy, immuno-logical and nutritional derangement, deterioration in liver function, risk of acute renal failure (hepatorenal syndrome), and increased susceptibility to infection. Relief of jaundice is achieved by:
- Endoscopic biliary stenting by ERCP.
- Percutaneous biliary drainage by PTC and internal stenting or insertion of an internal-external drainage catheter.
- Surgical biliary drainage by cholecystojejunostomy or choledoco-jejunostomy.

Relief of duodenal obstruction Surgical gastric bypass (gastrojejunostomy).

Relief of pain
- Oral morphine (oramorph or MST).
- Chemical ablation of the coeliac ganglia (percutaneous coeliac nerve block or thoracoscopic division of the splanchnic nerves are alternatives).

Curative treatment Radical surgical resection is the only hope of cure if patient is suitable.
- Pancreatoduodenectomy (Whipple's operation) for periampullary tumours and cancer of the pancreas confined to the head.
- Total pancreatectomy for extensive tumour.
- Distal pancreatectomy for tumours in the tail.

Adjuvant therapy For advanced disease, adjuvant chemotherapy (e.g. 5-flu-orouracil) improves prognosis.

Prognosis Poor; even in patients with resectable disease, the 5y survival is 12%.

Cancer of the liver, gall bladder, and biliary tree

Key facts

- Commonest tumours of the liver are metastatic (pancreas, colon, stomach, oesophagus, and breast).
- Thirty-five per cent of patients who die of malignant disease have hepatic metastases.

Clinicopathological features

Hepatocellular carcinoma (HCC)

- Ninety per cent of primary liver tumours, but <1% of all new cancers in UK.
- Common in Africa and Asia; commoner in men than women.
- Risk factors:
  - Cirrhosis, especially due to chronic viral hepatitis (HBV/HCV) or alcohol.
  - Aflatoxin exposure, contraceptives, and androgens.
- Arises from liver parenchymal cells, spreads via local invasion, via portal vein invasion to other sites in the liver, or via hepatic vein invasion to distant metastases (e.g. lung).
- Commonest presentation—rapid deterioration in pre-existing cirrhosis.

Cholangiocarcinoma

- Usually arises in the extrahepatic biliary tree, but may be intrahepatic.
- Typical sites are distal CBD, common hepatic duct, confluence of hepatic ducts ('Klatskin tumour').

Adenocarcinoma of the gall bladder

- Gallstones are found in 70% of cases.
- Associated with ulcerative colitis and primary sclerosing cholangitis.
- Often diagnosed incidentally as unexpected finding during or after cholecystectomy for 'benign' disease causing right upper quadrant pain.
- May present as a gall bladder mass or obstructive jaundice due to local invasion of the common hepatic duct.
- Spread is direct into liver tissue (possibly resectable), to hilar lymph nodes, or blood-borne (incurable).

Ampullary carcinoma

- Typically small and presents relatively early due to the early onset of painless obstructive jaundice.
- Best prognosis of all hepatobiliary cancers due to early presentation before local or lymphatic spread.

Other primary liver cancers

- Fibrolamellar carcinoma (FLC).
  - Usually affects younger patients (3rd and 4th decades).
  - Does not occur on a background of liver disease.
  - Presents as a large vascular mass.

- Angiosarcoma.
  - Less than 1% of liver tumours (most common sarcoma of the liver).
  - Associated with exposure to arsenicals, vinyl chloride, anabolic steroids, and contraceptives.

Diagnosis and investigations
- AFP >500ng/mL highly suggestive of HCC, even in cirrhosis.
- Ultrasound scan often identifies site and cause of biliary obstruction; good assessment of liver parenchyma.
- Needle biopsy to confirm diagnosis of HCC.
- ERCP. Diagnosis of ampullary and bile duct carcinoma; allows biopsy or brush cytology of distal tumours; allows therapeutic stenting.
- MRCP. Diagnosis of proximal tumours or where ERCP not possible.
- PTC. Diagnosis of intrahepatic biliary tumours, therapeutic stenting, or external drainage of proximal biliary tumours.
- CT scan. Assessment of local spread (including blood vessels), lymph nodes, metastases.

Treatment
Curative
- Surgery offers the only cure for primary liver or biliary cancers.
- Patients suitable for resection must:
  - Be fit for major surgery.
  - No evidence of metastases or involved lymph nodes (rare).
  - Tumours technically suitable for complete resection (rare).
- Surgical options for resection include:
  - Partial hepatectomy (HCC).
  - Liver transplantation (HCC associated with chronic hepatitis).
  - Radical cholecystectomy (adenocarcinoma of gall bladder).
  - Radical excision of bile duct with reconstruction (cholangiocarcinoma).
  - Pancreaticoduodenectomy (Whipple procedure) (distal cholangiocarcinoma or ampullary carcinoma).

Palliative
- Endoscopic or percutaneous stenting for unresectable cholangiocarcinoma or ampullary carcinoma.
- Chemotherapy is of minimal benefit in any primary liver or biliary cancers.
- Embolization. Percutaneous thermal or radiofrequency ablation (HCC).

Prognosis
- *HCC.* 5y survival 44% if surgically resectable.
- *Cholangiocarcinoma.* Median survival 9 months.
- *Adenocarcinoma of gall bladder.* 5y survival <5%.

About 20% of these tumours are resectable at the time of diagnosis.

Acute variceal haemorrhage

Key facts Mortality rate of first variceal bleed with established PH is 30%.

Causes and features

See 📖 p. 294 for differential diagnosis. Typical variceal bleeding is:

- Rapid onset, copious dark red venous blood with little mixing with food.
- Features of established PH, e.g. caput medusa.
- Features of developing hepatic encephalopathy (ingested blood provides an extremely protein-rich 'meal').

Emergency management

Resuscitation (see Fig. 8.1)

- Establish large calibre IV access. Give crystalloid fluid up to 1000mL if tachycardic or hypotensive. Only use O –ve blood if the patient is *in extremis*; otherwise wait for cross-matched blood if transfusion needed.
- Catheterize and place on a fluid balance chart.
- Send blood for FBC (Hb, WCC), U&E (Na, K), LFTs (albumin), cross-match (at least 3U if haematemesis large), clotting.
- Always consider alerting HDU/ITU; variceal bleeds can deteriorate extremely rapidly.
- Monitor pulse rate, BP, and urine output (urinary catheter).
- Insertion of a Sengstaken–Blakemore gastro-oesophageal tube may be a life-saving resuscitation manoeuvre. Usually only inserted without a prior gastroscopy if the patient is known to have varices and has life-threatening bleeding. Key points are the following.
  - If the patient needs a 'Sengstaken' tube, they need to be on ITU.
  - Most patients need sedation or a GA for the tube to be inserted.
  - The tube is inserted and the gastric balloon blown up first and traction applied gently until the tube becomes fixed; this alone may stop the bleeding if the varices are gastric.
  - If bleeding continues, the oesophageal balloon is blown up to a pressure around 20–30mmHg.
  - The oesophageal balloon must be deflated regularly to prevent oesophageal necrosis.

Establish a diagnosis

- Urgent OGD is the investigation of choice (at least within 24h).
  - May require ongoing resuscitation with anaesthetist present.
  - *Never* biopsy suspected varices.
  - Therapeutic interventions, including sclerotherapy and banding, are up to 90% successful at controlling acute bleeds and preventing further interventions.

Early treatment
- Give IV PPI (e.g. omeprazole 40mg); stop all NSAIDs.
- Give IV vasopressin, somatostatin, or octreotide to lower oesophageal variceal pressure.
- Blood transfusion if large volume haematemesis or drop in Hb.
- Ensure that the appropriate surgical team knows of the patient in case surgical intervention is required.
- Consider giving FFP to correct clotting abnormalities.

Definitive management

Considered for failed endoscopic treatment and ongoing bleeding.
- Transjugular intrahepatic portosystemic shunt formation (TIPS) (intrahepatic shunt). May be performed to rapidly reduce the portal pressure, but has the risk of inducing portal encephalopathy.
- Extrahepatic shunt. In portacaval shunts, encephalopathy occurs in 50% of survivors and the procedure is now seldom performed.
- Oesophageal transaction.
  - Left gastric vein devascularization.
  - Extremely high mortality.
  - Low incidence of encephalopathy, but high incidence of recurrent bleeding.

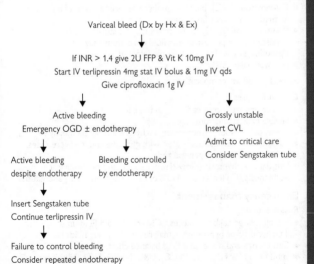

Fig. 8.1 Management of acute variceal haemorrhage.

Acute pancreatitis

Causes and features

Inflammatory process with cascade of release of inflammatory cytokines (TNFα, IL2, IL6, platelet-activating factor (PAF)) and pancreatic enzymes (trypsin, lipases, co-lipases) initiated by pancreatic injury, but which may develop into full blown MODS or SIRS (see 📖 p. 138).

Causes
- Gallstones (60%).
- Alcohol (30%).
- Hyperlipidaemia.
- Hypercalcaemia (hyperparathyroidism, multiple myeloma).
- Direct damage (trauma, ERCP, post-surgery, cardiopulmonary bypass).
- Toxins:
  - Drugs, e.g. azathioprine, oestrogens, thiazides, isoniazid, steroids, NSAIDs.
  - Infection, e.g. viral (mumps, CMV, hepatitis B), mycoplasma.
  - Venom (scorpion, snake bites).
- Idiopathic.

Classification/complications
- Oedematous (70%). May be simple or associated with phlegmon formation; transient fluid collections common.
- Severe/necrotizing (25%). Necrosis may be sterile or infected. Persistent large peripancreatic fluid collections may form ('pseudocyst'), which may become infected.
- Haemorrhagic (5%).

See 📖 p. 138 for complications of SIRS.

Clinical features
- Severe epigastric pain radiating to the back.
- Severe nausea and vomiting.
- Fever, dehydration, hypotension, tachycardia (may be frankly shocked).
- Epigastric tenderness associated with guarding and in severe cases, rigidity which may be generalized.
- Left flank ecchymosis (Grey–Turner's sign) and periumbilical ecchymosis (Cullen's sign), 1–3% of cases haemorrhagic pancreatitis.

Emergency management

Resuscitation
- Establish large calibre IV access. Give crystalloid fluid up to 1000mL if tachycardic or hypotensive; may require ongoing fluids IV.
- Catheterize and place on a fluid balance chart.
- Send blood for FBC (Hb, WCC), U&E (Na, K), LFTs (bilirubin, albumin), amylase, group and save, clotting.
- Monitor pulse rate, BP, and urine output (urinary catheter).
- Consider insertion of a central line and manage patient in HDU if haemodynamically unstable or fails to respond to early resuscitation.
- Assess the severity of the attack by the Glasgow Imrie criteria (see Box 8.1).

Box 8.1 Glasgow Imrie criteria

Three or more positive criteria within 48h of admission = severe attack (mnemonic: PANCREAS):

- **P**aO$_2$ <8kPa.
- **A**ge >55y.
- **N**eutrophils/WCC >15 000 × 10^9/L.
- **C**orrected calcium <2mmol/L.
- **R**aised blood urea >16mmol/L.
- Elevated **E**nzymes, AST>200U/L, LDH >600U/L.
- **A**lbumin <32g/L.
- **S**ugar, blood glucose >10mmol/L.

Establish a diagnosis

- *Serum amylase >1000U.* Diagnostic, but may be normal even in severe cases; elevated amylase may occur in a wide range of other acute abdominal events (intestinal ischaemia, leaking aneurysm, perforated ulcer, cholecystitis).
- *Serum lipase.* Remains elevated longer than serum amylase; more specific, but less sensitive.
- *AXR (non-specific findings).* Absent psoas shadows, 'sentinel loop sign' (dilated proximal jejunal loop adjacent to pancreas because of local ileus), 'colon cut-off sign' (distended colon to mid-transverse colon with no air distally); may show gallstone, pancreatic calcification.
- *CT may be required.* Shows pancreatic oedema, swelling, loss of fat planes; may show haemorrhagic or necrotic complications.
- *Ultrasound scan.* Must be done within 48h of admission to identify gallstones in the bile duct.[1]

Early treatment Urgent ERCP and stone extraction are indicated for proven bile duct stones causing obstruction and pancreatitis.

Definitive management

Identify/prevent complications

- IV antibiotics (e.g. IV imipenem tds), sometimes started in moderate to severe cases even without evidence of infected necrosis.
- CT scan identifies development of pancreatic phlegmon, early fluid collections, necrosis, or haemorrhage.
- CT-guided pancreatic aspiration to identify infected necrosis.
- Early low volume enteral feeding is increasingly used to reduce the risk of stress ulceration and bacterial translocation causing sepsis.

Treatment of early complications

- Consider treating all severe cases on HDU/ITU for optimized fluid balance, respiratory, cardiovascular, and renal support.
- Proven infected necrosis. Surgical debridement may be required, but is associated with a poor prognosis.
- Acute pseudocysts rarely need drainage unless very large.

Overall outcome Mortality is associated with pancreatic necrosis and the presence of sepsis, including MODS.

Reference

1 UK Working Party on Acute Pancreatitis (2005). UK guidelines for the management of acute pancreatitis. *Gut* **54**, iii1–iii9.

Abdominal wall

Abdominal wall hernias

No disease of the human body, belonging to the province of the surgeon, requires in its treatment a better combination of accurate anatomical knowledge with surgical skill than hernia in all its varieties.

Sir Astley Paston Cooper (1804)

Definition of a hernia The abnormal protrusion of a viscus or part of a viscus through a weakness in its containing wall.

Aetiology
- *Congenital.* Associated with a developmental disorder, such as persistent processus vaginalis (infantile inguinal hernia) or failure of complete obliteration of umbilical opening (infantile umbilical hernia).
- *Acquired.* Weakness of the abdominal wall due to ageing or previous surgery; risk increases in conditions where there is ↑ intra-abdominal pressure, such as heavy lifting, chronic cough, straining on urination or defecation, abdominal distension, ascites, pregnancy, etc.

Composition of a hernia
- *Sac.* Peritoneal lining of a hernia; may be complete or incomplete as in sliding hernia (◻ p. 346).
- *Neck of the sack.* At the level of the defect in the abdominal wall where the hernia emerges.
- *Contents.* Bowel or omentum.

Behaviour
- *Reducible.* Contents can be fully restored to the abdominal cavity, spontaneously or with manipulation.
- *Incarcerated.* Part or all of the contents cannot be reduced due to a narrow neck and/or adhesions; there is a risk of strangulation.
- *Obstructed.* Contains an obstructed bowel loop due to kinking; usually goes on to strangulation.

Groin hernias rank third, after adhesive obstruction and cancer, as the most common cause of bowel obstruction in the west. In tropical Africa, strangulated external hernia is the commonest cause of intestinal obstruction.
- *Strangulated.* Blood supply to the contents of the sac is cut off; the tight neck of the peritoneal sac is the usual site of strangulation.

Pathological sequence Venous and lymphatic occlusion → oedema and ↑ venous pressure → impeding arterial flow → bowel necrosis and perforation.

▶ If not diagnosed and managed early, bowel infarction can result and lead to serious complications like peritonitis and septic shock.

Key revision points—general considerations in assessing a patient with a hernia

History
- Is it a hernia? (history of reducibility)
- Site?
- Simple or complicated? Complicated if:
  - Incarcerated: patient can't reduce it anymore.
  - Obstructed: symptoms of bowel obstruction.
  - Strangulated: acute and severe pain, bowel obstruction, and patient is generally unwell.
- Any risk factors? (heavy lifting, COPD, constipation, BPH, previous surgery).

Physical examination
- Confirm the diagnosis and type (reducibility, cough impulse, anatomical location).
- Always examine both sides in suspected groin hernias.
- Any scars? (recurrent or incisional hernia)
- General examination is essential to look for predisposing factors like bowel pathology and BPH.

Decision making
Is surgery warranted? (symptomatic, ↑ risk of strangulation as with narrow neck, patient mobility and fitness for surgery).

Inguinal hernia

Key facts
- It has been estimated that worldwide, >20 million repairs of inguinal hernia are carried out each year and in the UK 100 000.
- Commonest type of abdominal hernia; ♂:♀, 8:1.
- Abdominal contents protrude through the inguinal canal.
- Classified to indirect and direct according to its (surgically determined) relationship to the inferior epigastric artery (see Table 9.1).
- Coexistence of direct and indirect hernias descending either side of the epigastric artery produces a 'pantaloon hernia'.

Clinical features
- Most have no symptoms until a lump is noticed in the groin.
- Ache or dragging sensation, especially towards the end of the day.
- Some can relate the onset of the pain and bulge to a specific activity (e.g. lifting).

Diagnosis and investigations
If the diagnosis is uncertain, investigations are of some help.
- *Ultrasound.* Least invasive and cheap, but may lead to false results.
- *CT and MRI.* Highly accurate, but CT involves substantial radiation.
- *Herniography* (intraperitoneal contrast injection and subsequent X-ray). Aids in the diagnosis in cases of groin pain when no hernia can be felt; rarely performed.

Treatment
- Patients with symptoms or have had episodes of irreducibility or bowel obstruction documented should be offered repair.
- Elderly, immobile patients or those with high morbidity for operation may be safely observed if asymptomatic or mildly symptomatic (annual risk of incarceration is 2–3 per 1000 patients per year).
- A groin truss is of limited symptomatic benefit for non-surgical patients.

Technical aspects
- Repair may be performed by open surgery or via the laparoscopic approach (either transperitoneal or in the pre-peritoneal space).
- General or local anaesthesia if done via the open approach.
- Tension-free reinforcement of the transversalis fascia (TVF) layer (usually with non-absorbable mesh); in open repairs, this lies in front of the TVF and in laparoscopic, behind it).
- Mesh may be fixed in place by sutures (open) or 'tacking' devices (laparoscopic approach).
- Avoid heavy lifting and straining for first to second week post-op.
- Lifetime recurrence of combined mesh repairs is approximately 1–2%.
- Laparoscopic approach is recommended for recurrent and bilateral hernias and should be carried out by experienced surgeons in well-equipped units (NICE guidelines).

Table 9.1 Comparison between indirect and direct inguinal hernias

	Indirect	Direct
Age	Any age, but usually young	Uncommon in children and young adult
Aetiology	Congenital (patent processus vaginalis)	Acquired weakness in abdominal wall
Relationship to inferior epigastric artery	Lateral	Medial
Descending to scrotum	Often	Rarely
Occluding the internal ring	Controls it	Does not control it
Neck	Narrow	Wide
Strangulation	More likely	Rare
Treatment	Infant—herniotomy (ligation and excision of the sac) Adult—open mesh repair, laparoscopic repair	Open mesh repair, laparoscopic repair

Key revision points—anatomy of the inguinal canal

- The inguinal canal is the oblique passage through the lower abdominal wall. It runs from deep to superficial, from the internal to the external inguinal rings.
- The inguinal canal transmits the spermatic cord (round ligament in the female) and the ilioinguinal nerve.
- Contents of the spermatic cord are:
  - Three vessels (testicular artery, cremasteric artery, artery to the vas).
  - Three nerves (genital branch of genitofemoral, autonomic supply to the testicle, ilioinguinal nerve).
  - Three structures (vas, pampiniform venous plexus, testicular lymphatics).
  - Three coverings (external spermatic fascia, cremasteric fascia, internal spermatic fascia).
- The **deep ring** is formed through the transversalis fascia and lies 1–2cm above the inguinal ligament, midway between the symphysis pubis and the anterior superior iliac spine.
- The **superficial ring** is a V-shaped defect in the aponeurosis of external oblique, above and medial to the pubic tubercle.
- Direct inguinal hernias pass through a weakness in the transversalis fascia in the **Hesselbach's triangle** area (bounded by inguinal ligament inferiorly, inferior epigastric artery laterally, and lateral border of the rectus muscle medially).

Femoral hernia

Key facts
- Commoner in women than men.
- Occurs through tissues of femoral canal.
- Has a high risk of strangulation due to the neck of the sac having bony and ligamentous structures limiting it on three sides.
- Approximately 30% of femoral hernias present as emergencies; 50% of these require bowel resection for strangulation and ischaemia.

Clinical features
- Appears below and lateral to pubic tubercle, medial to femoral pulse.
- May be asymptomatic until incarceration or strangulation occurs.
- May be mistaken for an upper medial thigh swelling.

Diagnosis and investigations
- Differential diagnosis includes:
  - Low presentation of inguinal hernia.
  - Femoral canal lipoma.
  - Femoral lymph node.
  - Saphena varix (compressible, disappears when lying flat, palpable thrill on coughing or percussion of the saphenous vein).
  - Femoral artery aneurysm (pulsatile).
  - Psoas abscess (fluctuant and lateral to femoral artery).
- Ultrasound scanning may help with the differential diagnosis. If there is significant doubt, exploration is usually indicated due to the high risk of complications in untreated femoral hernia.

Treatment
- All should be repaired because of great risk of strangulation; truss has no place in the management.
- Once the hernia is reduced, the femoral canal should be narrowed by interrupted sutures to prevent recurrence; care must be taken not to narrow the adjacent femoral vein. There are two main approaches.

Low approach (infrainguinal)
- Incision below inguinal ligament approaching femoral canal from below.
- Has the advantage of not interfering with the inguinal structures, but provides little or no scope for resecting any compromised small bowel and so is best reserved for elective surgery.

High approach (inguinal)
- Incision above the inguinal ligament approaching femoral canal from above by dissecting through the posterior wall of the inguinal canal.
- Requires repair of the inguinal canal on closure, but offers excellent access to the peritoneal cavity should small bowel surgery be required and is the usual approach in emergency presentations.

Key revision points—anatomy of the femoral canal

- Lies medial to femoral vein within femoral sheath.
- Contains loose areolar tissue and a lymph node known as the lymph node of Cloquet.
- The femoral ring is the abdominal opening of the femoral canal. The increased diameter of the true pelvis in females proportionally widens the femoral canal.
- Boundaries to the femoral ring are:
  - Anteriorly, inguinal ligament.
  - Medially, lacunar ligament.
  - Posteriorly, pectineal ligament.
  - Laterally, femoral vein.
- An aberrant obturator artery branch of inferior epigastric may cross the lacunar ligament and can cause haemorrhage during surgical repair.
- Femoral hernia repair (open) involves suture-plication of the inguinal and pectineal ligaments or placement of a mesh plug that is fixed in position in the defect with non-absorbable sutures.

Umbilical and epigastric hernias

Key facts
These hernias are sometimes referred to collectively as ventral hernias.
- Umbilical hernias can be divided into:
  - *True umbilical hernias*. Occur through the umbilical cicatrix and are almost always congenital in origin; those present at birth may close spontaneously before the age of 3; more common in Afro-Caribbean races.
  - *Paraumbilical hernias*. Occur through the periumbilical tissues and are always acquired; common in obese and parous women.
- Epigastric hernias are defects in the linea alba somewhere between the xiphisternum and umbilicus at sites of penetration of the linea alba by nerves and vessels; they may be small or extensive.

Clinical features
Umbilical hernia
- Small, centrally placed within the umbilicus.
- Often contains pre-peritoneal fat and rarely contains bowel/omentum.
- May be painful, but rarely strangulates.

Paraumbilical hernia
- Variable in size, up to moderate.
- Paced eccentrically and distorts the shape of the umbilicus.
- May contain bowel or omentum.
- Often painful and occasionally strangulate.

Epigastric hernia
- Variable, up to large defects.
- Always placed in the midline although when large, may lie to one side.
- Most frequently contains only pre-peritoneal fat.
- Moderate risk of strangulation.

Diagnosis and investigations The diagnosis is rarely in doubt. If there is concern that a palpable lump may be a lipoma or subcutaneous tissue growth, then a CT scan can usually confirm the diagnosis.

Treatment
- Congenital umbilical hernias should only be repaired if they persist beyond the age of 2–3y.
- Surgical repair is offered for symptomatic hernias or those with a high risk of complications.

Principles of repair
- Identify edges of hernial sac and reduce hernia.
- Small defects are usually repaired by an overlapping sutured repair using non-absorbable suture, e.g. 0 Prolene, without reinforcements; larger defects or recurrent hernias may be repaired with mesh (usually polypropylene-based, e.g. Prolene).
- Laparoscopic repair is increasingly being used.

Incisional hernias

Key facts
- Incisional hernias are very uncommon outside the abdomen.
- Up to 10% of midline laparotomy wounds suffer herniation to some degree. Factors that predispose to incisional herniation include:
  - Wound infection.
  - Steroid use, anaemia, or malnutrition at the time of original surgery.
  - Incisional hernias are probably slightly less common after muscle splitting or transverse incisions, compared to midline laparotomies.
  - Poor surgical techniques in abdominal closure increase the risk.
- The peak time of presentation is up to 5y after surgery.

Pathological features
The hernia occurs through the tissues in which the incision is made. Typically, the sac is made up of peritoneum, eventrated scar tissue, and subcutaneous scar tissue.

Clinical features
- The hernia may vary from a few cm to a near complete defect in the anterior abdominal wall through which all the mobile viscera regularly protrude.
- The risk of strangulation is maximal in small- to medium-sized defects.

In large and very large defects, the viscera are often permanently herniated and if this has been the case for a long period, they 'lose the right of abode' within the true abdominal cavity. This means that the remaining lateral abdominal wall tissues chronically retract and there may be insufficient room for all the viscera within the revised abdominal cavity when the tissues are re-approximated.

Diagnosis and investigations
When assessing incisional hernias, ask yourself the following.
- What is the risk of complications/strangulation?
- Is it likely that the contents of the hernia can be reduced fully?
- Is the patient able to undergo the anaesthesia necessary for the surgery required?
- Is there a risk of compromise to respiratory function if a very large incisional hernia is reduced and repaired?

Treatment
- Small defects (<4cm). Simple sutured repair.
- Medium and large defects (>4cm). A mesh is placed between the posterior rectus sheath and the rectus muscle fibres. If below the umbilicus, the mesh is placed in the pre-peritoneal space. After the mesh is fixated, the anterior rectus sheath is closed.
- Laparoscopic repair is increasingly being used. The use of an 'underlay' intraperitoneal mesh enhances the repair, but also creates the potential for bowel adhesions or fistula formation.

Polytetrafluoroethylene (PTEF) mesh is recommended to reduce adhesive complications.
- Unfit patients or patients unwilling to have surgery. A custom-made support corset is often useful.

Other types of hernia

These types are rare, but clinically significant.

Spigelian
- Occurs under the lower edge of the linea semilunaris and protrudes along the lateral border of the rectus sheath.
- Typically difficult to diagnose in the supine position.
- Ultrasound and CT scan may help to confirm the diagnosis.
- Has a high risk of complications.
- Repair is via direct sutured repair of the rectus sheath.

Obturator
- Occurs through the obturator canal from the lateral wall of the pelvis with the sac protruding into the medial upper thigh.
- Symptoms include pain or abnormal sensations in the distribution of the obturator nerve in the skin of the inner medial thigh.
- Diagnosis is often very difficult and is usually made by CT scan.
- A high proportion present with complications of bowel obstruction due to the sac being hidden within the adductor muscles compartment.
- The neck is narrow and prone to strangulation.
- Repair can be via exposure of the sac in the medial thigh or, more commonly, at laparotomy for complications.

Lumbar
- Occurs through either the inferior or superior lumbar triangles (bounded by the lumbar muscles, lumbosacral fascia, and bony features of the posterior abdominal wall) or, rarely, through lumbar incisions.
- Usually contain retroperitoneal fat and rarely bowel.
- May be repaired by direct suture or mesh repair for larger defects.

Perineal
- Spontaneous perineal hernias occur through the greater or lesser sciatic foramina and are exceptionally rare.
- Present with acute complications and are diagnosed only at surgery.
- Post-operative perineal hernias occur through the pelvic floor muscles and do so usually as a result of surgical procedures (particularly after abdominoperineal resection of the rectum).
- Repair may be via sutured closure of the defect or, more commonly, filling of the defect with prosthetic material (mesh) or biological tissue (muscle flap).

Sliding
- The sac is formed partly by a retroperitoneal structure.
- It is thought that the structure slides down the canal pulling its overlying peritoneum with it hence the name 'hernia-en-glissade'.

Littre's hernia The hernia sac contains a Meckel's diverticulum.

Richter's hernia Only part of the circumference of the bowel is strangulated.

Rectus sheath haematoma

Key facts

Result from haemorrhage from any of the vascular network within the rectus sheath that is formed by terminal branches of the superior and inferior epigastric arteries.

Clinical features

- Presents with a sudden localized abdominal pain ± a tender mass.
- A history of major or minor blunt trauma may be elicited.
- Some patients report events that cause sudden contraction of the rectus muscle, such as coughing, sneezing, or any vigorous physical activity; it may also develop spontaneously in anticoagulated patients.
- Pain typically increases with contraction of the rectus muscles and a tender mass may be palpated and remains unchanged when the rectus muscle is contracted.

Diagnosis and investigations

- Can be confused with conditions that present with unilateral abdominal pain like appendicitis.
- Hb level and coagulation profile should be checked.
- Ultrasonography may help in the diagnosis; CT is diagnostic.

Treatment

- Small and stable haematomas may be observed without patient hospitalization.
- Bilateral or large haematomas need hospitalization; blood transfusion and reversal of coagulation may be needed.
- Angiographic embolization is required infrequently, but may be necessary in case of haematoma enlargement, free bleeding, or clinical deterioration.
- Surgical ligation of bleeding vessels is indicated if angiographic treatment fails or the patient becomes haemodynamic unstable.

Groin disruption

Key facts

- Also called 'Gilmore's groin' or 'sports hernia' (although hernia is rarely present).
- An overuse syndrome that results in muscular imbalances of the pelvis and abdominal wall muscles.
- Common in male athletes, especially in sports that require repetitive twisting and turning at high speeds (e.g. soccer, tennis, ice hockey).

Pathological features

It has distinctive features that include a torn external oblique aponeurosis, a torn conjoined tendon, a dilated superficial inguinal ring, and a dehiscence between inguinal ligament and conjoined tendon.

Clinical features

- Unilateral groin pain that is often insidious and gradually worsens and is felt 'deep' in the groin area.
- Some patients may identify a distinct provocative event like kicking or a sudden change in direction while playing.
- Pain is almost always absent at rest.
- Physical findings are non-specific. The external inguinal ring may be dilated and tender. Valsalva manoeuvres and resisted adduction may elicit pain and are useful provocative tests.

Diagnosis and investigations

- The differential diagnosis includes osteitis pubis, adductor tendinopathy, and pubic instability or fracture.
- Radiographic findings are usually normal, but helpful in ruling out other conditions. Therefore, it is a clinical diagnosis that is confirmed intra-operatively.

Treatment

- These patients are managed conservatively initially due to the difficulty in making a diagnosis.
- If symptoms persist, surgical repair is indicated and should be carried out by a surgeon who is experienced in managing groin disruption.
- Mesh reinforcement is often utilized during the repair.
- This is followed by 2–4-week rehabilitation programme.

Acute groin swelling

Causes of chronic testicular swelling are discussed on 📖 p. 366.

Causes and features

- *Incarcerated groin hernia* (inguinal or femoral). May or may not be associated with intestinal obstruction; often red, hot, and tender.
- *Acute epididymo-orchitis* (in males). Tenderness is particularly over the spermatic cord and the epididymis.
- *Torsion of the testis.* May present with pain in the groin, but unless the testicle is undescended, the tenderness is primarily over the scrotum (and testis). Testicle is tender, swollen, and high riding. Elevation of the scrotum, unlike epididymitis, makes the pain worse.
- *Iliopsoas abscess.* Tenderness primarily below the inguinal ligament; may be fluctuant, associated tenderness in the RIF due to underlying pathology.
- *Acute iliofemoral lymphadenopathy* (e.g. from infected toenail). Tender diffuse swelling; often multiple palpable lumps (nodes).
- *Acute saphena varix.* Compressible, cough thrill.
- Acute complications of *femoral artery aneurysm.*

Emergency management

Resuscitation

- Establish IV access; consider giving crystalloid fluid if there is a suspicion of a complicated hernia or an iliopsoas abscess.
- Catheterize and place on a fluid balance chart if hypotensive.
- Send blood for FBC (Hb, WCC), U&E (Na, K).
- Group and save and clotting if arterial disease or abscess formation is suspected.

Establish a diagnosis

▶ Torsion of the testis is a true surgical emergency and should not wait for a diagnosis short of exploration.
Colour flow Doppler assessment may be able to confirm the presence of a hyperaemic testis, but unless it is immediately available, it should not delay operation.

▶ If there is a strong clinical history in a young male, immediate operation remains the diagnostic investigation of choice.
- If an iliopsoas abscess is suspected, abdominopelvic CT scanning is the investigation of choice.
- Rigid sigmoidoscopy and biopsy only if not unstable.
- Flexible endoscopy may be indicated, but carries a risk of perforation.

Definitive management

Incarcerated groin hernia

- Repair is indicated for all patients except those considered unfit for any surgical procedure or those declining treatment.
- It may not be possible to establish if the hernia is inguinal or femoral preoperatively; if so, it is safest to approach as if for an inguinal hernia.

- Femoral hernias may be approached via an infrainguinal or transinguinal dissection (see 📖 p. 342).
  - Infrainguinal approaches may be limited in exposure if there is necrotic bowel within the hernia requiring resection.
  - A transinguinal approach will involve repair of the inguinal canal as well, but offers an almost unlimited exposure of the femoral canal from above and allows plenty of exposure for bowel resection.
- Inguinal hernias should be approached through a conventional incision. Repair may require a mesh although there is an increased risk of infection if there is an associated bowel resection.
- Anaesthesia may be general or local with sedation.

Psoas abscess The underlying cause should be identified as a matter or priority. Incision and drainage of the groin collection may be indicated, but only as part of the overall treatment.

Torsion of the testis
- Once identified, the affected testis should assessed; if non-viable, a simple orchidectomy is performed and if viable, an orchidopexy.
- If the diagnosis is confirmed, the contralateral testicle should be fixed by orchidopexy to prevent subsequent torsion.

Epididymo-orchitis Antibiotics PO (e.g. ciprofloxacin 500mg od) for 14 days or IV if severe.

Urology

Symptoms and signs in urology

Symptoms

Pain

- May be located over the site of pathology, e.g. testes.
- May radiate in accordance with innervation of the structure involved.
  - *Kidney pain.* In the renal angle (between the lower border of the 12th rib and the spine).
  - *Ureteric pain.* Between the renal angle and the groin.
  - *Bladder pain.* In the suprapubic region.
  - *Prostatic pain.* In the perineum, but may radiate along the urethra to the tip of the penis.
- May be related to function, e.g. suprapubic pain exacerbated by bladder filling.

Haematuria (macroscopic)

- Frequently a sinister symptom of malignant disease, especially the bladder when it is normally painless.
- When associated with painful voiding, it is usually due to bladder infection or stones.

Lower urinary tract symptoms

- Refers to a group of symptoms that typically affect the ageing male.
- Often caused by bladder outflow obstruction related to prostatic enlargement.
- Includes symptoms related to both voiding and storage.
- Voiding symptoms. Poor urine flow, hesitancy, post-micturition dribbling.
- Storage symptoms. Frequency, nocturia, urgency, urge incontinence.
- International prostate symptom score (IPSS) is a validated questionnaire to estimate the patient's perception of severity of symptoms.

Urinary incontinence

- Affects women more commonly than men.
- *Stress incontinence.* Urine leakage that occurs at times of increased intravesical pressure, e.g. during coughing, sneezing, lifting.
  - Results from incompetence of urethral sphincter and bladder neck mechanism; usually related to pregnancy and childbirth.
- *Urge incontinence.* Urine leakage that occurs in association with a strong desire to void.
  - Urine leaks from the bladder before the patient is able to reach a toilet.
  - Usual cause is overactivity of the detrusor muscle.
  - May be idiopathic or secondary to other bladder disease.
  - Stress and urge incontinence frequently coexist.
- *Insensible urine leakage.* Occurs without any associated symptoms.
  - Urine leaks from the bladder continuously and the patient is sometimes unaware.

- *Causes.* Overflow incontinence from chronic retention, fistulation (commonly between bladder and vagina), gross sphincter disturbance resulting from surgery or neurological disease.

Male sexual dysfunction
- Erectile dysfunction (ED), commonly known as impotence.
  - Inability to attain and maintain an erection adequate for satisfactory sexual intercourse.
  - There are degrees of ED.
  - Men with incomplete ED respond more satisfactorily to treatment.
  - The majority of cases have an organic basis.
  - All cases have a degree of psychogenic involvement.
  - Twenty per cent of cases are primarily psychogenic.
- Premature ejaculation.
  - More common in younger men.
  - Invariably has a psychogenic basis.
  - Often associated with performance anxiety.
- Loss of libido.
  - Loss of normal sex drive.
  - Either psychogenic or related to hypogonadal states.

Haemospermia
- Presence of blood in ejaculate.
- Rarely associated with significant pathology.

Signs

Inspection
Examination of the penis must include retraction of the foreskin (if possible) and inspection of the glans and external meatus for signs of infection, inflammation, or tumour.

Palpation
- Tenderness in the renal angle or a palpable loin mass may indicate renal pathology.
- Suprapubic dullness to percussion is an indication of a bladder mass or full of urine.
- Check for testicular asymmetry, masses, or tenderness (underdevelopment, tumours, and infection).
- Intrascrotal mass may include the testis (e.g. hydrocele) or be separate from it (e.g. epididymal cyst).
- Do a digital rectal examination to determine the size, consistency, regularity, and symmetry of the prostate.

Investigations of urinary tract disease

Laboratory investigations

Urinalysis

- Dipstick analysis for blood, leucocytes, protein, nitrites, and glucose.
  - Nitrites, blood, and leucocytes—infection.
  - Blood—microscopic haematuria.
  - Protein, leucocytes—intrinsic renal disease.
- Microbiology, cytology for presence of urinary infection or malignant cells. Midstream urine (MSU) specimens are required for bacteriological culture; take care to avoid contamination particularly in women.
- Matched urine and serum biochemistry to assess glomerular function, e.g. matched osmolarities, sodiums, and potassiums.

Blood

- Serum creatinine levels. Provides a crude assessment of overall renal function.
- Creatinine (Cr) clearance (requires 24h urine collection and measurement of serum creatinine).

$$\text{Cr clearance (mL/min)} = u \times v/p$$

where u is urine Cr concentration, v is 24h urine volume, p is plasma Cr concentration.

- Serum prostate-specific antigen (PSA). Indicator of prostate disease.
  - Interpreted according to age-specific reference range.
  - High levels are found in benign prostatic hyperplasia, prostate cancer, acute retention, and urinary infection.
- Sex hormone measurements. Occasionally useful in the assessment of male sexual dysfunction and infertility.

Radiology investigations

Ultrasound

- *Renal and bladder scans.* For haematuria and urinary tract infection (UTI).
- *Transrectal ultrasound scan.* Measures prostate accurately and allows systematic biopsy for detection of cancer.
- *Scrotal ultrasound.* Evaluates acute scrotum from a suspected testicular cancer.

Intravenous urogram (IVU)

- Provides greater functional information than ultrasound.
- Provides superior imaging of the ureter.

CT

- Pre- and post-contrast scans provide some functional information with regard to arterial and venous blood flow and excretory function of the kidneys.
- Vital for the staging of renal, bladder, and testicular cancers.

MRI
- Provides greater accuracy than CT in assessment of the prostate capsule and seminal vesicles.
- Sensitive test for the presence of bone metastases.

Isotope bone scan
- Demonstrates abnormal area of bone turnover.
- A useful screening test for the presence of bone metastases.
- Plain films are taken to aid interpretation if the site or pattern of hot spots is indeterminate.

Isotope renography
- Provides anatomical and functional information about the kidneys.
- Dimercaptosuccinate (DMSA) scan provides an image of functioning renal parenchymal tissue.
- ^{99m}Tc-mercaptoacetyltriglycine (MAG3) renogram provides dynamic information regarding excretion from the kidneys and determines whether or not obstruction is present.

Endoscopy

Flexible cystoscopy
- Examines urethra and bladder.
- Performed using local anaesthetic gel.
- There is limited potential for intervention.

Rigid cystoscopy Under GA, permits biopsy and resectoscope allows resection of tissue.

Ureteroscopy
- Rigid and flexible ureteroscopes provide access to the ureter and pelvicalyceal system.
- Allows the passage of instruments and laser fibres for the treatment of stones and upper tract tumours.

Urinary tract stones

Key facts
- Prevalence of stones in the population is around 3%; ♂ > ♀.
- The commonest reason for emergency urological admissions.
- Peak presentation in the summer months.
- Most common age of presentation of urinary calculi is 20–50y.
- Ninety per cent of urinary calculi are radio-opaque.

Aetiology
- Metabolic. Hyperparathyroidism, idiopathic hypercalciuria, disseminated malignancy, sarcoidosis, hypervitaminosis D.
- Familial metabolic causes. Cystinuria, errors of purine metabolism, hyperoxaluria, hyperuricuria, xanthinuria.
- Infection.
- Impaired urinary drainage, e.g. medullary sponge kidney, pelviureteric junction (PUJ) obstruction, ureteric stricture, extrinsic obstruction.

Pathological features
Calcium stones
- Seventy-five per cent of all urinary calculi.
- Usually combined with oxalate or phosphate, are sharp, and may cause symptoms, even when small.

Triple phosphate stones ('struvite stones')
- Compounds of magnesium, ammonium, and calcium phosphate.
- Fifteen per cent of all calculi.
- Commonly occur against a background of chronic urinary infection and may grow rapidly.
- 'Staghorn' calculi (fill the calyceal system) are a form of struvite.

Uric acid stones
- As a consequence of high levels of uric acid in the urine.
- Five per cent of all urinary stones; radiolucent.

Cystine stones
- Relatively rare; 1–2% of all cases.
- Difficult to treat due to extremely hard consistency.

Other stones Xanthine, pyruvate, and other stones; 1% of all calculi.

Clinical features
- 'Ureteric/renal colic'. Severe, intermittent, stabbing pain radiating from loin to groin.
- Microscopic or, rarely, frank haematuria.
- Systemic symptoms such as nausea, vomiting, tachycardia, pyrexia.
- Loin or renal angle tenderness due to infection or inflammation.
- Iliac fossa tenderness if the calculus has passed into the distal ureter.

Investigations
- Basic tests.
  - Raised WCC and CRP suggest superadded infection (should be confirmed by MSU); raised Cr suggests renal impairment.

- Stones often visible on plain abdominal X-ray ('kidneys/ureters/bladder' (KUB)).
- Serum calcium, phosphate, and uric acid.
- 24h urine for calcium, phosphate, oxalate, urate, cystine, and xanthine.
- Advanced tests.
  - Non-contrast spiral CT is the gold standard for locating stones and assessing evidence of complications.
  - IVU will locate stones and show any proximal obstruction.
  - Renal ultrasound scan for hydronephrosis.

Treatment

Acute presentations (renal colic, ureteric obstruction)

- Analgesia, e.g. diclofenac 100mg PR; antiemetic, e.g. metoclopramide 10mg IV; IV fluids.
- Small stones (<0.5cm) may be managed expectantly as most will pass spontaneously.
- Emergency treatment with percutaneous nephrostomy and/or ureteric stent insertion is necessary if either pain or obstruction is persistent.

Elective presentations

- *Extracorporeal shock wave lithotripsy (ESWL).*
  - Focused, externally generated electrohydraulic or ultrasonic shock waves.
  - Targeted onto the calculus using ultrasound, X-ray, or a combination.
  - Causes stone disintegration and the fragments are then voided.
- *Percutaneous nephrolithotomy (PCNL).*
  - For stones in the renal pelvis or calyces and occasionally for stones in the upper ureter.
  - Percutaneous track into the renal pelvis using fluoroscopic guidance.
  - Nephroscope is inserted and the calculus visualized.
  - Removed either in total or, if large, following fragmentation.
- *Endoscopic treatment.*
  - Ureteroscope is inserted and the stone visualized.
  - Stone is fragmented using ultrasound, electrohydraulic intracorporeal lithotripsy, or laser.
- *Open nephrolithotomy/ureterolithotomy.* For large staghorn calculi or complex stones, e.g. above ureteric stricture.

Prevention of recurrence

- Increase oral fluid intake and reduce calcium intake.
- Correct metabolic abnormalities.
- Treat infection promptly.
- Urinary alkalization, e.g. sodium bicarbonate 5–10g/24h PO in water (mainly for cystine and urate stones).
- Thiazide diuretics (for idiopathic hypercalciuria).

Obstruction of the ureter

(See Fig. 10.1)

Key facts Ureteric obstruction leads to hydronephrosis (ureteric and pelvicalyceal dilatation).

Pathological features Hydronephrosis can be unilateral or bilateral.

Unilateral
- Extramural.
  - Aberrant vessels at the PUJ.
  - Extrinsic tumour. Carcinoma of the cervix, prostate, large bowel, or retroperitoneal endometriosis.
  - Idiopathic retroperitoneal fibrosis.
  - Post-radiation fibrosis.
  - Retrocaval ureter.
  - Abdominal aortic aneurysm.
- Intramural.
  - Transitional cell carcinoma of the renal pelvis or ureter.
  - Urinary calculi.
  - Ureteric stricture.
  - Aperistaltic segment. Almost always congenital.

Bilateral
- All causes of unilateral obstruction may cause bilateral hydronephrosis.
- Congenital posterior urethral valve.
- Congenital or acquired urethral stricture.
- Benign enlargement of the prostate.
- Locally advanced prostate cancer.
- Large bladder tumours.
- Gravid uterus.

Clinical features
- Loin pain.
- Fever and/or rigors (if complicated by infection).
- Symptoms and signs of renal failure (if obstruction longstanding).

Investigation and diagnosis
- Serum biochemistry and haematology.
- MSU.
- KUB X-ray/IVU.
- Ultrasound scan and/or CT scan.
- Isotope renogram.
- Retrograde pyelogram.

Complications
- Infection, pyonephrosis.
- Hypertension.
- Renal failure.

Treatment

▶▶ *Emergency presentation*

- Emergency treatment is indicated if there are signs of infection, established renal failure, uncontrollable symptoms.
- Treatment is drainage of the kidney via a percutaneous nephrostomy or retrograde ureteric stent.

Elective presentation

- Definitive treatment is directed at the underlying cause. Possible interventions include:
  - Treatments of calculi (see 📖 p. 358).
  - Ureteric stenting (unilateral or bilateral).
  - Ureterolysis and ureteric transfer (for retroperitoneal fibrosis).
  - Prostatic resection.
  - Bladder drainage using a urethral or suprapubic catheter.
- In cases where renal function cannot be restored, a nephrectomy is performed to avoid infective complications.

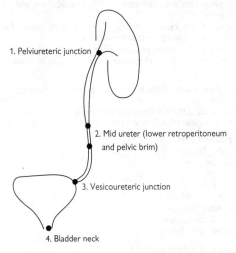

1. Pelviureteric junction

2. Mid ureter (lower retroperitoneum and pelvic brim)

3. Vesicoureteric junction

4. Bladder neck

Fig. 10.1 Commonest sites of renal stone impaction. 1, pelviureteric junction; 2, pelvic brim; 3, vesicoureteric junction.

Benign prostatic hyperplasia

Key facts

- Benign prostatic hyperplasia (BPH) is a non-malignant enlargement of the prostate gland. There is an increase in both stromal and glandular components.
- Incidence of BPH is about 25% in age 40–60y, 40% in over 60s.
- Commonest cause of lower urinary tract symptoms (LUTS) in middle-aged and elderly men.

Pathological features

Aetiology is largely unknown. Possible factors include:

- Androgens. No BPH in those who have had early castration.
- Oestrogens. Increased oestrogen:testosterone ratio with age.
- Growth factors, e.g. high concentration of TGFα in BPH.

Clinical features

Symptoms

- Storage symptoms, such as frequency, urgency, nocturia, and incontinence.
- Voiding symptoms, including hesitancy, poor stream, intermittency, terminal dribble, and abdominal straining.
- Superimposed infection may cause dysuria and haematuria.
- Incomplete emptying and chronic or acute retention of urine.

Signs

- Smooth enlargement of the prostate detected by digital rectal examination.
- Possible palpable bladder if chronic retention.
- Always examine for neurological signs in those with LUTS.

Complications of BPH

- Intractable LUTS.
- Haematuria.
- UTI.
- Stone formation.
- Acute retention of urine.
- Chronic retention of urine.
- Overflow incontinence.
- Obstructive renal failure.

Diagnosis and investigations

- Prostate symptom score to assess severity.
- Digital rectal examination and serum PSA measurement to assess for features of malignancy.

Basic investigations

- Serum creatinine, urinalysis in all patients.
- Urine flowmetry and residual volume estimation in those considered for intervention.

Advanced investigations
- Cystoscopy. To exclude bladder disease.
- Transrectal ultrasound ± guided biopsy. If concern over underlying malignancy.
- Renal ultrasound, invasive urodynamic studies.

Treatment
Recommended for those with LUTS that are impacting on quality of life or those with complications.

Medical treatment
- Patients with mild symptoms and no complications may be observed (watchful waiting).
- α-adrenergic antagonists. Relax smooth muscle of prostatic urethra to decrease outlet resistance; side effects include dizziness and hypotension (especially postural).
- 5α-reductase inhibitors. Block conversion of testosterone to dihydrotestosterone (DHT) and shown to cause involution of BPH; side effects include loss of libido and erectile dysfunction.
- Combination drug therapy with both the above agents. May reduce the clinical progression and decrease the need for surgery.

Surgical treatment
- Reserved for those with any of the complications or symptoms not responding to medical therapy.
- Surgical options include:
  - Transurethral resection of the prostate (TURP), the most commonly performed procedure for BPH in the UK.
  - Open retropubic prostatectomy.
  - Transurethral incision in the prostate (TUIP).
  - Bladder neck incision.
  - Laser 'prostatectomy'.
  - Microwave thermotherapy ablation of the prostate.

Key revision points—anatomy of the prostate
- Three glandular zones:
  - Peripheral (70%), most prone to carcinoma formation.
  - Central (25%), most prone to BPH.
  - Transitional (5%), most prone to BPH.
- Blood supply:
  - Arterial supply is triple, mainly inferior vesical, some from inferior rectal and internal pudendal.
  - Venous drainage, extensive plexus beneath capsule.
- Innervation:
  - Autonomic, extensive from inferior hypogastric plexus as a capsular plexus supplying prostate, seminal vesicles, and urethra, which also supplies the penile structures (glands, corpora, and urethra).
  - Somatic, from pudendal nerve (S2, 3, 4) to supply external urethral sphincter.

Stricture of the urethra

Key facts
- Classified according to site and aetiology, e.g. post-inflammatory bulbar stricture or traumatic membranous stricture.
- Graded according to length and (in the anterior urethra) degree of fibrosis of corpus spongiosum (spongiofibrosis).
- Any part of the urethra may be involved.
- The propensity for stricture recurrence parallels the severity (grade).

Aetiology
- Trauma.
  - Pelvic fracture.
  - Falls astride, e.g. on bicycle crossbar.
  - Urinary tract instrumentation/surgery.
- Infection.
  - *Neisseria gonorrhoea* and *Chlamydia trachomatis*.
  - Catheter-associated UTI.
- Lichen sclerosis et atrophicus.

Pathological features
- Annular narrowing by scar tissue composed of dense collagen and fibroblasts, which may extend into corpus spongiosum.
- Lichen sclerosus (balanitis xerotica obliterans (BXO)) consists of dermal sclerosis with epidermal atrophy; urethral lesions are usually confined to the meatus and fossa navicularis.

Clinical features
- History of urethritis, trauma, or urinary tract instrumentation.
- LUTS, divergent or diminished stream, straining to void, urgency, frequency.
- Haematuria ('initial' or 'terminal', i.e. at the beginning or end of the stream).
- UTI (often recurrent).
- Urinary retention, acute or chronic.
- Overflow incontinence.

Complications
- Urinary tract calculi formation.
- Infection, including UTI, prostatitis, epididymitis, and (rarely) Fournier's necrotizing fasciitis.
- Renal failure secondary to chronic obstruction.

Diagnosis and investigations
- Urinalysis (microbiology, biochemistry, and cytology).
- U&E.
- Uroflowmetry and measurement of post-void residual bladder volume.
- Voiding cystourethrogram with or without retrograde urethrogram.
- Endoscopy.

- Ultrasound scan (transperineal or endoluminal) to assess extent of spongiofibrosis.
- Magnetic resonance tomography.

Treatment

Initial

- Treat infection before surgical treatment.
- For acute urinary retention, severe symptoms, or renal failure, temporary suprapubic catheterization.

Definitive

- All urethral reconstructive surgery has an 'attrition rate'.
- Initial internal urethrotomy may cure up to 30%, but repeat procedures are rarely successful and may cause progression.
- Urethroplasty may be used for some cases.
  - Short strictures are excised and the urethra primarily re-anastomosed.
  - For longer or complex strictures, pedicled flap reconstruction or graft reconstruction is used; the graft or flap may be applied as an onlay (to augment the native urethra) or as a tube.
  - For free grafts, buccal mucosa is currently favoured.
  - More complicated repairs are best managed with staged repairs.
- Perineal urethrostomy may be required.

Scrotal swellings

Major causes

Intratesticular lesions
- Malignant testicular tumours.
- Benign intratesticular lesions. Simple intratesticular cyst or epidermoid cysts and benign teratoma (especially in the prepubertal testis).

Inflammatory lesions
- Acute epididymo-orchitis or viral orchitis.
- Chronic tuberculous epididymo-orchitis, schistosomal epididymitis, sperm granuloma.

Traumatic lesions
- Scrotal haematoma.
- Haematocele (haematoma within tunica vaginalis).
- Testicular haematoma (within tunica albuginea testis).

Derangement of testicular, adnexal, or cord anatomy
- Epididymal cysts or spermatocele of the epididymis.
- Varicocele (varicosities of the pampiniform plexus).
- Inguinal hernia (patent processus vaginalis in children).
- Hydrocele (vagina = within tunica vaginalis or cordal).
- Late (missed) or prenatal torsion of the spermatic cord.
- Persistence of embryological vestigial structures.
  - Müllerian duct remnant (appendix testis).
  - Wolffian duct remnants (appendix epididymis, vas aberrans of Haller, paradidymis).

Miscellaneous
- Acute idiopathic scrotal oedema.
- Cutaneous lesions, e.g. sebaceous cysts.
- Henoch–Schönlein purpura.

Clinical features/diagnosis

- ▶ Testicular tumours:
  - Firm intratesticular or progressively enlarging lesions are tumours until proven otherwise.
  - Do not be misled by painful testicular swelling following relatively trivial trauma; tumours may present this way.
- Tuberculous epididymitis may occur with or without evidence of pulmonary, systemic, or other genitourinary involvement.
- Hydroceles, patent processus vaginalis, and large spermatoceles are transilluminable, may be fluctuant, and are usually confined to the scrotum.
- Varicocele. Often associated with subfertility or dragging discomfort that worsens on standing and settles when recumbent. More obvious as a fluctuant swelling with the patient standing. A cough impulse may be felt. Ipsilateral testis may be atrophied. Examine the abdomen to exclude an associated renal tumour.

- Inguinal hernias tend to be intermittent, associated with groin discomfort, and when 'out', the examining hand cannot 'get above' the swelling in the cord/inguinal canal. A history of longstanding enlargement is typical.

Investigations

- Urinalysis for M,C,&S.
- Blood tests. Consider tumour markers (AFP, β-HCG), inflammatory markers (CRP, WCC).
- Ultrasound scanning of the scrotal contents has several important uses.
  - Distinguishes intratesticular from paratesticular swellings, solid from cystic lesions, cellulitis from abscess, etc.
  - Can examine impalpable testes, e.g. within large hydroceles.
  - Can identify rupture of the tunica albuginea testis.
  - Examination of the abdomen can identify renal mass associated with varicocele or ascites with hydrocele/scrotal oedema, etc.
  - Colour flow Doppler ultrasound can identify hyperaemia, underperfusion, and varicocele.

Treatment

Testicular tumours, acute epididymo-orchitis (see 📖 pp. 382, 388).

- Suspected paratesticular tumours are approached surgically in the same way as testis tumours. Surgery may be conservative with benign testicular and paratesticular tumours.
- Sperm granuloma may be excised or epididymectomy may be performed. Reassurance may be all that is required in many cases. Recurrence rates after surgery are high.
- Epididymal cysts/spermatocele may be aspirated, but recurrence is common. Excision risks loss of epididymal patency, is associated with risk of recurrence, and should probably be discouraged in men who have not completed their family.
- Hydroceles. Treat if symptomatic. Procedures usually reconfigure the serosal remnant of tunica vaginalis so as to allow lymphatic drainage via scrotal lymphatics. Reduction, inversion (Jaboulay), or imbrication (Lord's) of the tunica vaginalis is used.
- Embryological remnants. No treatment if asymptomatic.
- Varicocele. Treat if symptomatic, associated with infertility, or with failure of testicular growth. Venous embolization and retroperitoneal ligation (laparoscopic or open) of the testicular vein have similar results. Minimally invasive treatments are preferable. Gubernacular veins and other collaterals may account for failures. Open surgical ligations via an inguinal incision can deal with these.
- Acute idiopathic penoscrotal oedema of childhood usually settles with conservative treatment. Antihistamines and antibiotics are frequently prescribed, but there is little evidence to support this.

Disorders of the foreskin

Phimosis (see Fig. 10.2a)
Key facts
- Narrowness of the preputial opening, preventing retraction and exposure of the glans.
- May be physiological in infants and young children and will resolve.
- Pathological phimosis is secondary to scarring such as BXO or following monilial balanoposthitis.
- Pathological phimosis may be associated with discomfort, UTI, balanoposthitis, and (perhaps) carcinogenesis.

Clinical features
- In childhood, physiological phimosis may be identified by absence of scarring of the preputial tip and by pouting of the inner layer of the prepuce when a gentle attempt is made to retract it.
- A whitish sclerotic preputial tip and no pouting characterize BXO.
- Parents may complain of ballooning of their child's foreskin or of recurrent balanoposthitis. In adults, the diagnosis is obvious.

Treatment
- Physiological phimosis needs no treatment.
- Early BXO may be treated by application of topical steroid cream.
- Surgical treatment of phimosis includes circumcision and dorsal slit.

Paraphimosis (see Fig. 10.2b)
Key facts/diagnosis
- The retracted foreskin acts as a constricting ring, reducing lymphatic and venous drainage of tissues distal to the ring (glans, inner layer of foreskin). Subsequent oedema makes reduction more difficult.
- Involved tissues typically appear odematous and inflamed with progression to infection, ulceration, and necrosis if left untreated. Can occur in normal penises.

▶▶ Treatment
- *Early cases.* Gentle manual compression of the oedematous tissues within a saline-soaked swab will allow reduction of the foreskin after a few minutes without anaesthesia.
- *Established cases.* LA penile block or anaesthesia may be necessary. Hyaluronidase can be injected under the constriction.
- *Neglected/severe cases.* A relaxing dorsal incision may be made through the constriction and the tissues immediately proximal and distal to it. Subsequent circumcision is often offered.

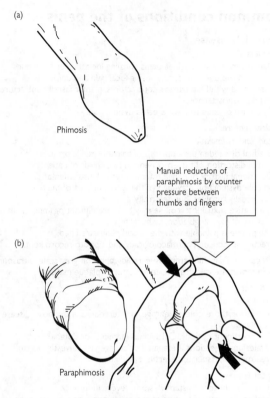

(a)

Phimosis

Manual reduction of
paraphimosis by counter
pressure between
thumbs and fingers

(b)

Paraphimosis

Fig. 10.2 (a) Phimosis. (b) Reduction of an acute paraphimosis.

Common conditions of the penis

Peyronie's disease

Key facts
- Damage to tunica albuginea penis, forming inelastic penile plaques mostly in the dorsal midline, causing local pain and deformity.
- Associated with Dupuytren's contractures, plantar fascial contractures, and tympanosclerosis.
- One-third of patients have erectile dysfunction.

Clinical features
History and examination
- Gradual or sudden development of palpable penile plaques with painful distortion of the erect penis in two-thirds of patients.
- Occasional history of penile trauma, urethral instrumentation.
- Erectile dysfunction may involve the whole or part of the penis.
- Pain usually resolves, but deformity does not.
- Penetrative sexual intercourse may be more difficult or impossible because of pain, angulation, or buckling.
- The plaque is palpable with the flaccid penis stretched.
- Erection is induced pharmacologically and a photo record kept.

Investigations Plain film soft tissue radiography or grey-scale ultrasound may demonstrate calcification, an indicator of plaque maturity.

Treatment
Medical
Indicated for those able to engage in intercourse and whose disease is still evolving.
- Oral treatment options. Colchicine, vitamin E, or Potaba®.
- Intralesional injections. Verapamil or collagenase (investigational).
- Treatment of associated erectile dysfunction.

Surgical
Indicated for those with stable lesions, severe deformity.
- *Plication techniques.* Plication of the tunica opposite the deforming plaque.
- *Grafting techniques.* The plaque is excised and the defect grafted.
- *Prosthesis insertion within corpora cavernosa.* Generally reserved for patients with severe erectile dysfunction refractory to medical therapy.

Priapism

Key facts Abnormally sustained erection unrelated to sexual stimulation. It is classified as high flow (arterial) or low flow (veno-occlusive).

Low flow priapism
- Congestion secondarily reduces arterial blood flow, leading to local hypoxia, acidosis, and hypercapnoea.
- Causes include:
  - *Drugs* (intracavernosal prostaglandin and papaverine, psychotropics, e.g. trazodone, chlorpromazine).

- Abnormal blood viscosity (sickle cell, myeloma, leukaemia, thalassaemia, total parenteral nutrition).
- Neurological disease, e.g. spinal or cerebrovascular disease.
- Miscellaneous, e.g. infiltration by solid tumour.
- Characterized by painful persistent erection, not involving the glans and corpus spongiosum.

High flow priapism

- Most commonly follows blunt trauma to penis or perineum, but has been caused by intracavernosal injection or revascularization.
- The mechanism is arterio-cavernosal fistula with unregulated arterial inflow and increased venous outflow.
- Characterized by partial, painless swelling of the glans and corpus spongiosum.

Investigation

- Colour Doppler ultrasonography or cavernosal blood gases.
- pH <7.25, pO_2 <30mmHg, pCO_2 >60mmHg suggest low flow.
- FBC and differentials; Hb electrophoresis.

Treatment—low flow

- Correct underlying abnormalities, e.g. sickle cell (rehydration, O_2, transfusion), myeloma (plasmapheresis).
- Oral β-agonists, e.g. terbutaline 5mg + further 5mg 15min later.
- Intracavernosal phenylephrine.
- Corpora cavernosa aspiration (up to 50mL) + manual pressure.
- Surgical techniques augment venous drainage of the corpora cavernosa.

Treatment—high flow

Selective pudendal arteriography and embolization.

Erectile dysfunction

Key facts
- Erectile dysfunction (ED) is the inability to achieve or maintain an erection satisfactory for sexual intercourse.
- Distinct from premature, retrograde, or delayed ejaculation.
- Causes include:
  - *Psychogenic.* Anxiety, depression.
  - *Drugs.* Antihypertensives, recreational drugs, tobacco, alcohol.
  - *Vascular.* Hypercholesterolaemia, atheroma, diabetes mellitus (DM).
  - *Metabolic/endocrine.* Azotaemia, hypercholesterolaemia, hypogonadism, hyperthyroidism, hyperprolactinaemia, DM.
  - *Neurological.* Parkinson's disease, CVA, spinal injury, neurological damage following pelvic surgery, pelvic fracture, autonomic neuropathies.
  - *Penile.* Cavernositis, Peyronie's disease, previous priapism.

Clinical features
- Specific validated questionnaires have been developed as investigational tools and can be used in practice.
- The presence of morning erections strongly suggests psychogenic cause.
- Small testicles, lack of secondary sexual characteristics suggest an endocrine cause.
- Lack of lower limb pulses suggests possible vascular cause.
- Neurological deficits in S2, 3, 4 distributions suggest neurological cause.

Investigations and diagnosis
- Check blood glucose, lipids and serum electrolytes, hormone profiles (testosterone, FSH/LH, prolactin), thyroid function for underlying cause.
- Dynamic cavernosometry confirms if there is a true vasculogenic cause (venous or arterial).
- Angiography demonstrates arterial anatomy if revascularization is contemplated.

Treatment
- Psychotherapy or specialist sexual counselling for psychogenic causes.
- Oral phosphodiesterase-5 inhibitors—sildenafil (Viagra™), vardenafil, tadalafil.
- Apomorphine sublingual.
- Intracavernosal—prostaglandins, α-blockers, papaverine.
- Intraurethral—prostaglandin.
- Vacuum devices-induced pseudoerection.
- Prosthesis.

Adenocarcinoma of the kidney

Key facts
- Accounts for 2% of all cancers.
- Incidence is 2–5 per 100 population.
- ♂:♀, 3:1.

Clinical features
- May be asymptomatic at presentation, the tumour being detected during imaging of the abdomen for an unrelated condition (e.g. CT scan or ultrasound scan).
- Symptoms include painless haematuria, groin pain, awareness of a mass arising from the flank.
- Chest symptoms and bone pain may be present with metastases to these sites.
- Positive family history or clinical evidence of neurological or ocular disease should raise the possibility of von Hippel–Lindau disease (VHL).
- Renal carcinomas are often small and may be multiple.
- Local spread often includes spread via intravascular invasion into the renal vein and inferior vena cava.

Diagnosis and investigations
- Blood tests. Hb and ferritin to check for anaemia (iron-deficient); electrolytes and Cr to check for overall renal function. Raised corrected calcium and alkaline phosphatase suggest possible bony metastases.
- Diagnostic and staging investigation of choice is a pre- and post-IV contrast-enhanced CT scan of abdomen and chest (delineates size, local extent, local invasion, likely sites of possible metastases).
- Isotope bone scan if there is clinical or biochemical evidence of bony metastases.

Treatment
Surgery
- Recommended as the only curative treatment except in the very elderly, extensive (inoperable) local invasion, and the presence of metastases.
- May be via open or laparoscopic approach.
- Radical nephrectomy is recommended for large tumours.
- Partial nephrectomy may be suitable for peripheral tumours <4cm in size.
- Resection of the primary cancer is occasionally appropriate with the presence of metastasis (the deposit must be solitary and itself amenable to complete local resection, e.g. in the liver or lungs).

Medical therapy
- Used for metastatic disease.
- Biological therapy can be with immune modulators such as interferons and interleukins. Partial response rates of 15–20% can be achieved, but the treatment carries significant morbidity. This is reserved for patients with a good performance status.

- Chemotherapy is rarely used as the tumours are not chemosensitive.
- Hormonal therapy (androgens and tamoxifen) may have some benefit.
- Radiotherapy is useful to palliate painful bony metastases.

Prognosis

- The outcome following nephrectomy is unpredictable.
- Tumours that are pathologically confined to the kidney confer a good prognosis. Adverse risk factors include extracapsular spread, invasion of the renal vein, lymph node involvement.
- Cure is likely if the tumour is <4cm in diameter and if there are no adverse pathological features.
- Periodic radiological follow-up is recommended in most cases so that locally recurrent or metastatic disease can be detected at an early stage.

Key revision points—anatomy of the kidney

Usually five segments (apical, anterior superior, anterior inferior, posterior and inferior), each supplied by its own artery.
- Fascial coverings.
  - Perirenal, anterior and posterior layers, enclosing kidney and perirenal fat.
  - Lateral conal fascia, formed from anterior and posterior perirenal fascia; fused with transversalis and iliac fascia laterally.
- Blood supply.
  - Arterial supply, direct from the aorta; renal arteries also give supply to the renal pelvis and upper ureter and adrenal gland.
  - Venous drainage, direct to inferior vena cava; left renal vein also drains the left gonadal vein.
- Common anatomical variants.
  - Unilaterally absent kidney (1 in 1200).
  - Pelvic kidney (1 in 2500).
  - Joined (horseshoe) kidney (1 in 400).

Transitional cell tumours

Key facts
- Transitional cell tumours (TCT) may affect any part of the urinary epithelium (renal pelvis, ureter, bladder, or very rarely, urethra).
- TCT have a spectrum of disease from benign superficial 'papilliferous' growths to frankly invasive transitional cell carcinoma (TCC); progression may occur from benign to more malignant forms with time.
- TCC of the bladder. Fifth commonest cause of cancer deaths and the commonest form of bladder cancer in the UK; ♂:♀, 3:1.
- TCC of the upper urinary tract is similar in spectrum of disease and management to bladder tumours, but much less common.
- TCT is associated with:
  - Exposure to aromatic hydrocarbons, e.g. workers in the petrochemical, industrial dye, rubber industries, chimney sweeps.
  - Smoking (especially in women).
- Risk is probably due to excretion of carcinogenic products excreted and concentrated in the urine and tumours are more likely in locations exposed to urine for the longest periods, i.e. bladder.

Pathological features
- The majority (70%) are superficial in nature at diagnosis, being confined to the mucosa.
- Invasion into the lamina propria, muscle, and perivesical fat can occur with lymphatic and distant spread occurring in advanced cases.
- TCC *in situ* is pre-invasive and associated with a high risk of muscle-invasive disease if not adequately treated.
- TCC must be differentiated from other forms of bladder cancer.
  - *Squamous cell carcinoma.* Usually caused by chronic irritation due to schistosomiasis infestation (bilharzia), indwelling catheter, repeated previous surgical interventions.
  - *Adenocarcinoma.* Rare; presents in middle age and is usually located in the dome of the bladder in association with the urachus.

Clinical features
- The majority of cases present with painless haematuria.
- Other features are painful micturition, renal colic due to blood clot, disturbance of urinary stream, retention of urine.

Diagnosis and investigation

Urine cytology May reveal malignant cells; if there are malignant cells, TCC or carcinoma *in situ* will probably be present.

Cystoscopy
- Usually carried out using a fibre optic flexible cystoscope and local anaesthetic gel.
- Images the bladder and urethra; suspect lesions usually require transurethral resection under GA for diagnosis.

Transurethral resection
- Usually carried out using a rigid endoresectoscope under GA.
- Permits resection of all or part of the tumour using a diathermy 'loop', with the tumour resected piecemeal; resection may be carried out into deep tissue (the muscle wall of the bladder beneath the tumour).
- Subsequent pathological examination will determine the histological grade and the pathological stage, e.g. depth of invasion.
- Following resection, bimanual examination determines whether or not a residual mass is present.

Upper tract imaging
- Used to identify and assess pelviureteric tumours.
- IVU or ultrasound scan.
- Ultrasound scan permits examination of the renal cortex and will detect tumours of 1cm diameter in the pelvicalyceal system, ureter, and bladder.
- Bladder tumour may show as a filling defect in the cystogram phase.

Local staging MRI and CT scanning to detect local or systemic spread.

Treatment
Superficial TCT
- Remove; completed by endoscopic resection.
- Recurrence is common and regular endoscopic surveillance with check cystoscopy is performed.
- Intravesical chemotherapy reduces the risk of tumour recurrence (single dose of mitomycin C instilled after resection of the tumour).
- For multiple or recurrent TCC, six intravesical treatments are given.

Carcinoma in situ
- Requires thorough therapy to prevent invasive TCC.
- Immunotherapy with intravesical BCG is effective in 60% of cases.
- Needs close endoscopic surveillance with regular bladder biopsy.

Invasive TCC
- Muscle-invasive tumours are of high grade and the prognosis is poor.
- Curative therapy can be offered with radical cystectomy (combined with a urinary diversion via an ileal conduit) or radical radiotherapy.

Squamous cell and adenocarcinoma
- Radical cystectomy provided general condition allows.
- Usually resistant to radiotherapy and chemotherapy.

Prognosis
- Approximately 30% develop muscle-invasive disease.
- The 5y survival rate for muscle-invasive bladder cancer is 40–50%.
- Metastatic TCC is poor prognosis with a median survival of 13 months.
- Systemic chemotherapy with cis-platinum-containing regimes provides a long-term response in 15% of cases.

Adenocarcinoma of the prostate

Key facts

- Most commonly diagnosed cancer affecting men in the western world.
- Approximately 30 000 new cases diagnosed annually in the UK with 10 000 deaths.
- Peak incidence in eighth decade.
- Approximately 40% of cases present with early disease; 20% of cases have metastases at presentation.

Clinical features

- The majority of men present with LUTS (📖 p. 354).
- Bone pain, pathological factures, and features of hypercalcaemia are occasional presenting features due to metastases.
- May be diagnosed by digital rectal examination; areas of firmness or palpable nodules are suggestive of malignant change.

Diagnosis and investigations

- *Serum PSA.* Can be used as a screening test; high sensitivity, but low specificity; elevated age-specific levels are an indication to consider prostate biopsy.
- *Transrectal ultrasound (TRUS).* Permits detailed imaging of the prostate. Systematic needle biopsy is performed guided by the ultrasound images with antibiotic prophylaxis; graded using the Gleason grading system which assigns a numerical score to adverse features from a minimum of 2 to a maximum of 10.
- *Pelvic MRI.* Used to detect the presence of extracapsular extension or the presence of pelvic lymphadenopathy (suggests spread).
- *Laparoscopic node biopsy.* May be performed to sample enlarged nodes prior to considering radical treatment.
- *Isotope bone scan.* Will detect the presence of bone metastases.

Treatment

Localized disease (confined to prostate)

Patients with a life expectancy of <10y

- Active monitoring with treatment deferred until there is evidence of disease progression (rising serum PSA).
- Hormonal therapy or α-blocker treatment offered for troublesome LUTS.
- TURP is considered for severe symptoms with features of obstruction.

Life expectancy of >10y

- Counselled in detail about radical treatment aimed at cure.
- The options are as follows:
  - *Radical prostatectomy.* Operation to remove the prostate and seminal vesicles; complications include incontinence (severe in 3%) and ED (40–50% of cases).
  - *External beam radiotherapy.* Radiation is delivered at a radical dose of 55–70Gy in 20–25 fractions over a 4–5-week period; complications include cystitis, proctitis, and ED.

- *Brachytherapy*. Radioactive seeds placed into the prostate using TRUS guidance; a relatively new technique and long-term follow-up data are lacking.

Locally advanced disease (spread beyond the prostate)

- Incurable and treatment is therefore palliative.
- Eighty per cent are androgen-dependent. Hormone therapy reduces androgenic drive to the prostate cancer cell using two methods:
  - *Luteinizing hormone-releasing hormone (LHRH) agonists*. Given by 3-monthly depot injections, suppresses testosterone production by the testes; side effects include hot flushes, lethargy, loss of sexual function.
  - *Anti-androgens*. Given orally, act as competitive inhibitors at the level of the androgen receptor, reduce androgenic stimulus to the prostate cancer cell without reducing serum testosterone levels; side effects include gynaecomastia and nipple tenderness (60%), potency is sometimes preserved.

Metastatic disease

Treated with hormonal therapy using LHRH analogues. Addition of an anti-androgen provides a secondary response in some cases of PSA relapse. Pain from bone metastases usually responds to radiotherapy.

Hormone-resistant disease

- All prostate cancers will eventually become hormone-resistant.
- Chemotherapy is appropriate for patients who have a good performance status.
- Palliative radiotherapy and bisphosphonates are used for bony metastases.

Prognosis

- Localized prostate cancer. Excellent prognosis with 70–90% 10y disease-specific survival figures.
- Locally advanced, non-metastatic disease. Median survival of 7y.
- Metastatic disease. Median survival of 2–3y.
- Once the state of hormone-resistant disease has been reached, the median survival is 6–12 months.

Carcinoma of the penis

Key facts
- Rarest of the urological cancers.
- Occurs primarily in older men.

Clinicopathological features
- Over 95% are squamous cell carcinoma.
- Usually affects the glans, but may involve the shaft.
- Associated with chronic infection of the penis, particularly in the presence of phimosis.
- Early cases present with a painless ulcer, nodule, or 'warty' outgrowth on the penis that may also involve the foreskin.
- Advanced disease presents with a fungating mass, usually ulcerated. Inguinal lymphadenopathy may be present on examination. Nodes are often reactive rather than being metastatic and antibiotics should be given prior to further assessment.

Diagnosis and investigations
- Biopsy lesion to confirm the diagnosis.
- Pelvic and abdominal CT scanning provide further evidence of nodular involvement in cases with positive inguinal nodes.

Treatment
- If primary tumour confined to glans, treatment involves either partial amputation or radiotherapy.
- Superficial lesions can be treated by excision of the glans followed by glans reconstruction.
- More advanced carcinomas require total penectomy. Inguinal and iliac lymph node dissections are considered.

Prognosis
- Early stage penile cancer has a high cure rate with either surgery or radiotherapy.
- Long-term survival is sometimes seen even in cases of lymph node involvement.

Testicular Tumours

Testicular tumours

Key facts
- Commonest malignancy in men between the ages of 18 and 40.
- Annual incidence 6 per 100 000 males per year.
- Associated with testicular maldescent.
- Increased risk is associated with higher levels of exogenous oestrogens, either prenatally or in childhood.
- Increased level of awareness has led to more tumours being detected on self-examination, particularly amongst younger men.

Pathological features
- Common types are seminoma and non-seminomatous germ cell tumours (NSGCT; previously called 'teratoma'). Lymphoma is a rare testicular tumour.
- Seminoma.
  - Peak incidence 30–40y.
  - Lymphatic spread more common than haematogenous.
  - Lymphatic spreads to iliac and para-aortic nodes.
- NSGCTs.
  - Peak incidence 20–30y.
  - Haematogeneous spread most common to lungs, brain, and liver.
- Lymphomas. Peak incidence over 60y.
- Marsden staging (after investigations and treatment).
  - Stage 1, confined to testis.
  - Stage 2, abdominal nodal spread.
  - Stage 3, nodal disease outside the abdomen.
  - Stage 4, extralymphatic spread.

Clinical features
- The usual presentation is with a painless testicular mass.
- Typical features are irregular, firm, fixed, and does not transilluminate.
- Palpate the abdomen for intra-abdominal masses (either para-aortic node masses or hepatomegaly).
- Check for supraclavicular lymphadenopathy and signs of lung or neurological disease.

Diagnosis and investigation
▶ Any clinically suspicious mass requires urgent testicular ultrasound scan. Typical features are a non-homogeneous mass with increased vascularity.
- *Serum tumour markers, B-HCG and AFP.* Increased levels suggest metastatic disease in NSGCTs, but may be normal in localized or metastatic disease; very rarely elevated in seminoma even if metastatic.
- *CT scan of abdomen and chest.* To assess presence of metastases.
- *CT brain, bone scan.* Only if clinically indicated.

Treatment

- Orchidectomy is carried out at the earliest opportunity; this is performed via an inguinal approach so that the spermatic cord can be clamped prior to mobilization of testis.
- Seminoma is radiosensitive and even widespread local disease responds well to radiotherapy.
  - *Stage 1.* May be treated by orchidectomy only, orchidectomy + prophylactic iliac and para-aortic radiotherapy, or orchidectomy + prophylactic chemotherapy.
  - *Stages 2/3/4.* Orchidectomy + radiotherapy to involved node groups ± chemotherapy.
  - Visceral metastases are treated with a combination of chemotherapy and radiotherapy.
- NSGCT is chemosensitive and even widespread metastatic disease responds well.
  - *Stage 1.* Orchidectomy.
  - *Stages 2/3/4.* Orchidectomy + chemotherapy; if lymphadenopathy is still present following chemotherapy, a retroperitoneal lymph node dissection is performed.

Prognosis

- Cure rates >95% for stage 1 tumours.
- Metastatic disease also has excellent long-time survival rates with combination therapy.

Haematuria

Causes and features

May be microscopic or macroscopic.
- *UTI*. Commonest cause; usually associated with LUTS, particularly cystitis.
- *Renal stones*. Often associated with pain (renal colic).
- *Malignancy* (TCT, renal adenocarcinoma, prostate adenocarcinoma). Most likely to be macroscopic, often with few other acute symptoms.
- *Post-interventional*. For example, post-TURP, post-cystoscopy, post-catheterization.
- *Renal disease*. For example, glomerulonephritis, vasculitis; usually causes microscopic haematuria, is often asymptomatic, and rarely presents as an emergency.

Complications
- Suprapubic colicky pain or acute retention of urine suggests clots in the bladder/urethra.
- Cardiovascular collapse is rare.

Emergency management

Resuscitation
- Establish large calibre IV access if the bleed is large; give crystalloid fluid up to 1000mL if tachycardic or hypotensive.
- *Do not* catheterize without seeking senior advice if there is any suggestion of lower urinary tract pathology or post-interventional bleeding.
- Irrigation ('3-way') catheters may be used to relieve acute symptoms of clot colic or clot retention, but should be placed by experienced staff.
- Send blood for FBC (Hb, WCC), U&E (Na, K), group and save, clotting.

Establish a diagnosis
- *Full clinical examination*. Particularly check the prostate on PR exam.
- *Ultrasound kidney*. To identify renal tumours, cysts.
- *Cystoscopy* (usually rigid, may be flexible). To identify bladder tumours.
- *CT scan abdomen*. If renal tumour is suspected.

Early treatment
- Ensure all clotting abnormalities are corrected.
- Ensure fluid balance is correct; promote an active diuresis to prevent clot formation and retention.
- Transfuse blood only if Hb <8g/dL or the patient is symptomatic or high risk.
- Start antibiotics according to local protocol if infection is suspected (before cultures are available).

Definitive management

Transitional cell tumours Transurethral resection will control symptoms, establish a diagnosis, and start treatment (see 📖 p. 382).

Renal stones (see 📖 p. 358)
- May pass spontaneously.
- May need endoscopic removal, lithotripsy, or percutaneous treatment.

Post-interventional Flexible cystoscopy may be required.

Acute urinary retention (AUR)

Causes and features

Defined as a painful inability to pass urine.

Local causes

- Prostatic enlargement (BPH or carcinoma) (see 📖 p. 362). Often acute-on-chronic retention.
- Post-urological surgery, e.g. post-TURP, clot impaction.
- Bladder or urethral stone impaction.
- Pressure on bladder, e.g. late pregnancy, faecal impaction.
- UTI.

General causes

- Pharmacological, for example:
  - Anticholinergic side effects of many drugs.
  - Anaesthetic drugs.
  - Alcohol intoxication.
  - α-sympatheticomimetics.
- Post-non-urological surgery:
  - Precipitated by recent catheterization.
  - Abdominal surgery with lower abdominal pain.
  - Epidural or spinal anaesthesia.
- Loss of normal neurological control:
  - Spinal injury (trauma, 'slipped disc', neurological disease).
  - Epidural/spinal anaesthesia.

Symptoms

- Suprapubic pain, inability to pass urine despite desire.
- May dribble urine in small volumes, especially if there is underlying chronic retention.
- Palpable/percussible bladder strongly suggests pre-existing chronic retention/lower urinary tract disease.

Signs

- Prostatic enlargement on PR examination.
- Check for signs of neurological disease.

Emergency management

Resuscitation

- Give analgesia (e.g. morphine 5–10mg IV); it will also help relaxation and may aid spontaneous micturition.
- A warm bath may aid micturition in drug-induced retention.
- Catheterize if retention persists. ► Seek senior advice before starting if there are concerns about local pathology as a cause or if there is a history of previous surgical instrumentation of the urethra.
- Suprapubic catheterization may be required for known or suspected urethral disease or failed urethral catheterization (see 📖 p. 210).
- Document initial urine volume passed after catheter inserted; large volumes suggest underlying chronic retention.

- Send urine for M,C,&S.
- Send blood for FBC (Hb, WCC), U&E (Na, K), Cr.

Establish a diagnosis
- Check medications, especially recent changes.
- Cystoscopy may be required.
- Review full clinical examination, including neurological findings and rectal examination.

Early treatment
- Monitor renal function, especially if there is underlying chronic retention; renal function may deteriorate even after relief of the obstruction.
- Monitor fluid balance in first 48h if there is associated chronic retention; a secondary diuresis may occur.
- Start antibiotics according to local protocols if there is evidence of a UTI.

Definitive management
Prostatic disease (see p. 362)
- TURP may be required.
- α-blocker may enable successful trial of voiding.

Acute testicular pain

Causes and features

This is an acute emergency in men of childbearing age. Torsion of the testicle must be dealt with immediately to preserve testicular function. It is the commonest cause for referral for acute testicular pain.

Torsion of the testicle

Key facts

- Occurs due to anatomical variants in testicular anatomy, e.g. 'bell clapper' testicle with pronounced meso-orchium allowing rotation within the tunica vaginalis.
- Peak age of incidence 12–18y.
- Torsion initially causes venous obstruction, but with prolonged increased venous pressure, arterial compression occurs and the testicle rapidly develops irreversible ischaemia and necrosis.
- Testicular salvage depends on the degree of torsion and time spent torted. Speed of presentation, diagnosis, and treatment are all important. Torsion greater than 360° lasting longer than 24h results in near universal complete or severe atrophy.
- Spermatogenic cells are more susceptible to ischaemia than Leydig cells. Subfertility may occur even if the testicle is macroscopically normal after treatment.

Features

- Sudden onset of moderate to severe, constant, unilateral scrotal pain, often with nausea, vomiting, and abdominal pain.
- May have been preceding episodes of intermittent pain that suddenly resolved.
- The testis is globally tender, high in the scrotum, may have a transverse axis, and be slightly enlarged. If it is infarcted, scrotal wall oedema and tenderness may be present. Absence of ipsilateral cremasteric reflex is the most reliable sign.

Torsion of the testicular appendages

- Occurs in testicular appendix 'hydatid of Morgagni' or epidydmal appendages (e.g. cysts, ductal remnants).
- Similar features and symptoms to testicular torsion.
- The 'blue dot sign' is said to be pathognomonic when present.
- The testis and epididymis may be non-tender and the cremasteric reflex should be preserved.

Acute epididymo-orchitis

- Peak incidences vary according to cause, ages 35y and >55y.
- Common organisms include *Chlamydia trachomatis*, *Neisseria gonorrhoea* in the young (sexually-transmitted infections (STI)).
- *Escherichia coli* and *Proteus* occur in chronic bladder outflow obstruction or urinary tract instrumentation.
- One-third of male adolescents with mumps develop orchitis, which is unilateral in 80%; a third of these testes atrophy.

Features
- Gradual onset of pain (hours or days).
- Dysuria, urethral discharge, and pyrexia are common.
- Tenderness and induration are localized to the epididymis and spermatic cord in epididymitis.
- Cremasteric reflex is preserved.
- Prehn's sign (relief of pain with scrotal elevation).

Idiopathic scrotal oedema
- Often less painful and tender than appears.
- Swelling is mostly cutaneous and normal size and texture testicle may be palpable with care.

Acute inguinal lymphadenopathy
- May occur secondary to lower limb, buttock, or perineal infections.
- Rarely part of systemic infection of lymphatic disorder.

Emergency management

Resuscitation Give analgesia (e.g. morphine 5–10mg IV).

Establish a diagnosis

▶▶ Immediate surgical exploration is indicated for all cases where the diagnosis of torsion is considered possible and the history is short (i.e. testicular viability is still at issue).
- Testicular colour duplex ultrasound. May be used if *immediately* available or where symptoms have been present for days and testicular viability is unlikely if torted.
- Send MSU, urethral swab, chlamydia serology if suspected infection.

Definitive management

If a torted testicle is found at surgery:
- A viable testicle is detorted and fixed.
- A clearly non-viable testicle is excised.
- The opposite testicle is fixed (orchidopexy) to prevent the opposite side torting in future.

Torsion of testicular or epididymal appendage Excise appendage.

Epididymo-orchitis
- Suspected STI, e.g. ceftriaxone 250mg IM single dose, doxycycline 100mg PO bd 7 days.
- Suspected UTI-related—ciprofloxacin 500mg PO bd 10–14 days.
- Scrotal elevation, local ice therapy, and oral NSAIDs may help.
- Abscess formation may require drainage or orchidectomy.
- Treatment of acute viral orchitis is symptomatic.

Colorectal surgery

Ulcerative colitis

Key facts

- An acute and chronic inflammatory disease originating in the colonic columnar mucosa.
- Precise aetiology is unknown, but an environmental trigger combined with a genetic predisposition (family history) are factors.
- Often precipitated by an apparent acute GI infection; peak age of diagnosis is the late teens and twenties, but may present in late adulthood.
- Commonest in white Anglo-Saxon Caucasians.

Pathological features

- Granular, hypervascular, and mildly oedematous mucosa with loss of vascular pattern seen at endoscopy.
- Acute neutrophil infiltration of the colonic mucosa and submucosa; mucosal crypt abscesses with goblet cell mucin depletion.
- With more severe inflammation, there are multiple aphthous ulcers, which may become confluent with only islands of inflamed mucosa and granulation tissue remaining ('pseudopolyposis').
- Transmural inflammation may occur in severe disease secondary to the widespread loss of mucosa and subsequent severe inflammation.
- Chronic 'burnt-out' disease leads to a pale, featureless, ahaustral pattern to the colon.
- Disease tends to be present in the distal colon and rectum and spread proximally with increasing extent of disease.

Clinical features

- *Proctitis*. Commonest presentation. Rectum 'always' involved unless already on topical treatment. Symptoms of urgency and frequency of defecation due to rectal irritability; bloody mucus mixed with loose stools (frank bloody diarrhoea rare).
- *Left-sided colitis*. Disease up to the splenic flexure. Symptoms of rectal irritation plus extensive bloody mucus in stools, often leading to bloody diarrhoea; mild associated systemic features.
- *Pancolitis*. Disease involving the entire colon. May be associated with mild secondary inflammation of the terminal ileum ('backwash ileitis'). Diarrhoea predominant feature; systemic features common (fever, malaise, anorexia, tachycardia). May be associated with anaemia (due to blood loss), hypoalbuminaemia, and hypokalaemia (due to mucus loss).

Diagnosis and investigations

Basic tests

↑ WCC and CRP; ↓ Hb and albumin, especially during episodes of inflammation. AXR may show oedematous colonic mucosa ('thumbprinting'), but is unreliable for diagnosis or extent of disease. Proctosigmoidoscopy usually shows erythematous, granular, or frankly ulcerated rectal mucosa with mucus and blood. Biopsies should be taken before starting treatment. Always send stool M,C,&S and test for parasites and cysts in any acute presentation to exclude infectious causes.

Advanced tests

Extent of disease is best assessed with colonoscopy and biopsies; will also usually exclude colonic Crohn's disease.

Treatment

See 📖 p. 418 for management of acute severe colitis.

Medical treatment

Principles are to reduce inflammation and prevent complications. Acute derangements in blood results should be corrected (e.g. blood transfusion for severe anaemia, potassium supplementation, nutritional support for hypoalbuminaemia).

Proctitis

- Topical steroids—Predsol® suppositories.
- Topical 5-aminosalicyclic acid (5-ASA) suppositories.

Left-sided colitis

- Topical steroids—Predsol® foam enemas (penetrate up as far as the splenic flexure).
- Topical 5-ASA foam enemas.
- May require systemic steroid treatment (prednisolone).

Pancolitis

- Topical steroids or 5-ASA treatments for local symptoms.
- Usually need systemic treatment, e.g. oral steroids (prednisolone), 5-ASA treatment.
- Oral immunosuppressives, e.g. azathioprine, 6-mercaptopurine.
- Systemic affectors of lymphocyte function, e.g. cyclosporin A, anti-TNFα (infliximab)

Surgical treatment

Surgery is indicated for acute colitis that fails to respond to treatment (see 📖 p. 418) and for chronic colitis when:

- Chronically symptomatic despite maximal medical therapy.
- Medical therapy controlling symptoms, but associated with unacceptable side effects, e.g. osteoporosis, immunosuppression.
- Recurrent exacerbations affecting growth or development in adolescents.
- Confirmed diagnosis of either high grade dysplasia or dysplasia-associated lesion or mass (DALM), or carcinoma of colon.

Surgical treatment may be:

- Proctocolectomy (removal of colon and rectum) with ileoanal pouch formation (see 📖 p. 402).
- Panproctocolectomy (removal of colon, rectum, and anus) with end ileostomy formation (permanent).
- Total abdominal colectomy (removal of colon) with ileostomy (used when the patient is too unwell for major pelvic surgery, e.g. for acute severe colitis).

Crohn's disease

Key facts

- A chronic inflammatory non-caseating, granulomatous disease affecting any part of the GI tract.
- Associated with several extraintestinal disorders (see Box 11.1).
- Precise aetiology is unknown, but products from the bacterial flora combined with a genetic predisposition (family history) are factors.
- Peak age of onset of symptoms is the teens and early twenties, but diagnosis is often several years later.
- Commonest in white Anglo-Saxon Caucasians.

Pathological features

- Commonly focused in the terminal ileum and caecum, but may affect the anus, colon, or entire small bowel.
- Anal Crohn's disease is not common, but may be severe and associated with active small bowel disease.
- Colonic Crohn's disease is a long-term risk factor for colorectal cancer formation.
- Affected bowel looks blue-grey, thickened, with spiral surface vessels and encroachment of the mesenteric fat around the bowel ('fat wrapping').
- Transmural inflammation in the form of lymphoid aggregates, particularly in the subserosal tissues ('Crohn's rosary'), mucosal crypt ulceration, and fissuring ulceration.
- Mucosal thickening and serpiginous longitudinal ulceration combine to give the appearance of 'cobblestoning'.
- Perforation, fistulation, and abscess formation are occasional 'fistulizing' sequelae of transmural inflammation.
- Extensive fibrosis and smooth muscle hyperplasia may occur, giving rise to stenosis.

Clinical features

- *Inflammatory features.* Fever, malaise, abdominal pain (often RIF), change in bowel habit (usually diarrhoea without blood), and weight loss. Children and adolescents may have failure to thrive or have retarded growth. Rectal bleeding is rare except in Crohn's colitis.
- *Fistulizing features.* Para-enteric abscess formation often with a tender abdominal mass, fistula formation (ileocolic, ileoileal, ileocutaneous); rarely free perforation with features of peritonitis.
- *Stenosing features.* Colicky abdominal pain, weight loss due to poor food intake ('food fear'), palpable or visible distended small bowel loops.
- *Anal disease.* Atypical severe anal fissures, fistula in ano, anal mucosal thickening, and discoloration.

Diagnosis and investigations

Basic tests

↑ WCC and CRP; ↓ Hb and albumin, especially during episodes of inflammation.

Advanced tests

- In acute presentations, an abdominal CT may show an inflammatory mass, abscess formation, localized or free perforation.
- In subacute or chronic presentations, small bowel disease may be shown by a small bowel contrast study (shows mucosal irregularity and narrowing) or a white cell scan showing ileal 'hot spots'.
- Crohn's colitis is diagnosed by endoscopy and biopsy.
- Anal disease may require, EUA, anal ultrasound, or MRI scanning for assessment.
- OGD and biopsies may show features of Crohn's in gastric mucosa.

Treatment

Medical treatment

Principles are to reduce inflammation and control complications. Acute derangements in blood results should be corrected.

- Systemic (5-ASA) drugs are first-line acute and long-term treatment.
- Systemic steroids (hydrocortisone, prednisolone) control acute exacerbations of inflammation and steroids with very high first pass metabolism (budesonide) can be used chronically.
- Immunosuppressives (azathioprine, 6-mercaptopurine) are used as maintenance therapy and anti-TNFα antibodies (infliximab) may be effective in fistulizing complications.
- Dietary manipulation (elemental diet) may reduce inflammatory factors.

Surgical treatment

Principles are to deal with septic complications, relieve significant bowel obstruction, and remove as little bowel as possible. Indications for surgery include the following.

- *Acute.* Free perforation, severe haemorrhage, acute severe colitis, complete intestinal obstruction.
- *Subacute.* Inflammatory mass, subacute obstruction, abscess formation, symptomatic fistulation.
- *Chronic.* Steroid dependency or complications, growth retardation, cancer treatment or prevention.

Box 11.1 Extraintestinal manifestations of Crohn's disease

Associated with disease activity
- Pyoderma gangrenosum
- Erythema nodosum
- Primary biliary cirrhosis

Independent of disease activity
- Ankylosing spondylitis
- Polyarthritis
- Chronic active hepatitis

Other forms of colitis

Key facts and pathological features

Various insults of widely differing origin may give rise to colitis other then idiopathic inflammatory bowel disease.

Acute infective colitis
- Typically caused by pathological variants of normal enteric organisms, e.g. enteropathogenic *E. coli*; only rarely progresses to acute severe colitis.
- Typhoid colitis (*Salmonella typhi*) (rare in the UK). Typified by acute bloody diarrhoea, but few if any colonic mucosal neutrophils on biopsy due to bone marrow suppression.

Clostridium (C.) difficile-*related colitis*

Caused by *C. difficile* infestation. Associated with antibiotic use, particularly third generation cephalosporins (even a single dose), prolonged inpatient stay. Toxin A produced by the organism causes acute severe inflammation in the mucosa.

Clinical picture may be varied.
- *C. difficile diarrhoea.* Foul green liquid without bloody stools.
- *Acute C. difficile colitis.* Caused by progressive rapid mucosal loss, acute neutrophil infiltration, and inflammation.
- *Pseudomembranous colitis.* Exudate and slough forms grey-white 'plaques' of material on the denuded colonic surface called pseudomembranes. May rapidly progress to acute severe 'invasive' colitis, especially in the immunocompromised or acutely unwell. Typified by secondary infections associated with mucosal loss.

Neutropenic colitis

Occurs in the severely immunocompromised with neutropenia and/or neutrophil dysfunction. Caused by multiple, normally non-pathogenic, enteric organisms colonizing the colonic mucosa.

Radiation colitis

Acute, transient colitis caused by mucosal injury secondary to external beam radiotherapy. May progress to chronic mucosal damage, haemorrhagic telangectasia, and possible stricturing after months or years.

Ischaemic colitis

Commonest in the upper left colon where the collateral blood supply between the middle and inferior colic arteries is poorest. Usually precipitated by an acute occlusion of part or all of the inferior mesenteric artery. May progress to infarction, but often presents with acute onset bloody diarrhoea and abdominal pain; may settle spontaneously although occasionally forms an ischaemic stricture.

Clinical features

Broadly similar, independently of the underlying cause. Typical features are vague abdominal pain, mild fever (absent in neutropenic colitis), diarrhoea (may be bloody, especially in ischaemic, radiation, severe pseudomembranous, and typhoid colitis). Cessation of diarrhoea, except with treatment, suggests acute severe colitis is developing and should be investigated urgently.

Diagnosis and investigations

Depending on the suspected cause:

- Stool sent for C. difficile toxin (CDT), three samples.
- Stool for M,C,&S (if atypical infective causes possible, also send for cysts, parasites, and ova (C,P,&O)).
- Plain abdominal radiograph may show thickened colonic haustrae.
- CT abdomen often shows typical mucosal thickening in colitis and may be diagnostic for pseudomembranous colitis.
- Flexible endoscopy (usually flexible sigmoidoscopy) with biopsy.

Treatment

Medical treatment

- *Acute infective colitis.* Antibiotics only if severely symptomatic.
- *C. difficile diarrhoea/colitis.* Oral vancomycin up to 200mg PO daily or metronidazole 400mg tds; treatment may be as for pseudomembranous colitis if severe.
- *Pseudomembranous colitis.* Oral vancomycin up to 200mg PO daily or metronidazole 400mg PO tds; adjuvant systemic treatment may be added in severe cases, e.g. IV vancomycin or tigicycline.
- *Neutropenic colitis.* Broad-spectrum antibiotics, bone marrow support.
- *Radiation colitis.* Symptomatic treatment only; anti-diarrhoeals.
- *Ischaemic colitis.* Supportive treatment; anticoagulation may be appropriate if the underlying cause is thromboembolic.

Surgical treatment

Rarely indicated. Any form of colitis may progress to acute severe colitis and require emergency colectomy (see p. 418). Indications are:

- Failure to respond to maximal medical therapy with life-threatening colitis (usually requires perioperative ITU support).
- Complications of colitis. Uncontrollable bleeding, perforation (especially in ischaemic or neutropenic colitis).

Key revision points—colorectal resections

Anastomosis of the colon/rectum may be in several ways.

- Hand sewn. Either end to end or end to side, usually single layer of sutures (dissolvable), either interrupted or continuous.
- Stapled colonic. By mechanical stapler ('linear stapler'), usually side to side.
- Stapled colorectal. By mechanical stapler ('endoluminal stapler'), end to end.
- Defunctioning (loop) ileostomy typically for rectal anastomosis when:
  - Below the peritoneal reflection.
  - Comorbidities (diabetes, age, previous DXT, acute illness).

Colorectal polyps

'Polyp' is a purely descriptive term and any growth from the lining of the large bowel can be described as a polyp. Polyps may be predominantly raised with a stalk attachment (pedunculated), flat and spreading over the surface of the bowel wall (sessile), or occasionally a combination of the two.

Key facts and pathological features

Polyps may arise for many different reasons.

Juvenile polyps

Mucin-filled cystic swellings of the lower rectal mucosa. Rarely part of a hereditary syndrome (juvenile polyposis) with multiple juvenile polyps throughout the colon; small increased risk of colorectal cancer.

Hamartomatous polyps

Polyps containing excessive amounts of the normal architectural components of the bowel wall, usually isolated. May be part of a hereditary syndrome (Peutz–Jeghers syndrome, with polyps characterized by extensive branched growth of the muscularis mucosa); small increased risk of colorectal and other GI cancers.

Hyperplastic polyps

Small sessile polyps formed from normal elongated mucosal crypts. Only associated with risk of colorectal cancer if numerous ('hyperplastic polyposis').

Adenomatous polyps

- True neoplastic polyps formed by excessive growth of the colorectal epithelium; divided by the morphology of the glandular tissue into tubular, tubulovillous, and villous types.
- May be sessile, pedunculated, or mixed.
- Thought to be the precursor of most colorectal cancers; the risk of cancerous change within an adenomatous polyp increases with size (particularly >1cm), villous morphology, and sessile form.
- Majority are sporadic (either isolated or in small numbers), although occasionally part of a hereditary syndrome.

Familial adenomatous polyposis (FAP)

Caused by an autosomal dominant defect in the *APC* gene on chromosome 5. Characterized by between dozens and thousands of adenomatous polyps in the colorectum and an increased risk of polyp formation in the stomach and duodenum. The risk of cancerous transformation in any given polyp is similar to that in normal polyps, but the overall risk is very high due to the vastly increased number present.

Associated with:

- Desmoid formation, particularly in the abdominal tissues.
- Multiple osteomata, fibromata, and thyroid inflammation (called Gardner's syndrome).

Hereditary non-polyposis colorectal cancer (HNPCC)

A range of abnormalities of the mismatch repair (MMR) genes that predispose adenomas to acquire multiple genetic defects and so progress more rapidly than normal to cancer, although the overall rate of adenoma formation is similar to that in normals.

Clinical features

Most polyps are asymptomatic, although symptoms may occur with increasing size and with proximity to the anus. Typical symptoms are:
- *Bleeding*. Usually low volume, dark red, often flecks or mixed with stool.
- *Mucus discharge*. White, clear, or watery; commonest with large villous adenomas and may cause hypokalaemia and hypoproteinaemia if the villous adenoma is large with copious mucus discharge.
- *Prolapse*. If pedunculated and low in the rectum polyps, may prolapse out of the anus.

Diagnosis and investigations

- Most polyps are diagnosed by colonoscopy.
- Most patients with polyps require further follow-up investigations to keep them under surveillance for future polyp formation; the frequency and length of follow-up depends on the number, size, and histology of the polyp.[1]
- Hereditary polyposis syndromes may be investigated by genetic mutation analysis.

Treatment

Medical treatment

- Colonoscopic polypectomy (see 🕮 p. 36). Simple, is carried out for pedunculated polyps larger than 1–2mm; others may be removed by EMR/ESD (see 🕮 p. 403).
- Patients with FAP require regular gastroscopy and upper GI surveillance to identify premalignant polyps.

Surgical treatment

- Surgical excision is required for polyps that are too large or unsuitable for colonoscopic removal and in which there is a risk of current or future malignant change; for colonic polyps this means either resection or open excision.
- Rectal polyps may be removed by transanal microsurgery (see 🕮 p. 403).
- FAP is usually treated by proctocolectomy (usually with ileoanal pouch formation) or colectomy and ileorectal anastomosis before early adulthood; other polyposis syndromes may also be treated by prophylactic colectomy.

Reference

1 Atkin WS, Saunders BP (2002). Surveillance guidelines after removal of colorectal adenomatous polyps. *Gut* **51** (Suppl. V), v6–v9.

Colorectal cancer

Key facts
Colorectal cancer (CRCa) is the second commonest tumour and commonest GI malignancy. One in 18 of the population will suffer CRCa; ♂:♀ ≈ 3:1. Peak age of incidence 55–75y, but is increasing in younger ages.

Pathological features
The predominant type is adenocarcinoma (mucinous, signet ring cell, and anaplastic subtypes). Classified as well, moderately, or poorly differentiated. Predisposing factors include:
- Polyposis syndromes (including FAP, HNPCC, juvenile polyposis).
- Strong family history of colorectal carcinoma.
- Previous history of polyps or CRCa.
- Chronic ulcerative colitis or colonic Crohn's disease.
- Diet poor in fruit and vegetables.

Morphology
CRCa may occur as a polypoid, ulcerating, stenosing, or infiltrative tumour mass. The majority (75%) lie on the left side of the colon and rectum (rectum, 45%; descending-sigmoid, 30%; transverse, 5%; right-sided, 20%). Three to five per cent have a synchronous carcinoma at time of diagnosis.

Clinical features
Rectal location
- *PR bleeding.* Deep red on the surface of stools.
- *Change in bowel habit.* Difficulty with defecation, sensation of incomplete evacuation, and painful defecation (tenesmus).

Descending-sigmoid location
- *PR bleeding.* Typically dark red, mixed with stool, sometimes clotted.
- *Change in bowel habit.* Typically increased frequency, variable consistency, mucus PR, bloating, and flatulence.

Right-sided location
Iron deficiency anaemia may be the only elective presentation.

Emergency presentations
Up to 40% of colorectal carcinomas will present as emergencies.
- Large bowel obstruction (colicky pain, bloating, bowels not open).
- Perforation with peritonitis.
- Acute PR bleeding.

Diagnosis and investigations
Elective diagnosis By PR examination or rigid sigmoidoscopy for rectal carcinoma. Colonoscopy is the preferred diagnostic investigation (alternatives are barium enema and CT colonography).

Emergency presentations Commonly diagnosed by abdominal CT scan. Single contrast enema may be used when the diagnosis of large bowel obstruction is possible and CT scanning is unavailable. Acute PR bleeding is sometimes investigated by urgent colonoscopy.

Staging investigations

- Assessment of the presence of metastases (liver, lung, or para-aortic). Thoracoabdominopelvic CT scanning is gold standard; CT PET scan may be used to evaluate equivocal lesions.
- Assessment of local extent. For colonic carcinoma, CT scanning is adequate; for rectal cancer, pelvic MRI and TRUS are commonly used.
- Assessment of synchronous tumours. If not diagnosed by colonoscopy or barium enema, one of these two tests is usually performed to identify synchronous tumours.
- Tumour marker (CEA) is of no use for diagnosis or staging, but can be used to monitor disease relapse if raised at diagnosis and falls to normal after resection.

Pathological staging

Duke's (approx. % 5y survival)	*TNM*
- A, confined to bowel wall only (75–90) - B, through bowel wall (55–70) - C, any with +ve lymph nodes (30–60) - D, any with metastases (5–10)	- T1–4, stages of invasion of bowel wall - N0/1/2, no/up to 4/more than 4 lymph nodes involved - M0/1, metastases not present/present

Treatment

Potentially curative treatment

Suitable for technically resectable tumours with no evidence of metastases (or metastases potentially curable by liver or lung resection).

- Surgical resection (with lymphadenectomy) is the only curative treatment. Typical operations:
  - Right/transverse. Right/extended right hemicolectomy.
  - Left. Left hemicolectomy.
  - Sigmoid/upper rectum. High anterior resection.
  - Lower rectum. Low anterior resection/abdominoperineal resection (APER).
  - Anorectal. APER.
- Preoperative (neoadjuvant) chemoradiotherapy may be used in rectal cancer to increase the chance of curative resection.
- Adjuvant chemotherapy (5-FU based) is offered for tumours with positive lymph nodes or evidence of vascular invasion.
- Hepatic or lung resection may be offered to patients with suitable metastases and a clear resected/resectable primary tumour.

Palliative treatment

For unresectable metastases or unresectable tumours.

- Chemotherapy may effectively extend life expectancy with a good quality of life.
- Obstructing tumours may be endoluminally stented with self-expanding metal stents or transanally ablated if rectal.
- Surgery reserved for untreatable obstruction, bleeding, or severe symptoms.

Restorative pelvic surgery

Low/ultralow anterior resection

Anterior resection = removal of part or all of the rectum and anastomosis of the left colon to the remaining stump of tissue.

- Low anterior resection refers to a join that takes place below the level of the peritoneal reflection. i.e. to a short stump of rectum.
- Ultralow anterior resection refers to a join that takes place on to the top of the anal canal, i.e. no native rectum remains. The anastomosis may be stapled or sewn by hand.

The lower the level of the anastomosis, the higher the risk of complications of anastomosis, particularly anastomotic leakage (see 📖 p. 420). Most low and almost every ultralow anastomosis will have a temporary loop ileostomy formed to reduce the risk of major septic complications and consequences of leakage, but cannot prevent them.

Indications

- Rectal carcinoma.
- Rectal adenoma untreatable by other means (very rare with transanal endoscopic microsurgery (TEMS)).
- Severe or complex anorectal sepsis (including rectovaginal fistula).

Ileoanal pouch formation

For operations that remove all the colon and rectum, but do not require removal of the anus, a permanent stoma can be avoided by the formation of an ileal pouch. Formed from a side-to-side double fold of ileum ('J' pouch) or three folds sewn together ('W' pouch), joined either by hand or by staples to the upper anal canal (ileoanal anastomosis). A temporary loop ileostomy is often formed for the same reasons as for a low anterior resection (above).

Indications

- Ulcerative colitis not responding to medical management.
- FAP or multiple colorectal polyposis.
- Crohn's disease of the colon (controversial).
- Multiple colonic tumours including the rectum.

Complications of pelvic anastomosis (anterior resection and ileoanal pouch)

- *Leakage.* Occurs in up to 15% of cases; highest in the lowest anastomosis. Typically presents as fever, abdominal pain, and tachycardia (see 📖 p. 420).
- *Bleeding.* Uncommon; usually settles with supportive treatment.
- *Ischaemia.* The proximal bowel involved in the anastomosis may become ischaemic. This may present as a leak, bleeding PR, or fever and tachycardia. Diagnosis is by careful flexible sigmoidoscopy. May resolve spontaneously; progressive ischaemia results in perforation and death if not corrected by surgery.
- *Stenosis.* Narrowing of the anastomosis or bowel used to form it is an occasional late complication. Presents with difficulty in defecation and small volume frequent stools. Treatment is dilatation under anaesthetic; very rarely requires re-operation.

Minimally-invasive colorectal surgery

Transanal endoscopic microsurgery (TEMS)

Large calibre operating protoscope with operating microscope allows microsurgery within the rectum.

Indications
- Excision of large adenomas of the rectum (up to the rectosigmoid junction) in a single specimen either by mucosectomy (or occasionally full thickness).
- Excision of early rectal carcinoma (only if <3cm size, early tumour (T1), no adverse features or in elderly/comorbid patients) by single specimen full thickness excision.
- Repair of a rectovaginal fistula.

Advantages Include entirely endoscopic technique, very low risk of pararectal/pelvic sepsis, single complete specimen for histological assessment, may avoid more radical surgery.

Complications Include bleeding (rarely requires active treatment), infection in the pelvic tissues (rare, presents with deep pelvic pain, fever, tachycardia, and disturbance of bowel habit; treat with IV antibiotics).

Laparoscopic surgery

Several variants now exist. All use the same principles: minimal incisions, avoidance of exposure of viscera, light anaesthetic techniques with minimal opiates, and often enhanced recovery post-operatively.

Typical Indications
- Any colorectal resection can be performed by laparoscopic surgery.
- Rectopexy for prolapse.
- Combined treatment of large/extensive colonic polyps.
- Formation of some stomas.

Two newer variants have been used:
- *SILS.* Single incision laparoscopic surgery; one larger port for camera and instruments used at the umbilicus.
- *LESS.* Combined laparoscopic and endoscopic single site surgery; combines laparoscopic mobilization and handling with endoluminal endoscopic techniques to remove very large lesions.

Advanced polypectomy

Several advanced endoscopic techniques are used to remove large and often sessile colonic polyps.
- *EMR.* Endoscopic mucosal resection; excision (usually piecemeal) of (presumed) adenoma with use of submucosal fluid injection to facilitate snaring of the polyp.
- *ESD.* Endoscopic submucosal dissection; attempted complete excision of (presumed) adenoma using submucosal injection and endoscopic diathermy 'knife'.

Diverticular disease of the colon

Key facts

Colonic diverticula are acquired outpouchings of colonic mucosa and overlying connective tissue through the colonic wall.

- Tend to occur along the lines where the penetrating colonic arteries traverse the colonic wall between the taenia coli.
- Associated with hypertrophy of the surrounding colonic muscle with thickening of the colonic mucosa. This is probably due to the underlying pathological process, which is high pressure contractions of the colon, causing chronic pressure on the colonic wall.
- Peak age of presentation is 50–70y, but diverticular disease is increasing in frequency and occurring at a progressively younger age.

Clinical and pathological features

Asymptomatic

The majority of diverticular disease is found incidentally on barium enema examination.

Painful diverticular disease

Intermittent LIF pain may be due to diverticular disease, but irritable bowel syndrome commonly coexists and may be the cause of symptoms.

Acute diverticulitis

Rapid onset of LIF pain, nausea, fever, frequently with loose stools. Usually febrile with moderate tachycardia and LIF tenderness. Colonic wall shows acute neutrophil infiltration around the inflamed diverticulum and in the subserosal tissues.

Bleeding diverticular disease

Usually spontaneous in onset with no prodromal symptoms. Presenting with large volume dark red, clotted rectal blood. Due to rupture of a peridiverticular submucosal blood vessel. Not typically associated with inflammation.

Complications

Pericolic/paracolic mass/abscess

Acute diverticulitis may progress to persistent pericolic infection with thickening of surrounding tissues and the formation of a mass. If this suppurates, a pericolic abscess forms. Enlargement and extension of this into the paracolic area leads to a paracolic abscess. The features are those of acute diverticulitis with a swinging fever, fluctuating tachycardia, unresolving abdominal pain, and a tender LIF mass.

Peritonitis

Perforation of a pericolic or paracolic abscess usually leads to purulent peritonitis. Direct perforation of the acute diverticular segment leads to faeculent peritonitis. The features are of acute diverticulitis with high fever, severe abdominal pain, and generalized guarding and rigidity.

Diverticular fistula

Acute infection with paracolic sepsis may drain by perforation into adjacent structures. This is typically the posterior vaginal vault in women or the bladder in either sex. Colovesical fistula leads to recurrent UTI caused by enteric organisms with bubbles and debris in the urine. Colovaginal fistula leads to faeculent per vagina (PV) discharge.

Stricture formation

Chronic or repetitive inflammatory episodes may lead to fibrosis and narrowing of the colon. A history of recurrent diverticulitis with recurrent colicky abdominal pain, distension, and bloating suggests stricture formation.

Diagnosis and investigations

- Elective diagnosis is usually by double contrast barium enema. Colonoscopy is a relatively poor investigation to assess number and extent of diverticula.
- Hb, WCC, CRP during acute episodes of inflammation.
- CT scanning is the test of choice to identify complications, including abscess formation and perforation.
- Double contrast barium enema is used to assess for possible stricture formation.
- Colonoscopy is indicated if there is any suggestion of coexistent malignancy.

Treatment

Medical treatment

- High fibre diet, high fluid intake, and stool softeners to reduce intracolonic pressure.
- IV antibiotics (amoxycillin 500mg IV tds, metronidazole 500mg IV tds, gentamicin IV od) during acute infective exacerbations.
- Recurrent infective episodes *may* be prevented by a 6-week course of oral antibiotics (e.g. ciprofloxacin 500mg PO od).
- Significant paracolic abscesses may be drained by radiological guidance.

Surgical treatment

- Resection is indicated for:
  - Acute inflammation failing to respond to medical management.
  - Undrainable paracolic sepsis.
  - Free perforation.

The affected region should be resected (segmental colectomy). The ends may be re-anastomosed if they are healthy and the patient's general condition is suitable. If not, a proximal end colostomy and oversewing of the distal end is usual (Hartmann's type resection).

- Stricture may be treated by elective resection or balloon dilatation.
- Diverticular fistula may be treated by elective resection to prevent recurrent infections.

Rectal prolapse

Key facts

Rectal prolapse may be partial thickness (usually just mucosa) or full thickness involving all the layers of the rectal wall. Full thickness may be contained within the rectum (internal prolapse also called intussusception). Commonest in post-menopausal women, multiple vaginal deliveries, associated with chronic straining and chronic disorders of defecation (which cause weakness of the pelvic floor and sphincter complex), and slow transit constipation. Occasionally occurs in children suffering constipation (usually self-limiting).

Pathological features

Mucosa involved in prolapse undergoes chronic changes.
- Typically glandular branching and occasional gland misplacement.
- Thickening of the muscularis mucosae and excess submucosal collagen deposition.
- Mucosal inflammation and focal ulceration may also occur. Extensive mucosal ulceration associated with mucosal prolapse may result in an appearance called 'solitary rectal ulcer'.

Clinical features

- *Mucosal prolapse.* Discharge of mucus and small volume faecal staining, pruritus ani, and occasionally small volume bright red rectal bleeding.
- *Internal full thickness prolapse.* Sensation of rectal fullness/mass, incomplete defecation, dissatisfaction after defecation and repeated defecation.
- *External full thickness prolapse.* External prolapsing mass after defecation (usually requiring manual reduction), mucus and faecal soiling, occasional bright red rectal bleeding (may be large volume if prolapse becomes ulcerated).

Diagnosis and investigations

- Rigid sigmoidoscopy may show features of mucosal inflammation, particularly the anterior rectal mucosa.
- Prolapse may be demonstrable on straining in clinic.
- Defecating proctogram may be performed to confirm the diagnosis if it is unclear and surgery is contemplated. Proctogram required to confirm the diagnosis of internal prolapse if suspected. May also demonstrate associated problems of pelvic floor and rectocele.
- Colonic transit studies may be used if there is suspected slow transit constipation and resection is possible.

Treatment

Medical treatment

- Avoidance of straining and adaptation of defecatory habit (biofeedback).
- Avoidance of constipation (stool softeners and bulking agents, rather than stimulants).

Surgical treatment

Mucosal prolapse
- Recurrent banding or dilute phenol injection of excess mucosa.
- Mucosal excision.
- Stapled anopexy (also called procedure for prolapse and haemorrhoids (PPH)) sometimes used.

Full thickness prolapse (internal or external)
Surgery indicated for failure of control of symptoms. Choice of operation depends on age and extent of prolapse.
- Delorme's perineal rectopexy (mucosal excision with sutured plication of the excessively long rectal muscle tube in an effort to shorten it to prevent prolapse). Ideal for very frail and elderly, but least successful with highest recurrence rate of all surgical procedures.
- Altmeier's perineal rectal resection (mucosal and rectal muscle tube excision with sutured perineal anastomosis). Avoids abdominal operation, but has increased morbidity due to perineal anastomosis.
- Transabdominal rectopexy (mobilization of the rectum and suturing to the presacral fascia). May be done via a laparotomy or laparoscopically. May be just to ventral surface of the rectum with suspensory mesh (ventral mesh rectopexy). Highest success rate for prevention of recurrence of prolapse. May be combined with a sigmoid resection if there is marked associated constipation on transit studies.

Key revision points—anorectal physiology
- The internal anal sphincter is smooth muscle and under involuntary control of the pelvic autonomic system. Relaxants include nitric oxide donors (e.g. GTN) and calcium antagonists (e.g. diltiazem).
- The external anal sphincter is skeletal muscle and under voluntary control of the pudendal nerve (S2, 3, 4). Relaxation (by temporary partial paralysis) may be achieved by botulinum toxin injection.
- Defecation is a complex sensorimotor process that requires intact pelvic autonomics, sacral spinal nerves, and pelvic floor muscle function.

Pilonidal sinus disease

Key facts

Single or multiple sinuses ('pits') that exist in the midline of the buttock clefts. Usually contain hair, inspissated secretions, and debris. Commonest in men, dark-haired, hirsute people, especially eastern Mediterranean races. Probably caused by local trauma, causing retention of hairs within initially normal midline pits. May be precipitated by long periods seated, e.g. lorry drivers, computer operators.

Pathological features

Typified by chronic inflammation. Once inflammation has started, sinuses often extend and may become interlinked. Lateral tracks may run out into the neighbouring buttock tissue.

Clinical features

- *Irritative features.* Intermittent discharge and inflammation with pain and swelling.
- *Acute sepsis.* Acute abscess formation is common with swelling, pain, and erythema; may discharge spontaneously or may cause fistulation with sinuses appearing in the lateral buttock tissue.
- *Chronic sepsis.* Usually follows unresolved acute sepsis either after spontaneous discharge or surgical drainage.

Diagnosis and investigations

- Ensure the patient is tested for occult diabetes mellitus.
- Very extensive sinus formation and fistulation may be assessed by MRI scanning of the natal cleft and buttocks.

Treatment

Medical/non-surgical
- Shaving of local hairs and washing of accessible cavities (usually by a partner or family member) may control local symptoms.
- Intermittent courses of antibiotics may be required for septic episodes.
- Formed pilonidal abscess or collection requires surgical drainage (under local or general anaesthetic).
- Recurrent acute sepsis or persistently symptomatic chronic sepsis usually requires surgical treatment.

Surgical
Principles of surgical treatments are:
- Excision of all sinus openings.
- Obliteration of all infected or chronically inflamed tissue.
- Obliteration of the natal cleft by flattening (thought to be most important in the prevention of recurrence by reducing the risk of further hair implantation).

Surgical options are:
- Primary excision with laying open of wound and closure by secondary intention is very rarely used, except in extensive recurrent disease; it requires daily dressings for many weeks or months.
- Tension-free apposition of the skin edges (may be by lateral flaps, e.g. Karyadakis or Bascom procedures, or by plastic surgical flaps, e.g. rhomboid, rotational, or Z plasty flaps).

Key revision points—anatomy of the large bowel
- Main features of large intestine structure:
  - Complete layer of circular smooth muscle throughout, but incomplete bands of longitudinal muscle (taeniae coli) in colon (complete in rectum).
  - Fatty appendages along taeniae (appendices epiploicae).
  - Folded internal mucosal appearances (haustrations).
  - 'Segmented' external appearances (sacculations).
- Four main arterial (and lymph node) territories (used for resections):
  - Ileocolic and right colic arteries (from SMA): last terminal ileal loop, caecum, and ascending colon.
  - Middle colic artery (from SMA): transverse colon up to the splenic flexure.
  - Left colic (from IMA): splenic flexure and descending colon.
  - Superior rectal artery (from IMA): rectum and upper anal canal.
- Autonomic nerve supply:
  - Sympathetic, mainly from greater splanchnic nerves via SMA and IMA plexuses.
  - Parasympathetic, from vagus via SMA and IMA plexus from caecum to splenic flexure and from pelvic parasympathetics (S2, 3, 4) via hypogastric plexuses and retroperitoneal nerves from splenic flexure to upper anal canal.

Fistula-in-ano

Key facts

A fistula is an abnormal connection of two epithelial surfaces and the two surfaces joined in fistula in ano are the anorectal lining and the perineal or vaginal skin. Very common, especially in otherwise fit young adults. May occur in the presence of Crohn's disease; minor association with obesity and diabetes mellitus, very rarely due to trauma or ulceration of anorectal tumours.

Pathological features

Commonest cause is sepsis arising in an anal gland that forces its way out through the anal tissues to appear in the perianal or in women, vaginal skin (cryptoglandular theory of fistula in ano). Often presents initially as an acute perianal abscess. The tissues through which the track pushes determines the classification of fistulas (see Fig. 11.1).

Clinical features

- *Acute perianal abscess.* Rapid onset of severe perianal or perineal pain. Swelling and erythema of the perianal skin with fever and tachycardia.
- *Recurrent perianal sepsis.* Recurrent intermittent sepsis typified by gradual build-up of 'pressure' sensation and swelling in the perianal skin and eventual discharge of bloodstained purulent fluid.
- *Chronic perianal discharge.* Persistent low grade sepsis of the track with chronic discharge of seropurulent fluid via a punctum that is usually clearly identified by the patient.

Diagnosis and investigations

Diagnosis and investigation should aim to confirm the presence of a fistula and identify the course of the track to determine the type of fistula:

- Examination of the perineum and rectal examination may reveal a palpable fibrous track.
- EUA with probing of any external opening to aid identification of the course of the track.
- Endoanal ultrasound (sometimes with hydrogen peroxide injected into the track) identifies the course of the track.
- MRI scanning is probably the most sensitive method of determining the course of the track and identifying any occult perianal or pelvic sepsis.
- Flexible sigmoidoscopy if associated colorectal disease, e.g. Crohn's disease, is suspected.

Treatment

Medical treatment

- Antibiotics may reduce symptoms from recurrent sepsis, but cannot treat the underlying fistula.
- Medical treatment of inflammatory bowel disease may dramatically reduce symptoms from associated fistulas.

Surgical treatment

Principles of surgical treatment are as follows:

- Drainage of any acute sepsis if present.
- Prevention of recurrent sepsis. Usually by insertion of a loose seton suture, e.g. silastic sling.
- Low fistula in ano. Lay open track, remove all chronic granulation tissue, and allow to heal spontaneously (fistulotomy); little risk of impairment of continence due to minimal division of sphincter tissues.
- High fistula in ano:
  - Remove fistula track and close the internal opening (core fistulectomy and endorectal flap advancement).
  - Slowly divide the sphincter tissue between the fistula and the perianal skin (cutting seton); low risk of incontinence.
  - Fill the fistula with fibrin glue.

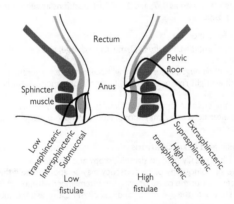

Fig. 11.1 Classification of fistula-in-ano.

Haemorrhoids

Key facts

Broad term, often incorrectly used to refer any perianal excess tissue. True haemorrhoids are excessive amounts of the normal endoanal cushions that comprise anorectal mucosa, submucosal tissue, and submucosal blood vessels (small arterioles and veins). Commonest age of onset is in young adulthood. Associated with constipation, chronic straining, obesity, and previous childbirth. May become ulcerated and inflamed if recurrently prolapsing.

- If confined to the tissue of the upper anal canal, they are referred to as 'internal'.
- If extend to the tissues of the lower anal canal, they are referred to as 'external'.
- Typically occur in the same location as the main anal blood vessel pedicles (described as 3, 7, and 11 o'clock positions as seen in the supine position).

Clinical features

- *Features of irritation.* Pruritus ani, mucus discharge, and perianal discomfort.
- *Features of damage to mucosal lining.* Recurrent post-defecatory bleeding—bright red, not mixed with stools, on paper or splashing in the toilet pan.
- *Features of prolapse.* Intermittent lump appearing at anal margin, usually after defecation, may spontaneously reduce or require manual reduction.

Diagnosis and investigations

- Diagnosis is usually by rigid sigmoidoscopy and proctoscopy.
- Flexible sigmoidoscopy or colonoscopy may be appropriate if there is concern about the cause of symptoms; *remember*—haemorrhoids rarely start over the age of 55y and it is often best to assume another cause until proven otherwise in these cases.

Treatment

Medical treatment Avoidance of constipation and straining; bulking or softener laxatives.

Surgical treatment

- Banding or excessive tissue. Best for prolapse symptoms (not possible for external components due to excellent nerve supply of lower anal canal).
- Dilute phenol injections (5% in almond oil). Best for bleeding symptoms.
- Haemorrhoidal devascularization procedures (e.g. arterial ligation 'HALO' either Doppler ultrasound-guided or blind). For failed topical treatments and surgery not indicated/desired.
- Stapled anopexy (also called PPH). Sometimes used for circumferential prolapsing haemorrhoids.

- Haemorrhoidectomy for large external haemorrhoids or haemorrhoids failing to respond to conservative treatment. Associated with a small risk of impaired continence and anal stenosis.

Key revision points—anatomy of the anus
- Lower third of the anal canal is somatic tissue in origin—stratified squamous epithelium; very sensitive (pudendal and distal sacral nerves); relatively poor blood supply and healing.
- Upper third of the canal is visceral tissue in origin—columnar epithelium; insensitive; excellent blood supply and healing.

Acute anorectal pain

Causes and features

Fissure-in-ano Acute severe, localized, 'knife-like' pain in the anus during defecation. Often associated with deep throbbing pain for minutes or hours afterwards due to pelvic floor spasm. Blood on the paper when wiping (small volume, red-pink streaks or spots).

Haemorrhoids Usually acutely prolapsed and inflamed with associated perianal lump, soreness, and irritation. May bleed, often profuse, bright red.

Perianal abscess Gradual onset, constant localized perianal pain. Associated swelling with tenderness and possible discharge. May have associated systemic features of fever, malaise, anorexia.

Perianal haematoma Usually sudden onset; acutely painful with associated perianal swelling (dark red coloured).

Rectal prolapse Acute full thickness rectal prolapse, occasionally causes pain. Obvious large perineal lump, dark red blue with surface mucus and occasionally some surface ulceration.

Emergency management

Establish a diagnosis

- Good inspection and careful digital rectal examination is usually all that is required.
- Rigid sigmoidoscopy may be painful and is often unnecessary.
- Flexible sigmoidoscopy is rarely indicated.

Early treatment

- Give adequate analgesia; opiates may be necessary.
- Topical treatment is highly effective; cool pads, topical local anaesthetic gels.

Definitive management

Fissure-in-ano Mainstay of acute treatment is analgesia and anal sphincter muscle relaxants, e.g. topical GTN 0.2% ointment, diltiazem 2% ointment. Local anaesthetics are helpful early in treatment.

Haemorrhoids May require bed rest with continued topical treatment until swelling resolves and spontaneous reduction begins. Acute haemorrhoidectomy is almost always best avoided due to the risk of over-excision of anal tissue. Minimal anal dilatation under GA is rarely necessary.

Perianal abscess Incision and drainage is a surgical emergency, particularly if the patient is diabetic or immunosuppressed.

Perianal haematoma Incision to allow decompression of acute haematoma may be necessary, often done under topical LA.

Rectal prolapse Swelling may be reduced by cool packs, elevation, and sometimes icing sugar applied to the swollen mucosa as a dessicant! Very rarely requires emergency surgery.

Acute rectal bleeding

Causes and features

Acute rectal bleeding is broadly divided into regions of the colon from which it comes and the blood is typically different according to the origin.

Anorectal

Bright red blood, on the surface of the stool and paper, after defecation.
- Haemorrhoids.
- Acute anal fissure.
- Distal proctitis.
- Rectal prolapse.

Rectosigmoid

Darker red blood, with clots, in surface of stool and mixed.
- Rectal tumours (benign or malignant).
- Proctocolitis.
- Diverticular disease.

Proximal colonic

Dark red blood mixed into stool or altered blood.
- Colonic tumours (benign or malignant).
- Colitis.
- Angiodysplasia.
- NSAID-induced ulceration.

Upper GI bleeding occasionally produces dark red rectal bleeding, but it is usually associated with significant haemodynamic instability when sufficiently large.

Features (signs)

- Tachycardia and hypotension suggests substantial loss.
- LIF tenderness suggests diverticular inflammation with bleeding.

Emergency management

Resuscitation

- Establish large calibre IV access; give crystalloid fluid up to 1000mL if tachycardic or hypotensive.
- Catheterize and place on a fluid balance chart if hypotensive.
- Send blood for FBC (Hb, WCC), U&E (Na, K), LFTs (albumin), group and save, clotting.

Establish a diagnosis

- Rigid proctosigmoidoscopy should be performed in all cases to exclude a simple anorectal cause.
- Urgent flexible sigmoidoscopy and colonoscopy may be undertaken. It is higher risk than elective endoscopy, but may confirm an origin and may allow therapeutic intervention (adrenaline injection, heater probe coagulation, argon plasma coagulation (APC)).
- Urgent selective mesenteric arteriography for obscure or persistent bleeding; needs active bleeding of 0.5mL/min.

- Urgent gastroscopy should be used to exclude massive upper GI bleeding if suspected.

Early treatment Consider blood transfusion if major bleed (persisting haemodynamic instability despite resuscitation, Hb <8g/dL).

Definitive management

Anorectal causes Most can be controlled by local measures, such as injection, coagulation, or packing.

Acute colitis
- IV or PO metronidazole if thought to be infective until organism identified.
- IV hydrocortisone 100mg qds if thought to be ulcerative or Crohn's colitis.
- Surgery may be necessary whatever the aetiology if bleeding persists (subtotal colectomy and ileostomy formation).

Diverticular disease
- IV antibiotics (cefuroxime 750mg tds + metronidazole 500mg tds).
- Angiographic embolization if bleeding fails to stop and patient not critically unstable for time in radiology.
- Surgery is high risk, but may be unavoidable. If the location is known, a directed hemicolectomy may be performed (on-table colonoscopy may be used). If not, a subtotal colectomy is safest.

Angiodysplasia
- Colonoscopic therapy (injection, heater probe, APC) is ideal.
- Angiographic embolization may be possible.
- Right hemicolectomy is occasionally unavoidable.

Undiagnosed source
Rarely, the patient remains unstable with active bleeding and no cause can be reliably confirmed. Surgical options to deal with this include:
- On-table colonoscopy with washout via colostomy to locate bleeding source.
- Formation of mid-transverse loop colostomy and subsequent targeted hemicolectomy.
- 'Blind' hemicolectomy (left if significant diverticular disease present; right if no other cause obvious and angiodysplasia is likely).

Acute severe colitis

Causes and features

Any cause of colitis may progress to acute severity. Common causes include:

- Severe ulcerative colitis (UC; usually pancolitis); occasionally, acute severe colitis is the presentation of UC with no prior history;
- Acute infective colitis (e.g. Salmonella, *C. difficile*, amoebae, parasites);
- Neutropenic colitis;
- Pseudomembranous colitis (*C. difficile*-related);
- Progressive Crohn's colitis (usually with a clear prior history).

Symptoms

- Diarrhoea (usually bloody with urgency and frequency). 'Constipation' may be an ominous feature, suggesting acute colonic dilatation.
- Abdominal pain (generalized).
- Malaise, anorexia, and fever (systemic inflammatory features).

Signs

- Fever, tachycardia, possible hypotension.
- Abdominal tenderness; peritonism suggests perforation.

Complications

Any acute severe colitis may develop any of these complications.

- Haemorrhage.
- Hypokalaemia.
- Hypoalbuminaemia;.
- Perforation (localized or generalized).

'Toxic dilatation' is a term used to describe the situation of acute severe colitis with colonic dilatation usually associated with reduced bowel frequency and impending perforation.

Fulminant severe colitis is defined as: tachycardia >120bpm or stool frequency >10 times/24h or albumin <25g/dL.

Emergency management

Resuscitation

- Establish large calibre IV access; give crystalloid fluid up to 1000mL if tachycardic or hypotensive.
- Catheterize and place on a fluid balance chart if hypotensive.
- Send blood for FBC (Hb, WCC), U&E (Na, K), LFTs (albumin), group and save, clotting.

Establish a diagnosis

- Send 'hot' stools for M,C,&S as well as microscopy for C,P,&O. Even known colitics may catch acute infective colitis.
- Plain AXR (looking for colonic dilatation) and erect CXR (looking for free gas).
- Rigid sigmoidoscopy and biopsy only if not unstable.
- Flexible endoscopy may be indicated, but carries a risk of perforation.

Early treatment
- Give IV hydrocortisone if the diagnosis of UC is likely; if infective colitis is suspected, consider withholding steroids until the M,C,&S results are back.
- Blood transfusion if anaemic.
- Surgery if peritonitis or free gas on CXR (the operation for any acute colitis is usually total abdominal colectomy and end ileostomy formation).

Definitive management

Acute ulcerative colitis
- IV hydrocortisone 100mg qds, converted to oral prednisolone if responding to treatment.
- IV cyclosporin if fulminant/not responding to IV steroids.
- Surgery for failure to respond to medical treatment or acute complications of haemorrhage or perforation.
- Regular blood investigations and plain abdominal radiography to monitor treatment.

Infective colitis
- IV or PO metronidazole until organism identified.
- Salmonella, *C. difficile*—metronidazole.
- Surgery for failure to respond to medical treatment or acute complications of haemorrhage or perforation.

Neutropenic colitis
- IV antibiotics.
- Bone marrow support.
- Surgery for failure to respond to medical treatment or acute complications of haemorrhage or perforation.

Post-operative anastomotic leakage

Causes and features
Any intra-abdominal anastomosis may leak. Highest risk of leak occurs with oesophageal and rectal anastomosis and lowest with small bowel anastomosis (see Table 11.1).

Anastomotic leakage may present as one of several clinical pictures.

▶▶ Peritonitis
Acute severe generalized abdominal pain with generalized guarding and rigidity. Fever, tachycardia, and tachypnoea are common. Diagnosis is usually clinical, but may require CT scanning if unsure.

Intra-abdominal abscess (see 📖 p. 308)
Swinging fever and tachycardia, commonly around 5–7 days post-operatively. Localized tenderness related to the anastomosis may be present. Diagnosis should be sought by CT scanning.

Enteric fistula
A fistula between the anastomosis and the wound or another organ may occur. Usually occurs as a result of a subclinical leak and abscess formation that discharges through a pathway of low resistance. Often presents late as an apparent wound infection that discharges with enteric content. Diagnosis made by CT scanning or occasionally, fistulography if presents very late.

▶ Cardiovascular complications
⚠ Sepsis originating from an initially subclinical leak may present with apparent cardiovascular complications, e.g. AF, SVT, chest pain, and sinus tachycardia. A wise precautionary rule is, 'Any acute post-operative disturbance of physiology in a patient with an intra-abdominal anastomosis is due to leak until proven otherwise.'

Emergency management
Resuscitation
- Establish large calibre IV access; give crystalloid fluid up to 1000mL if tachycardic or hypotensive.
- Catheterize and place on a fluid balance chart if hypotensive.
- Send blood for FBC (Hb, WCC), U&E (Na, K), LFTs (albumin), group and save, clotting.
- Give appropriate analgesia if not on an epidural or PCA.

Establish a diagnosis
- Acute peritonitis needs no diagnostic investigation. Emergency re-look laparotomy should be organized immediately.
- CT scanning with IV and PO contrast is the investigation of choice for all other suspected leaks.
- For rectal anastomoses, a water-soluble contrast study may delineate a leak.

Table 11.1 Risk factors associated with increased risk of leak

Patient factors	Disease factors	Operative factors
Chronic malnutrition Immunosuppression	Unprepared bowel, e.g. obstruction	Poor blood supply or bowel ends
High dose steroid use Diabetes mellitus	Local or generalized sepsis Metastatic malignancy	Tension on bowel ends

Early treatment
- Give IV antibiotics (e.g. IV cefuroxime 750mg tds + metronidazole 500mg tds).
- Monitor fluid balance hourly.

Definitive management
▶▶ *Peritonitis*
Always requires surgical intervention unless the patient is deemed unfit. Prepare for theatre. Ensure blood results from resuscitation are available. Stoma care review is not always necessary and often not practical or useful.

Once the leak has been identified, options for management include:
- Dividing the anastomosis, closing the distal end, and forming the proximal end into a stoma;
- Emptying the bowel (lavage) and forming a proximal defunctioning stoma;
- Re-forming or repairing the anastomosis (only suitable for fit patients with minimal contamination and an otherwise healthy anastomosis);
- Placing a large drain(s) next to the anastomosis.

Intra-abdominal abscess
- Radiologically guided drainage and antibiotics, provided patient does not become peritonitic or show signs of secondary complications.
- Open surgical drainage if inaccessible or unresponsive to radiological drainage.

Enteric fistula
- Usually managed by antibiotics. May close spontaneously; if fails to close, surgical repair may be required.
- Treat as for abscess or peritonitis if either develops.

Paediatric surgery

Principles of managing paediatric surgical cases

Key facts
- Children are not small adults.
- Children come in different sizes; always obtain a weight before starting treatment.
- Fluids and drug doses depend on body weight.
- Babies and children have different differential diagnoses from adults.
- Children often differ from adults in physiology and anatomy (see Table 12.1).
- Babies and young children have difficulty communicating symptoms.

Special problems with babies
- Thermoregulation is impaired (immature sweating, high surface area to body weight increases rate of heat loss). Prone to hypothermia.
- Minimal glycogen stores. Prone to acute hypoglycaemia.
- Principal breathing pattern is diaphragmatic. Prone to breathing difficulties with abdominal distension.
- Immature body physiology. Much less biological functional reserve than adults; acute disturbances of physiology more serious with less room for error.
- May not metabolize drugs as expected.

Intravenous fluids
Maintenance fluids (see Box 12.1)

Box 12.1 Paediatric fluid regimen
- 4mL/kg/h total fluid for each of the first 10kg of weight (0–10kg).
- 2mL/kg/h total fluid for each of the next 10kg of weight (11–20kg).
- 1mL/kg/h total fluid for each subsequent kg of weight (over 21kg)

- Always calculate fluid and sodium requirements according to weight.
- Remember to add glucose, especially for neonates.
- Adjust the fluid regimen according to clinical setting for neonates and premature babies.

Resuscitation fluids
- Crystalloids or colloids can be given as resuscitation fluids.
- Mild dehydration—10mL/kg bolus; repeat as necessary.
- Moderate dehydration—20mL/kg bolus; repeat as necessary.

Table 12.1 Basic physiological parameters in children

	Neonates	Adolescents
Blood volume (mL/kg)	80	30–40
Oral fluid intake (mL/kg/day)	150	30–40
Daily Na$^+$ intake (mmol/kg)	2–3	1–2
Daily K$^+$ intake (mmol/kg)	2–3	1
Systolic BP (mmHg)	40–50	100–120
Resting pulse rate (bpm)	120–160	70–80

Acute abdominal emergencies—overview

Key facts

- Whatever the cause (see Fig. 12.1), these typically present with signs and symptoms of either peritonitis or intestinal obstruction.
- Features of peritonitis are often difficult to elicit in babies.
- Cardinal features of obstruction are:
  - Vomiting.
  - Abdominal distension.
  - Failure to pass meconium.
  - Pain.

Vomiting in children

- Vomiting is common in newborns and is often entirely benign. May be due to:
  - Overfeeding.
  - Rapid feeding.
  - Air swallowing (inadequate winding).
- Vomiting may be due to metabolic causes (inborn errors of metabolism, acidosis) or infections (UTI, chest infection, meningitis).
- Bile-stained vomiting should never be ignored.

Abdominal distension
Most pronounced in distal obstruction and less so in proximal causes of obstruction.

Failure to pass meconium

- Term babies should pass meconium within 36h.
- Babies with proximal obstruction or atresia may still pass meconium.

Pain
May be difficult to assess in babies. Typical features are going off feeds, lethargy, erratic heart rate.

Diagnostic features

History

- Family/genetic history for cystic fibrosis (CF). Meconium ileus.
- Premature birth. Necrotizing enterocolitis.
- Time of onset related to birth. The more proximal the obstruction, the earlier the presentation.

Examination

- Blood in vomit or stool may indicate necrotic bowel.
- Degree of distension. Most pronounced with distal obstruction.

Investigations

- Plain AXR may show diagnostic features.
  - *'Double bubble sign'*. Duodenal atresia or malrotation.
  - *'Ground glass'*. Meconium ileus.
  - *Multiple loops of small bowel*. Distal obstruction.
  - *Intramural gas* ('pneumatosis intestinalis'). Necrotizing enterocolitis.
  - *Free air*. Intestinal perforation.
- *Abdominal ultrasound*. Abdominal mass. Intussusception, tumour, duplication cyst.

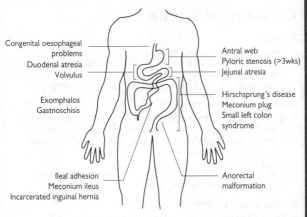

Fig. 12.1 Causes of acute abdominal emergencies in babies and infants.

Oesophageal atresia

Key facts

- Congenital abnormality of the formation of the upper aerodigestive tract (UADT), resulting in partial or complete interruption of the oesophageal lumen (see Fig. 12.2).
- Often associated with other congenital abnormalities (VACTERL).

Clinicopathological features

- May be diagnosed on prenatal ultrasound. Features include maternal polyhydramnios, absent stomach bubble, associated abnormalities.
- Post-natal diagnosis relies on features of persistent salivary drooling, regurgitation of all feeds, and cyanosis with feeding.
- Failure to pass NGT into stomach.
- Tracheo-oesophageal fistula in isolation unusual. Presents with recurrent aspiration/chest infections.

Diagnosis and treatment

- Plain AXR and thorax. NGT coiled in oesophagus.
- Presence of stomach gas suggests tracheo-distal oesophageal fistula.
- Plain X-ray spine. Associated congenital abnormalities.
- Echocardiography. Associated cardiac abnormalities.

Medical treatment

- Nurse head-up.
- NBM and continuous Replogle (oro-oesophageal) tube.
- Antibiotics for possible aspiration pneumonia.

Surgical treatment

- *Isolated atresia.*
  - Gastrostomy for feeding + continuous drainage of upper pouch.
  - Delayed closure of defect (may require interposition graft if a long segment involved).
- *Atresia with tracheo-oesophageal fistula.* Ligation of fistula and primary closure of oesophageal defect.
- *Isolated tracheo-oesophageal fistula.* Ligation of fistula (through neck).

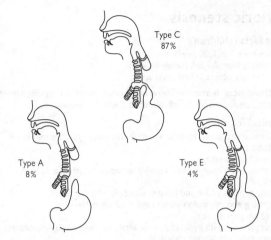

Fig. 12.2 Classification of oesophageal atresia. Type C (III), distal fistula; type A (I), atresia without fistula; type E (V), H-type fistula.

Pyloric stenosis

Key facts (children)

- Incidence 3 in 1000 live births.
- Increased familial risk (family history).
- It typically occurs in first born boys ($\circlearrowleft$:$\circlearrowleft$, 4:1).

Pathological features There is hypertrophy of the pyloric smooth muscle in early infancy, which occurs at about 3–6 weeks.

Clinical features

- Classical projectile, forceful vomiting (secondary gastritis may cause bloodstaining).
- Persisting vomiting.
- Sometimes a history of excessive positing and gastro-oesophageal reflux.
- Baby appears active and hungry, especially after vomiting.
- Small, green, starvation stools passed infrequently.
- Weight gain is poor.
- Dehydration with hypochloraemic alkalosis gradually supervenes in untreated, established condition.
- Baby usually looks well in early state.
- Dehydration, pallor, underweight only in advanced condition.
- Epigastric fullness with left-to-right gastric peristaltic wave.
- Test feed is usually performed to palpate a pyloric 'tumour' (see Box 12.2).

Diagnosis and investigations

- If pyloric 'tumour' is felt, no radiological investigations are necessary prior to surgery.
- Ultrasound shows thickened (>4mm), elongated (>16mm) pyloric muscle and increased muscle to lumen ratio with decreased movement of fluid through narrow canal (term infants).
- Barium meal (rarely necessary) shows an enlarged stomach, increased gastric peristalsis, and elongated, narrowed pyloric canal.
- Electrolytes and capillary blood gases ($\downarrow Na^+$, $\downarrow K^+$, $\downarrow Cl^-$, base excess, and pH).

Treatment

- Resuscitation with IV rehydration.
- Correct hypovolaemia with 10mL/kg 0.9% saline.
- Correct hypochloraemic alkalosis and hypokalaemia (may take 24–48h)—0.45% sodium chloride/5% dextrose with added potassium chloride at a rate of 120–150mL/kg/24h.
- NGT drainage to prevent aspiration of vomited secretions.

Surgical treatment

- Pyloromyotomy (division of pyloric muscle fibres without opening of bowel lumen).
  - Done via right upper quadrant incision, periumbilical, or laparoscopically.

- Caution not to open mucosa and avoid the prepyloric vein ('of Mayo').
- Start feeding within 4–6h post-operatively and increase to full volume by 24h.

Box 12.2 How to perform a test feed
- Undress baby (leaving loose nappy) and place on carer's lap with head elevated.
- Sit opposite baby and carer; position baby so head is to examiner's right.
- Begin feeding (breast or bottle). With active suckling, the abdominal wall relaxes.
- Palpate with left hand (middle finger).
- Begin above umbilicus and feel into RUQ under liver edge.
- Wait to feel appearance of olive-sized, firm, mobile lump in angle between liver edge and upper right rectus muscle (contracted pyloric muscles).
- As stomach inflates with air and milk, pylorus becomes more difficult to feel—aspiration of NGT may help.

Malrotation and volvulus

Key facts and clinical features (neonates)

Malrotation
- This can present at birth or soon after and symptoms are due to rotation of the small bowel, leading to duodenal obstruction.
- 'Ladd's bands' are occasionally the cause of the obstruction.
- Proximal duodenal distension leads to bile-stained vomiting.
- The caecum may be in an abnormally high or midline position.

Volvulus
- Twisting, in clockwise direction, of malrotated, non-fixed midgut loop on its narrow-based mesentery through 360° or more.
- Results in obstruction of superior mesenteric blood vessels.
- Signs. Sudden onset of abdominal pain, bile vomiting, progression to shock, passage of blood per rectum.
- May be less dramatic; most dangerous in newborn period because of delay in diagnosis and rapid development of gut ischaemia.
- Older children may present insidiously or as rapid onset of shock with less prominent other symptoms.

Diagnosis and investigations

▶▶ If in doubt, operate. Viability of twisted bowel is very time-dependent—delays in diagnosis can be very serious.

- *Plain AXR.* 'Double bubble' sign with some distal gas.
- *Barium meal.* Obstruction of second part duodenum, non-rotation of duodenum/jejunum, and corkscrew appearance of proximal small bowel loops; absent C loop of duodenum.
- *Ultrasound scan.* Reversed relation of superior mesenteric artery and vein.
- *Doppler ultrasound.* Absent or abnormal small bowel blood.

Treatment
- Resuscitation, including decompression with NGT.
- Prompt surgery to avoid irreversible bowel damage.
- Laparotomy may reveal:
  - Obstructed, but viable bowel.
  - Patchy ischaemic changes.
  - Established necrosis.
- Resection of ischaemic gut may risk 'short gut syndrome'.
- 'Second look' laparotomy (24–48h) allows reassessment prior to resection.

Intussusception

Key facts (children)
- Incidence approximately 2 per 1000 live births.
- Peak age of presentation at 3–10 months.
- ♂:♀, 2:1.
- Fewer than 10% have a clear focal pathological cause that starts the intussusception ('apex'; older children are more likely to have an apex).

Clinicopathological features
- Invagination/telescoping of the proximal bowel (called the intussusceptum, e.g. terminal ileum/ileocaecal valve) into the distal bowel (called the intussuscepiens, e.g. caecum/ascending colon).
- May be due to enlargement of lymphatic patches of Peyer ('idiopathic').
- Pathology at the apex may be:
  - Meckel's diverticulum.
  - Polyp.
  - Lymphoma.

Clinical features
- Classic triad of features is:
  - Abdominal pain (associated with pallor, screaming, and restlessness).
  - Palpable sausage-shaped mass (mid-abdominal or right upper quadrant).
  - Passage of 'redcurrant jelly' stool (rectal examination may reveal bloody mucus and the lead point may rarely be palpable).
- Typically, the infant is relatively settled between bouts of pain.
- Signs of shock (lethargy, poor feeding, hypotonia) require urgent fluid resuscitation.
- Features of obstruction (distension and vomiting) may occur.

Diagnosis and investigations
- *Ultrasound* (diagnostic test of choice). Intussusception in cross-section ('doughnut' or 'target' sign).
- *Plain X-ray*. May show soft tissue mass, small bowel obstruction, free air indicating perforation.
- *Air (or rarely gastrograffin) contrast enema*. Diagnostic and may be therapeutic (see below).

Treatment
- Immediate IV fluid resuscitation to correct fluid losses and to restore fluid, electrolyte, and acid/base balance.
- Maintenance fluid replacement and replacement of continued losses (vomiting or nasogastric losses). Reduction only attempted once fluid balance restored.
- Analgesia and sedation (morphine 0.2mg/kg) will aid process of reduction.
- Antibiotics and NGT.

Methods of reduction

Radiological reduction

- Air enema therapeutic in 75% of cases.
- Usually performed in radiology department under screening control.
- Surgeon should be present.
- Evidence of irreducible obstruction or perforation mandates immediate halt.
- Partial or incomplete reduction may warrant repeat attempt after 4–6h.
- Informed consent includes risk of perforation.

Surgical reduction

- Laparotomy indicated without enema if evidence of peritonitis or perforation.
- Manual reduction by retrograde squeezing and gentle proximal traction.
- Resection and anastomosis if bowel viability is in doubt (~10% require resection).
- Post-reduction septic shock may occur with release of bacterial products from viable, but damaged bowel segment.
- Most recover rapidly with resumption of oral feeding in 24–48h and discharge home in 4–5 days.

Complications

- Recurrence rate is 5–7% in non-operative cases and about 3% for operative reduction.
- Morbidity is low, but delayed diagnosis, inadequate resuscitation, and failure to recognize ischaemic or perforated bowel account for 1% mortality.

Hirschsprung's disease

Key facts (neonates/children)
- Incidence 1 in 5000 live births.
- Commoner in males.

Pathological features
- Due to incomplete migration of neural crest cells into the hindgut, resulting in distal aganglionosis and failure of coordinated peristaltic waves, abnormal anorectal relaxation, and loss of recto-anal inhibitory reflexes.
- May involve:
  - Just the anorectal junction (ultrashort segment), presents in adult life.
  - The rectum and recto-sigmoid (short segment. 70%), presents in infancy or early childhood.
  - Extensive colonic involvement (long segment), rare.
- The proximal (normal) bowel becomes progressively distended due to build-up of faecal matter.

Clinical features
- There is failure to pass meconium within 24–48h, abdominal distension, and bile vomiting.
- It may be associated with Down's syndrome.
- It may present late with poor weight gain, offensive diarrhoea, or enterocolitis.

Diagnosis and investigations
- Radiograph shows dilated colon to level of 'transition zone' to aganglionic bowel.
- Contrast enema shows less distensible rectum and may indicate transition zone.
- Suction rectal biopsy confirms diagnosis; thickened nerve fibres and aganglionisis (↑ AChE (in older children) shows failure of anal relaxation on rectal balloon distension (loss of recto-anal inhibitory reflex).
- Anorectal manometry (in older children) shows failure of anal relaxation on rectal balloon distension (loss of recto-anal inhibitory reflex).

Treatment
- Resuscitation and analgesia.
- Decompression of the colon with regular saline rectal wash-outs.
- If decompression is not achieved or there is total colonic involvement, a defunctioning stoma is necessary.
- Definitive surgery is to remove the aganglionic bowel and bring normally innervated bowel to the anus (pull-through technique— Soave, Swenson, or Duhamel types).
  - It is usually performed as a one-stage procedure without a covering stoma.
  - The pull-through can be performed transanally or abdominally.
  - Laparoscopy assists in establishing a level and mobilizing the colon/rectum.

Complications
- Constipation.
- Enterocolitis can affect 20–50% of children pre- and post-operatively (uncommon >5y of age unless an obstructive component exists).

Further reading
Langer JC (2004). Hirschsprung's disease. *Curr Probl Surg* **41**: 949–88.
Swenson O (2002). Hirschsprung's disease: a review. *Pediatrics* **109**(5): 914–8.
Teitelbaum DH, Coran AG (2003). Primary pull-through for Hirschsprung's disease. *Sem Neonatol* **8**(3): 233–41.

Rare causes of intestinal obstruction

Duodenal atresia
- Caused by failure of development or canalization of the duodenal canal.
- May be complete (i.e. entirely separate proximal and distal duodenum) or partial (e.g. an hourglass narrowing or web obstruction in the second part of the duodenum).

Diagnostic features
- Bile-stained vomiting occurs from birth.
- Epigastric fullness on examination.
- Look for features of associated Down's syndrome.
- Plain AXR. 'Double bubble sign' with no distal gas.

Management
- Resuscitation.
- Surgical bypass (duodenoduodenostomy bypass).

Jejuno-ileal atresia
- Caused by probable *in utero* vascular insult to mesenteric vessels.
- May occur in a single or multiple segments and may be short segments or long stretches of small bowel involved.

Diagnostic features
- Bile-stained vomiting from birth.
- Prominent abdominal distension, especially with distal atresia.
- Features of obstruction.

Investigation and management
- Resuscitation.
- Contrast enema may be helpful to exclude other diagnoses.
- Surgical anastomosis between atretic ends.

Meconium ileus
- Caused by the presence of impacted, abnormally thick meconium within the normal lumen of the small bowel.
- Pathognomonic of CF, but only 15% of CF present as meconium ileus.

Diagnostic features
- May be identified during antenatal ultrasound examination ('bright spots' in bowel) or family history with antenatal testing.
- Presents in neonatal period with features of distal obstruction: Vomiting, distension, failure to pass meconium, mass in RIF (meconium-obstructed bowel loops).

Investigation and management
- Resuscitation, IV fluids, NGT.
- Plain AXR.
- Contrast enema may be diagnostic and therapeutic.
- Surgical removal of meconium (may involve a temporary ileostomy).
- Immunoreactive trypsin and commonly associated CF genes (δF508).

Anorectal malformations

Incidence, approximately 1 in 5000 live births. Caused by failure of the correct septation of the hindgut cloaca or failure of formation of the anorectal canal (and associated pelvic floor structures).

- Low anomalies traverse a normal levator muscle.
- High anomalies end above the levator and are commonly associated with a fistula (bladder, urethra, vagina).
- Malformations may be part of a syndrome or linked to chromosomal abnormalities (VACTERL).

Diagnostic features

Condition should present at the neonatal check with recognition of an absent or abnormally placed anus and the failure to pass meconium with associated abdominal distension if a diagnosis has been missed. It may take up to 24h before meconium passes through the fistula.

Investigations and management

- Lateral prone X-ray of pelvis at 24h (assists in level assessment and sacrum).
- Perineal, renal ultrasound, and echocardiography (for associated abnormalities).
- Contrast loopogram 1 week after stoma formation (position of fistula/renal anomalies).
- Prophylactic antibiotics if vesicoureteric reflux is demonstrated.

Surgical treatment

- Low lesions (perineal fistula). Single stage perineal approach (anoplasty or dilatation).
- All other lesions. Defunctioning colostomy.
- Posterior sagittal anorectoplasty (PSARP). At 1–6 months and colostomy closure thereafter.

Prognosis

- Low anomalies often have relatively good function with a tendency to constipation in later life.
- High anomalies often have impaired function with up to 80% lifetime chance of soiling/incontinence.

Abdominal wall defects

Exomphalos (omphalocele)

Key facts
- Incidence 1 in 7000 births.

Clinicopathological features
- Herniation of the abdominal viscera through an umbilical defect that is covered by a membrane (unless ruptured).
- *Exomphalos minor.* The defect is <5cm and only the bowel is herniated.
- *Exomphalos major.* The defect is >5cm and bowel, liver, and other abdominal organs lie in the hernial sac.
- May present antenatally with an abnormal scan or raised maternal serum alpha-fetoprotein (AFP); in post-natal presentation, there is an obvious defect.

Diagnosis and investigations
- Investigations directed at identifying the associations (see Box 12.3). Check blood sugar.
- All newborn babies should have cardiac imaging prior to further management.

Treatment
- Parents may opt for termination in antenatally detected defects with associated major cardiac or chromosomal anomaly (mortality ~80%).
- Post-natal management involves protection of sac, insertion of NGT, IV access, and fluid management.
- Minor exomphalos should be suitable for reduction and primary closure of umbilical defect.
- Major exomphalos may be associated with underdeveloped abdominal cavity, precluding primary reduction. Epithelialization of the sac can be encouraged with application of silver sulphadiazine paste, resulting in a large ventral hernia that is suitable for delayed closure at ~1y of age.

Surgical treatment
- Primary reduction of smaller defects. Excision of sac, closure of umbilical defect (linear or purse string), and closure of umbilical skin.
- If the sac is ruptured in a larger defect. Application of silo or tissue flap.

Box 12.3 Associations of exomphalos
- Chromosomal abnormality (trisomy 18, 13, 21).
- Cardiac and renal anomalies found in up to 40%.
- Pulmonary hypoplasia caused by abnormal diaphragm function.
- Beckwith–Wiedemann syndrome: exomphalos, macroglossia, gigantism hyperinsulinism in infancy, renal/hepatic tumours.
- Pentalogy of Cantrell: exomphalos, sternal cleft, ectopia cordis, anterior diaphragmatic hernia, ventricular septal defect.

Gastroschisis

Key facts
- Incidence 1 in 7000 births (increasing).

Clinicopathological features
- There is a defect to the right of the umbilicus with protrusion of the stomach, small bowel, and large bowel.
- Associated with young maternal age and antenatal smoking or recreational drug use.
- Most present antenatally with an abnormal scan or raised maternal serum AFP.
- Antenatal diagnosis allows planned delivery (no evidence to recommend Caesarean section).
- Extraintestinal associated anomalies are uncommon.
- Intestinal atresia found in 10–20%.

Diagnosis and investigations
Associated anomalies are rare. No formal investigations are required.

Treatment
Management of gastroschisis at birth
- Planned vaginal delivery as close as possible to neonatal surgical unit.
- Standard neonatal resuscitation (clean, dry, stimulate, facial O_2, etc.).
- Cling film wrap to protect herniated bowel against trauma, contamination, heat loss, drying, and fluid loss (ensure mesentery not on tension).
- Insertion of NGT to decompress stomach.
- Fluid balance must include considerable evaporative losses from gut.
- Broad-spectrum antibiotics.

Non-surgical treatment Manual reduction and non-sutured closure of defect.

Surgical treatment
- If possible, the defect is delineated and closed.
- If herniated contents are unable to be reduced, the application of a 'silo' to cover gut and delayed closure once the gut is reduced (7–10 days).

Necrotizing enterocolitis (NEC)

Key facts
- Range of intestinal inflammation, ranging from mild mucosal injury to full thickness necrosis and perforation.
- Perforated NEC associated with 40% mortality in neonates.

Clinicopathological features
- Associated with:
  - Premature delivery.
  - Formula milk feeds.
  - Hypoxia.
  - Systemic sepsis.
  - 'Micro-epidemic' outbreaks in neonatal units.
- Typically affects premature babies on ventilatory support.
- Features of vomiting, distension, bloody mucus passing PR.
- May shows signs of severe sepsis/shock (tachypnoea, poor perfusion, temperature instability).

Diagnosis and investigations Plain AXR. Pneumatosis intestinalis, portal venous gas, free gas if perforation, dilated, thick-walled (oedematous) bowel.

Treatment
Medical
- Fluid resuscitation.
- IV antibiotics.
- Bowel rest and TPN.

Surgical treatment
- Indicated by complications (perforation, failure to respond to medical treatment, abdominal mass, systemic sepsis).
- May include:
  - Peritoneal drainage.
  - Bowel resection (usually with stoma formation).

Complications
- Septicaemia.
- Enteric fistulation.
- Peritonitis.
- Adhesions.
- Enteric stricture.
- Short gut syndrome.
- Death.

Inguinal hernia and scrotal swellings

Inguinal hernia

Key facts
- Childhood inguinal hernias derive from a persistent processus vaginalis and are invariably indirect.
- ♂:♀, 7:1.
- Right-sided hernias (60%) are commoner than the left (25%); 15% are bilateral.
- Higher incidence of complications (incarceration) than adult hernias.

Clinical features
- Usually noticed as a painless swelling, variable in size in the inguinoscrotal or labial area.
- More prominent when the baby cries and may disappear intermittently.
- Bowel entrapment causes pain and irreducibility leads to strangulation, intestinal obstruction, perforation, and peritonitis.
- Ovarian entrapment may occur in females.
- Bile vomiting in a young infant should always prompt examination of the inguinoscrotal area.
- Cardinal feature is a swelling in the groin above which the examining fingers cannot define the inguinal canal ('cannot get above').
- Asymmetrical thickening of the spermatic cord in the presence of a history compatible with a hernia is strongly suggestive of the diagnosis.

Treatment
- Prompt surgical treatment is important in premature/young infants to avoid risks of complications.
- Herniotomy alone is adequate. No need to repair the walls of the canal; usually a simple, straightforward day case procedure.
- Acute surgery can be very difficult when it is irreducible or strangulated or in very young infants.

Hydrocele
- Congenital fluid-filled processus vaginalis and tunica vaginalis.
- Communicates with the peritoneal cavity in children.
- Scrotum is usually smoothly enlarged and sometimes bluish in colour and the testis is often surrounded by the hydrocele.
- Occasionally acquired due to trauma, infection, or testicular tumour.
- Simple hydroceles may resolve spontaneously up to age of 18 months; surgical intervention is deferred until 18 months.
- At operation, ligation of the patent processus vaginalis and drainage of the fluid are adequate; there is no need to excise the hydrocele wall.

Varicocele
- Due to a dilated pampiniform venous plexus of the spermatic cord.
- Onset usually after puberty.
- Has the feel of a 'bag of worms' during palpation of the cord.

- Indications for treatment include discomfort (aching), cosmesis, and concern about fertility. The procedure is carried out by high ligation of the plexus, either by open or laparoscopic surgery.
- Beware an acute left varicocele in childhood due to obstruction of the left renal vein by tumour (nephroblastoma).
- Treatment may be surgical ligation or radiologically-guided embolization.

Idiopathic scrotal oedema

- Aetiology unknown; possibly due to an acute allergic reaction.
- Characterized by painless, red, unilateral scrotal swelling extending to the groin and the perineum.
- Rapidly resolves spontaneously; the clinical diagnosis precludes the need for investigation.

Other childhood hernias

Umbilical hernia

Key facts
- Persistence of the physiological umbilical defect beyond birth.
- Usually close spontaneously (especially in premature infants).
- Have a low incidence of complications (incarceration/strangulation).

Clinical features Usually noticed as a painless, intermittent swelling at the umbilicus.

Treatment
- Delay repair beyond age 4 in Caucasian children; beyond age 8 in Afro-Caribbean children.
- Simple sutured closure of defect in surgery required.

Epigastric hernia

Key facts
- Defect in the midline linea alba between the umbilicus and the xiphoid process.
- Very rarely closes spontaneously.
- Have a low incidence of complications (incarceration/strangulation).

Clinical features Usually noticed as a painless, intermittent swelling above the umbilicus.

Treatment Simple sutured closure of defect required.

Prepuce (foreskin) and circumcision

Key facts

- One of the commonest reasons for referral to a paediatric surgical clinic.
- Prepuce (foreskin) is initially fused to the glans penis. Preputial 'adhesions' lyse spontaneously as part of normal development.
- Separation of the prepuce from the glans is gradual; 80% of newborns, 50% of 1y-olds, and 10% of 5y-olds will have a non-retractable prepuce.

Non-retractable foreskin

Clinical features

- Only rarely causes problems which include dysuria, frequency, spots of blood, ballooning, and spraying.
- Very occasionally causes recurrent balanitis with redness, soreness, and cellulitis. Preputial 'cysts' are often present—these are collections of subpreputial smegma and are part of normal development.

Treatment

- Often only reassurance and advice are needed.
- Leave the foreskin alone if asymptomatic.
- Frequent bathing and hygiene and gentle attempts at retraction.
- Hydrocortisone 1% topically relieves symptoms and may speed separation.
- Topical or rarely, oral antibiotics only for recurrent balanitis.
- Persisting symptoms warrant retraction and separation using LA or under GA.

Phimosis

Defined as a non-retractable foreskin with associated scarring that will not resolve spontaneously.

Clinicopathological features

- May be congenital (uncommon) or acquired (usually age 5+) secondary to inflammation.
- Commonest cause balanitis xerotica obliterans (BXO); foreskin looks pale, thickened, and scarred.
- Additional symptoms to those of a non-retractable foreskin are retention of urine, paraphimosis, obstruction, and back pressure on the upper urinary tract. Consider an ultrasound scan and ascending urinary tract infection, in which case antibiotics are indicated.

Treatment

- Circumcision.
- Dorsal slit of foreskin.
- Preputioplasty (prepuceplasty).
- Non-surgical treatment using Plastibel is occasionally used in neonates.

How to examine a child's foreskin

- Try to ensure the boy is happy and relaxed, lying on examination couch or parental knee.
- Normal foreskin often appears long and 'redundant'.
- Gently hold tip of prepuce between finger tips, lift forward, and spread wide open. Preputial orifice usually demonstrated.
- If retraction attempted, perform gently to show pouting of mucosa.
- Blanching of skin below preputial opening—normal.
- Tight, white contracted preputial orifice indicates fibrotic phimosis ('muzzling').

Undescended testis

Key facts

- Testicular descent from the fetal abdominal site into the scrotum is normally complete by birth.
- Absence of a scrotal testis (cryptorchidism) may be due to agenesis (rare), intra-abdominal arrest, incomplete descent (intracanalicular), or ectopic descent (inguinal, perineal, crural, penile).
- Incidence 2–4% of newborn boys, falling to 1.5% at 6 months.
- Commoner on the right side.

Clinical features

- Undescended testis can be noted at the post-natal check, by parents, or by the GP.
- Rarely presents acutely as torsion (tender mass in inguinal region).
- A retractile testis is one that can be brought down into the scrotum with gentle manipulation, but retracts into the superficial inguinal pouch, either spontaneously or with minor pressure (see Box 12.4).

Diagnosis and investigations

- No investigations are required in palpable undescended testis.
- Chromosomal studies and HCG stimulation test may be requested in bilateral impalpable testes.
- Ultrasound may help locate an impalpable testis.
- Diagnostic laparoscopy is definitive and allows further management.

Treatment

- Testis should be brought to the scrotum at 1–2y of age to avoid secondary damage due to trauma, torsion, and increased ambient temperature.
- Hormone manipulation is ineffective in true undescended testis.
- Intracanalicular or ectopic testis should be managed by one-stage orchidopexy.
- Intra-abdominal testis can be brought down by one- or two-stage orchidopexy (50–90% success).
- Laparoscopy for bilateral impalpable testes.
- Scrotal position facilitates self-examination to detect signs of neoplastic change (~4 times normal in an abdominal testis).

Complications

- Post-operative atrophy of the testis (<2%) unless intra-abdominal position (10–50%).
- Retraction.

Box 12.4 How to exclude retractile testis

- A cooperative, relaxed little boy is essential. Examine on carer's knee or lying down.
- Control inguinal canal with finger pressure (prevents retraction of testis).
- Palpate tissues superficial to external inguinal ring, working down to scrotum.
- Try to manipulate testis into scrotum—then release.
- True retractile testis should remain in scrotum briefly.
- About 95% true retractile testes descend spontaneously before puberty and require no follow-up (~5% apparently retractile testes become 'ascending').

Indications for orchidopexy

- Maximize sperm production.
- Prevent testicular torsion.
- Repair of associated inguinal hernia.
- Cosmesis.
- Reduce chance of malignancy development and improve self-examination success.

Solid tumours of childhood

Neuroblastoma
- Commonest solid abdominal tumour of childhood.
- Spectrum of tumours derived from neuroblasts found in the adrenal gland, along the sympathetic chain, or extra-adrenal sympathetic tissues.
- Aggressive tumour with early spread to lymph glands, liver, bone (cortex or marrow), orbits, and skin.
- Presents as painless large, abdominal mass in children <2y.
- May present as weight loss, hypertension, or metastatic disease.
- Urinary HMMA, HVA elevated.
- CT scan. Optimal investigation for suspected neuroblastoma.
- Treatment by combination of chemotherapy, surgery, and radiotherapy.
- Survival of between 30 and 90%, depending on the site and stage at presentation.

Nephroblastoma (Wilms' tumour) of kidney
- Fast-growing tumour of the kidney.
- Ranges from benign mesoblastic nephroma of infancy to poorly differentiated, malignant nephroblastoma in the older child.
- Malignant tumours frequently metastasize to regional lymph nodes, liver, and lungs.
- Usually presents as a large, relatively painless abdominal mass in an otherwise well child.
- Treatment by combination of chemotherapy, surgery, and radiotherapy according to histology and spread at diagnosis.
- 5y survival:
  - Early stage, 90%.
  - Disseminated disease, 30%.

Rhabdomyosarcoma
- Tumour of striated muscle origin from the bladder, vagina, prostate, parameningeal tissue, and limbs.
- Haematuria, vaginal bleeding, and the appearance of grape-like cysts (sarcoma botryoides) at the vaginal introitus.
- Variable histology (embryonal is most favourable), which determines the prognosis.
- Survival of up to 70% from surgery and chemotherapy.

Hepatoblastoma
- This presents as a right hypochondrial mass extending across the midline.
- Chemotherapy may render initially inoperable tumours resectable.
- Depending on staging, size, and histology, survival of up to 70% is possible.

Neck swellings

Key facts

- Childhood neck lumps may be due to embryological abnormalities as well as the same spectrum of conditions in adults (📖 pp. 222–226).
- Embryological abnormalities may relate to:
  - Descent of the thyroid from the foramen caecum of the tongue → thyroglossal cysts (📖 p. 222).
  - Formation of 2nd, 3rd, and 4th branchial arches and clefts → branchial cysts (📖 p. 224).
  - Formation of lymphatic vessels and veins → cystic hygroma and cavernous haemangiomata.
- ▶ Lymphadenopathy is very common in children, but typically 'waxes and wanes'.
- ▶▶ If lymphadenopathy persists for longer than 2 months and measures >2cm diameter, it should be biopsied.

Causes and clinicopathological features

Thyroglossal cyst (📖 p. 222).

Branchial cysts (📖 p. 224).

Lymphadenopathy

- The neck contains large numbers of lymph glands draining areas of potential infection in the mouth, nose, fauces, and ears.
- Common causes of lymphadenopathy include upper respiratory tract infection, middle ear infections, tonsillitis, parotitis, dental abscess, atypical mycobacterial infection.
- Malignant lymphadenopathy is much less common.
  - May be primary lymphoma.
  - Secondary deposits, e.g. from neuroblastoma.

Salivary gland swellings

- May be due to duct obstruction (stones or duct stenosis), infection (mumps), autoimmune disorders (recurrent parotitis), neoplasia (adenoma).
- Commonest in the submandibular, sublingual, and parotid glands.

Skin lesions

- *Dermoid cysts.* Usually in the midline above the hyoid bone and are rarely infected.
- *Sebaceous cysts.* Epidermal origin with a small central punctum; may occur anywhere, but most commonly on the scalp or back of the neck.

Lymphovascular lesions

- *Haemangiomas.* Can be mixed capillary or cavernous haemangiomas or haemangioendotheliomas within the neck and parotid area; may grow rapidly in size and lead to high output cardiac failure or even carotid steal syndrome.
- *Cystic hygroma (lymphangioma).* Commonly in the posterior triangle of the neck.

Treatment

- Excision of dermoid cysts, sebaceous cysts, thyroglossal cysts, thyroid neoplasms, salivary gland enlargements, lymph gland enlargements (biopsy).
- Haemangioma. Supportive measures (intubation, steroids, interferon, and emergency surgical intervention).
- Cystic hygroma. Sclerosant injection (OK 432—streptococcal derivative), effective in lymphangiomas with few large cysts.

Differential diagnosis of neck lump

Neck lumps may be lateral or midline.

Lateral
- Lymph node
- Branchial sinuses and cyst
- Cystic hygroma
- Sternomastoid tumour
- Haemangioma
- Lymphangioma
- Submandibular gland
- Parotid gland
- Neoplasm

Midline
- Submental lymph nodes
- Thyroglossal cyst
- Thyroid swelling
- Dermoid cyst

Neck swellings by cause

Congenital
- Thyroglossal cysts
- Branchial cyst
- Cystic hygroma
- Haemangioma
- Dermoid cyst

Acquired
- Reactive lymphadenopathy
- Infective lymphadenopathy
- Secondary tumour deposits

Anatomy related to neck lump surgery

- Incisions should be parallel with skin creases (Langer's lines).
- Subcutaneous closure should be meticulous (e.g. removable 4/0, 5/0, or 6/0 continuous subcuticular monofilament).
- Facial nerve. Passes between the two lobes of parotid gland.
- Lingual nerve. Swerves around submandibular duct.
- Thoracic duct. Enters junction of left subclavian and jugular veins.

Paediatric orthopaedic

Developmental dysplasia of the hip (DDH)

DDH covers a spectrum of abnormalities from a mildly underdeveloped stable hip to well-established dislocation and/or acetabular dysplasia in the older child. The incidence is 1–2 per 1000 newborns in the UK. It is bilateral in 20%. It was previously called congenital dysplasia of the hip (CDH), but as it may also be acquired after birth, the term was changed. Early detection is important.

Risk factors

- Family history. First-degree relative.
- Breech presentation at or after 36 weeks of gestation.
- Foot abnormalities. Congenital talipes calcaneovalgus and metatarsus adductus.
- Oligohydramnios.
- Children with syndromes.
- Torticollis.

Clinical features

- *Barlow test (dislocatable hip)*. It tests if a hip is unstable. Take the baby's leg between your thumb and index finger and place your other fingers onto the buttock. Flex and adduct the hip. Posterior-directed force is applied in line with the shaft of the femur. In case of instability, the femoral head then subluxes or dislocates which you can palpate in the buttock.
- *Ortolani Sign (dislocated hip)*. Now abduct the leg. If the hip is dislocated and reducible, you will feel the femoral head moving into the joint. This often does not produce a palpable clunk.
- *Irreducible hip*.
  - Shortened leg.
  - Limited hip abduction.
  - Asymmetry of skin creases can be present; many children with normal hips have asymmetry of thigh and buttock skin creases.

Abnormal findings can prove easy to miss if the dislocations are bilateral.

Screening

All children with risk factors and an abnormal neonatal clinical hip examination have a hip ultrasound. The majority of hips are fully developed at full term plus 6 weeks. Therefore, the ultrasounds of those children with risk factors, but normal clinical findings, are done at that point. Those children with obvious clinical abnormalities on hip examination have the ultrasound done earlier.

Paton RW *et al.* reported in 2009 that there is no association between postural and fixed talipes equinovarus and DDH.[1] Since it can be difficult for non-paediatric orthopaedic surgeons to differentiate the different foot abnormalities, it is continued to scan the hips of children with club feet. Evidence shows that there is no advantage of universal baby hip screening over selective at risk screening.

Radiology

- Ultrasound is the investigation of choice. Baby hip ultrasound was pioneered by Dr Graf from Austria. It is more accurate than radiographs. It visualizes the cartilage and allows dynamic testing of the hip joint. A Graf alpha angle of $\geq 60°$ is classed as normal.
- Radiographs are taken in children who present late, usually after the age of 6 months.

Treatment

- *0–6 months of age*. A Pavlik harness is applied. This is a soft harness which flexes the hips and knees and directs the legs away from the body midline, thereby directing the femoral heads towards the hip joints. It allows limited hip movements. It is used until the hips normalize, which can take several months; it works 90% of times.
- *6–18 months*. If the harness is unsuccessful or if a child is older than 6 months, they need a closed or open reduction of the hip joint and hip spica cast immobilization. Some children need a hip adductor tendon release in the groin and occasionally, a femoral osteotomy. A removable hip abduction brace is used after spica removal.
- *≥ 18 months*. These children usually need an open reduction of the hip joint, a hip adductor release, and a femoral $\pm$ pelvic osteotomy and hip spica immobilization. A hip abduction brace is normally not necessary after hip spica removal because of the improved bone alignment.

Reference

1 Paton RW, Srinivasan MS, Shah B, et al. (1999). Ultrasound screening for hips at risk in developmental dysplasia: is it worth it? *J Bone Joint Surg Br.* **81**: 255–8.

Slipped upper femoral epiphysis (SUFE)

This is reported to have an incidence of 4–7 per 100 000 population. It is caused by the displacement of the femoral epiphysis (growth plate) in relation to the femoral neck. It is the commonest cause of a limp in a boy aged 12–14 or girl aged 11–13 (growth spurt at puberty). In this age group, it must be actively excluded in a limping child.

Risk factors

- Obesity. Classic is the limping, obese, 13y-old boy with knee pain.
- Rapid growth.
- Hormone disturbances. Hypothyroidism, renal rickets, pituitary deficiency, growth hormone deficiency, and treatment with it).
- Male—♂:♀, 3:1.
- Side affected. Left > right.

Classification

This is usually classified by the ability to weight bear on presentation.
- 'Unstable' slips cannot walk due to pain and present like a fracture.
- Diagnosis is easy.
- 'Stable' slips can weight bear, though usually with a limp.
- Presentation is usually late, i.e. after 2–3 weeks of limping.
- Fifty per cent will have no pain; pain is commonly referred to the knee.

▶ Any child with knee pain must have their hip examined.
  A summary of presentation and prognosis can be seen below.

Clinical features

- There will be an obvious limp, usually in an overweight child, commonly male.
- The affected limb will be shorter and lies in external rotation.
- Abduction is limited; when the hip is flexed, it will rotate externally— *this sign is almost diagnostic of the condition.*

Radiology

Anteroposterior and lateral views of *BOTH* hips should be insisted on. The slip is often easier to see on the *lateral* view. The slip is in an inferior and posterior direction (down and backwards). Widening of the physis may be a sign of impending slip (i.e. 'pre-slip').
- *Klein's line giving Trethowan's sign.* If you draw a line on the superior aspect of the femoral neck, it should cut through the femoral head; if it does not, it is diagnostic of a SUFE (see Fig. 13.1).

Management

The acute slip (i.e. <3 weeks history) can be managed by gentle manipulation and cannulated screw fixation in the reduced position. This is controversial, however, as any manipulation may damage the already damaged epiphysis and possibly cause avascular necrosis.

Standard treatment is stopping the slip from worsening and the slip is usually pinned *in situ* (where it is with no manipulation) with one cannulated screw percutaneously.

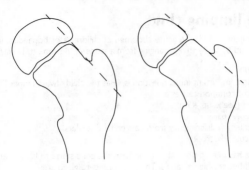

Fig. 13.1 Normal (left) and Abnormal, i.e. SUFE (right) Klein's lines.

Deformed epiphysis can remodel by up to 60°. Residual deformity can be corrected via an osteotomy once the epiphysis has fused if there is a functional deficit.

The condition can be bilateral in some cases. This is much more likely if there is an underlying endocrine disorder. Some surgeons advocate prophylactic pinning of the unaffected side, but this is controversial.

Complications
- Avascular necrosis of femoral head.
- Chondrolysis. Rapid progressive loss of cartilage; joint space narrowing is seen on X-ray.
- Subtrochanteric fracture. If pins entry point placed too low.
- Late osteoarthritis. Estimated 10%.

Further reading
Aronsson D, Loder RT, Breur GJ, Weinstein SL (2006). Slipped capital femoral epiphysis: current concepts. *J Am Acad Orthop Surg* **14**: 666–79.

The limping child

The limping child is the acute abdomen of children's orthopaedics. It can be caused by many things, ranging from a stone in the shoe to leukaemia.

History

The most important initial question is, 'Has the child always limped?' If so, the most common causes are:
- DDH (see 📖 p. 458).
- Cerebral palsy.
- Limb length discrepancy from congenital disorders.
- Muscular dystrophy.

If there has been a normal gait and then the child starts to limp, then the possibilities are highly varied. The main points to glean are:
- How long, what side, and what causes it? Is it constant or intermittent?
- Are there any associated complaints?
- Is there a history of trauma?
- How is the child's general health?
- What is the child's past medical and birth history?

Remember, what causes an older child to limp will cause a younger child to refuse to weight bear. This will be perceived as more serious by the parents and therefore, these patients will present much earlier.

Examination

- *Look at the child walking.* Decide on whether there is a limp! This is often a symptom used by parents (and grandparents) to make sure that you take their complaint seriously and a limp may not be the problem at all.
- *What type of limp is it?*
  - *Short leg.* Limb length discrepancy.
  - *Antalgic.* Less time on affected than unaffected limb due to pain.
  - *Trendelenberg.* Pelvis dips and trunk sways on affected side due to weak hip abductors.
  - *Bizarre.* Usually psychological, e.g. completely stiff leg.
- *Tailor examination to history.* Inspect limbs from hips to toes. Skin discoloration may be indicative of infection. Try to use distraction techniques to get the true picture.
- *Tenderness?* Bony tenderness with swelling and bruising is a clinical fracture. Infected areas will be painful and usually red, hot, or swollen.
- *Joints.* Concentrate joint examination as appropriate, but always examine hips if knee pain present. Put all joints through full passive range of motion.
- *Limb lengths?* Assess individual leg lengths with patient lying on the couch with legs straight. Look for level of heels and malleoli. If one leg is short, assess if discrepancy is within femur or tibia by flexing both hips and knees together. Look at the legs from the side to see if the front of the lower legs is at different levels (if yes—femoral shortening) and/or if the front of the thighs are at different levels (if yes—lower leg shortening).

- *Lymphadenopathy?* From generalized infection, local infection, or blood disorder.
- *Full systemic examination must also be performed.*

Remember common things are common! The age of the patient is a very useful screen (see Table 13.1).

Investigations
- *X-ray.* Always X-ray hips if no localizing signs. If one limb appears to be involved, especially in the younger patient, then X-ray the whole limb. Otherwise, X-ray bones/joints as appropriate from the clinical examination.
- *Blood tests.* FBC, U&E, G, LFTs, CRP, ESR useful as full general screen.

Management Dependent on diagnosis reached.

Further reading
Sawyer JR, Kapoor M (2009). The limping child: a systematic approach to diagnosis. *Am Fam Physician* **79**(3): 215–24. Available at: ⌖ http://www.aafp.org/afp/2009/0201/p215.html

Table 13.1 Screening using age of the patient

Young (0–5y)	Child (5–10y)	Adolescent (10–15y)	All ages
DDH	Perthes' disease	SUFE	Septic arthritis
Septic hip	Irritable hip	AVN of femoral head	Cellulitis
Limb length discrepancy	Juvenile rheumatoid arthritis	Overuse syndromes	Stress fracture
Occult fracture			Non-accidental injury (NAI)
			Neoplasia
			Neuromuscular disease

The child with a fracture

Accidents are part of normal life! Some, usually the more severe, result in a fracture. In a city of 1 million inhabitants, there would be around 3000 children's fractures annually.

Most childhood fractures are minor, almost half affecting the forearm. They are weather-dependent, increasing in good weather when climbing (and falling) is common.

Clinical features

- *A clear history of trauma* and a complaint of pain are present in all, but a small number of patients. In a young child, however, the pain may not be localized and instead of crying, they may present with pseudoparalysis of a limb, limp, or refusal to weight bear.
- *Look for external signs of injury.* Bruising, due to a thick subcuticular fat layer is not a constant feature. Palpate for tenderness unless there is a clear deformity. Remember to examine the normal limb first and when examining the affected side, start away from the injury. This will gain the child's confidence. If you're going to do something that hurts them, tell them rather than saying, 'This won't hurt'. If you lie to them, you will lose their trust and make examination impossible.
- *Neurovascular status.* Check the distal capillary refill and pulses as well as distal neurology in the form of power and sensation. Document all findings. It is good practice and also helps if there are any medicolegal issues about treatment.
- *Investigation.* Though a fracture is a clinical diagnosis, this can sometimes be difficult in the child. A low threshold for X-rays should always be adopted. The joint above and below any injury must be visualized with two perpendicular views being standard practice.
- *Analgesia.* Always splint an obvious fracture and give analgesia before X-rays. If a limb is clearly deformed (hence fractured), then a plaster should be applied before the X-ray. Radiographs of deformed limbs out of splintage are unacceptable. This is also the case for adults!
- *Unnecessary X-rays.* Try to avoid 'comparison' views of the normal side if you are unsure about radiological features. With growing bones, ossification centres and epiphysis interpretation can be difficult. If you are unsure about a feature, show the X-ray to a senior.
- *Fractures.* The classical fracture in a child is the greenstick injury. This is when there is a fracture of one cortex and a plastic deformation (i.e. a bend, not break) of the other at the same level. Even complete fractures tend to displace far less in children as the periosteum in children is highly structural, thick, and strong. It will hold the fracture in rough approximation. In adults, the periosteum is a very weak component of bone, hence the wider displacement.

Management

- Fractures usually unite. If there is a minor greenstick fracture with little symptoms and no risk of displacement, then there is no need to apply a plaster cast. However, this is not normally acceptable to parents once they know their child has a broken limb.

- In undisplaced, stable, greenstick fractures of the forearm, a fibreglass removable cast can be placed and the parents simply remove this in 4 weeks' time with no need to be followed up in a clinic.
- Normally the joint above and below the fracture needs to be immobilized. Often this is safer in children to 'slow them down' anyway. The fracture should be monitored in the fracture clinic. If a plaster is placed, then clear plaster instructions, in the form of a printed sheet, should be given to the parents. An example is shown in Box 13.1.

Box 13.1 Plaster instructions

Return to the Accident and Emergency Department or Plaster room if your child complains of any of the following:
- Numbness or pins and needles in the affected limb.
- Restricted movement or tight swelling of the fingers or toes.
- If the fingers or toes go white or blue.
- If there is local itching, pain, or burning in the plaster.
- A strong foul smell is coming from the plaster.
- The plaster becomes soft or loose.

Also, if the plaster is rubbing or digging in, this will irritate the skin and cause blistering.
- Do NOT place anything down the plaster if it is itching. This will cause skin damage or blisters and may cause an infection.
- Do NOT get the plaster wet.

- If the fracture is displaced or angulated, then it may require manipulation or, less commonly, open reduction and fixation under GA.
- *Angulation,* if close to the joint and in the plane of motion of the joint, is very well tolerated. Remodelling of the bone will occur; a 15° angulation in a child <6y old and 10° angulation in a child 6–10y old is acceptable orthopaedically, though is often not accepted by the parents! Rotational displacement will not remodel and needs correction.

Non-accidental injury (NAI)

Definition

Physical violence towards a baby or child. It is one part of child abuse which may occur in isolation or in combination with other forms of child abuse, including neglect, emotional abuse and/or sexual abuse. It denotes an injury that cannot be explained by an accident and where responsible adults do not have a viable explanation of how the injury occurred.

Incidence

- The National Society for the Prevention of Cruelty to Children (NSPCC) reported in 2011 that 46 700 children were at risk of abuse in the UK.
- It is estimated that 4 million children a year are abused in some manner in the USA.
- It happens in all socio-economic classes, but is more common in the deprived. Twins, preterm babies, and special needs children are also at increased risk.
- The majority of NAI fractures occur under 2y of age (80% of children with NAI fractures are under 18 months of age). The majority of accidental injuries occur in children over 5y of age (85%).

Suspicious features

- Inexplicable delay from time of injury to medical advice being sought.
- No convincing explanation of mechanism of injury.
- Patterns of soft tissue injury, e.g. bruising in the shape of fingers or objects (belt, buckles) or in unusual areas (back, away from bony prominences), bites, and burns.
- Unusual fractures or fracture patterns, e.g. rib fractures, non-linear skull fractures, transverse fractures of long bones, scapula, lateral clavicle, and vertebral fractures.
- Fractures of differing ages on a radiograph.
- No fracture in isolation is pathognomonic of NAI.
- Rib, humeral, femoral, and skull fractures have the highest probability for abuse. Rib fractures are present in 5–27% of children who are abused. Diaphyseal fractures are four times more common than metaphyseal fractures in NAI.
- Metaphyseal corner and bucket handle fractures. They are only present in a minority of children who present with NAI (the reported rates vary widely, 11–50%). Many references refer to them as pathognomonic or specific for NAI. However, a similar appearance can occur with other conditions (e.g. severe osteogenesis imperfecta, rickets, scurvy).
  - Corner fracture. A small piece of bone is avulsed due to shearing forces on the growth plate.
  - Bucket handle fracture (same as corner fracture). The fragment is larger and seen face on as a disc or bucket handle.
- Two or more fractures are present in 66–74% of abused children, but only in 16% of non-abused children.

- Periosteal reactions are common features in NAI; a very strong grip may cause such a reaction.
- Always keep NAI in mind when dealing with any child with trauma.

Examination

- A thorough history (this should be witnessed) and total body inspection and examination from head to toes is mandatory. Enquire about a history of fractures and deafness and look for blue sclera (osteogenesis imperfecta). Examination of genitalia should only be done by experts.
- Note how the child interacts with the carer/parent.
- Good communication and contemporaneous medical note writing is essential since every case of child abuse will be submitted to court.

Management

- Contact consultant in charge, departmental child protection lead, and/or hospital child protection team (paediatric consultant on call, child protection practitioner).
- Hospital admission if NAI is suspected, even if the medical condition does not require it.
- Skeletal survey (skull, chest, abdomen, upper and lower limbs). This will be organized by paediatric team if NAI is suspected.
- Blood tests (FBC, clotting screen, bone profile, calcium, phosphate, alkaline phosphatase, copper, caeruloplasmin, magnesium, fasting 25-hydroxyvitamin D, and parathyroid hormone).
- Every hospital has a policy dealing with safeguarding of children.

Differential diagnoses

- Osteogenesis imperfecta.
- Haemophilia.
- Birth trauma.
- Rickets.
- Leukaemia.
- Scurvy (mimics NAI).

Legg–Calvé–Perthes disease

Definition

Idiopathic avascular necrosis of the proximal femoral epiphysis, first described independently by Legg, Calvé, and Perthes. The cause is unknown. The epiphyseal changes can lead to permanent deformity and osteoarthritis in adult life. The diagnosis is made on X-rays.

Key facts

- Age of onset most commonly between 4 and 10y of age. If both hips look to be at the same stage, consider multiple epiphyseal dysplasia.
- ♂:♀, 5:1.
- 10–12% bilateral; the disease is usually at different stages.
- Females have poorer prognosis.
- Early onset up to age of 7y; late onset from age of 8y. The overall prognosis is better in the early group.

Pathology/radiology

- Waldenström described four radiographic stages—ischaemia, fragmentation, reossification, remodelling.
  - *Ischaemia.* Compromise of blood supply of the femoral head. The articular cartilage still grows as it is nourished by the joint fluid, resulting in increased joint space and apparent mild joint subluxation on X-ray (Waldenström's sign); the head ceases to enlarge.
  - *Fragmentation/resorption.* New bone is laid down on the dead trabeculae, causing increased bone density. Subchondral fractures may occur, causing a black subchondral line (crescent sign). The hyperaemia and revascularization causes bone lysis and rarefication, giving a fragmented appearance on the X-rays.
  - *Reossification (healing phase).* The head is plastic and if it is not concentrically contained within the acetabulum, it will become deformed.
  - *Remodelling.* The plasticity is lost and the femoral head shape will remain. The normal internal architecture will return, but inside an altered shape if this has occurred. Deformity will lead to arthritis.
- With non-operative treatment, revascularization and reossification takes 2–3y to complete in most cases.
- Herring's lateral pillar classification. Now generally used at presentation (Catterall in the past). Groups A, B, C; a B/C group added later.
  - *Group A.* The lateral column of the proximal femoral epiphysis is of normal height.
  - *Group B.* The height is reduced, but >50% of the height on the other side.
  - *Group C.* The height is reduced to <50% compared to the other side.
  - *Group B/C.* Lateral pillar is narrowed (2–3mm) or poorly ossified with approximately 50% height.

- Stulberg classification. Describes the end stage of the disease at skeletal maturity.
  - I. Normal spherical femoral head.
  - II. Round femoral head and fitting within 2mm of a circle on both anteroposterior and lateral radiographs.
  - III. Out of round by >2mm on either radiograph.
  - IV. Flat head and matching flat acetabulum (aspherical congruency).
  - V. Flat head with non-matching acetabulum (aspherical incongruency).
- Catterall classification (grades 1–4; 1, 25% head involvement; 2, 50%; 3, 75%; 4, >75%). Superseded by lateral pillar classification. He described five head-at-risk signs (Gage's sign—V-shaped lucency at lateral epiphysis, horizontal growth plate, lateral calcification, subluxation, metaphyseal cystic changes). Foster reported poor reliability for head-at-risk signs.

Clinical features

- Painless limp is common.
- There may be pain in groin, inner thigh, and/or only in the knee.
- Again, every child with knee pain must have their hip examined.
- Reduced hip abduction and internal rotation might be examined.

Management

- Overall very controversial.
- Annamalai et al. (2007)[1] showed a great deal of variability in the UK in the decision-making process and treatment.
- Non-operative symptomatic relief for the majority of patients. Physiotherapy/exercises; observation and serial radiographs.
- Largest multicentre centre conducted in America by Herring et al.[2,3] comparing non-operative management with operative management (either femoral varus or pelvic osteotomy) for early and late onset groups.
  - Early onset group. No difference in outcome between non-operative management, femoral varus, or pelvic osteotomy.
  - Late onset group. Improved outcome for lateral pillar groups B and B/C with either femoral varus or pelvic osteotomy over non-operative group; no difference for groups A and C.
- Containment surgery has been advocated by others when the femoral head extrudes from the acetabulum irrespective of age (the femoral head is maintained within the depth of the acetabulum with femoral osteotomy, pelvic osteotomy, or both combined).

Bracing is not used by the majority of paediatric orthopaedic surgeons as part of management of Legg–Calvé–Perthes disease.

References

1 Annamalai et al. (2007). Perthes disease: a survey of management amongst members of the British Society for Children's Orthopaedic Surgery (BSCOS). *J Child Orthop* **1**(2): 107–13.
2 Herring JA, Kim HT, Browne R. Legg-Calvé-Perthes Disease. (2004). Part I: Classification of radiographs with the use of the modified lateral pillar and Stulberg classifications. *J Bone Joint Surg Am* **86-A**: 2103–20.
3 Herring JA, Kim HT, Browne R. Legg-Calvé-Perthes Disease. (2004). Part II: Prospective multi-center study of the effect of treatment on outcome. *J Bone Joint Surg Am* **86-A**: 2121–34.

Motor development

Most children develop at roughly the same pace. Development is easier to understand if you realize that it will spread from head to feet, i.e. cephalocaudal.

Maturation of the nervous system occurs so that a child is able to do things more distally, the older they become. Fig. 13.2 summarizes this with some common 'milestones' of development.

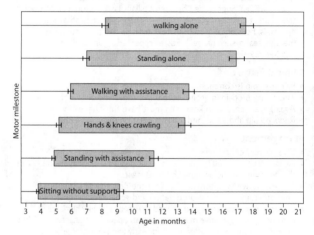

Fig. 13.2 WHO Multicentre Growth Reference Study Group (2006). WHO motor development study: windows of achievement for six gross motor development milestones. *Acta Paediatrica Supplement* **450**: 86–95.

Club foot or congenital talipes equinovarus (CTEV)

Club foot is a congenital condition that presents at birth and may be isolated or part of a more widespread congenital disorder. Its incidence is approximately 1 in 1000 live births in the UK with a ♂:♀ ratio of 2:1. The cause is unknown.

It occurs with other neuromuscular disorders such as:

- Arthrogryphosis.
- Myotonic muscular dystrophy.
- Myelomeningocele and other spinal dysraphisms (spina bifida).
- Cerebral palsy.

▶ Always perform a thorough examination of the hip and back to rule out other disorders/syndromes that might be associated with a club foot.

Clinical features

The hindfoot is plantar flexed (equinus) and in varus. There is midfoot and forefoot cavus and forefoot adduction. The forefoot looks supinated, but is actually pronated in relation to the midfoot. Overall, the foot is turned and twisted inwards so that the sole is facing towards the midline and backwards. In the true clubfoot deformity, the deformity is fixed to a varying degree. In the positional clubfoot deformity, the deformity is passively correctable and usually does not require any treatment.

Management

The cornerstone of treatment is to create a supple foot that is plantigrade that will allow the child to function well.

Treatment has been revolutionized by the use of the Ponseti method of casting which can be performed in the outpatients. This is often run by specialist nurses/physiotherapy practitioners who work closely with the paediatric orthopaedic team.

Serial casts are applied that stretch the contracted tissues back to normal in a defined order. First, you correct the adduction and cavus, which also corrects the hindfoot varus and finally, the equinus. About 80% of clubfeet need a percutaneous Achilles tendon tenotomy to correct the equinus.

The initial casting period goes over about 6 weeks with weekly cast changes. At the end of this period, the Achilles tenotomy is performed if necessary, followed by a further 3 weeks in cast. Thereafter, the feet are immobilized 23h/day with boots on a bar for 3 months and then only during the night until the age of 4–5y. Some children require a tibialis anterior tendon transfer when they are about 4–5y old because of a dynamic supination deformity. Recurrences are usually the result of non-compliance or if the child has a syndromic clubfoot.

Flat feet (pes planus)

There are always one or two children in every orthopaedic paedi-atric new patient clinic with flat feet. The children rarely complain of symptoms and the appearance and referral is often sparked by the parents.

Clinical features

Like all paediatric consultations, take an accurate neonatal, birth, and fam-ily history to look for associated problems. The cornerstone is whether the foot deformity is flexible (vast majority) or rigid.

▶ Flexible flat feet correct fully once the big toe is extended and the arch reforms and when the child stands on tip toes.

Ensure you examine the ankle and Achilles tendon as this often causes a 'compensatory' flat foot due to the stiffness and is easily remedied by physiotherapy.

Natural history

The majority of children form normal foot arches by the age of about 3y. In some, the arches never form and they remain flatfooted.

Management

Flexible flat feet generally need simple reassurance and the patient can be discharged. Some children with more severe flat feet benefit at times from the use of insoles since insoles improve the mechanical leg alignment. This applies, for example, to children who present with knee pain and moder-ate to severe flat feet where the feet are in a pronated position when standing. Tight Achilles tendons need physiotherapy.

Rigid flat feet are associated with an underlying abnormality such as:
• Congenital vertical talus (from birth).
• Tarsal coalition. Fusing of some part of the tarsal bones via scar or bone (often adolescents).
• Inflammatory joint disease.

Treatment is centred on the underlying disorder, i.e. tarsal coalition is often treated by offloading the area with orthotics and if this fails, attempts can be made to surgically resect the fibrous or bony coalition.

The osteochondritides

These conditions result in avascular necrosis of epiphyseal bone, similar to Legg–Calvé–Perthes disease, but less common. In general, they are troublesome rather than serious. Some are self-limiting.

Features

Most lead to aching and muscle spasm. Radiographic changes occur in the affected epiphysis, with varying degrees of density change and fragmentation.

Epiphyses commonly affected are:
- Lateral condyle of the humerus (Panner's disease).
- Carpal lunate (Kienbock).
- Carpal scaphoid (Preiser).
- Head of metatarsal (Freiberg).
- Tarsal navicular (Kohler).
- Patella (Larsen–Johanssen).
- Vertebral epiphyseal plates (Scheuermann).
- Vertebral body (Calvé).

Management

Usually symptomatic with limitation of activities and anti-inflammatory medication.

Traction apophysitis

An apophysis is a traction epiphysis which may undergo partial avulsion with avascular change followed by subsequent repair. These changes can be the result of trauma, overuse, or rapid growth. The commonest are:
- *Osgood–Schlatter's disease*. Apophysitis of the tibial tubercle into which the patellar tendon inserts.
- *Sever's disease*. Apophysitis of the apophysis at the posterior aspect of the calcaneum where the Achilles tendon inserts.

Clinical features

The patient is usually an adolescent who presents with aching, swelling, and/or pain.

Radiology

Radiographs show fragmentation of the tibial tuberosity/calcaneal apophysis.

Treatment

Explanation of the condition; limitation of activities; anti-inflammatory medication. Plaster immobilization for 4–6 weeks can be helpful in severe cases. Temporary use of a cushioned heel support for Sever's disease can be helpful.

Osteochondritis dissecans of the knee

- Avascular necrosis of the subchondral bone, resulting in softening of the articular cartilage and bone that may become loose and separated from the rest of the femoral condyle. The cause is unknown, but it is thought that it might be the result of repetitive minor trauma.
- Most lesions are located on the lateral side of the medial femoral condyle, but any joint can be affected.
- Children between 5 and 15y of age are most commonly affected with the majority occurring in teenage boys.

Clinical features

- Non-specific knee pain.
- If the fragment has become loose, the patient will report crepitance, popping, giving way, and/or locking.

Natural history

In children and adolescents, spontaneous healing over about 18 months is the usual outcome. Patients with more advanced lesions have an increased risk to develop early osteoarthritis.

Investigations

- *Radiographs.* The tunnel view will show the lesion the best.
- *MRI.* The scan shows extent of the lesion and, if there is detachment, with fluid interposition between fragment and underlying bone.

Management

- Activity restriction for the majority of cases.
- Unstable lesions require arthroscopic stabilization.

Major trauma

Management of major trauma

Key facts

- Trauma is the leading cause of death in the first four decades of life, but three people are permanently disabled for every one killed.
- Death from injury occurs in one of three time periods (trimodal).
  - *First peak.* Within seconds to minutes. Very few can be saved due to severity of their injuries.
  - *Second peak.* Within minutes to several hours. Deaths occur due to life-threatening injuries.
  - *Third peak.* After several hours to weeks. Deaths from sepsis and multiple organ failure.
- The 'golden hour' refers to the period when medical care can make the maximum impact on death and disability. It implies the urgency and not a fixed time period of 60min.

The advanced trauma life support (ATLS) system

- Accepted as a standard for trauma care during the 'golden hour' and focuses on the 'second peak'.
- Emphasizes that injury kills in certain reproducible time frames in a common sequence: loss of airway, inability to breathe, loss of circulating blood volume, expanding intracranial mass.
- The primary survey (ABCDEs) with simultaneous resuscitation is emphasized.

Prehospital care and the trauma team

- Effort is made to minimize scene time, emphasizing immediate transport to the closest appropriate facility (scoop and run).
- Hospital is informed of the impending arrival of the casualty.
- Trauma team usually comprises an anaesthetist, 'general' surgeon, orthopaedic surgeon, and A&E specialist, A&E nurses, and radiographers.
- Information from paramedics should include **M**echanism of injury, **I**njuries identified, vital **S**igns at scene, and any **T**reatment administered (MIST).
- Triage is the process of prioritizing patients according to treatment needs and the available resources (those with life-threatening conditions **and** with the greatest chance of survival are treated first).

Management

Primary survey

Identify and treat life-threatening conditions according to priority (ABCDE).

Airway maintenance with cervical spine protection

- Protect spinal cord with immobilization devices or using manual in-line immobilization. Protect until cervical spine injury is excluded.
- Access airway for patency. If patient can speak, airway is not immediately threatened.
- Consider foreign body and facial, mandibular, or tracheal/laryngeal fractures if unconscious. Perform chin lift/jaw thrust. Consider nasopharyngeal/oropharyngeal airway.

- If patient unable to maintain airway integrity, secure a definitive airway (orotracheal, nasotracheal, cricothyroidotomy).

Breathing and ventilation
- Administer high-flow O_2 using a non-rebreathing reservoir.
- Inspect for chest wall expansion, symmetry, respiratory rate, and wounds. Percuss and auscultate chest. Look for tracheal deviation, surgical emphysema.
- Identify and treat life-threatening conditions: tension pneumothorax, open pneumothorax, flail chest with pulmonary contusion, massive haemothorax.

Circulation with haemorrhage control
- Look for signs of shock.
- Hypotension is usually due to blood loss. Think: chest, abdomen, retroperitoneum, muscle compartment, open fractures ('blood on the floor and four more').
- Control external bleeding with pressure.
- Obtain IV access using two 12G cannulae. Send blood for cross-match, FBC, clotting, U&E.
- Commence bolus of warmed Ringer's lactate solution; unmatched, type-specific blood only for immediate life-threatening blood loss.
- Consider surgical control of haemorrhage (laparotomy, thoracotomy).

Disability
- Perform a rapid neurological evaluation. AVPU method (**A**lert, responds to **V**ocal stimuli, responds only to **P**ainful stimuli, **U**nresponsive to all stimuli), Glasgow coma scale (GCS).
- After excluding hypoxia and hypovoleamia, consider changes in level of consciousness to be due to head injury.

Exposure/environment control
- Undress patient for through examination.
- Prevent hypothermia by covering with warm blankets/warming device. Use warm IV fluids.

Adjuncts to primary survey
- Monitoring. Pulse, non-invasive BP, ECG, pulse oximetry.
- Urinary catheter (after ruling out urethral injury).
- Diagnostic studies. X-rays (lateral cervical spine, AP chest, and AP pelvis), ultrasound scan, CT scan, diagnostic peritoneal lavage.

Secondary survey
Begin only after primary survey is complete and resuscitation is continuing successfully.
- Take history. AMPLE (**A**llergy, **M**edication, **P**ast medical history, **L**ast meal, **E**vents of the incident).
- Perform a head-to-toe physical examination.
- Continue reassessment of all vital signs.
- Perform specialized diagnostic tests that may be required.

Thoracic injuries

Key features
- Thoracic injuries account for 25% of deaths from trauma.
- Fifty per cent of patients who die from multiple injuries also have a significant thoracic injury.
- Open injuries are caused by penetrating trauma from knives or gunshots. Closed injuries occur after blasts, blunt trauma, and deceleration. (Road traffic accidents (RTAs) are the most common cause.)

Management—primary survey
Identify and treat major thoracic life-threatening injuries.

Tension pneumothorax
- A clinical diagnosis. There is no time for X-rays.
- Patient has respiratory distress, is tachycardic and hypotensive.
- Look for tracheal deviation, decreased movement, hyperresonant percussion note, and absent breath sounds over affected hemithorax.
- Treat with immediate decompression. Insert a 12G cannula into the second intercostal space in the mid-clavicular line. Follow this with insertion of an underwater seal chest drain into the fifth intercostal space between the anterior and mid-axillary line.

Open pneumothorax
- Occlude with a three-sided dressing.
- Follow by immediate insertion of an intercostal drain through a separate incision.

Flail chest
- Results in paradoxical motion of the chest wall. Hypoxia is caused by restricted chest wall movement and underlying lung contusion.
- If the segment is small and respiration is not compromised, nurse patient in HDU with adequate analgesia. Encourage early ambulation and vigorous physiotherapy. Do regular blood gas analysis.
- In more severe cases, endotracheal intubation with positive pressure ventilation is required.

Massive haemothorax
- Accumulation of >1500mL of blood in pleural cavity.
- Suspect when shock is associated with dull percussion note and absent breath sounds on one side of chest.
- Simultaneously restore blood volume and carry out decompression by inserting a wide bore chest drain.
- Consider need for urgent thoracotomy to control bleeding if there is continued brisk bleeding and need for persistent blood transfusion. Consult with a regional thoracic centre.

Cardiac tamponade
- Most commonly results from penetrating injuries, but blood can also accumulate in pericardial sac after blunt trauma.
- Recognize by haemodynamic instability. Hypotension, tachycardia, raised JVP, pulsus paradoxus, and faint heart sounds.
- If critically ill with suspected tamponade, perform 'blind' pericardiocentesis and call cardiothoracic or general surgeons to consider emergency thoracotomy.
- If unwell, but responding to treatment, arrange urgent transthoracic echo or focused abdominal ultrasound in A&E.

Management—secondary survey

Perform a further in-depth examination. In stab injuries, expose the patient fully and position them so that you can assess front, back, and sides of the chest for any wounds missed in the primary survey.

An erect CXR looking for the following injuries.

Simple pneumo-/haemothorax Treat with a chest drain if large or symptomatic or in any patient likely to undergo GA.

Pulmonary contusion Most common potentially lethal chest injury. Risk of worsening associated consolidation and local pulmonary oedema. Treat with analgesia, physiotherapy, and oxygenation. Consider respiratory support for a patient with significant hypoxia.

Tracheobronchial rupture
- Suspect when there is persistent large air leak after chest drain insertion. Seek immediate (cardiothoracic) surgical consultation.
- Thoracic CT scan usually diagnostic.

Blunt cardiac injury (myocardial contusion/traumatic infarction)
- Suspect when there are significant abnormalities on ECG or echocardiography.
- Seek cardiological/cardiothoracic surgical advice.

Aortic disruption
- Patients survive immediate death because the haematoma is contained.
- Suspect when history of decelerating force and where there is widened mediastinum on CXR.
- Thoracic CT scan is diagnostic.
- Consider cardiothoracic surgical referral.

Diaphragmatic rupture
- Usually secondary to blunt trauma in restrained car passengers (seat belt compression causes 'burst' injury commonly on the left side).
- Suspect in patient with a suitable history and a raised left hemidiaphragm on CXR.
- Penetrating trauma below the fifth intercostal space can produce a perforation.
- Thoracoabdominal CT scan usually diagnostic.

Abdominal trauma

Key features

- Abdominal injuries are present in 7–10% of trauma patients. These injuries, if unrecognized, can cause preventable deaths.
- Blunt trauma. Most frequent injuries are spleen (45%), liver (40%), and retroperitoneal haematoma (15%). Blunt trauma may cause:
  - Compression or crushing, causing rupture of solid or hollow organs.
  - Deceleration injury due to differential movement of fixed and non-fixed parts of organs, causing tearing or avulsion from their vascular supply, e.g. liver tear and vena caval rupture.
- Blunt abdominal trauma is very common in RTAs where:
  - There have been fatalities.
  - Any casualty has been ejected from the vehicle.
  - The closing speed is >50mph.
- Penetrating trauma. These may be:
  - Stab wounds and low velocity gunshot wounds. Cause damage by laceration or cutting; stab wounds commonly involve the liver (40%), small bowel (30%), diaphragm (20%), colon (15%).
  - High velocity gunshot wounds transfer more kinetic energy and also cause further injury by cavitation effect, tumble, and fragmentation; commonly involve the small bowel (50%), colon (40%), liver (30%), and vessels (25%).

Management—primary survey

- Any patient persistently hypotensive despite resuscitation, for whom no obvious cause of blood loss has been identified by the primary survey, can be assumed to have intra-abdominal bleeding.
- If the patient is stable, an emergency abdominal CT scan is indicated.
- If the patient remains critically unstable, an emergency laparotomy is usually indicated.

Management—secondary survey of the abdomen

History

- Obtain from patient, other passengers, observers, police, and emergency medical personnel.
- Mechanism of injury. Seat belt usage, steering wheel deformation, speed, damage to vehicle, ejection of victim, etc. in automobile collision; velocity, calibre, presumed path of bullet, distance from weapon, etc. in penetrating injuries.
- Prehospital condition and treatment of patient.

Physical examination

- Inspect anterior abdomen which includes lower thorax, perineum, and log roll to inspect posterior abdomen. Look for abrasions, contusions, lacerations, penetrating wounds, distension, evisceration of viscera.
- Palpate abdomen for tenderness, involuntary muscle guarding, rebound tenderness, gravid uterus.

- Auscultate for presence/absence of bowel sounds.
- Percuss to elicit subtle rebound tenderness.
- Assess pelvic stability.
- Penile, perineum, rectal, vaginal examinations, and examination of gluteal regions.

Investigations

Blood and urine sampling Raised serum amylase may indicate small bowel or pancreatic injury.

Plain radiography Supine CXR is unreliable in the diagnosis of free intra-abdominal air.

Focused abdominal sonography for trauma (FAST)
- It consists of imaging of the four Ps. Morrison's **p**ouch, **p**ouch of Douglas (or **p**elvic), **p**erisplenic, and **p**ericardium.
- It is used to identify the peritoneal cavity as a source of significant haemorrhage.
- It is also used as a screening test for patients without major risk factors for abdominal injury.

Diagnostic peritoneal lavage (DPL)
- Mostly superseded by FAST for unstable patients and CT scanning in stable patients. Useful, when these are inappropriate or unavailable, for the identification of the presence of free intraperitoneal fluid (usually blood).
- Aspiration of blood, GI contents, bile, or faeces through the lavage catheter indicates laparotomy.

CT
- The investigation of choice in haemodynamically stable patients in whom there is no apparent indication for an emergency laparotomy.
- It provides detailed information relative to specific organ injury and its extent and may guide/inform conservative management.

Indications for resuscitative laparotomy Blunt abdominal trauma. Unresponsive hypotension despite adequate resuscitation and no other cause for bleeding found.

Indications for urgent laparotomy
- Blunt trauma with positive DPL or free blood on ultrasound and an unstable circulatory status.
- Blunt trauma with CT features of solid organ injury not suitable for conservative management.
- Clinical features of peritonitis.
- Any knife injury associated with visible viscera, clinical features of peritonitis, haemodynamic instability, or developing fever/signs of sepsis.
- Any gunshot wound.

Vascular injuries

Key features

- Wounds that involve vascular structures of the extremity are a significant cause of morbidity and mortality in the traumatized patient.
- Motor vehicle accidents and falls are the most common causes of blunt injury.
- Stab wounds cause most of the upper extremity vascular injuries, while gunshot wounds cause the majority of lower extremity vascular injuries in penetrating vascular injury.
- Blunt trauma causes more morbidity than penetrating injuries due to associated fractures, dislocations, and crush injuries to muscles and nerves.

Management—primary survey

- Apply direct pressure to open haemorrhaging wound.
- Carry out aggressive fluid resuscitation.
- A rapidly expanding haematoma suggests a significant vascular injury.
- Realign and splint any associated fracture. Immobilize dislocated joint.
- Seek surgical consultation.

Management—secondary survey

- Begin only after primary survey is complete and resuscitation is continuing successfully.
- Identify limb-threatening injuries.
- Look for hard or soft signs of vascular injury:
  - 'Hard' signs are massive external blood loss, expanding or pulsatile haematoma, absent or diminished distal pulses, and a thrill or audible continuous murmur.
  - 'Soft' findings are history, if active bleeding at the accident scene, proximity of penetrating or blunt trauma to a major artery, small non-pulsatile haematoma, and neurological deficit.
- Measure distal systolic Doppler pressures of the injured arm or leg and compare with uninjured brachial systolic pressure. An index of <1.0 is a predictor of arterial injury.
- Presence of hard signs requires immediate operative intervention or arteriography when limb is viable and active bleeding is absent. Intraoperative arteriography helps in planning the operative approach. Some minimal arterial injuries can be managed non-operatively. Embolization can be used to manage selected arterial injuries.

Principles of operative management

- Obtain proximal and distal control prior to exposing the injury.
- Inspect the injured vessel and debride as necessary.
- Remove intraluminal thrombus by using Fogarty catheter.
- Flush lumen with heparinized normal saline solution.
- Consider temporary intraluminal shunting if limb is ischaemic and there is a delay (if revascularization is anticipated).

- The type of vascular repair depends on the extent of damage. Techniques used are lateral repair, patch angioplasty, end-to-end anastomosis, interposition graft, or bypass graft.
- Use systemic anticoagulation if there is no contraindication.
- Consider intraoperative completion arteriography.
- Ensure completed vascular repair is free of tension and covered with viable soft tissue.
- In patients with combined vascular and orthopaedic injuries, perform arterial repair first to restore circulation before orthopaedic stabilization. Where there is massive soft tissue injury, debride all non-viable tissue.
- Anticipate development of compartment syndrome. Perform fasciotomies to decompress all four compartments of the leg.

Head injuries

Causes and features

- Most common reasons for head injuries—falls, RTAs, and assaults.
- About 80% of head injuries are mild, 10% moderate, and 10% severe.
- Up to half of the deaths from trauma under the age of 45 are due to a head injury. Sequelae are common in survivors.

Management—primary survey

- Maintain adequate oxygenation and BP. This avoids potentially devastating secondary brain injury.
- Determine consciousness level on the AVPU or GCS (see Table 14.1; use a standard head injury proforma).
- Involve anaesthetist to provide appropriate airway management in patients with GCS <8 or AVPU = P or U.
- Avoid systemic analgesia until full neurological assessment made.

Management—secondary survey

- Fully assess the head and neck including:
  - Examination of skull vault.
  - Looking for signs of base of skull fractures (haemotympanum, 'panda' eyes, cerebrospinal fluid (CSF) otorrhoea or rhinorrhoea, Battle's sign).
  - Repeated monitoring of vital signs.
  - Repeated assessment of conscious level (GCS or AVPU).
- Follow guidelines when transferring patients to the neurosurgical unit. Ensure resuscitation and stabilization of patient is complete before transfer.
- Give verbal advice and a written head injury advice card to patients who are being discharged from A&E.

Indications for CT scanning in head injuries

- GCS <13 at any point since the injury; GCS = 13 or 14 at 2h after the injury.
- Suspected open or depressed skull fracture.
- Any sign of basal skull fracture.
- Post-traumatic seizure.
- Focal neurological deficit.
- More than one episode of vomiting.
- Amnesia for greater than 30min of events before impact.
- Age ≥65y, coagulopathy, dangerous mechanism of injury, provided that some loss of consciousness or amnesia has been experienced.

Indications for neurosurgical referral in head injuries
- Major intracranial injury (extradural haematoma, moderate or larger subdural haematoma, intracerebral haematoma).
- Progressive focal neurological signs.
- Definite or suspected penetrating head injury.
- A CSF leak or base of skull fracture.
- Persisting coma (GCS ≤8) after initial resuscitation or deterioration in GCS score after admission.

Indications for admission in head injuries
- Patients with new, clinically significant abnormalities on imaging.
- Patient has not returned to GCS = 15 after imaging, regardless of the imaging results.
- Patient fulfils the criteria for CT scanning, but this cannot be done within the appropriate period, either because CT is not available or because the patient is not sufficiently cooperative to allow scanning.
- Continuing worrying signs, e.g. persistent vomiting, severe headaches.
- Other sources of concern, e.g. drug or alcohol intoxication, other injuries, shock, suspected non-accidental injury, meningism, CSF leak.

Table 14.1 Glasgow coma scale*

Feature	Scale	Score
Eye opening (E)	Nil	1
	In response to pain	2
	In response to speech	3
	Spontaneous	4
Motor response (M)	Nil	1
	Extension	2
	Abnormal flexion	3
	Flexion away from pain	4
	Localizes pain	5
	Obeys commands	6
Verbal response (V)	Nil	1
	Sounds	2
	Inappropriate words	3
	Confused sentences	4
	Orientated fully	5

* Minimum score, 3; maximum score, 15.

Reproduced from Teasdale, G. and Jennett, B. (1974). *The Lancet*, **304**: 7872, with kind permission from Elsevier.

Orthopaedic surgery

Examination of a joint

- Applying a systematic approach will avoid missing vital clues.
- Always begin with a history, followed by examination.
- The classical orthopaedic triad of 'look, feel, and move' applies.[1]
- Remember to examine the patient as a whole, not just the joint!

Ask

- Is the joint painful?
- Is there a specific area of tenderness?
- Does the pain radiate?
- Is the joint swollen?
- Can the joint be moved actively?
- Has there been an injury to the joint?

Look

- Remember, always compare unaffected with affected side.
- Is there any swelling? If so, is it an effusion, synovitis, or bony deformity?
- Are there any colour changes? Bruising or erythema?
- Is there any skin involvement, i.e. rheumatoid nodules at elbow, psoriatic plaques?
- Are there any scars? If so, are they traumatic, surgical, or infective?
- Look for muscle wasting, generally around the joint and specifically in the whole limb.
- Examine the patient as a whole for clues to the disease process at the joint.

Feel

- Always gain verbal consent and explain what you are doing to the patient.
- Examine the unaffected or least painful side prior to examining the affected side.
- Is the joint hot, cold, or moist?
- Is there any local tenderness? Look at the patient's face, not the joint.
- Is the joint swollen? An effusion can occur after trauma (haemarthrosis) or with infection (septic arthritis). Does the fluid shift with sweeping? Is synovitis present (non-movable fluid feel), or is it a bony swelling?

Move

- Compare affected with unaffected side.
- Test active movements first before passive. This gives an idea of the patient's pain and reduces further discomfort.
- Ask the patient to move the joint through a full range of movement.
- Look for pain (patient's face) and limitation of movement.
- Is the limitation mechanical (blocked by loose body, meniscal tear, contracture) or restrictive (resisted by the patient due to pain)?
- *Shoulder.* Flexion, extension, abduction, internal and external rotation.

- *Elbow.* Flexion, extension, pronation, and supination (ensure humerus at patient's side).
- *Wrist.* Flexion, extension, radial and ulnar deviation, pronation, and supination.
- *Metacarpophalangeal joint* (MCPJ). Flexion, extension, abduction, and adduction.
- *Proximal interphalangeal joint* (PIPJ) and distal interphalangeal joint (DIPJ). Flexion and extension.
- *Thumb.* Flexion, extension, abduction, adduction, and opposition.
- *Hip.* Flexion, extension, internal and external rotation.
- *Knee.* Flexion and extension.
- *Ankle.* Plantar and dorsiflexion, eversion and inversion.
- *Cervical spine.* Flexion, extension, and lateral rotation and flexion.
- *Lumbar spine.* Flexion, extension, and lateral rotation and flexion.
- Muscle power is graded via the MRC system (see 📖 p. 492).
- Always get the patient to walk to test gait if the problem is lower limb.

Special tests

These depend on the individual joint examined and are numerous for each joint!

They normally involve either:
- Tests of instability, for example:
  - Collateral testing in the knee, elbow, or finger joints.
  - Cruciate ligament testing (anterior draw, Lachmans).
  - Apprehension tests (shoulder instability).
- Or provocation tests that aim to locate the cause of intra-articular pain, for example:
  - Grind tests (thumb base osteoarthritis, knee meniscal injury).
  - Meniscal provocation tests (McMurray's test).

Reference

1 Soloman L, Warwick D, Nayagam S (Eds) (2010). *Apley's system of orthopaedics and fractures,* 9th Edn. Hodder Arnold, London.

Examination of the limbs and trunk

Develop your own system that you feel comfortable with. Always compare affected with unaffected side. Make allowances for the dominant side.

Look

Is there any swelling, deformity, asymmetry, muscle wasting, twitching (fasciculation), scars, skin colour changes, rashes?

Feel

Is there any tenderness, temperature changes, solid or fluid swellings, muscle bulk?

Move

- Move each joint through its full active and passive range.
- Is the limb tone normal, reduced (flaccid or floppy), or increased (rigidity)? Is there any spasm? Are there any joint contractures?
- Is the rigidity through whole movement or only initially (spasticity)?
- Is the alteration in movement from a neuromuscular disorder, a mechanical block, or pain from the joint?

Power (MRC grading)

- Grade 0, no movement.
- Grade 1, flicker of movement only.
- Grade 2, movement with gravity eliminated.
- Grade 3, movement against gravity.
- Grade 4, movement against resistance.
- Grade 5, normal power.

Test all muscle groups within their relevant myotomes according to the patient's history.

Coordination

- Ask the patient to touch their nose with their index finger with their eyes open and then shut. Compare side to side.
- Alternatively, ask the patient to put their right heel on to their left knee and run it down their shin and vice versa. Note whether these movements are smooth or jerky.
- Romberg's test. Stand with feet together and eyes shut. Positive result will cause the patient to become unstable or fall; be prepared!

Reflexes

- Biceps jerk, C5/6.
- Abdominal, T8–T12.
- Triceps jerk, C6/7.
- Knee jerk, L2/3/4.
- Brachioradialis, C5/6.
- Ankle jerk, S1/2.
- Plantar response. Normal flexor, abnormal extensor (Babinski's sign).
- Clonus at ankle (normal two beats or less).

Grading
- 0, absent.
- 1, hypoactive.
- 2, normal.
- 3, hyperactive, no clonus.
- 4, hyperactive with clonus.

Sensation

Explain what you are about to do clearly to the patient and perform the test with their eyes closed. Compare symmetrical sides of the body at the same time. Map out the abnormalities.

- Pinprick, light touch, and temperature tested in a dermatomal pattern.
- Vibration sense tested with a 128MHz low-pitched tuning fork on a bony prominence. Start distal and if abnormal, move from proximal.
- Proprioception (joint position sense) tested by moving the metatarsophalangeal joint (MTPJ) of the hallux, up and down; the patient confirms the correct movement.

Fracture healing

Fracture healing occurs as either primary or secondary bone union.

- Secondary bone healing produces *callus*. It occurs when fractures are immobilized with 'relative stability' (some minimal movement at fracture site, e.g. a plaster cast). It involves two simultaneously occurring, but distinct, processes: intramembranous and endochondral ossification, producing periosteal bony callus and fibrocartilagenous bridging callus, respectively.
- Primary bone healing does not produce callus. It occurs when fracture fragments are reduced 'anatomically' and 'interfragmentary compression' is achieved with 'absolute stability'. There is no motion between fracture surfaces (e.g. compression plating techniques or lag screw fixation).

Secondary bone healing (callus)

Initial phase: haematoma and inflammation

- Torn vessels at fracture site bleed, producing a haematoma and subsequent clot.
- The size of the haematoma depends upon the blood supply to the bone and the violence of the injury; it can continue to expand during the first 36h.
- Injured tissue and platelet activation causes an inflammatory cascade via the release of growth factors and various cytokines.
- Inflammatory cell migration to the haematoma occurs (macrophages, fibroblasts, osteoclasts, chondroblasts).
- Fibroblasts and chondroblasts organize the haematoma into collagen and granulation tissue, with new capillary ingrowth (angiogenesis).
- Osteoclasts and macrophages remove dead bone and tissue, respectively.
- This stage usually lasts up to 1 week.

Second phase: callus formation (soft and hard)

- Cell (osteoblasts) proliferation and differentiation results in callus formation.
- Intramembranous (or periosteal) hard callus forms peripherally, with endochondral (fibrocartilagenous/bridging) soft callus forming alongside. A third type 'medullary callus' forms later if the above fails.
- The amount and type of callus produced is dependent upon local factors such as the type of fracture, proximity of the bone ends, amount of haematoma, and is inversely proportional to the amount of movement present.
- Soft callus is calcified by chondroblasts and subsequently resorbed by chondroclasts.
- New blood vessels invasion into the callus brings osteoblastic type cells, resulting in ossification into woven bone.
- By this point, the fracture will have united and be pain-free.
- This stage lasts 1 week to 4 months.

Third phase: remodelling
- Woven bone is resorbed by osteoclasts and osteoblasts replace this with lamellar bone, which is very hard and dense.
- Final remodelling occurs when swelling around the fracture site decreases; trabeculae can be seen crossing the fracture site on radiographs and the medullary canal is recreated.
- Remodelling is most marked in children and follows the mechanical forces applied to the bone in a physiological environment.
- This process is identical in both primary and secondary bone healing and can last for several years.

Primary bone healing (absolute stability)
- The inflammatory response is much reduced.
- Areas of direct contact undergo some activity.
- Any gaps are invaded with blood vessels and cells differentiate into osteoblasts, laying down woven and lamellar bone (gap healing).
- Osteoclasts acting as 'cutting cones' pass directly across the fracture site, leaving channels that are filled with blood vessels and allowing osteoblasts to fill them with lamellar bone.
- No callus is formed and union takes much longer to achieve, with the strength of the healing process being borne by the mechanical properties of the fixation device.
- Remodelling occurs as above.

Factors adversely affecting fracture healing
- Degree of local trauma (bone loss, soft tissue trauma and interposition, neurovascular injury, open fractures).
- Inadequate reduction and immobilization.
- Infection.
- Location of fracture. Which bone and where on bone i.e. metaphysis versus diaphysis (see below)?
- Disturbances of ossification, e.g. metabolic bone disease, osteoporosis, local pathological tumour.
- Age, poor nutrition, smoking, drugs (especially NSAIDs), diabetes.

How long do fractures take to unite?
Perkins rules
- Fractures of cancellous (metaphyseal) bone (e.g. those around joints) will take 6 weeks to unite.
- Fractures of cortical (diaphyseal) bone (e.g. shafts of long bones) will take 12 weeks to unite.
- Fractures of the tibia (because of poor blood supply) will take 24 weeks to unite.
- Time to union for children equals the age of the child in years plus 1, e.g. tibial fracture in a 2y-old child will unite in 3 weeks. Common sense needs to be applied when applying the rule to fractures of cancellous bone in older children.

Delayed union

Defined as a failure of union to occur in 1.5× the normal time for fracture union.

Non-union

Defined as a failure of union to occur within twice the normal time to fracture union. However, expect open fractures to normally take twice the normal Perkins rule.

- *Hypertrophic non-union.* Excess mobility or strain at fracture site. There is a good blood supply with healing potential. Appears as large callus (elephant's foot pattern) on X-rays. Usually requires stabilization to allow callus progression.
- *Atrophic non-union.* Due to poor blood supply resulting from initial injury or surgical intervention. There is poor healing potential. Usually require stabilization and biological augmentation to heal.

Further reading

Soloman L, Warwick D, Nayagam S (Eds) (2010). *Apley's system of orthopaedics and fractures.* 9th Edn. Hodder Arnold, London.

Ramachandran M (2007). *Basic Orthopaedic Sciences: The Stanmore Guide.* Hodder Arnold, London.

Reduction and fixation of fractures

Caveat. A fracture is a soft tissue injury with an associated broken bone. Treat the soft tissues with utmost respect to ensure fracture healing.

Modern fracture reduction and treatment was pioneered by the AO group and centres around four key principles:[1]

- Fracture reduction and fixation to restore anatomical relationships.
- Stability by fixation or splintage as the personality of the fracture and the injury dictates.
- Preservation of the blood supply to the soft tissue and bone by careful handling and gentle reduction techniques.
- Early and safe mobilization of the part and patient.

Fracture reduction can be achieved by closed[2] (indirect) or open (direct and indirect) methods. Maintenance of the reduction may also be achieved via closed methods which can be non-surgical (plaster or brace) or surgical (intramedullary nail, external fixation, Kershner (K) wires), or via open methods such as rigid internal fixation with plates and screws.

Casting

- Application of a plaster of Paris (or modern alternatives) cast over appropriate padding to stabilize a reduced fracture.
- Typically involves splinting of joints either side of a long bone fracture to provide additional rotational stability.
- Simplest and cheapest to apply.
- Lowest risk of septic complications.
- It will provide pain relief.
- 'Half casts' or 'backslabs' can be utilized to immobilize a fracture prior to definitive management.
- Complications include problems with cast (pressure areas, loosening and breakdown of cast), thromboembolic events, coverage of wounds.
- It is a very involved process, requiring regular follow-up to ensure maintenance of reduction.

Cast bracing

- Stabilization of a fracture across a joint with a cast, but the joint itself is left free to move by the incorporation of a hinge across it.
- Has the advantage of allowing early movement of the joint without the use of weight bearing, e.g. tibial shaft fractures.

Internal fixation

Indications

- *Intra-articular fractures.* To prevent or reduce the incidence of osteoarthrosis.
- *Unstable fracture patterns.*
- *Neurovascular damage.* Fracture stability must be achieved before the delicate repair of vessels or nerves takes place. If not, these repairs may be damaged.
- *Polytrauma.* Multiple injuries better managed by fixation to facilitate nursing care and to allow early mobilization.

- Elderly patients tolerate immobilization and prolonged bed rest poorly (fractured neck of femur).
- *Fractures of long bones* (e.g. forearm, femur, tibia). Rehabilitation is facilitated more quickly with internal fixation after anatomical reduction.
- *Failure of conservative therapy* (loss of acceptable alignment).
- *Pathological fractures.*

Methods

Compression plates and screws, locking plates and screws, Kershner (K) wires, intramedullary nails, tension band wiring.

Complications

- Infection which increases with the size and increased time of exposure required.
- Nerve and vessel injury.
- Non-union (increased with iatrogenic soft tissue and periosteal injury).
- Implant failure and subsequent fracture through a bony defect if the implant is removed.

External fixation

Indications

Temporizing measure for:
- Open fractures (commonly tibia or femur) associated with significant soft tissue damage or nerve and vessel injury.
- Highly comminuted or unstable fractures and fracture dislocations.
- Life-saving splintage procedure in pelvic fractures.
- Initial stabilizing device for any fracture where 'damage limitation' surgery may be appropriate in the multiply injured patient (damage control orthopaedics).
- Definitive treatment of periarticular fractures (pilon and tibial plateau).
- As a salvage option in the face of mal-union, non-union, or significant bone loss.

Methods

- Pin-and-rod construct most commonly used (tibia–pelvis).
- Modern systems incorporate ring fixators with pins and rods (hybrid).
- Circular fixators (Ilizarov) can be used for definitive fracture fixation or as a salvage option.

Complications

- Pin site infection and possible osteomyelitis.
- Nerve, vessel, ligament, and tendon injury (good understanding of cross-sectional anatomy required).
- Over-distraction, resulting in non-union.

Locking plates

- Modern implants in which the screw heads are threaded and engage and lock into threads in the plate holes.
- These act as 'internal, external fixators' where forces are transmitted from bone to screw to plate.

- The locking plate provides *angular stability* and is much stronger than a normal plate as all screws act in unison.
- Advantages are:
  - Excellent holding power as all locked screws have to fail at once for construct to fail. Thus, excellent choice of fixation in osteoporotic fractures.
  - Spares periosteal blood supply as does not rely on compression of plate on bone.
  - They can be placed percutaneously (avoiding stripping soft tissue and blood supply from a fracture site).
  - They do not require contouring.
  - The screws are usually self-drilling and self-tapping.

References

1 Ruedi TP, Murphy WM (2000). *AO principles of fracture management*. Thieme Medical Publishers, New York.
2 McRae R, Esser M (2008). *Practical fracture treatment*, 5th edn. Churchill Livingstone, Edinburgh.

The skeletal radiograph

This is the most important investigation in orthopaedics, but does not substitute for accurate history and examination. Always remember a fracture is a clinical, not a radiological diagnosis.

Evaluation

Have a system. The following is only one example:

- Note the history, race, occupation, handedness, pastimes, age, sex, and recent laboratory results of the patient.
- Accurate history and clear requests to be documented on X-ray forms. Always write the side in full, e.g. 'right'.
- Always take two views at 90° to each other (orthogonal).
- Examine the film carefully.
- Most hospitals use computer-based X-ray viewing systems but if using a viewing box, have a bright spotlight and magnifying glass available.
- When describing the lesion, think of side, anatomical site, nature, displacement, and soft tissue components.
- Keep it simple.
  - A. Adequate views and alignment.
  - B. Bones.
  - C. Cartilage (soft tissues).
- Look for cortical/medullary changes, periosteal reactions, deformity, soft tissue swelling, and cortical breach (definition of a fracture).
- Supplement radiological findings with further biochemical investigations, bone scanning, and biopsy if indicated.

Radiological features

Osteoporosis

- The most common form of bone disease.
- Characterized by low bone mass and deterioration of the microarchitecture of bone tissue with consequent increase in bone fragility and susceptibility to low trauma fractures.
- Affects middle-aged and elderly women, predisposing them to fractures of the distal radius, femoral neck, and vertebral bodies.
- Localized osteoporosis follows disease, e.g. after joint fusion.
- The cortices are thin with reduced medullary trabeculae, i.e. the bone is essentially normal; there is just too little of it.

Osteomalacia

There is reduced mineralization of osteoid.

- The trabeculae are blurred.
- Symmetrical transverse or oblique cortical defects appear (Looser's zones, pseudofractures).
- In children, changes are most marked at the metaphysis (rickets).

Hyperparathyroidism

There is bone resorption. Best place to see it is in the phalanges of the hands in the subperiosteal cortex. Note generalized cortical striations. Usually diagnosed with parathyroid hormone levels after incidental finding of raised calcium levels.

Diffuse increase in density

Think of neoplasia, fluorosis, sarcoidosis, bone dysplasia (osteopetrosis).

Abnormalities of bone modelling

Developmental disorders, e.g. osteochondrodysplasia, are often present from birth. Look for abnormalities of the eyes, heart, and ears. Thorough assessment by biochemical and genetic specialist required.

Local abnormalities may occur in congenital disorders, e.g. endochon-dromatosis (Ollier's disease), fibrous dysplasia, neurofibromatosis, or acquired disorders, e.g. Paget's disease.

Solitary lesions

Always think of sepsis, primary bone tumours, or secondary metastasis. Location and age are important, e.g. an epiphyseal lesion in a child may be a chondroblastoma and a subarticular lesion in a young adult may be a giant cell tumour. The older the patient, the more likely it is a metastasis.

Describing a fracture

- First check details match patient (i.e. date of X-ray, patient age, side, hospital number).
- Ensure the appropriate X-ray is taken with two views at 90° to each other (e.g. an X-ray of an ankle, rather than the whole lower leg).
- Which bone is fractured?
- Where is the fracture in the bone? Joint (intra-articular), proximal, middle, or distal third, or metaphysis (flares at end of bones), diaphysis (shaft), physis (growth plate), and epiphysis (end part of bone) in children.
- What is the pattern? Transverse, oblique, spiral, comminuted or multifragmentary, segmental.
- Is there displacement? Quantify this (e.g. 50% of bone width or completely 'off ended' >100%).
- Is there any angulation? Which direction (varus, valgus, recuvartum)?
- If a joint is involved, comment on whether it is 'in joint' or dislocated.
- Other things to look for are gas in soft tissues (suggests open fracture or gas-forming infection), foreign bodies (metal, glass, grit), fluid in joints (e.g. lipohaemarthrosis in knee suggests fracture), fat pad signs in the elbow (suggest fracture and are prominent due to blood in joint).
- A ring-like structure (e.g. the bony pelvis) rarely fractures in only one place; if you find one fracture, look hard for another one!
- Comment on implants if present and the proximity and involvement of this to fracture (periprosthetic fractures of a total hip replacement (THR) or total knee replacement (TKR)).
- *Pitfalls.* Is it a fracture? Structures that may be mistaken for fractures include suture lines between bones, vascular channels, and physes in immature skeletons. Anatomic structures are more likely to be symmetrical, if not midline.

Further reading

Raby N, Berman L, de Lacy G (2005). *Accident and emergency radiology: a survival guide*, 2nd edn. Saunders, London.
Nicholson DA, Driscoll P (1995). *ABC of emergency radiology*. BMJ Books, Wiley, England.

Injuries of the phalanges and metacarpals

Thumb

Mechanism Direct blows to thumb, forced opposition of the thumb.

Extra-articular

- *Metacarpal shaft fractures.* Undisplaced can be managed in cast. Displaced fractures require reduction and fixation, either open or closed.
- *Metacarpal base fractures.* Often displaced or angulated due to deforming forces of the tendon attachments. If fractures undisplaced, can manage with closed reduction and immobilization in cast. For displaced/significantly angulated fractures, closed reduction with K wire fixation or open reduction with internal fixation (ORIF) is required.

Up to 30° of angulation can be accepted due to the vast range of movements at the base of thumb.

Intra-articular (± fracture dislocation)

- *Bennett's fracture dislocation.* Volar/ulnar fragment left behind due to strong ligament attachments; remaining distal metacarpal dislocates proximally and dorsally. Treatment involves closed reduction and K wire fixation to either carpus (trapezium) and/or index finger metacarpal. Open reduction is rarely needed.
- *Rolando fractures.* Multifragmentary fracture, at least three parts in a 'T' or 'Y' pattern ± dislocation. Treatment depends on degree of fragmentation. Reduction and K wire fixation or external fixation should be considered. ORIF only if large fragments.

Thumb dislocation

- At the MCPJ, usually results in ulnar collateral ligament (UCL) injury (gamekeeper's thumb).
- Tear of the UCL can be partial or complete, with adductor aponeurosis stuck in the joint (Stener lesion), preventing reduction.
- Partial tears (stable) are immobilized in cast for 6 weeks.
- Complete tears (unstable or Stener Lesion) require surgical repair.
- Chronic tears are treated with tendon reconstruction of UCL or MCPJ fusion.

Metacarpal fractures

Mechanism Usually 'punch' injury ('Friday night' or 'boxer's' fracture). The little finger most commonly affected. Remember to check for rotational deformity as this is not an acceptable deformity.

Metacarpal neck fractures

Accept up to 15° angulation in index/middle and 35° in ring/little fingers. Most treated conservatively (neighbour strapping). Reduction and pinning or ORIF if significant angulation.

Metacarpal shaft fractures

Check for rotation. Transverse or unstable fractures (especially ring and little fingers), treat with ORIF or K wire fixation. Undisplaced fractures can be treated conservatively (neighbour strapping). Similar degrees of angulation to neck fractures can be accepted.

Metacarpal base fractures (± subluxation)

Always get a true lateral X-ray of hand to assess for subluxation. These are usually stable fractures and can be treated conservatively in cast for 3 weeks. If subluxed (little finger akin to Bennett's fracture), treatment involves closed reduction and K wire fixation to carpal bone for 4 weeks.

Distal phalanx fractures

Mechanism Crush injury that is comminuted and often compound. Tuft type fractures.

Treatment

Wound toilet, simple nail bed repair if needed, and primary suture or Steri-strip® with pressure dressing. Wound inspection at 48h and as required. Can be dealt with in A&E department. Antibiotics if open.

Mallet finger

- Sudden flexion injury of distal phalanx (i.e. stubbing finger), resulting in either avulsion of extensor tendon insertion with flake or large fragment of bone, but can be purely tendinous.
- Small fragments or purely tendinous types are treated in 'mallet splint' (extension) for 8 weeks continuously, followed by 2–4 weeks just at night. If large fragment, fixation can be undertaken if unable to maintain in splint.

Proximal and middle phalanx fractures

Mechanism Direct blow or twisting injuries.

Treatment

- Dependent on fracture configuration. Check for rotational deformity.
- Undisplaced stable fractures are treated with neighbour strapping for 2–3 weeks with early mobilization.
- If unstable, rotated, severely angulated, or involving the joint, consider closed reduction and K wire fixation or ORIF with mini-fragment screws ± plate. Stable fixation to allow early mobilization is the goal.

PIP joint dislocations

- Dorsal dislocation is the most common. It is associated with avulsion of volar plate or fracture of volar base of middle phalanx.
- Dislocations require reduction under ring block.
- If stable, they can be treated with extension blocking splint with PIPJ flexed for 4–6 weeks.
- If unstable or associated with significant fracture, they require either manipulation under anaesthesia (MUA) and K wiring, ORIF, or volar plate arthroplasty.

Immobilization for hand injuries (Edinburgh position)

To prevent stiffness, the metacarpal joint should be immobilized in 90° of flexion and the PIPJ in extension with the wrist extended at 30°. This places the ligaments on maximal stretch whilst immobilized.

Further reading

Soloman L, Warwick D, Nayagam S (Eds) (2010). *Apley's system of orthopaedics and fractures*, 9th edn. Hodder Arnold, London.

Wrist injuries

Scaphoid fractures[1]

Mechanism Fall on to the outstretched hand with forced dorsiflexion.

Examination
- Fullness in the anatomical snuffbox means an effusion.
- Tenderness on the volar surface of the scaphoid, i.e. the tubercle, is more predictive than snuffbox tenderness (dorsal) which is unreliable.
- Wrist movement, particularly pronation followed by ulnar deviation, may be painful.
- Pain on compression of the thumb longitudinally or on gripping may be present.
- However, clinical examination is highly variable and skill-dependent.

Investigation (radiographs)
'Scaphoid series' films (PA wrist in ulnar deviation, lateral wrist in neutral; PA in 45° pronation and ulnar deviation; and AP with 30° supination and ulnar deviation). False negative rate of <5%. Fractures are usually of the waist, but may be more proximal.

Treatment
- Below elbow, cast in neutral position (RCTs show that the thumb does not need to be included)[2] for 8 weeks, but the fracture may take 12 weeks to unite. At 12 weeks, remove plaster regardless of symptoms.
- If initial X-rays negative, but clinical suspicion persists, cast the wrist and repeat films in 2 weeks.
- Displacement of >1mm or angulation requires ORIF with compression screw.
- Proximal pole fractures are relative indication for fixation as high chance of non-union.

Complications
- *Non-union.* ↑ with proximal fractures due to blood supply running from distal to proximal in the bone. If not united at 12 weeks, proceed to ORIF (compression screw) ± bone grafting.
- *Avascular necrosis.* ↑ with proximal and displaced fractures (see above). Treatment is by internal fixation and bone grafting which may need to be a 'vascularized' graft.
- *Degenerative change.* May occur after non- or mal-union. Treated by limited wrist fusion (four corner fusion, scaphoidectomy, and radial styloidectomy).

Other carpal fractures
- The most common is *hamate fracture*. The hook is fractured by direct blow to the palm of the hand or repeated direct contact (e.g. motorcyclists, golfers, racquet sports, and cricketers).
- Treatment is usually excision, but internal fixation may be attempted if the fragment is large.

Ligamentous injuries of the wrist

- Common; difficult to diagnose so easily missed.
- If left untreated, they can cause long-term disability.
- The proximal row of carpal bones forms an intercalated segment, i.e. they are connected and work together as a unit. Injury may occur to the ligaments connecting the bones.

Scapholunate ligament

Common in isolation or in association with fractures (especially distal radius). 'Terry Thomas' sign, i.e. increase in the space between scaphoid and lunate on a clenched fist PA view. Acute ruptures may be repaired, but chronic injuries may require reconstruction or fusion.

Lunotriquetral ligament

Less common; acute repair may be successful, but chronic injuries require lunotriquetral fusion.

Carpal dislocations

Complete ligamentous injury may allow the carpus to dislocate.

- Occurs either with the lunate remaining in place, a *perilunate dislocation*, or the carpus staying in place and the lunate moving, a *lunate dislocation*.
- On rarer occasions, the scapholunate ligament remains intact and the scaphoid fractures, resulting in a *trans-scaphoid perilunate dislocation*.

Treatment Severe injury requires reduction—best open as it allows formal repair of the disrupted ligaments, as well as stabilization of the carpus. If the scaphoid is fractured, it should be internally fixed as well.

Carpometacarpal fracture dislocation

- Usually as the result of a punch injury. Affects little or ring fingers.
- Commonly missed due to poor history and examination.
- Indicated by tenderness at the carpometacarpal base.
- Diagnosed with a *true* lateral (not the standard lateral oblique) X-ray (shows subluxation or dislocation at the carpometacarpal joint).

Treatment Unstable injury—reduce with traction and local pressure, then stabilize the joint with K wire fixation for 4 weeks.

Triangular fibrocartilage complex (TFCC) injury

TFCC and the ulnar small ligaments of the hand. An acute tear is usually peripheral and the result of trauma, including a fracture to the ulna styloid. It will present with ulna-based wrist pain in ulnar deviation with or without rotation.

Treatment If associated with a large ulnar styloid fracture, this can be internally fixed with a tension band wire technique. Arthroscopic debridement or repair of the tear has been attempted, but is technically demanding.

References

1 ℅ http://www.eatonhand.com.
2 Clay NR, Dias JJ, Costigan PS, *et al.* (1991). Need the thumb be immobilized in scaphoid fractures? A randomised prospective trial. *J Bone Joint Surg Br* **73**(5): 828–32.

Fractures of the distal radius and ulna

- Usually caused by a fall on to the outstretched hand.
- Very common. Approximately 1 in 6 of all fractures treated.
- Bimodal incidence. Peaks in childhood (6–10y) and early old age (60–70y).
- Scaphoid and ligamentous wrist injuries may also be present.

Classification

- Classification systems are the AO system[1] and the Frykman system.[2]
- Historical eponymous terms ('Colles', 'Smith's') are still used.
- To avoid confusion, stick to describing the fracture by anatomical methods, e.g. dorsally displaced fracture of the distal radius with shortening and ulnar deviation.
- In children, the fracture usually involves the epiphyseal region and these fractures are classified by the Salter–Harris system.[3] Salter–Harris type II is easily the most common injury of the distal radius.

Important radiological features to assess

- These parameters give an idea of the severity of the injury and thus the stability of the fracture; the more features, the more unstable.
- Dorsal cortex comminution.
- Intra-articular extension (radiocarpal and distal radioulnar joint (DRUJ)).
- Ulnar styloid fracture (suggests a TFCC injury which is a strong DRUJ stabilizer).
- Loss of radial inclination (normally approximately 22°).
- Loss of palmar tilt or dorsal angulation (normal tilt approximately 11°).
- Loss of radial height (approximately 11mm from distal ulna to tip of radial styloid).

Treatment[4]

Children

- Fractures of the distal radius. Usually treated by closed reduction (manipulation) and the application of a well moulded plaster.
- If very unstable in theatre (radial and ulnar complete fractures, displaced) or if the fracture has slipped position in plaster after manipulation, then internal fixation with percutaneous K wires or more rarely, open fixation with plates and screws may be used.

Adults

Fractures with dorsal displacement/angulation

- Undisplaced + stable. Below elbow plaster immobilization for 6 weeks.
- Displaced + stable. Closed reduction and plaster immobilization for 6 weeks.
- Displaced + unstable. Closed reduction and either percutaneous K wire fixation (two wires), external fixation, or ORIF with plates and screws.
- Complex intra-articular fractures or highly unstable patterns can now be successfully treated with modern anatomic pre-contoured distal radius locking plates.

Traditionally a difficult area to know the best treatment method.
- Take each case on its own merits. There are many patient and fracture factors to allow for.
- Dorsal comminution is a common problem and must be taken into account in the method chosen.
- Bone structural substitutes, e.g. Biobon, lack RCT data to back up their use and considerable expense.

Fractures with volar displacement ('Smith's fracture')
Unstable and are treated by a volar buttress plate (supports a fracture like a shelf, propping up or supporting the distal fragment).

Intra-articular fractures with volar displacement ('Barton's fracture')
Internal fixation is mandatory as it is a highly unstable fracture.

Ulnar styloid fractures
Do not often require fixation unless the fragment is large in which case, it may represent a TFCC injury (see 📖 p. 512) treated by internal fixation.

References
1 🔗 http://www.trauma.org/ortho/aoclass.html.
2 Frykman G (1967). Fracture of the distal radius including sequelae—shoulder–hand–finger syndrome, disturbance in the distal radio ulna joint and impairment of nerve function. A clinical and experimental study. *Acta Orthop Scand Suppl* **108**, 3.
3 Salter RB, Harris WR (1963). Injuries involving the epiphyseal plate. *J Bone Joint Surg Am* **45**, 587–632.
4 🔗 http://www.eradius.com/

Fractures of the radius and ulnar shaft

Mechanism
- Commonly a fall on to the outstretched hand or a direct blow injury.
- High energy may be involved, therefore look closely for neurovascular status and compartment syndrome.
- As displaced or angulated fractures affect the proximal (Monteggia) and distal (Galeazzi) radioulnar joints, it is essential to get orthogonal X-rays of the wrist and elbow.

Fracture types
Children
- Usually transverse fractures of the radius and ulna.
- May be angulated only with one of the cortices still intact ('greenstick fracture').
- Be aware of plastic deformation (no obvious fracture, but bowing of one or both bones).
- May sustain a fracture dislocation as in adults.

Adults
- Usually either a transverse or oblique fracture of the radius and ulna.
- Isolated ulna shaft fractures ('nightstick fractures' named after mechanism of defending direct blow from a policeman's nightstick or truncheon).
- Displacement and significant angulation are indications for fixation.
- Remember, the forearm is a 'force parallelogram' and that a fracture of only one bone will usually result in a dislocation of the other bone at the proximal or distal joints. These fracture dislocations are:
  - *Monteggia fracture.* Proximal ulnar fracture with dislocation of the proximal radial head.
  - *Galeazzi fracture.* Distal radial fracture with dislocation of the DRUJ.

Treatment
Children
- Greenstick fractures. Closed reduction and cast immobilization from wrist to above the elbow.
  - In-line traction is always the key to any initial reduction and often all that is required to realign, given patience.
  - Use minimal force. If the periosteal hinge is broken during reduction, the fracture may displace completely and become unstable.
- Plastic deformation needs to be corrected.
- Displaced fractures are often unstable and can be treated by ORIF with plates and screws, or flexible intramedullary nail fixation.
- Fracture dislocations (Monteggia and Galeazzi). Closed manipulation and cast immobilization (failed reduction may require open reduction).

Adults
- Usually impossible to achieve or maintain a closed reduction for adult forearm shaft fractures.

- Undisplaced fractures can be managed in an above elbow cast.
- Displaced fractures are treated with open reduction and compression plate fixation.
- 'Nightstick fractures' of the ulna are splinted by the intact radius so if undisplaced, then early protected motion with an elbow cast-brace is indicated.
- If the fracture is displaced (>50% displacement or >10°), open reduction and compression plate fixation should be used.
- Fracture dislocations. Treated with open reduction and internal fixation to accurately reduce and hold the associated dislocations.

Complications

- Mal-union or non-union. Close follow-up of closed, manipulated fractures. An X-ray at 1 and 2 weeks is mandatory to watch for slip of position. Mal-union can present with functional problems with forearm rotation.
- Non-union is normally treated by open reduction, debridement of the non-union site, and compression plate fixation with or without bone grafting.
- It is not usually necessary to remove metalwork from the radius and ulna unless they cause significant problems after the fracture has healed. Radial plate removal has been associated with a significant risk of neurovascular complications.

Fractures and dislocations around the elbow in children

- Second commonest injury in children (8% of childhood fractures).[1]
- Cause is usually a fall on to the outstretched hand. The result is related to age:
  - <9y, supracondylar fracture of the humerus.
  - >10y, dislocated elbow.
  - >60y, shoulder injuries.
- Salter–Harris injuries of the elbow occur through the lateral condyle and radial neck.

Supracondylar fractures

Types
- Based on the mechanism of injury, *extension type* (approximately 95%) and *flexion type* (5%).
- Classified using the modified *Gartland* system:[2]
  - Type I. Undisplaced.
  - Type II. Angulated/displaced, but posterior cortex is intact, acting as a hinge.
  - Type III. Complete displacement.
  - Type IV. Completely displaced and unstable in flexion and extension.

Treatment

Displaced supracondylar fractures (types III/IV) are an orthopaedic emergency, especially if complicated with an absent distal pulse. Do not delay.

- Assess neurovascular status and document beforehand.
- Reduce under GA by straight arm traction (up to 5min may be required).
- Then manipulate to correct rotation, varus/valgus tilt, and finally any extension deformity.
- Try to flex the elbow up past 90° with the forearm pronated (may be difficult due to anterior soft tissue swelling; the reduction technique itself can cause loss of the pulse in the flexed position).
- Displaced (type III/IV) fractures should be reduced and stabilized with K wires. Some advocate the same for type II injuries.
- Common configuration is two crossed condylar K wires, one medial (beware of ulnar nerve), and one lateral used to fix the fracture.
- An above elbow cast is then used to supplement fixations and wires are removed at 4 weeks.
- Long arm traction may be used as definitive treatment, but involves a long inpatient stay until the bone has united (usually 3 weeks).

Undisplaced fractures (type I) can be treated with a collar and cuff with or without plaster backslab.

Complications

Vascular

- Injury to the brachial artery is rare as the pulse usually returns after fracture reduction.
- Examination is the key. An absent pulse with a well perfused hand does not require any immediate vascular management; however, a pulseless cold hand or a pulse that is lost post-reduction and pinning does!
- True loss of the radial pulse may be due to:
  - *Vascular spasm*. Typified by good capillary refill after reduction, but slow return of the pulse. Failure of pulse return may be due to other injuries and requires a vascular surgical opinion. partial injury (endothelial flap) is treated by direct repair.
  - *Complete transection or disruption*. May be treated by direct repair or more often, interposition vein graft.
- Contracture. Untreated vascular injury will result in fibrosis and contracture of the forearm ('Volkman's ischaemic contracture'). This is a devastating and debilitating condition and should be avoidable with early (<12h) exploration and/or repair or vascular damage.

Neurological

- Neuropraxia is commonest with gradual recovery. May involve the:
  - Radial nerve.
  - Anterior interosseous (branch of medial nerve).
  - Median and rarely, ulnar nerves.

Mal-union

- Incorrectly reduced fractures will not remodel and can lead to cubitus valgus and a 'gunstock deformity'. Much less common with K wire fixation.
- Recurvatum common following cast management of type II/III; remodels poorly.

Lateral condyle fractures

Types

Classified according to Milch, depending on how much of the intra-articular surface is involved:

- *Type I*. Fracture through growth centre of capitellum (Salter–Harris type IV).
- *Type II*. Fracture medial to growth centre and can involve trochlea (Salter–Harris type II).

Treatment

- Displaced fracture. ORIF with either two cannulated screws or two K wires.
- The fragment is always considerably larger than expected from the X-ray due to the condyle being not fully ossified.
- If not reduced and fixed, the fragment will displace. This is due to the pull of the wrist extensors, arising from the lateral epicondyle. This will lead to a cubitus valgus deformity and can present in later life with an ulnar nerve palsy as it has been chronically stretched ('tardy' ulnar nerve palsy).

Medial condyle fractures

- Not to be confused with epicondyle fractures.
- These fractures occur in a similar pattern to the lateral condyle (type I and II).
- Treatment is essentially as described for lateral condyle fractures.
- The key is recognition of this injury as it is intra-articular and if missed, can be associated with valgus instability of the elbow and subluxation.

Epicondyle fractures

Medial epicondyle fractures Avulsion type injuries of the apophysis. High association with elbow dislocations. The fragment can remain undisplaced, displaced, or become trapped in elbow joint. Treatment is usually conservative in a long arm cast. Surgery is indicated for trapped fragments.

Lateral epicondyle fractures Essentially the same as medial; treated with a long arm cast unless fragment entrapped in joint.

Radial head and neck fractures

- Usually result from a valgus force to the elbow, associated with dislocation or fractures (Monteggia).
- Fractures of the neck are often angulated, displaced, or both.
- Head fractures are of the Salter–Harris type.
- Fractures associated with dislocation happen at the time of injury or as a result of reduction (radial head pushed into ulno-humeral joint).

Treatment

- <30°. Angulation acceptable; sling is provided and early mobilization.
- 30–60°. Reduction should be attempted, but ongoing debate.
- >60°. Reduction is required under GA, usually stable; once reduced, do not require any further fixation.
- Occasionally open reduction is required.
- Intra-articular fractures that are displaced may require fixation with K wires or screws.

Olecranon fractures

Can often be difficult to spot. The proximal epiphysis appears between 8 and 10y. Isolated fractures do occur, but are more commonly associated with fracture dislocations of radial neck.

Treatment

- Undisplaced fractures require a cast in extension (removes pull of triceps) for 4 weeks.
- Displaced fractures require ORIF with tension band wiring.

References

1 Wenger DR, Pring ME (2006). *Rang's Children's Fractures*, 3rd edn. Lippincott, Williams and Wilkins, Philadelphia.
2 Wilkins KE (1997). Supracondylar fractures: what's new? *J Paediatr Orthop B* **6**(2): 110–16.

Fractures of the humeral shaft and elbow in adults

Humeral shaft fractures

Mechanism

- Usually as a result of a fall with direct blow or torsional forces.
- Can be low energy (osteoporotic) or high energy (younger age group).
- X-rays of joints (above and below) important to rule out intra-articular extension. High energy injuries, especially to rule out floating elbow or shoulder.
- Remember to evaluate neurovascular status (radial nerve at risk).

Types

- Transverse, oblique, spiral, multifragmentary.
- Distal third fractures associated with radial nerve palsy, known as Holstein–Lewis fracture.

Treatment

Conservative management Is the mainstay.

- Initial sugar tongue cast or hanging cast for 1–2 weeks, then convert to functional brace until union (usually by 3 months); requires regular clinic evaluation.
- Can accept 20° anterior/posterior angulation, 30° varus/valgus angulation, 15° rotations, and 1–3cm of shortening.
- Remember to mobilize elbow and shoulder or will stiffen!

Surgical treatment Indicated if there is an open fracture, vascular injury, associated intra-articular fracture, floating joint (proximally or distally), pathological fracture.

- Relative indications include multiple injuries, inability to maintain reduction closed, segmental fractures, or transverse fractures in young athletes.
- ORIF with plate and screws is commonly used. Locking plates can be utilized if poor bone quality.
- Intramedullary nailing is an alternative, good for pathological or segmental fractures, or medically labile patients due to small exposure. It is associated with shoulder pain and rotator cuff dysfunction.

Humeral condylar fractures

Mechanism

Usually due to impaction injury (the olecranon driven into the humerus via a direct fall and the condyle usually splits into a 'T'- or 'Y'-shaped pattern). Pattern depends upon bone quality and angle of flexion at time of injury. Careful neurovascular evaluation required.

Types

- Intercondylar fracture (most common). The fracture line extends from the articular surface to the supracondylar region in a 'T'- or 'Y'-shaped pattern.
- Supracondylar.

- Isolated medial or lateral condyle fracture.
- Isolated capitellum fracture.

Treatment
Intercondylar
- Intra-articular fractures. Thus principles are open anatomical reduction with absolute stability, providing stability to allow early mobilization.
  - Posterior approach with either a triceps spilt or if more complex, a trans-olecranon osteotomy to visualize the articular surface.
  - Fixation by plate and screw constructs (reconstruction plates). Compression across the intra-articular segments may be required. Newer pre-contoured distal humerus locking plates more commonly used.
- Can be difficult to treat if heavily comminuted and the bone quality is poor.
  - An option is conservative management in cast, but early mobilization to try to maintain as much function as possible ('bag of bones' technique).
  - Non-union is not uncommon following these fractures and sometimes salvage surgery in the form of elbow replacement may be considered.
  - In the elderly with a low fracture pattern, primary elbow replacement is sometimes used.

Supracondylar
- Conservative management in a cast if undisplaced or highly comminuted in elderly. Mobilize at 2 weeks in hinged brace. Cast. Discontinue when healed (6–8 weeks).
- ORIF if displaced. 90/90 plating was the classical method (medial and posterolateral), but now utilize pre-contoured, bicolumnar locking plates. Again stable fixation with early mobilization is the goal.

Transcondylar
- A very distal fracture and within the joint capsule.
- Management follows same principles as of supracondylar type.

Capitellum
- *Radiographs.* The capitellum aligns with radial head on AP and lateral views. Classification dependent on size of fragment (best seen on lateral).
  - Type I is a large osseous fragment, often involving the trochlea.
  - Type II is a thin articular fragment with little osseous composition.
  - Type III is multifragmentary.
- *Treatment.* Type I requires ORIF. A common technique is headless compression screws from a posterior to anterior direction. Type II is usually not amenable to fixation and is excised, as are the loose components of type II injuries.
- Kocher's approach (interval between anconeus and extensor carpi ulnaris) often used.

Olecranon fractures

Mechanism A fall on to the point of the elbow, but can occur as a fall on to the outstretched hand where the triceps avulses the olecranon process.

Colton classification

- *Type I.* Undisplaced (<2mm separation, able to extend elbow against gravity).
- *Type II.* Displaced (subtypes—IIA, avulsion; IIB, oblique/transverse; IIC, comminuted; IID, fracture-dislocation).

Treatment

- Undisplaced. Place in a cast at 90°. At 4 weeks, begin mobilization.
- Displaced. ORIF with tension band wire technique.
- Comminuted. Plate and screw ± bone graft. Newer pre-contoured locking plate available.

Radial head fractures

Mechanism Fall on to the outstretched hand, forearm in pronation.

Mason classification

- *Type 1.* Minimally displaced.
- *Type 2.* Displaced.
- *Type 3.* Comminuted and displaced.

Treatment

- *Type 1* (<3mm displacement). Sling or half cast for 1–2 weeks, then mobilization (aspiration of the joint haematoma acutely can give pain relief and injection of local anaesthetic can rule out any mechanical block).
- *Type 2* (displaced, mechanical block to motion or part of more complex injury pattern). ORIF with compression screw and/or mini-plate.
- *Type 3* (too comminuted to allow ORIF). Radial head replacement indicated. Excision considered at a later stage and contraindicated if other destabilizing ligamentous injuries.

Complications of elbow fractures

- Joint stiffness (rotational).
- Degenerative joint disease (osteoarthritis).
- Heterotopic ossification.
- Neurovascular injury and its sequelae.

References

1 Colton CL (1973). Fractures of the olecranon in adults: classification and management. *Injury* **5**: 21–9.
2 Sarmiento A, Zagorski JB, Zuch GA, *et al.* (2000). Functional bracing for the treatment of fractures of the humeral diaphysis. *J Bone Joint Surg Am* **82-A**: 478–86.

Dislocations and fracture dislocations of the elbow

Mechanism
- *Simple*. No bony component.
- *Complex*. Associated bony injury.
- *Posterior and posterolateral*. Most common type; fall on to an outstretched hand with the elbow in extension or slight flexion (with supination and valgus forces).
- *Anterior* (rare). Fall on to a flexed elbow or as a direct blow from behind ('side swipe injury').
- *Divergent* (rare). Radius and ulna separated proximally.

Associated fractures (complex injury)
- Elbow stability dependent on bony and ligamentous component integrity—radial head, coronoid, olecranon, medial and lateral collateral ligaments.
- Coronoid fractures. Occur as distal humerus is driven against it during subluxation, dislocation, or instability. Any injury to coronoid suggests an episode of instability.
- Regan and Morrey classification.
  - Type 1, tip fractured (consider anterior capsule injury).
  - Type 2, <50% of the process.
  - Type 3, >50% of the process.

Treatment
- Aim to reduce under GA to allow thorough assessment of stability.
- In-line traction. Supinate forearm (clears coronoid); flex elbow from an extended position whilst pulling olecranon in an anterior direction.
- Check elbow stability once reduced and X-ray to confirm.
- If stable, collar and cuff at 90° for 7–10 days with early motion.
- If unstable (redislocates), place forearm in pronation if lateral collateral ligament disrupted or supination if medial collateral ligament disrupted, and immobilize in above elbow cast for 2–3 weeks.
- If there are associated injuries, then most fractures will require ORIF to aid the stability and allow early mobilization. This may include radial head prosthetic replacement.

The 'terrible triad'
- Posterior elbow dislocation associated with radial head fracture, coronoid process fracture, and lateral collateral ligament tear.
- The elbow will require surgical stabilization via ORIF of coronoid and anterior capsular repair, ORIF or replacement of radial head, lateral collateral ligament repair.

Complications
- Neurovascular injury.
- Compartment syndrome.
- Chronic elbow instability.

- Articular cartilage damage.
- Heterotopic calcification.
- Stiffness (especially extension). Early motion at 1 week to try to prevent this.

Further reading

Ring D, Jupiter JB (1998). Fracture-dislocation of the elbow. *J Bone Joint Surg Am* **80**(4): 566–80. [Current concepts review]

Fractures around the shoulder

Clavicle

Mechanism Fall or direct blow to lateral shoulder (5–10% of all fractures).

Types
- Occurs in the middle (75%), lateral (20%), or medial (5%) third.
- The pattern of lateral third fractures depends on relationship and integrity of the coracoclavicular ligaments, and involvement of the acromioclavicular joint.
- Medial third fractures are assessed with displacement and involvement of sternoclavicular joint in mind.

Treatment
- *Middle third.* Virtually all can be treated conservatively with a broad arm sling (not a collar and cuff). Indications for ORIF (plate and screws) are open fractures, significant neurovascular injuries, skin tenting, floating shoulder. Fractures with >100% displacement and 2cm of shortening have better outcomes with ORIF.
- *Lateral third.* Undisplaced can be treated non-surgically; however, the presence of displacement suggestive of coracoclavicular ligament disruption will require fixation with either plate and screw constructs, hook plate, or ligament reconstruction (Weaver–Dunn procedure).
- *Medial third.* Most are undisplaced and treated conservatively in a sling. Displacement, especially posterior, into the root of the neck may warrant surgery.

Complications
- *Metalwork.* Failure or subcutaneous irritation.
- *Non-union.* Associated with displacement and shortening.
- *Acute complications.* Neurovascular injury (including brachial plexus injury), neurovascular compression (costoclavicular syndrome), pneumothorax from bony penetration of the pleura.

Scapula

Mechanism Direct trauma, usually a high velocity injury such as an RTA. Always have a high clinical suspicion of other possible injuries such as rib fracture, pulmonary contusion, and pneumo/haemothorax; 20–40% have ipsilateral clavicle fractures.

Treatment
- Simple (no involvement of the glenoid (glenohumeral joint)). Adequate analgesia (very painful injury; may require HDU admission) and early mobilization.
- Complex (involving the glenoid and glenoid neck). May need ORIF after further imaging such as CT/MRI scanning.
- Floating shoulder will require ORIF of clavicle.

Proximal humerus

Mechanism Young—high energy injury; elderly—low energy falls. Full neurovascular assessment (especially axillary nerve) is essential, alongside pre-injury function (aids management decision).

The Neer classification[1]

Based on Codman's fracture lines along old physeal scars; four segments or parts. A fracture part is considered when it is >1cm displaced or >45° angulated. Thus defined as 1-, 2-, 3-, or 4-part fractures.

Treatment

- Undisplaced or impacted. Collar and cuff with early pendular mobilization.
- Displaced. Usually requires ORIF by 'locking' plate, proximal humeral intramedullary nails or cannulated screws, and K wires with or without tension band wiring.
- Severely comminuted fractures (4-part), especially including fracture dislocations, have a high rate of avascular necrosis; usually treated with hemiarthroplasty and soft tissue reconstruction of the rotator cuff to the prosthesis.

Complications Non- and mal-union, avascular necrosis of the humeral head, and osteoarthritis of the shoulder joint are the commonest. High velocity injuries may also cause neurovascular injuries, particularly of the brachial plexus.

Paediatric humeral fractures

- Usually occur at the surgical neck or through and around the proximal humeral epiphysis.
- May be indicative of a non-accidental injury.
- Most require no treatment apart from collar and cuff with mobilization as for adults. Remodelling potential is good in this area.

Reference

1 Neer CS (1970). Displaced proximal humeral fractures. I. Classification and evaluation. *J Bone Joint Surg Am* **52-A**: 1077–89.

Dislocations of the shoulder region

See Fig. 15.1.

Sternoclavicular joint

- Uncommon injury.
- *Mechanism.* Indirect force to lateral shoulder or direct impact on medial end of clavicle.
- *Types.* Usually dislocates anteriorly; posterior dislocation is rare. The deformity is at the medial clavicle.
- *Complications.* Tracheal and oesophageal compression may occur with posterior dislocation. Careful assessment is required.

Treatment

- *Anterior dislocation.* Treated symptomatically with a sling, analgesia, and early mobilization.
- *Posterior dislocation with tracheal compression.* Requires closed reduction or open if this fails (with cardiothoracic surgical help).

Acromioclavicular joint (ACJ)

- Usually an injury of second to fourth decade, more common in males.
- *Mechanism.* Fall or direct impact on to the point of the shoulder.
- *Rockwood classification.*[1] Six types with increasing numbers relating to increasing severity of ligamentous disruption (acromioclavicular and coracoclavicular) and displacement.
  - Type I. Sprained acromioclavicular ligament (no displacement).
  - Type II. Acromioclavicular ligaments disrupted, ACJ subluxed.
  - Type III. Acromioclavicular and coracoclavicular ligaments disrupted (>100% displacement).
  - Type IV. Both ligaments disrupted with posterior displacement.
  - Type V. All ligaments torn and massively displaced.
  - Type VI. All ligaments torn and inferior displacement (very rare).

Treatment

- *Types I and II* (and some III). Broad arm sling and early mobilization when pain allows. Persistent pain or functional limitation is treated by reconstruction of the coracoacromial ligament.
- *Type III and above.* Acute repair indicated. Soft tissue reconstruction better than hook plate.

Anterior dislocation of the glenohumeral joint[2,3]

Mechanism Traumatic event, leading to forced abduction and external rotation (fall on to the outstretched arm).

Associated features

- *Young.* Ninety per cent have traumatic injury to bony and/or soft tissue restraints in the shoulder—the Bankart lesion (anteroinferior glenoid labrum tear, with or without a glenoid rim fracture), Hill–Sachs lesion (impression fracture as the anterior glenoid impacts on humeral head).
- *Rotator cuff tears.* Approximately 30% of those >40y and 80% of those >60y will have a tear.
- *Greater tuberosity fractures.* Common over the age of 50y.

Clinical findings
- History of injury and whether had previous dislocations.
- The shoulder looks 'square' as the deltoid is flat and a sulcus can be visible where the humeral head may be.
- The patient supports the arm which is abducted and very painful.
- Assess neurovascular status (axillary nerve).
- X-rays (AP and axillary or scapular 'Y' lateral views) show the humeral head anterior and inferior to the glenoid. Used to exclude a fracture of the humerus or glenoid.

Treatment
- Reduce as an emergency in A&E.
- Give IV morphine 5–10mg + inhaled N_2O (IV midazolam 5mg is usually unnecessary).
  - Simplest, extremely reliable method is gentle, continued straight line traction with the arm abducted about 10–20° from the trunk. May take 10–15min, but patience is the key, not force.
  - Avoid rotation (such as in a 'Kocher's manoeuvre') as this is dangerous and may cause fracture of the humerus.
  - Countertraction can be placed across the trunk with a broad sheet.
- Alternative technique is patient prone on the trolley, arm hanging freely down and weighted (e.g. 3L bag of saline) ('Stimson's technique').
- If there is an associated humeral neck fracture, then the reduction should be done under GA.
- Place the arm in a collar and cuff sling under the clothes. Repeat the X-ray to confirm reduction and that there has been no iatrogenic fracture.
- Always document the neurological status (axillary nerve) before and after reduction.
- Follow-up in clinic mandatory to assess for associated injuries.

Posterior dislocation of the glenohumeral joint
Mechanism Rare. Due to forced internal rotation or direct blow to the anterior shoulder (e.g. after an epileptic fit or electric shock). Common to be missed.

Features
- The arm is held internally rotated and no external rotation is possible.
- The humeral head should be palpable posteriorly.
- AP X-rays may show the humeral head as a 'light bulb' shape (internally rotated), but this is not diagnostic of posterior dislocation.
- Lateral X-ray shows the dislocation.

Treatment
- In-line traction method (as above), but consider GA if difficult—avoid excessive force.
- May be very unstable; occasionally the 'broomstick' plaster may be used.

Recurrent dislocation of the shoulder

- Usually due to a Bankart lesion or capsular redundancy (stretched and floppy).
- Commonest in young age of first dislocation (90% recurrence if <20y, 60% if 20–40y, <10% if older than 40y).

Treatment—surgery

- Repair and fixation of the anterior 'Bankart lesion'.
- May be done open or arthroscopically.
- Capsular laxity is treated by capsular shift, an overlapping 'pants-over-vest' procedure to improve proprioceptive joint sensation.

References

1 Bucholz RW, Court-Brown CM, Heckman JD, Tornetta P (Eds) (2009). *Rockwood and Green's fractures in adults*, 7th edn. Lippincott, Williams, and Wilkins, Philadelphia.
2 Robinson CM, Dobson RJ (2004). Anterior instability of the shoulder after trauma. *J Bone Joint Surg Br* **86-B**, 469. [review]
3 http://www.wheelessonline.com/orthoo/43.htm.

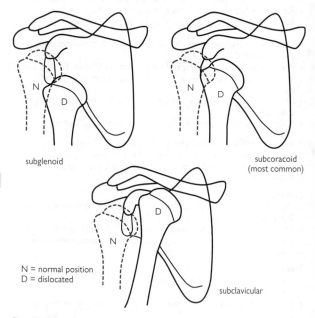

subglenoid

subcoracoid (most common)

N = normal position
D = dislocated

subclavicular

Fig. 15.1 Types of shoulder dislocation. Reproduced with permission from Collier, J. et al. (2006). *Oxford Handbook of Clinical Specialties*, 7th edn. Oxford University Press, Oxford.

Fractures of the ribs and sternum

Mechanism

- Single rib fractures occur as a result of direct injury such as a fall.
- Fractures of the lower ribs can occur with coughing.
- Sternal fractures occur with direct injury, e.g. contact with steering wheel or by restraint by a seat belt.
- High velocity (RTA) or large crush injuries can result in a 'stove-in' chest with a flail segment, i.e. multiple rib fractures, each fractured at two sites.

Treatment

- *Single rib fracture.* Symptomatic with analgesia.
- *Multiple rib fracture.* If ≥3 ribs involved, should admit for observation overnight, but treatment symptomatic with analgesia and chest physiotherapy.
- *Sternal fracture.* Symptomatic treatment, but observe for associated injuries (see below).
- *Flail chest or extensive multiple rib fractures.* Potentially life-threatening injury and may present with severe respiratory distress.
  - Flail segments move paradoxically, preventing adequate ventilation.
  - Multiple fractures restrict respiratory effort, severely impairing ventilation.
  - Treat with high flow O_2 and analgesia. CPAP and even IPPV may be required.

Complications[1]

Incidence of complications rises dramatically if the injury involves:

- >3 ribs.
- First, second, or third ribs.
- Sternum.
- Scapula.

They are all indicators of high energy transfer injury.

Cardiac tamponade

- Bleeding into the pericardial cavity causes severe haemodynamic shock and may be the cause of a cardiac arrest at presentation.
- Diagnosis is by high clinical suspicion, muffled heart sounds, raised JVP, and no signs of a tension pneumothorax.
- Treat by immediate pericardiocentesis with transfer to cardiothoracic unit for repair of the defect.

Pneumothorax

- Usually due to direct pleural injury by bone fragments during injury.
- Often associated with haemothorax.
- Signs are respiratory distress, absent breath sounds, hyperresonant percussion note (pneumothorax), or shock.

- Tension pneumothorax is life-threatening and requires immediate decompression via a 16G needle placed into the second anterior intercostal space, followed by definitive chest drain placement.
- If in any doubt, always treat first on clinical grounds rather than wait for investigations (X-rays, etc.).

Reference

1 American College of Surgeons (2008). *Advanced trauma life support (ATLS) for doctors, student manual*, 8th edn. American College of Surgeons, Chicago.

Fractures of the pelvis

Mechanism
- *Age <60y.* High energy—RTA or falls at work (building sites) or sport (horse riding).
- *Age >60y.* Low energy (insufficiency fracture)—fall from standing height.

The force required to fracture the pelvis in the young is considerable and as a result, the morbidity and mortality can be as high as 20%. It is the main cause of death in multiple trauma patients.

Types
- The pelvis is a ring consisting of two innominate bones and the sacrum.
- Anteriorly are the ligaments of the symphysis pubis and posteriorly, the ligaments to the sacrum (sacrospinous, sacrotuberous, and sacroiliac).
- An isolated break at any part is generally stable (the ring will not separate).
- Two breaks in the ring make it unstable (able to displace or open). Remember this can be due to a fracture or ligament disruption!
- Young and Burgess classification (descriptive):[1]
  - AP compression (impact from the front or rear).
  - Lateral compression (impact from side).
  - Vertical shear (usually a fall from height).
  - Combined mechanical (mixture of all of the above).

Assessment
- ATLS approach.
- Mechanism of injury important as gives insight into degree of injury.
- Assessment and documentation of other injuries is mandatory.
- Look for neurological, gastrointestinal, and genitourinary injury.

Treatment
Initial treatment of all pelvic fractures should include ATLS protocols. Once stable, an AP pelvis X-ray supplemented with inlet and outlet views are required.

A CT is helpful to assess the posterior pelvic structures that can be obscured on a plain X-ray.

Single ring fracture (stable)
- Check for an occult sacroiliac ligament injury (local bruising and tenderness with pain on stressing the joint); this suggests the injury could be unstable.
- Fractures of both superior and inferior pubic rami on the same side are a single break in terms of ring stability.
- Other stable patterns include ilium fractures into sciatic notch or sacrum.
- *Remember* that if a significant single break in the ring is present, there is a chance that concurrent ligamentous injury exists. Thus, a CT scan is often required prior to mobilization to confirm stability.

- Isolated fractures of the ilium, ischium, or pubis are normally treated with bed rest, analgesia, and early mobilization as soon as the pain allows.
- Fractures that extend to the acetabulum (joint) require further investigation to plan treatment, but are usually stable if isolated.
- Simple pubic rami fractures in the elderly (osteoporotic) can be treated conservatively with bed rest and early rehabilitation.

Multiple ring fractures (unstable)

Unstable fractures are liable to massive haemorrhage within the soft tissues of the pelvis. This is mostly because the pelvic ring is grossly displaced during the injury and tearing of the extensive posterior pre-sacral venous plexus occurs. A patient's entire blood volume can be lost, hence the high mortality rate.

Establish haemodynamic control
- Approach patient according to ATLS guidelines (ABCDE).
- Haemorrhage is leading cause of death with pelvic injuries.
- Tachycardia and hypotension suggest bleeding.
- Establish at least two large calibre IV infusions and commence resuscitation with warm crystalloid 2000mL, and then reassess.
- Send blood for urgent cross-match of 4–6U. O –ve blood is given if no response to initial fluid challenge.
- Continued bleeding must be controlled by reducing the pelvic volume. This may be achieved by:
  - Pelvic binder or binding a bedsheet tightly around the pelvis and internally rotating the hips—very effective as an emergency procedure.
  - Application of an external pelvic fixator is a more definitive solution, but should be done in the trauma theatre.
- Laparotomy is contraindicated unless there are life-threatening intra-abdominal injuries that must be treated since this effectively 'decompresses' the pelvis again superiorly.
- Urethral injury occurs, especially with anterior compression bony injuries. If there is blood at the urethral meatus, perineal bruising, haematuria, or a high riding prostate on rectal examination, then catheterization should only be performed by an experienced urologist (very often suprapubically). Investigation for injury is with a retrograde urethrogram or IVU once the patient is stable.

Definitive management
- Significant AP compression mechanism can result in an 'open book' pelvis. Severe subtypes of the lateral compression or vertical sheer fractures are very unstable and associated with other injuries.
- Once ATLS stabilization is complete, CT scanning is required to define the fracture and plan treatment.
- External fixation is excellent to temporarily control unstable fractures and manage definitively. It can help to control haemorrhage in a haemodynamically unstable patient.

- Once stable, liaise with local pelvic fixation centres to arrange definitive fixation if required.
- ORIF with screws and plates for the symphysis pubis of ilium fractures. Posterior pelvic instability involving the sacrum require screw fixation.

Complications

- Haemorrhage, shock, and death from exsanguination.
- Open fractures carry a 50% mortality and need to be treated aggressively by both orthopaedic and general surgical teams.
- Urogenital injury.
- Thromboembolism (35–50% develop DVT and 10% PE).
- Neurological injury.
- Paralytic ileus.
- Mal-union may lead to difficulty with pregnancy.
- Osteoarthritis.

Acetabular fractures

- Usually high energy injury in the young from RTA (dashboard impact) or fall from a height. Associated with hip dislocation.
- Assess as per all pelvic fractures (i.e. ATLS).
- X-rays required include AP pelvic views plus Judet views (45° internal and external views); CT is routine.
- Letournel–Judet classification. Fractures as posterior wall, posterior column, anterior wall, anterior column, or transverse.
- Non-surgical management is reserved for fractures that are undisplaced (except posterior wall as hip unstable) and do not involve the 'dome', the superior acetabular roof (weight bearing area).
- Surgical management, ORIF, in displaced dome fractures, fractures resulting in joint instability, or trapped intra-articular fragments.

Sacral fractures

- High energy injury in the young or low energy in the elderly.
- Assess as per all pelvic fractures (i.e. ATLS). Must assess for sacral nerve root injury.
- X-rays include AP pelvic (inlet and outlet views); CT is required as difficult to fully appreciate on X-ray.
- Denis classification. Alar lateral to foramen, involving the foramen, or central portion medial to foramen.
- Non-surgical management is reserved for fractures that are undisplaced or impacted.
- Surgical management if displaced or loose fragments impinging on nerve roots.

References

1 Burgess A, Young JWR *et al.* (1990). Pelvic ring disruptions: effective classification system and treatment protocols. *J Trauma* **30**(7), 848–56.

Further Reading

American College of Surgeons (2008). *Advanced trauma life support (ATLS) for doctors, student manual*, 8th edn. American College of Surgeons, Chicago.

Femoral neck fractures

Femoral neck fractures

Mechanism
- Commonest fracture in the elderly with an exponential increase in incidence with age.[1]
- The risk increases with decreasing bone mass (osteoporosis).
- In the elderly, usually result from a trip/fall onto side (low energy).
- Fractures in the young are usually a result of high energy trauma.

Classification
Fractures should be described anatomically:
- *Intracapsular fractures.* Occur within the joint capsule (proximal to the intertrochanteric line).
- *Extracapsular fractures.* Occur distal to the joint capsule (involving or distal to intertrochanteric line).
- It is then important to describe fractures as displaced or undisplaced.
- The relationship to the blood supply is key:
  - The femoral head receives its supply via the medial and lateral femoral circumflex arteries which form the extracapsular ring and give rise to the cervical arteries (the lateral being most important). There is also supply via the intraosseus nutrient vessels and the ligamentum teres.
  - Displaced intracapsular fractures disrupt their blood supply and have a high rate of avascular necrosis (AVN) of the femoral head and non-union.
  - Extracapsular fractures maintain the blood supply to the head (thus reduced AVN and generally heal well).
- Other classification systems are not generally required.
- *Subtrochanteric fractures.* Occur below the level of the lesser trochanter. May be through an area of pathological bone (metastasis) or high energy in young.

Assessment
- Inability to weight bear following a fall in the elderly is a common presenting feature.
- Consider medical cause of fall (stroke, MI, etc.).
- Other comorbidities essential to ascertain.
- Pre-injury level of function and home circumstances important.
- If the fracture is displaced (common), the leg will be shortened and externally rotated. Straight leg raise and hip movements are globally inhibited by pain. Neurological state important.
- Most fractures do not require any temporary stabilization; however, subtrochanteric fractures may benefit from a Thomas splint for pain relief.
- X-rays. AP pelvis and lateral of affected hip (long leg views if history of malignancy to look for metastases).
  - Displaced fractures are usually obvious.
  - Undisplaced, intracapsular compression fractures may be difficult to see on X-ray. If high clinical suspicion of fracture, then further investigation is warranted; isotope bone scan (highly sensitive, poor specificity), MRI (gold standard), or CT scan.

Treatment
The majority of hip fractures require surgical stabilization to allow early mobilization and prevent displacement. This will reduce the risks of long periods of immobilization and bed rest (pressure sore, DVT, etc.).

Intracapsular
- *Undisplaced impacted in the elderly.* Treated by early mobilization with analgesia; 15% late displacement rate, requiring operative intervention.
- *Undisplaced.* Treated by internal fixation with either cannulated screws or a 2-hole dynamic hip screw (DHS).
- *Displaced.* Treated by hemiarthroplasty.[2]
- Total hip arthroplasty can be used if symptomatic pre-existing arthritis or those with few comorbidities and high functioning (controversial).
- In children or young adults, reduction (open or closed) and fixation is employed.

Extracapsular
- Closed reduction on the traction table and open fixation with the use of a DHS.
- Intramedullary hip screw (IMHS) may be used in 4-part fractures.
- Subtrochanteric and reverse obliquity fractures require stabilization, utilizing an intramedullary nail or fixed angle plating system.

Complications
- Overall mortality in the elderly is 20% at 90 days. This is indicative of the fact that the fracture is more a marker of generally poor condition rather than due to acute surgical perioperative complications.
- AVN of the femoral head.
- Dislocation of arthroplasty.
- Loss of fixation.
- Non-union.
- Lower limb thromboembolic disease.

References
1 Parker MJ, Pryor GA, Thorngren KG (1997). *Handbook of hip fracture surgery.* Butterworth-Heinemann publications, Oxford.
2 Parker MJ, Khan RJ, Crawford J, et al. (2002). Hemiarthroplasty versus internal fixation for displaced intracapsular hip fractures in the elderly. A randomised trial of 455 patients. *J Bone Joint Surg Br* **84-B**: 1150–5.

Further Reading
Soloman L, Warwick D, Nayagam S (Eds) (2010). *Apley's system of orthopaedics and fractures,* 9th edn. Hodder Arnold, England.

Femoral shaft fractures

Mechanism

- High energy RTA in young adults (dashboard injury) or fall from height.
- Stress fractures.
- Low energy in elderly.
- Pathological (metastases).

Classification

- AO system can be used, but is complex.
- Anatomical description is the simplest:
  - Location (proximal, mid- or distal shaft, divide into thirds, or metaphyseal or diaphyseal).
  - Configuration (transverse, oblique, spiral, segmental, comminuted).
  - Number of fragments.

Associated injuries

- Polytrauma is common. Look for head, chest, and abdominal injuries.
- Ipsilateral femoral neck fracture (up to 5%).
- Pelvic and acetabular fractures.
- Knee joint injuries. Both bony or ligamental (e.g. anterior cruciate ligament (ACL) rupture).
- Soft tissue injury to skin, muscle, neurovascular structures.
- Sciatic nerve traction injury (uncommon).
- Bilateral femoral shaft fractures associated with 25% mortality.

Treatment

- *ATLS* (ABCDE).
- Establish two large calibre IV access and give 2000mL of crystalloid; initial haemodynamic compensation is common in the young and may hide a large blood loss. Can lose up to 4U (1500mL) of blood into tissues around a femoral fracture.
- Send blood for FBC, U&E, group and save.
- Realign and splint the leg with skin traction and a Thomas splint. This will help to control pain and haemorrhage.
- *An X-ray of a femoral fracture not in a splint should never be seen! Diagnose clinically; splint, then get the X-ray.*
- If an 'OPEN' fracture, photograph the wound, socially clean it, and place a betadine dressing over it, stabilize it. Commence IV antibiotics and tetanus toxoid if required.
- Full secondary survey, looking for associated injuries.

Children

- Nearly always heal and remodel.
- Age 0–2y. Treat in gallows (suspension) traction until callus seen (2–4 weeks) or Pavlik harness/hip spica.
- Age 2–6y. Treat with closed manipulation and hip plaster spica (allows discharge) or continuation of the Thomas splint.

- Age 6–14y. Options are a flexible intramedullary nail ('elastic' nail), ORIF with a plate and screws, or external fixation.
- Age >14y. Can consider locked intramedullary fixation.

Adults

- Non-operative treatment with traction if patient too sick for surgery (be aware of complications: pressure sores, DVT, etc.).
- Locked and reamed intramedullary nailing is the common treatment regime (provides rotational stability).
- Plate and screw construct can be used if there is distal metaphyseal extension. Usually much larger exposure.
- Temporizing external fixation is occasionally required in damage control scenarios. This can be exchanged for a nail once patient stable enough.

Complications

- Compartment syndrome.
- Fat embolus (1%) and possible ARDS.
- Infection (5% after open, 1% after closed nailing).
- Non-union.
- Thromboembolic disease.
- Neurological injury.
- Mal-union, rotation being the most symptomatic.
- Pressure sores, bronchopneumonia, UTI on conservatively treated patients.

Further reading

Metaizeau JP (2004). Stable elastic intramedullary nailing for fractures of the femur in children. *J Bone Joint Surg Br* **86-B**: 954–7. [Operative technique]

Wolinsky P et al. (2001). Controversies in intramedullary nailing of femoral shaft fractures. *J Bone Joint Surg Am* **83-A**: 1404–15. [Instructional course lecture]

Fractures of the tibial shaft

Mechanism

- High energy injuries in young as a result of RTA, sporting injury, fall from height.
- Direction of force dictates fracture pattern—torsional (spiral), direct blow (transverse or short oblique). Higher energy patterns suggested by multifragmentary fractures with or without bone loss.
- Soft tissue injuries common as tibia subcutaneous. Be aware of 'OPEN' fractures.

Assessment

- ATLS approach recommended.
- Inspect for angulation, deformity, and malrotation.
- Subcutaneous crepitation may be present or obvious open wound.
- Neurovascular status needs to be assessed and documented.
- Watch for 'compartment syndrome'. Presents as pain, uncontrolled by analgesia, and out of proportion to injury. Look for pallor, paraesthesia, and pulselessness (late signs). Passive dorsiflexion of joint distal to injury stretching the muscles in the affected compartment is usually diagnostic.
- Compartmental pressures can be measured; an absolute pressure of >40mmHg or <30mmHg difference between compartment and diastolic BP diagnostic.
- *This is a clinical diagnosis and requires immediate management via fasciotomies of affected compartments.*

Classification

- AO system can be used, but is complex.
- Anatomical description is the simplest:
  - Position (mid-shaft, junction of distal third, etc.).
  - Configuration (transverse, oblique, spiral, segmental, comminuted).
  - Number of fragments.
- Open injuries are normally classified additionally by the Gustillo–Anderson system.[1]

Treatment[2,3]

There is no one method of treatment that is appropriate for all fractures. There is a continual contentious debate about the pros and cons of different modalities. The best rule is to judge each fracture and associated soft tissue injury on an individual basis and treat appropriately.

Non-surgical (plaster of Paris)

- Used for undisplaced fractures and low energy displaced fractures in children that can be closed reduced.
- Long leg cast, with the knee flexed 20° and the ankle in neutral.
- Mobilize non-weight bearing on crutches, with X-rays weekly for the first 4 weeks to check alignment.
- Start weight bearing at 8 weeks in a weight bearing contact 'Sarmiento' cast.

- Union takes around 14–16 weeks.
- *Advantages*. Simple and avoids all operative risks.
- *Disadvantages*. Takes a long time; requires good follow-up and patient compliance. Stiffness at the knee and ankle is common and unstable injuries are very difficult to manipulate and control in plaster alone.

Cast bracing A variation of plaster where Sarmiento plaster is applied from day 1.

Surgical
- Indicated if unable to maintain closed reduction, i.e. >50% displaced, >10° angulated, >10° rotational deformity, >1cm shortening.
- Unstable fracture patterns. Multifragmentary and same level tibial fractures.
- Open fractures.

Locking plate fixation
- Mostly used for fractures near the joint surface.
- Plates used in the shaft have a high rate of infection and non-union caused by the large soft tissue exposure required.
- *Advantages*. Simple, quick, rapid mobilization, and avoids the need for plaster.
- *Disadvantages*. Risk of infection, non-union, and implant failure.

Intramedullary nailing
- Currently the treatment of choice in most centres, but requires increased operating time and experience.
- May be used in compound fractures, especially where soft tissue flaps are required since it gives relatively unlimited access to the tibia 'fix and flap'.[4]
- Best for mid-shaft fractures and is poor at controlling fractures within 5–10cm of the knee and ankle joints.
- *Advantages*. Early mobilization, quicker rehabilitation than closed methods, soft tissue undisturbed by technique, access for flaps easy.
- *Disadvantages*. Technically demanding, high rate of chronic anterior knee pain (site of nail insertion—not recommended for kneeling profession, e.g. carpet fitters).

External fixation
- Often used in compound fractures as it allows least disturbance of soft tissue. Can be placed in an extremely rigid configuration to allow stability. Rigidity can then be reduced sequentially in outpatients, if required.
- Tensioned wire circlage frames pioneered in Russia (Ilizarov) can be used for difficult fractures around the knee or ankle.
- *Advantages*. Technically simple (not Ilizarov); allows early mobilization, avoids further soft tissue damage.
- *Disadvantages*. Pin site infections common, but usually easily treated. Requires good nursing backup and patient compliance. Pin sites need to be planned carefully with plastic team if flaps used so as not to compromise soft tissue cover.

Open fractures

- Guided by the British Orthopaedic Association and British Association of Plastic, Reconstructive, and Aesthetic Surgeons Guidelines.[5]
- Recommend a multidisciplinary approach in a specialist centre, if possible.
- High energy patterns of fracture with soft tissue injury (skin loss, degloving, muscle damage or loss, arterial injuries) need to be acted upon promptly.
- Initially ATLS approach.
- Assessment of affected limb. Neurovascular status essential and repeated regularly.
- Give IV broad-spectrum antibiotics (within 3h of injury).
- Treat limb-threatening injuries immediately (vascular or compartment syndrome).[6]
- Remove gross contamination from open wounds, photograph, wrap in saline-soaked gauze and film dressing. Immobilize the whole affected limb in a splint. Tetanus status checked.
- Combined management approach to plan definitive treatment of fracture and soft tissues. Aim to do within 24h of injury if isolated open fracture.

References

1 Gustilo RB, Anderson JT (1976). Prevention of infection in the treatment of one thousand and twenty-five open fractures of long bones: retrospective and prospective analyses. *J Bone Joint Surg Am* **58-A**: 453–8.

2 Schmidt AH et al. (2003). Treatment of closed tibial fractures. *J Bone Joint Surg Am* **85-A**, 352–68. [Instructional course lecture]

3 Bhandari M et al. (2001). Treatment of open fractures of the shaft of the tibia. *J Bone Joint Surg B* **83-B**: 62–8. [Review]

4 Gopal S, Majumder S, Batchelor AG, et al. (2000). Fix and flap: the radical orthopaedic and plastic treatment of severe open fractures of the tibia. *J Bone Joint Surg Br* **82-B**: 959–66.

5 Standards for management of open fractures of the lower limb. (2009). BOA and BAPRAS. ◌ http://www.boa.ac.uk or ◌ http://www.bapras.org.uk

6 Elliott KG, Johnstone AJ (2003). Diagnosing acute compartment syndrome. *J Bone Joint Surg Br* **85-B**: 62–8. [Review]

Fractures of the ankle

- Commonest fracture of the lower limb.
- Usually low energy rotational force, resulting in simple to complex configurations.
- The talus rotates in the mortise and produces different patterns dependent on whether the foot is inverted or everted.
- Axial load causes fracture of the tibial plafond.
- The ankle should be thought of as a ring and stability is conferred by:
  - *Bones.* Medial and lateral malleoli and the talus (form 'mortise').
  - *Ligaments.* Laterally, the tibiofibular ligamentous complex (syndesmosis) and the lateral collateral ligaments (talofibula and calcaneofibular); medially the deltoid ligament.
- Remember that a fracture of the proximal fibula (at the knee) is associated with an ankle fracture or dislocation until proven otherwise.

Assessment

- Initially, ATLS approach.
- Inspect for bruising, swelling, obvious deformity, open wounds, skin tenting, signs of neurovascular compromise.
- Depending on the degree of injury, some patients may walk in for assessment.
- Remember to examine the whole fibula for proximal tenderness.
- Examine for medial tenderness. The medial injury may be ligamentous only, but this is enough to destabilize the ankle and allow talar shift.
- X-rays are mortise AP (15° internal rotation) and lateral views.

Classification

- AO/Danis–Weber system (based on level of fibula fracture):
  - Type A. Below the syndesmosis.
  - Type B. At the syndesmosis.
  - Type C. Above the syndesmosis.
- The Lauge–Hansen classification is more complex and based upon mechanism of injury. Foot supinated and adducted or externally rotated **or** foot pronated and abducted or externally rotated.
- A distal tibial fracture involving the joint is known as a pilon fracture.

Treatment

Displaced fracture/dislocation

- A displaced fracture dislocation is an orthopaedic emergency and is always clinically obvious. Displacement is often more than expected due to soft tissue swelling.
- Reduce the fracture immediately in A & E and apply a below-knee backslab before sending the patient for an X-ray. An X-ray of a dislocated ankle should never be seen!
- Check neurovascular status before and after reduction.
- Give plenty of analgesia ± sedation (usually done in resuscitation area).

Stable injuries
- Lateral malleolus only (Weber A or B) with no talar displacement (shift) in the mortise.
- Ensure no medial tenderness exists.
- These can be managed in a well fitting below-knee cast with the foot at 90° (neutral).
- Obtain a post-cast X-ray to ensure position acceptable.
- Regular follow-up and serial X-rays required to ensure reduction remains.
- Total of 6 weeks cast.
- Weight-bearing is allowed.
- Some simple Weber A fractures require just a supportive elasticated stocking.

Unstable injuries
- Minimal displacement (≤2mm) is acceptable in the elderly and treated by plaster as above.
- Weber B or C fractures with medial tenderness or talar shift.
- Initially placed into backslab for comfort, elevated, and iced (reduces swelling).
- If too swollen, skin closure is compromised, thus aim to do within first 24–48h.
- Check for significant blisters around areas of incision.
- ORIF is used with the lateral fracture reduced and held with a 'lag screw' and 'neutralization' plate and screw construct.
- The medial malleolus is fixed directly with two partially-threaded cancellous screws (compression) or if a small fragment, a tension band wire construct.
- A cast is applied following fixation and the patient remains in this non-weight bearing for up to 6 weeks.

Pilon fractures
- Intra-articular fractures of the tibial plafond due to axial force (high energy).
- Initial management is as for ankle fractures.
- Careful assessment for swelling, skin compromise, blisters, and neurovascular status.
- Standard AP and lateral X-rays required; often a CT is needed to define fracture pattern further and plan treatment.
- Non-surgical management only for undisplaced fractures.
- Surgical management is related to soft tissue status.
- External and internal fixation techniques are applicable.

Further reading

Vander Griend R, Michelson JD, Bone LB (1996). Fractures of the ankle and the distal part of the tibia. *J Bone Joint Surg Am* **78-A**: 1772–83. [Instructional course lecture]
ℛ http://www.blackburnfeet.org.uk/hyperbook/trauma/ankle_fractures/ankle_fractures_intro.htm.

Fractures of the tarsus and foot

Talus[1]

Mechanism

- Usually a fall from height or an RTA (high energy).
- Foot forcibly dorsiflexed against the tibia.
- Look for associated ankle fractures.
- Blood supply to the talus often compromised. Talus has limited soft tissue attachments, thus relies on extraosseous vessels, which are easily disrupted.

Assessment

- ATLS.
- Look for associated injuries.
- Look for compartment syndrome of foot.
- Neurovascular status.
- AP and lateral of ankle plus CT.

Classification

- By anatomical site, i.e. head, neck, body, or lateral process.
- 'Hawkins' classification for talar neck fractures (types I–IV, increasing levels of displacement and subluxation with increasing grade).

Treatment

- Body fractures. Treated surgically with ORIF unless undisplaced.
- Neck fractures:
  - *Undisplaced.* Strict non-weight bearing in below-knee plaster for 6 weeks.
  - *Displaced.* ORIF is required. If dislocated, urgent management required as soft tissue can be compromised.

Complications

- Avascular necrosis. Rate increases with displacement (10% in type I to 90% in type III).
- Osteoarthritis of tibiotalar and subtalar joints.
- Mal-union.

Calcaneum[2]

Mechanism

Axial load. Fall from height or RTA.

Assessment

- ATLS.
- Assess for associated injuries. Spinal (thoracolumbar) fracture and upper limb injuries.
- Swelling can be significant. Assess for compartment syndrome acutely.
- AP ankle and lateral plus axial Harris view.
- CT may be required.

Classification
- Extra- or intra-articular.
- Intra-articular fractures involve the subtalar joint and are classified by their 'Saunders' system.

Treatment
- Extra-articular or undisplaced intra-articular fractures.
  - Conservative. Elevation, ice, bed rest, and observation of soft tissues overnight.
  - Mobilize non-weight bearing with a removable splint to stop equinus at the ankle. Early subtalar passive mobilization should be initiated.
- Displaced intra-articular fractures. Operative treatment is still controversial. ORIF is usually delayed 10–14 days for swelling to resolve. Caution is exercised if patient a smoker, advanced age, complex patterns, multiple trauma, compensation, bilateral fractures.

Complications
- Wound breakdown.
- Mal-union.
- Subtalar arthritis.
- Peroneal tendon pathology.

Tarsometatarsal (TMT) fracture-dislocations (Lisfranc)[1]

Jacques Lisfranc de Saint-Martin described an amputation technique across the five TMT joints as a solution to forefoot gangrene secondary to frost-bite. This became known as the Lisfranc joint.

Mechanism and assessment
- Direct dorsal force (RTA) or indirect rotational injury to a plantar flexed and fixed forefoot (foot caught in a riding stirrup and rotation of body around it).
- The Lisfranc ligament runs from the base of the second metatarsal to the medial cuneiform. It is the only link between the first ray and the rest of the forefoot. The recessed base of the second metatarsal also provides bony stability.
- Disruption of the Lisfranc ligament, with or without a bony component, results in incongruity of the TMT joint.
- Neurovascular status and compartment syndrome must be assessed.
- AP, oblique, and lateral X-rays are required. Consider weight-bearing views.
- The medial cortex of second metatarsal should align with medial cuneiform. Look for 'fleck' sign, suggesting avulsion of Lisfranc ligament.
- These injuries are commonly missed so a high index of suspicion is required.

Treatment
- ORIF is required for all displaced injuries using screws, plates and screws, and supplementary wires.

Complications
- Foot compartment syndrome in acute injuries.
- Metatarsalgia.
- Post-traumatic arthritis.
- Purely ligamentous injuries have the worse outcome.

Metatarsal and phalanges

Mechanism
- Crushing or twisting injuries (e.g. the foot being run over).
- Fifth metatarsal fracture occurs after an inversion injury and can be mistaken for an ankle fracture if not examined correctly.
- Always be suspicious of compartment syndrome in severe crush injuries.

Treatment
- *Metatarsal fractures.* If minimal displacement or angulations, conservative treatment with mobilization as pain allows. Plaster only if mobilization is too painful. Multiple fractures may require reduction and fixation.
- Non-union of the fifth metatarsal sometimes requires ORIF with grafting if problematic (rare).
- *Phalangeal fractures.* Neighbour strapping.

References

1 ℘ http://www.orthoteers.co.uk/Nrujp~ij33lm/Orthfootfracfoot.htm.
2 Sanders R (2000). Displaced intra-articular fractures of the calcaneus. *J Bone Joint Surg Am* **82-A**: 225–50. [Current concepts review]

Injuries and the spinal radiograph

If a patient complains of central pain in the spinal column after trauma, always obtain radiographs. This should not delay resuscitation as a spinal fracture can be immobilized and life-threatening problems corrected first.

Spinal injuries can be associated with other injuries and the patient may not be able to communicate this to you because they are:
- Unconscious.
- Intubated.
- Shocked.
- Intoxicated.
- Anaesthetized distal to a cord lesion.

Common injuries associated with spinal trauma are:
- Bilateral calcaneal fractures—thoracolumbar fractures.
- Facial fractures—cervical fracture/dislocation.
- Severe head injury—cervical injuries, especially C1/C2.
- Sternal dislocation—thoracic spine fracture.
- Ankylosing spondylitis—cervical and thoracic fractures.
- Cervical fracture—10% rate of fracture at another level.

An awake, alert, oriented patient who can demonstrate a normal painless range of motion of the cervical spine does not need radiographic evaluation.

X-ray interpretation
- Develop a mental picture of the normal spinal radiograph. If you feel that the X-ray 'just doesn't look right', then it probably isn't!
- Try to develop a system and use this for every fracture you see, even when you know it will be normal. It gets you into the habit.
- A systematic approach has been shown to reduce the risk of missed spine injuries.

C-spine
- AP, lateral, and open mouth views for C1/C2 are required.
- You must be able to see from C1 to T1; if not, request further views (swimmer's view).
- Look at the bones and their alignment.
- On the lateral film, a smooth line should run down the anterior aspect of the vertebral body, the posterior aspect, the anterior aspect of the spinous process (spinolaminar line), and the posterior aspect of the spinous process.
- Look for any obvious steps between vertebral bodies (up to 25% displacement may suggest unifacet dislocation, >25% suggests complete facet joint instability) and angulation.
- Examine each vertebral body for integrity.
- Look at the facet joints for congruity (facet joint dislocations).
- Look at the distance between the spinous processes (increase suggests injury).
- Assess the soft tissues. Disc spaced for narrowing or widening.

- Assess the soft tissues anterior to the spine. This should be no more than 7mm at C3 and 3cm at C7. Any increase suggests swelling and thus injury.
- Look at the odontoid peg and its relationship to C1. Look for fractures and the gap in front of peg (usually <3mm).
- On the AP film, assess the vertebral body height and alignment.
- The interpedicular distances (increase may suggest fracture).
- Look for central alignment of the spinous processes. Beware the empty vertebrae; this may imply damage to the spinous process.
- Check the transverse processes; they become displaced when fractured.

Thoracolumbar spine
- AP and lateral views required.
- Thoracic spine is difficult to interpret; look for other clues such as multiple rib fractures.
- On the AP, look at alignment.
  - Vertebral body height.
  - Interpedicular distance. An absent or broken pedicular ring may suggest fracture of the posterior elements.
  - Central spinous process alignment.
  - Integrity of the transverse processes.
  - Disc height.
- On the lateral X-ray, assess alignment and look for steps.
  - Look at the vertebral body and check for anterior wedging (>50% loss of body height suggests instability).
  - Any bony fragments displaced into the vertebral canal posteriorly.
  - Check disc height.
  - Overall angulation of the spine (kyphosis in lumbar spine or increased kyphosis of thoracic).

Further imaging
- If a fracture is found on the X-rays that is deemed unstable or the films are difficult to interpret and there is a high suspicion of injury, a CT should be requested.
- A CT scan will assess the bony spine.
- If a soft tissue or spinal cord injury is suspected, an MRI will be required.

Signs that imply spinal instability
Denis divides the spine into three structural columns:
- *Anterior.* Anterior half of vertebral body and the anterior longitudinal ligament.
- *Middle.* Posterior half of vertebral body and posterior longitudinal ligament (PLL).
- *Posterior.* All structures posterior to the PLL (facet joints, pedicles, ligamentum flavum, spinous processes, and their interspinous ligaments).

With increasing column involvement, there is increasing instability, i.e. one-column injury usually stable, three-column injury highly unstable.

- Complete vertebral dislocation or translocation.
- Significant anterior wedging (>50%).
- Fractures in a previously fused spine, especially ankylosing spondylitis.
- Signs of movement. Malalignment, avulsion fractures, and evidence of paravertebral swelling.
- Increased interspinous or interpedicular distance.

Further reading

Raby N, Berman L, de Lacy G (2005). *Accident and emergency radiology: a survival guide*, 2nd edn. Saunders, London.

Spinal injuries

Any patient with major trauma arriving in A&E should be assumed to have a cervical injury unless proven otherwise. Remember that the **A** in the primary survey of ATLS resuscitation stands for airway with cervical spine control, i.e. it is top priority.[1]

- Cervical spine is the commonest area to have a major spinal injury.
- Other areas of concern are where mobile areas are at a junction with a less mobile one, e.g. C7/T1, T12/L1, and L5/S1 junctions.
- The main reason for delay in diagnosis of spinal injuries is failure to have a high clinical index of suspicion in all major trauma patients.

Principles of treatment

- Begin with ATLS approach and C-spine immobilization (rigid collar, lateral head supports, and strapping).
- Particular attention needs to be paid to this as some studies have suggested up to 25% of spinal cord injuries occur in the early management phase, after the initial injury!
- All trauma patients should be assumed to have a spinal injury until proven otherwise, especially in the presence of altered mental state or blunt head injury.
- A thorough primary and secondary survey needs to be performed, looking for mechanisms that would increase the risk of spine injury (RTA, motorcyclist, seat belt marks) and signs suggestive of other injuries (boggy swelling along the spine on log rolling).
- Until injuries of the spine have been deemed as stable, log rolling should take place to prevent any spinal cord injury from occurring.
- A full neurological examination is mandatory (if patient conscious).
- Once resuscitation and stabilization have occurred, appropriate radiological studies need to be undertaken.
- In the trauma setting, the ATLS manual now recommends CT scanning of the C-spine rather than a lateral X-ray. However, you must still be able to assess an X-ray if CT is unavailable!

Definitive management

Cervical spine

- *C1 (Jefferson fracture).*
  - If stable, semi-rigid collar or halo fixator.
  - If unstable, halo fixator or traction ± surgical fixation.
- *C2 (odontoid peg fracture).*
  - Type 1 (tip). Treat with semi-rigid collar.
  - Type 2 (waist). In elderly, consider cervical collar or C1/C2 fusion; in young patients, if undisplaced—halo fixator, if displaced—internal fixation or C/C2 fusion.
  - Type 3 (base and extends into body of C2). Stable, treat with cervical collar.
- *C3–C7.*

- Anterior compression fractures treated in semi-rigid collar or halo (if >25% loss anterior height or kyphosis >11°, may need operative fusion).
- Burst fractures (from axial load). Associated with cord injury; treatment with decompression and fusion may be required.
- *Facet joint dislocations.* Both unilateral and bilateral dislocations require reduction with progressive traction. Once reduced, unifacet dislocations are stable and treated in a cervical collar; bilateral dislocations require surgical stabilization.

Thoracolumbar injury

- Most common at T11–L2 as transitional segment (rigid to mobile).
- Up to 12% incidence of fracture at different spinal level.
- Denis classified into compression, burst, flexion-distraction, and fracture-dislocations, based on 3-column theory.
- Stable fractures (<50% loss of vertebral body height, <25% kyphosis, <50% spinal canal compromise) and neurologically intact are treated conservatively with a thoracolumbar spine orthosis (TLSO) for 3 months.
- Unstable fractures or neurological deficit require stabilization via fusion and decompression of spinal canal.

Sacral injury See Fractures of the pelvis, 📖 p. 532.

Spinal cord injury (SCI)

- Assess acutely as previously described (ALTS and so forth).
- Full neurological evaluation.
- Establish level of SCI. C5 or above requires intubation.
- Complete or incomplete lesions. Find motor level, then establish presence of sacral sensation (intact suggests incomplete).
- Look for other injuries and treat accordingly.
- Steroid use for SCI is controversial with a paucity of level 1 evidence.
- High dose methylprednisolone administered within 8h of injury and continued for 48h has been shown to improve outcomes.[2]
- Always adhere to local policy.

Neurogenic shock

- Neurological injury causing failure of descending sympathetic pathways of cervical and upper thoracic cord. Affects vasomotor tone and cardiac function.
- Results in vasodilatation and bradycardia (unopposed parasympathetic).
- Be careful of excessive fluid therapy to treat hypotension as may result in fluid overload.

Spinal shock

- Loss of muscle tone (flaccidity), loss of reflexes (areflexia), and anaesthesia following SCI.
- Duration variable (usually 48h).
- End defined by onset of spasticity below level of SCI.
- No recovery by 48h suggests complete cord injury and poor prognosis.

'Incomplete' spinal cord syndromes

If there is preservation of some modalities of cord function distal to the injury level, the cord lesion is referred to as 'incomplete'. Several recognized patterns exist.

Central cord syndrome

- Most common.
- Hyperextension injury to a spine with stenosis; usually age >50y.
- Weakness affects upper limbs > lower limbs. Deficits worst distal than proximal. Variable sensory loss.
- Due to vascular compromise to cord (anterior spinal artery supplies central cord).
- Recovery. Lower extremities, then bladder, then proximal upper limbs, and then hands.

Anterior cord syndrome

- Flexion injury.
- Poorest prognosis (10–20% recovery).
- Dense motor (paraplegia/quadraplegia) and sensory loss below level of injury. Affects spinothalamic and corticospinal tracts.
- Proprioception and vibration sense (posterior column) spared.

Brown–Sequard syndrome

- Penetrating trauma.
- Hemisection of the cord, giving ipsilateral motor (corticospinal), vibration and proprioceptive loss (posterior columns), and contralateral loss of pain and temperature (spinothalamic).
- Variable, but best chance of recovery.

Posterior cord syndrome

Proprioception and vibration sense lost, but intact motor power (rare).

References

1 American College of Surgeons (2008). *Advanced trauma life support (ATLS) for doctors, student manual*. 8th Edition. American College of Surgeons, Chicago.
2 Bracken MB (2009). Steroids for acute spinal cord injury. *The Cochrane Database of Systematic Reviews* Issue 1, Art. No.: CD001046.

Acute haematogenous osteomyelitis

This is a disease of growing bones. It is common in infants and children, but rare in adults unless they are immunocompromised or diabetic.

Aetiology
- Infants (<1y). *Staphylococcus (S.) aureus*, group B streptococci, and *Escherichia coli*.
- Children (1–16y). *S. aureus*, *Streptococcus (S.) pyogenes*, *Haemophilus (H.) influenzae*.
- Adults. *S. aureus*, *Staphylococcus (S.) epidermidis*.
- Sickle cell patients. *Salmonella* sp.
- Rare causes. *Brucella*, TB, spirochetes, and fungi.

Pathological features
The organisms settle near the metaphysis at the growing end of a long bone. The following stages typically occur.
- *Inflammation*. Acute inflammation with venous congestion.
- *Suppuration*. After 2–3 days, pus forms in the medulla and forces its way out to the periosteum.
- *Necrosis*. After 7 days, blood supply is compromised and infective thrombosis leads to necrosis and formation of a pocket of dead tissue (sequestrum).
- *Repair*. At around 10–14 days, new bone is formed from the subperiosteal layer that was stripped with the swelling (involucrum).
- *Discharge*. Involucrum can develop defects (cloacae), allowing discharge of pus and sequestrum to allow resolution. This can also be achieved by surgical release and debridement.

Clinical features
- Usually a child with a preceding history of trauma or infection (skin or respiratory).
- Fever, pain, and malaise develop after a few days.
- The child may be limping or refusing to weight bear.
- On examination, there may be localized swelling or redness of a long bone.
- Infants may present with a failure to thrive, drowsiness, or irritability.
- Neonates may present with life-threatening septicaemia in which obvious inflammation of a long bone develops or a more benign form in which the symptoms are slow to develop, but bone changes are extensive and often multiple.

Investigation
- Plain X-rays may be normal for the first 10 days. Do not be reassured!
- ^{99}Technetium bone scan is usually positive in the first 24–48h and is effective in confirming diagnosis early.
- ^{67}Gallium bone scan and ^{111}indium-labelled white cell scans are more specific, but generally not available in most units.
- MRI is very sensitive, but not specific and difficult for children.
- CT scanning can define extent of bone sequestration and cavitation.

X-ray features

- Soft tissue swelling is an early sign; look for displacement of fat planes.
- Patchy lucencies develop in the metaphysis at around 10 days.
- Periosteal new bone may be seen.
- Involucrum formation is only apparent at around 3 weeks.
- Sequestrum appears radiodense compared to the surrounding bone which is osteopenic.
- Normal bone density occurs with healing.

Laboratory tests results

- FBC. ↑ WCC, normally with a raised neutrophil count.
- ↑ ESR.
- ↑ CRP, but returns to normal quickly post-treatment.
- Blood cultures positive in 50% of cases (use to inform and adjust antibiotic therapy).
- Perform U&E, LFTs, and glucose.

Treatment

- Pain relief by bed rest, splintage, and analgesics.
- Give IV antibiotics according to local guidelines (after blood cultures and pus swab samples taken), e.g. flucloxacillin IV, then PO qds for up to 6 weeks, dose-adjusted according to age, clindamycin if penicillin-allergic, vancomycin if MRSA, ampicillin for *Haemophilus*.
- Surgical drainage of mature subperiosteal abscess with debridement of all necrotic tissue, obliteration of dead spaces, adequate soft tissue coverage, and restoration of an effective blood supply.

Complications

- Disseminated systemic infection, e.g. septicaemia, cerebral abscess.
- Chronic osteomyelitis.
- Septic arthritis.
- Deformity due to epiphyseal involvement.

Further reading

Lazzarini L, Mader JT, Calhoun JH (2004). Osteomyelitis in long bones. *J Bone Joint Surg Am* **86-A**: 2305–18. [Current concepts review]

Chronic osteomyelitis

Causes
- Occasionally following acute haematogenous osteomyelitis.
- Most common following contaminated trauma and open fractures.
- After joint replacement surgery.
- Primary chronic infections of bone.

Secondary to acute osteomyelitis
Features
- Sinus formation due to sequestra or resistant bacteria.
- Prevented by adequate treatment of the initial acute attack.

Treatment
- Conservative (simple dressings) may be appropriate (elderly). Recurrent attacks with spontaneous recovery may occur and surgery should be reserved for cases where an abscess forms.
- Chronic abscess. May require drainage, debridement of all necrotic tissue, and obliteration of dead spaces. May involve plastic surgery to achieve soft tissue cover and restoration of an effective blood supply.
- Closed suction drainage/irrigation systems can be effective, especially if irrigation fluid contains antibiotics. The disadvantage is that early blockage of the system can occur.
- Antibiotic (gentamicin)-impregnated beads or sponges deliver high local levels and may be beneficial in areas of poor blood supply, hence systemic antibiotic penetration.
- Unresolving cases may require amputation.

Secondary to trauma (open fractures)
- Prevention by early aggressive approach to compound fractures with debridement and lavage of contaminated tissue.
  - Excise all dead tissue widely and remove all devitalized bone fragments, i.e. with no soft tissue connections.
  - Copious lavage is necessary as *'the solution to pollution is dilution'* (≥10L is common).
  - Skeletal stabilization is mandatory.
  - IV antibiotics, e.g. IV cefuroxime ± metronidazole if anaerobes may be involved (soil).
- Treat established chronic infection as above with removal of internal foreign bodies, e.g. metalwork, and possible application of external fixation.

Secondary to joint replacement surgery
- Rare (≤1%), but is often a disaster for the elective patient.
- Prevention is better than cure. Dedicated laminar flow theatres, strict theatre discipline, and prophylactic IV antibiotics are mandatory.
- Fifty per cent will require surgical intervention.
  - Initial joint irrigation, debridement, and tissue sampling can be attempted if the prosthesis is still solid and not 'loose'.

- If grossly infected, the prosthesis must be removed, the surfaces debrided, and an antibiotic cement spacer placed on the raw bone ends to allow the soft tissue envelope to settle.
- Once inflammatory markers have settled (CRP is the best) and the clinical infection has resolved, second stage replacement of the spacer with a new prosthetic joint can go ahead. This may take 12 months and may not be possible.

Chronic osteomyelitis as an initial presentation

Brodie's abscess

- An isolated well-contained chronic abscess.
- Treatment. Operative drainage with excision of the abscess wall and antibiotics.

Tuberculosis

- Usually associated with other systemic features of the disease.
- May present acutely.
- Muscle atrophy develops and spontaneous discharge of a 'cold' abscess may lead to sinus formation and destruction of bone.
- Spinal TB may cause vertebral collapse, leading to acute neurology ('Pott's paraplegia').

Syphilitic osteomyelitis

- Associated with advanced, tertiary disease in adults. Features diffuse periostitis (with sabre tibia) or localized gummata with sequestra, sinus formation, and pathological fractures. X-rays show periosteal thickening with 'punched out' areas in sclerotic bone.
- Infants with congenital disease have epiphysitis and metaphysitis. X-rays show areas of sclerosis near the growth plate separated by areas of rarefaction.

Mycotic osteomyelitis

- Typically occurs in immunocompromised patients.
- Bone granulomas, necrosis, and suppuration present without worsening acute illness.
- Usually occurs as spread from primary lung infections such as coccidiomycosis, cryptococcosis, blastomycosis, and histoplasmosis.
- Treatment. Amphotericin B and/or surgical excision.

Further reading

Lazzarini L, Mader JT, Calhoun JH (2004). Osteomyelitis in long bones. *J Bone Joint Surg Am* **86-A**: 2305–18. [Current concepts review]

Septic arthritis

A condition due to infection of a joint space and its synovium. It is common in infants and children, but rare in adults unless they are immunocompromised or diabetic.

Aetiology

The infective organisms are the same as for acute osteomyelitis.

Pathological features.

- Primary seeding of the synovial membrane.
- Secondary infection from adjacent metaphysis or directly from epiphysis.
- In some joints, the metaphysis lies partly within the joint capsule (shoulder, elbow, hip, and ankle); osteomyelitis can break through metaphysis and into joint.
- Proteolytic enzymes are released from synovial cells and proteases from chondrocytes, causing destruction of the articular cartilage:
  - By 5 days, proteoglycans are lost from cartilage.
  - By 9 days, collagen is lost.

Clinical features

- Usually a child with a preceding history of trauma or infection (skin or respiratory).
- Acute onset with pyrexia and irritability.
- The child may be limping or refusing to weight bear.
- The affected joint is held still in position of maximal comfort (e.g. hip flexed, abducted, and externally rotated gives largest joint volume).
- Look for an erythematous, hot, swollen joint with an effusion.
- A neonate may present with none of the above, just irritable, lethargic, off feeds, and not moving affected limb.
- In the adult, the joint will be exquisitely painful, hot, red, and swollen, and they will usually not allow passive motion.

Investigation

- Plain X-rays may show joint space widening, joint subluxation or dislocation, and soft tissue swelling.
- Ultrasound scan can demonstrate effusion and guide aspiration.
- The mainstay of diagnosis is aspiration of the affected joint with immediate Gram stain and microscopy, followed by cultures and sensitivities.
- Always ask for the sample to be analysed for crystals and some septic-looking joints in adults are actually due to crystalopathies (gout or pseudogout).

Laboratory tests results

- FBC. ↑ WCC, normally with a raised neutrophil count.
- ↑ ESR.
- ↑ CRP, but returns to normal quickly post-treatment.

- Blood cultures positive in 50% of cases (use to inform and adjust antibiotic therapy).
- Perform U&E, LFTs, and glucose.

Treatment

- Septic arthritis is a surgical emergency and as such, rapid diagnosis, and management is required.
- Open (or arthroscopic) drainage of the affected joint with copious irrigation.
- Resuscitation and antibiotics.
- Re-exploration should be considered for those not settling.
- IV antibiotics, broad-spectrum, then tailored once culture results are available for 2 weeks, then oral for further 4 weeks.

Peripheral nerve injuries

Common; approximately 9000 people a year are admitted to hospital with an injury to a peripheral nerve.
- Causes include traction, trauma, inflammation, compression.
- The degree of injury depends on the mechanism (open or closed injury, acute or chronic), health of nerve prior to injury.

Pathological features

Seddon classification.

Neuropraxia

- Stretching or compression of the nerve which remains anatomically intact.
- Conduction block with normal conduction above and below.
- Focal demyelination occurs at the site of injury, which is repaired by the Schwann cells.
- Recovery is usually complete, occurring in days or weeks. There is no axonal degeneration.

Axontemesis

- The axon is divided, but the covering connective tissue component remains intact, i.e. the nerve cylinder remains.
- Usually a traction or severe crush injury.
- Axonal ('Wallerian') degeneration occurs distal to the injury and is followed by nerve regeneration (by sprouting from the severed nerve end) after 10 days.
- Nerve growth occurs at a rate of 1mm per day.
- Prognosis is generally good as the cylinder is intact, but the more proximal the lesion, the less the distal recovery.
- Sensation recovery is generally better than motor recovery, especially if the lesion is proximal and muscle wasting occurs whilst it is 'dennervated'.

Neurotemesis

- The nerve is completely divided or irreparably damaged with loss of apposition of the severed nerve bundles and their respective distal parts.
- Usually a high energy injury, penetrating trauma, severe traction, ischaemia, or high pressure injection injury.
- Minimal recovery is possible without operative intervention to repair or graft a new nerve to the injury.
- Surgical repair may allow axon regeneration to the correct end organ, but recovery will not be complete as often 'miswiring' occurs.

Diagnosis

- What is the injury? Is there an open wound, fracture, recent surgery, or prolonged immobility?
- Complete neurological examination. You must know the motor and sensory supplies of peripheral nerves! Use a pin or your finger

for sensory testing. Compare the area of normal and injured side sequentially.

- *Tips.* Anaesthetic skin looks shiny and does not sweat. Dennervated skin will not wrinkle in water.
- There are specific features of different levels of injury in peripheral nerves of the upper limb.
- Examination very soon after injury can be misleading as sensory loss may take time to appear.
- Diagnosis of a peripheral nerve injury is clinical, but can be supplemented with nerve conduction studies and electromyography (EMG).

Treatment

Closed injury

- Injuries in continuity. Neuropraxia and axontemeses (vast majority) can be expected to recover spontaneously, so exploration is not indicated.
- Compression injuries should have compressive forces removed, e.g. external such as plaster or internal such as carpal tunnel syndrome.
- Physiotherapy and splintage should be used whilst awaiting recovery; this will maintain functionality and prevent contractures.

Open injuries

- *Primary repair (suture).* Within 24h is ideal, but an uncontaminated operative field, adequate skin cover, and proper equipment (e.g. microscopes) must be present.
- *Delayed secondary repair.* Can be done at any time after injury once the soft tissues have healed (3–6 weeks acceptable). The nerve can be mobilized to allow a no tension repair after resection of the cut nerve stumps. Usually, however, a nerve graft has to be used to bridge the defect (sural nerve as a donor the commonest).

Further reading

Soloman L, Warwick D, Nayagam S (Eds) (2010). *Apley's system of orthopaedics and fractures.* 9th edn. Hodder Arnold, London.

Brachial plexus injuries

The brachial plexus is formed from the ventral rami of C5 to T1. It is subsequently divided into root, trunks, divisions, cords, and terminal branches. The lesion can be at any of the above levels.

Terminal branches arising from the root level (phrenic nerve (C3–5), dorsal scapular nerve (C5), and long thoracic nerve (C5–7)) are important to recognize as if they are spared, it suggests the lesion is post-ganglionic.

Causes

- *Child*. Obstetric, i.e. difficult deliveries with traction on the plexus.
- *Adult*. Almost all traumatic.
  - Usually closed, e.g. motorcycle accidents, falls, and traction injuries with forced abduction of the arm.
  - May be open, e.g. stab or gunshot wounds.
- Always look for associated injuries, e.g. head, neck, chest, abdominal, and vascular.

Types

- *Erb–Duchenne (upper)*. Involves C5 and C6; the arm classically hangs at the side with the arm flaccid, internally rotated, adducted, and the wrist flexed (waiter's tip position).
- *Klumpke's (lower)*. Involves C8 and T1; the hand is clawed due to intrinsic muscle paralysis and if the sympathetic trunk is involved, there is Horner's syndrome.

Try to localize the lesion to preganglionic (intraspinal) or post-ganglionic (extraspinal) by clinical means as described earlier. At the T1 level, look for signs of Horner's syndrome (ptosis, meiosis, ipsilateral anhydrosis), suggesting a preganglionic lesion.

If histamine is injected into the skin of the supplied area, vasodilatation, weal, and flare indicate a positive result and a preganglionic injury is present. If there is no flare, the lesion is postganglionic.

Anatomic level of injury should be delineated.

Treatment

Physiotherapy to prevent joint contracture and stiffness. If no return of function at 2 months, consider myelography or histamine tests to localize the injury level.

- Open injuries should be explored acutely, but not if there are more life-threatening injuries (which is usually the case). Primary repair may be possible in this group.
- Delayed surgery (if required at all) is normal for most patients.
- Preganglionic injuries are irreparable and should not be explored.
- Post-ganglionic injuries may be explored for up to 6 months post-injury. Secondary repair with nerve grafting can then be attempted if a clear lesion is isolated.

Prognosis

- If there are no EMG abnormalities at 3–4 weeks, prognosis is good with conservative treatment.

- Causalgic pain, Horner's syndrome, and the presence of root avulsion on myelogram (hence intraspinal lesion) indicate a poor prognosis.
- Recovery is generally very slow and often unsatisfactory.
- Salvage surgery with tendon transfers or shoulder arthrodesis may improve function and give better results than amputation.

Further reading

Birch R (1996). Brachial plexus injuries. *J Bone Joint Surg Br* **78-B**: 986–92. [Review]

Osteoarthrosis (osteoarthritis)

This is degenerative joint disease; it is a disease of cartilage, not the joint.
- It is limited to the joint itself and there is no systemic effect.
- It may involve any synovial joint, but is most common in the hip, knee, and hands.
- It is the most common form of arthritis with an estimated radiographic incidence in moderate to severe changes in 5 million people in the UK.[1]
- Approximately 2 million people visit their GP with osteoarthritis per year and it is predicted that there will be a 66% increase in the number of people with osteoarthritis-related disability by 2020.

Types

Primary osteoarthritis (idiopathic)
Mainly affects the following joints: distal interphalangeal, first carpometa-carpal, hips, knees, and apophyseal joints of the spine. Women are more affected than men and there may be a hereditary component, but the aetiology is unknown.

Secondary osteoarthritis
Affects previously damaged joints and is more common in weight-bearing joints. Both sexes are equally affected. Local causes are fractures, acquired or congenital deformities, joint injury (chondral lesions), diabetic neuropathy (Charcot joints), and avascular necrosis.

Clinical features
- Characteristic pain, swelling, and deformity.
- Dull, aching pain with morning stiffness of the affected joint.
- Pain becomes steadily worse throughout the day and may disturb sleep.
- Acute onset. Swollen, hot, and painful joint with raised inflammatory markers.
- Look for Heberden's nodes at the distal and Bouchard's nodes at the proximal interphalangeal joints.
- Physical symptoms may not correlate with the severity of the radiographic changes so judge each patient on an individual basis.

X-ray changes
- Loss of joint space.
- Subchondral bone sclerosis.
- Cyst formation (especially at the hip).
- Osteophyte formation.

Treatment
Relieve pain, improve mobility, and correct deformity in that order.

Medical
- Pain relief with simple analgesics (paracetamol, codeine), in combination with NSAIDs, helps control symptoms and increase

mobility. Beware of GI bleeding, especially in the elderly, and of worsening asthma.
- Radiant heat in the form of infrared light or a hot water bottle frequently helps.
- Weight loss, physiotherapy, and aids to daily living such as walking sticks, heel raises, raised chair, and household aids should all be in place before contemplating surgery.
- Joint injections of steroid and local anaesthetic may help in up to 50% patients.

Surgical treatment

This is indicated for pain relief, improved mobility, and correcting deformity *only* when conservative measures have failed.

Options include:
- *Osteotomy*. Realignment of a joint to unload an arthritic area.
- *Arthrodesis*. Permanent stiffening of a joint by excision and fusion to stop pain.
- *Excision*. Removal of the joint without fusion.
- *Arthroplasty*. Replacement of all or part of the joint surface by an artificial material.

Reference

1 ℘ http://www.arc.org.uk/about_arth/astats.htm.

Carpal tunnel syndrome

- Compression of the median nerve at the wrist.
- Boundaries of tunnel are: radially—scaphoid tubercle and trapezium, ulnarly—hook of hamate and pisiform, transverse palmar ligament, palmar aspect (roof).
- Contents—flexor tendons (flexor pollicis longus (FPL), flexor digitorum superficialis (FDS), flexor digitorum profundus (FDP)) and median nerve.
- Most common in middle age.
- Often bilateral, but when unilateral most commonly affects the dominant hand.

Aetiology

Remember, the commonest is idiopathic.

Compression of the tunnel wall

- Trauma, e.g. distal radial fracture.
- Rheumatoid arthritis (thickening of the surrounding synovium and tissues).
- Subluxation or dislocation of the wrist.
- Acromegaly (soft tissue thickening and enlargement).

Compression within the tunnel

- Fluid retention, e.g. pregnancy.
- Myxoedema.
- Space-occupying lesion, e.g. benign tumour.
- Chronic proliferative synovitis.

Changes in the median nerve

- Diabetic mellitus.
- Peripheral neuropathies.

Clinical features

Symptoms

- Aching pain and paraesthesia (pins and needles) over radial three-and-a-half fingers and palm.
- Pain typically at night and can disturb sleep.
- Relieved by shaking the hand.
- May notice dropping items (weak pinch grip), clumsiness.
- Can be made worse by activity.
- Atypical symptoms can be common.

Signs[1]

- Hand looks normal.
- Thenar muscle wasting if chronic and severe.
- Weakness of thumb abduction.
- Tinnel's test. Tapping over the nerve at the wrist in neutral produces symptoms.
- Phalen's test. Rest elbows on the table and passively flex the wrist. If symptoms appear within 60s, test is positive.
- Median nerve compression test. Extend elbow, supinate forearm, flex wrist to 60°, press on carpal tunnel. Positive if symptoms within 30s.

Investigations Nerve conduction studies are gold standard, but still show only 90% accuracy.

Treatment
Conservative
- Splintage.
- NSAIDs.
- Injection of corticosteroids.
- Avoidance of precipitating factors.

Surgical
- Surgical decompression.
- Use a tourniquet.
- Skin incision in line with ulnar border of the ring finger. This is to avoid the motor branch of the median nerve.
- Protect the nerve with a MacDonald's dissector and visualize the nerve directly throughout.
- Do not extend the skin incision beyond the wrist crease to protect the palmar cutaneous branch of the median nerve.

Complications
- Complex regional pain syndrome.
- Tender, hypertrophic scar giving pillar pain (pain in the heel of the scar on pressure).
- Neuroma of the palmar cutaneous branch.
- Recurrence.
- Bowstringing of flexor tendons.

Reference
1 Tetro AM, Evanoff BA, Hollstien SB, Gelberman RH (1998). A new provocative test for carpal tunnel syndrome: assessment of wrist flexion and nerve compression. *J Bone Joint Surg Br* **80(3)**: 493–8.

Ganglion

This is a degenerative mucinous cyst swelling that can arise from a tendon sheath or joint. It contains clear, colourless, gelatinous fluid.

Common sites
- Dorsum of the wrist, arising from the scapholunate ligament or midcarpal joint (70% of all cases).
- Radial aspect of the volar wrist normally from scaphotrapezial joint (20% of all cases).
- Base or DIPJ of finger.
- Dorsum of the foot.
- Around the knee.

Clinical features
- Slow growing, cystic lump commonly presenting as dorsal wrist pain.
- Increase and decrease in size.
- Firm, smooth, rubbery, and will usually transluminate.
- May be more obvious with wrist in palmar flexion.

Diagnosis
- Needle aspiration gives gelatinous fluid. If no fluid can be aspirated, then investigate further since a soft tissue tumour (including sarcoma) is possible.
- MRI scanning should be used if there is serious concern over a soft tissue tumour.
- Occult ganglia (no palpable lump) can yield symptoms in the wrist or foot. Ultrasound scan will confirm the diagnosis.

Treatment
- Fifty per cent will disappear spontaneously. Therefore, treat conservatively unless pressed by the patient.
- Aspiration may be curative in 50% of cases.
- Deliberately induced traumatic rupture often leads to recurrence.

Surgery
- Excision is not guaranteed success (recurrence approximately 10%; painful scar approximately 10%).
- Use a tourniquet.
- If not occult or excessively large, then local anaesthesia as day case procedure appropriate.
- Excise thoroughly and transfix the base to prevent recurrence.
- Volar wrist ganglia often surround or are very close to the radial artery!

Bone tumours

Diagnosis
The key to successful management of bone tumours is early detection and treatment; always having a clinical suspicion is essential!

Presenting features
- Pain. Persistent, at night, response to analgesics?
- Mass or swelling (? getting bigger, rate of progression).
- If there is a fracture, is there a history of trauma?
- Neurological symptoms.
- Systemic symptoms.
- Previous tumours, radio- or chemotherapy.
- Any family history.
- Watch for the 'red herring history' of trivial injury.

Examination
- Extract features of the mass/swelling and palpate for lymphadenopathy.
- Is it around a joint, is it deep to the fascia? Size, relationship to surrounding structures.

Radiological investigations
- A plain X-ray (AP and lateral) of affected area is mandatory.
- Where is lesion, what are effects on bone, is there a bone reaction (new bone, periosteal reaction, Codman's triangle, sunburst spiculation), is there a matrix?
- Once a diagnosis has been considered/made, further imaging is required; MRI scanning is usually gold standard.
- Accurately stage and assess local or systemic spread (CT, bony architecture; MRI, soft tissue or bony extensions).

Blood tests
Rarely diagnostic and often non-specific (e.g. ↑ alkaline phosphatase, ↑ ESR, ↑ Ca^{2+}).

Urgent referral
- Once a diagnosis is made, urgent referral (even before MRI is obtained in highly suspicious lesion) to local tumour services is required.
- They will advise and guide further local management and arrange definitive treatment if required.

Other considerations
- Angiography. Helps plan radical surgery and possible limb salvage.
- Open biopsy. Best to achieve histological diagnosis and required for treatment planning.
- Must be performed by the surgeon who is going to do the definitive surgery.
- The biopsy track must be excised as part of the definitive excision and placed to maximize the chance of limb salvage surgery.

Metastatic tumours

- Secondary metastases are the commonest tumours of bone (breast, prostate, lung, thyroid, and kidney primaries).
- Bone pain—worse at night and with weight bearing.
- Systemic symptoms (fatigue, weight loss, no appetite).
- History of cancer (personal or family).
- Pathological fractures common.
- If a patient is admitted with a history of pathological fracture with unknown primary, full examination should be performed to find source (breast, rectal, prostate, etc.).
- Blood tests, including calcium, phosphate, tumour markers (PSA, CEA, CA125).
- Bone scan, staging CT/MRI may be required.
- Treatment:
  - Treat electrolytes first if raised.
  - Internal fixation (ideally prophylactic before fracture occurs) allows early weight bearing and hopefully early discharge from hospital.
  - Radiotherapy for pain.
  - Manage in conjunction with oncologists.

Benign tumours

Osteochondroma ('exostosis')

- Most common benign tumour.
- A cartilaginous capped outgrowth of bone from the cortex, normally near an epiphysis. Lesion grows until skeletal maturity.
- Usually pain-free and present as lump. If painful, usually due to inflammation of overlying bursa.
- Usually solitary. Multiple lesions require close follow-up (hereditary).
- Any sudden increase in size may indicate malignant transformation to chondrosarcoma (<1%).

Chondroma

A non-calcified cartilaginous growth in the medulla (enchondroma) or cortex (ecchondroma) of tubular bones such as phalanges, metacarpals/tarsals.

Osteoid osteoma

- Occurs in young patients (5–30y).
- Progressive pain (night) of long bone, referred to other joints, classically relieved by NSAIDs.
- Commonly long bones (diaphysis), can be intra-articular, and a cause of painful scoliosis.
- Radiology shows a 'nidus' which is a small osteolytic area surrounded by a rim of dense sclerosis. Look for periosteal reaction.

Non-ossifying fibroma

- Fibrous tissue tumour which usually appears radiologically as an oval cortical defect with sclerotic rim. Common incidental finding on X-rays; usually needs no treatment.

- Treatment. Principles of treatment are simple local excision or removal by curettage if symptomatic or likely to cause pathological fracture (likely if >50% diameter of bone involved).
  - Cavities should be packed with bone graft or bone cement.
  - Internal fixation may be used once large tumours have been removed.
  - Difficult tumours should be managed in a 'bone tumour centre'.

Primary malignant tumours (rare)

All primary malignant tumours require a 'multidisciplinary team' (orthopaedic surgeon, oncologist, musculoskeletal radiologist, histopathologist).

Osteosarcoma

- Commonest primary bone tumour.
- Long bones of young adults (peak incidence 10–20y) or as a consequence of Paget's disease in the elderly (see 🕮 p. 582).
- Presents with progressive pain (rest/night) refractory to analgesia.
- Swelling, reduced joint movement, limp.
- ? Trivial sporting injury—not related to tumour development!
- X-ray features. Bone destruction, soft tissue invasion, radiating spicules of bone ('sunray' appearance), subperiosteal elevation with new bone formation ('Codman's triangle').
- MRI shows extent of tumour, skip lesions, soft tissue involvement.
- Metastasis via blood to the lungs and bone.
- Treatment:
  - Neoadjuvant chemotherapy followed by surgical resection and further chemotherapy.
  - Limb salvage surgery possible in about 90% (rare for pelvic tumours).
  - Local recurrence rate 5% (poor prognosis).
  - Radiotherapy may be used as an alternative in the elderly.
- 5y survival 60–70% (localized) or 25% (pelvic) with surgery; 20% if present with metastases.

Chondrosarcoma

- Commonest in older patients (30–75y).
- Usually occurs in a flat bone, e.g. ilium of pelvis, ribs, scapula.
- Location of presentation gives clues to type (scapula malignant and hand benign).
- May present *de novo* or arise from a pre-existing osteochondroma.
- Graded. Low to high (1, 2, 3, undifferentiated); 60% present grade 1.
- Metastasis is not common and is via blood.
- Local invasion is more usual, but is normally slow growing.
- High grade present with bone destruction and soft tissue mass.
- Treatment:
  - Low grade require wide resection. Local recurrence 20% at 10y.
  - High grade require wide resection ± amputation.
  - No real role for chemo- or radiotherapy unless undifferentiated or elderly).
  - 5y survival dependent on grade. Grade 1, up to 90%; grade 2, 60–70%; grade 3, 30–50%; undifferentiated, 10%.

Ewing's sarcoma
- Children and young adults (<20y).
- Pain, associated hot/erythematous swelling with associated pyrexia so that osteomyelitis may be suspected.
- Commonly pelvis, long bones, and scapula.
- ↑ ESR and ↑ WCC.
- X-rays show lytic bone destruction with periosteal reaction in multiple layers ('onion skin' appearance).
- MRI scan shows soft tissue involvement, which would not usually be the case in osteomyelitis.
- Metastasis to the lung is very fast and most people present with this.
- Treatment. Preoperative neoadjuvant chemotherapy (12 weeks) and then re-evaluate and re-stage.
- Isolated lesions managed with wide excision or amputation.
- Radiation can be used if metastases present.
- Response to chemotherapy predicts prognosis.
- Prognosis is still poor. Isolated extremity Ewing's approximately 65% 5y survival; metastatic disease at presentation <20% 5y survival.

Giant cell tumour (osteoclastoma)
- This is rare before the age of 20y.
- Usually benign, but may undergo malignant transformation (~10%).
- Rarely metastasizes; usually to lungs, but may be locally invasive.
- Treatment. Local excision and defect filled bone graft or cement.
- Recurrence is common (~20%), especially with malignancy.

Further reading
Excellent summaries of bone tumours can be found at: ♫ http://www.bonetumor.org/

Low back pain

- Very common condition in the UK; 60–80% of adults will be affected during their lifetime.
- Common cause of absence from work.
- In the majority of cases, it is a self-limiting condition requiring no surgical intervention.[1]
- Multifaceted condition with overlapping aetiology.
- Always consider neoplasia—metastasis, myeloma, osteoid osteoma.

Types of pain

Mechanical

- Pain (low back, buttock, and thigh), like 'toothache'.
- Rarely radiates below knee.
- Worse over course of day and with activity.
- Cannot get comfortable and wakes from sleep when turn.
- Acute pain from trivial movement which settles with rest.
- Typically midline and made worse by lordotic postures, e.g. bending and lifting (discogenic).
- Pain is from the annulus fibrosis layer of the disc when it is being stretched.

Nerve root entrapment

- Pain radiates down the leg from buttock to calf/foot.
- Commonly caused by a lumbar disc prolapse, compressing and irritating the nerve root as it exits the spinal foramina.
- Pain from spinal stenosis is worsened with extension (walking down a hill) and relieved with flexion (riding a bike).
- Radiation should match the sensory dermatome of the nerve root involved.
- Other features are pain on sneezing, coughing, and straining. Numbness or paraesthesia in the dermatome of the affected root may also be present.
- The earliest and most persistent feature of nerve root compression is loss of a tendon reflex, e.g. knee L3/4, ankle L5/S1.

Referred

May arise from retroperitoneal pathology (aortic aneurysm, pancreatic and biliary tree pathology, rectal pathology, renal stones, lymphadenopathy, and hip arthroses).

Psychosocial (yellow flags)

- The commonest cause for chronicity.
- A diagnosis of exclusion, i.e. exclude all other pathology before labelling people as 'neurotic'.
- Typical features of non-organic pain are pain on axial compression or pelvic rotation, non-dermatomal sensory loss, non-anatomical tenderness, cogwheel (give way) weakness, and overreaction (Waddell's signs).[2]

Common pathological (organic) causes

- *Mechanical* (80–90%).
  - Unknown cause. Muscle strain or ligamentous injury.
  - Degenerative disc or joint disease.
  - Vertebral fracture.
  - Congenital deformity (such as scoliosis, kyphosis, transitional vertebrae).
  - Spondylolysis.
  - Instability (spondylolisthesis).
- *Neurogenic* (5–15%).
  - Herniated disc.
  - Spinal stenosis.
  - Osteophytic nerve root composition.
  - Failed back surgery syndrome (such as arachnoiditis, epidural adhesions, recurrent herniation). May cause mechanical back pain as well.
  - Infection (such as herpes zoster).
- *Non-mechanical spinal conditions* (1–2%).
  - Neoplastic (such as primary or metastatic).
  - Infection (osteomyelitis, discitis, abscess—staphylococcal or TB).
  - Inflammatory arthritis (such as rheumatoid arthritis and spondyloarthropathies, including ankylosing spondylitis, reactive arthritis, enteropathic arthritis).
  - Paget's disease.
- *Coccydynia*. Pain in the coccyx may be due to lumbosacral disc disease.

Assessment

- History must distinguish between 'simple' back pain and that requiring urgent care.
- '*Red flags*' of serious spinal pathology.
  - Retention of urine or incontinence.
  - Onset over age 55 or under 20.
  - Symptoms of systemic illness (weight loss, fever).
  - Severe progressive pain (unrelenting).
  - Trauma.
  - A prior history of cancer.
  - IV drug use.
  - Prolonged immunosuppressant or steroid use.
- Examination must cover:
  - Palpation, movements, straight leg raising, femoral stretch test, power, sensation, reflexes.
- If signs of significant spinal pathology present (i.e. cauda equina), perianal sensation and PR examination must be performed.

Investigations

- Spinal X-rays (AP and lateral of affected level).
- CT scan good for assessing bony structures.

- MRI scan good for soft tissue problems (discs, spinal cord, nerve root involvement), but only relevant in planning, not in diagnosing treatment. Should be left for treating surgeon as it is often not required.

Treatment

Non-operative

- Majority of patients require non-operative treatment.
- Initial rest (1–2 days only).
- Analgesia (paracetamol, NSAIDs, muscle relaxants, opioids).
- Early mobilization with strong encouragement.
- Physiotherapy (massage, acupuncture, hydrotherapy).
- Counselling and psychosocial support.

Surgery

- Only a minority requires surgery. Should be clearly focused on proven pathology demonstrated by imaging where possible.
- Procedures used include:
  - Discectomy.
  - Chemonucleosis/percutaneous disc removal.
  - Nerve root decompression.
  - Spinal decompression.
  - Spinal fusion.

Cauda equina

- Surgical emergency.
- Cauda equina (horse's tail) is a collection of nerve roots (lower lumbar and sacral) at distal end of cord.
- It can present acutely, chronically, or following longstanding lower back problems.
- Causes include large central or paracentral disc herniation (L4/5 or L5/S1), spinal injury neoplasms, tumours, infections (abscess or TB), haematoma (iatrogenic).
- Key symptoms are dysfunction of bladder, bowel (and sexual function), saddle or perianal anaesthesia.
- Other symptoms include low back pain, radiation down one or both legs, sensory chances in lower limbs, weakness.
- Examination should be a thorough lower limb neurological assessment.
- Perianal sensation and anal sphincter tone (bulbocavernosus reflex) is essential.
- Imaging is required urgently if convincing clinical evidence exists. MRI is the modality of choice.
- Treatment once diagnosed is surgical decompression. Referral to an appropriate spinal centre, if not on site, is required urgently.
- Timing of surgery is controversial. Better outcomes are seen if performed <24h following onset.
- Outcomes are variable. If complete cauda equina (urinary retention or incontinence), the prognosis for recovery is poor.

References

1 Cohen SP, Argoff CE, Carragee EJ (2009). Management of low back pain. *BMJ* **338**: 100–6.
2 Lavy C, James A, Wilson-MacDonald J, Fairbank J (2009). Cauda equina syndrome. *BMJ* **338**: 881–4.

Paget's disease (osteitis deformans)

Key facts
- Described by Sir James Paget (1876).
- Incidence increases with age (>50y).
- Any bone may be involved. Commonest sites are spine, skull, pelvis and femur, tibia.
- Autosomal dominant.

Pathological features
- Increased osteoclastic bone resorbtion followed by compensatory bone formation, i.e. there is an overall increase in bone turnover.
- Three phases. Lytic, mixed (lysis and formation), and sclerotic.
- The bone is softer, but thickened and is liable to pathological fracture.

Clinical features
- Most are asymptomatic.
- Diagnosed via an incidental finding on X-ray or raised alkaline phosphatase whilst investigating other pathologies.
- Increased thickness of bone may be the only symptom or sign.
- Subcutaneous bones may be deformed, classically the tibia when it becomes 'sabre'-shaped.
- Pain may be present, but is unusual. It may represent high turnover at the time or more likely, a pathological fracture.
- In known Paget's patients, increase in pain must be taken seriously as it may be a marker of sarcomatous change in the bone.

Investigations
- Serum calcium and phosphorus are normal.
- Alkaline phosphatase is high (due to ↑ osteoblast activity).
- Urinary excretion of hydroxyproline is high (↑ bone turnover).
- Isotope bone scan shows 'hot spots' in affected areas.
- X-ray shows both sclerosis and osteoporosis. The cortex is thickened and the bones deformed. Pathological fracture is a feature and the normal bone architecture is lost with coarse trabecular pattern.

Complications
- Pathological fractures.
- Osteosarcomatous change (<5%; prognosis *very poor*).
- High output cardiac failure may develop due to the increased vascularity of Paget's bone. Functionally, the bone is acting as an arteriovenous fistula.
- Deafness. Bony deformation in the ear causes damage to cranial nerve.
- Osteoarthritis.
- Leontiasis ossea. Thickening of facial bones (rare).
- Paraplegia due to vertebral involvement (rare).

Treatment
- Most patients require no treatment.

- Fractures will heal normally, but bony deformity with a fracture can be a difficult challenge!
- Drugs that reduce bone turnover such as calcitonin or bisphosphonates are effective in relieving pain and may also relieve neurological complications such as deafness.

Further reading

http://www.paget.org/

The great toe

Hallux valgus ('bunions')[1,2]

- Medial prominence of the first metatarsal head, with lateral deviation of the great toe (hence valgus) due to the pull of the extensors.
- As time passes, a protective bursa develops over the metatarsal head (the 'bunion') and the great toe begins to crowd, or even overlap, its neighbours.

Causes

- Congenital. Often familial, related to metatarsus primus varus where the first metatarsal is angled more medially, i.e. splayed, than usual and is rotated.
- Acquired. The commonest form. Probably due to weak intrinsic muscles due to age. It is not proven to be related to shoes, but there is a higher incidence in shoe-wearing cultures.

Symptoms

- Commonly asymptomatic, even in cases of severe deformity.
- Pain typically at the site of the bunion due to pressure.
- Bursal inflammation.
- Nerve symptoms may be present (compression of digital nerve).
- As the disease advances, symptoms of joint pain may present due to osteoarthritis and subluxation of the joint.
- Lesser toe deformities may be present (hammer toes, calluses).

Investigations

- Weight-bearing AP and lateral views of the foot.
- Measurements of the extent of deformity are made to guide management.
- Commonly calculated are the hallux valgus angle (between long axis of first metatarsal and corresponding proximal phalanx) and the first/second intermetatarsal angle (between the long axis of first and second metatarsals).

Treatment

Conservative

- Correct footwear with a wider toe box and padding to protect bunion.
- This should always be tried and have failed before considering surgery.

Surgical

- *Exostectomy.* Removal of the bunion alone. This is simple, but does not remove the underlying deformity and the problem will recur.
- *Distal metatarsal osteotomy.* The bunion is removed and the metatarsal head or neck is cut. The distal fragment is then realigned anatomically and the fracture held with a K wire. There are many types or shapes of osteotomy described, but the commonest eponyms are Mitchell's, Wilson's, and Chevron. This is only suitable for smaller deformities.
- *Proximal metatarsal osteotomy.* This is an osteotomy just proximal to the base of the metatarsal and the metatarsocuneiform joint. Larger

bony deformities can be corrected this way. It may be combined with a distal soft tissue release where the lateral constraints by the MTPJ are also released through a small separate dorsal excision.

- *Excision arthroplasty*. Removal of the metatarsal head (Mayo) or base of the proximal phalanx (Keller) can be attempted, but is fraught with long-term complications and is only an operation for the elderly.
- *Arthrodesis*. This is suitable for severe deformity and degenerative change and is tolerated well by males. Females may have a problem with footwear (have to wear flat shoes after). It is normally reserved for salvage surgery.

Hallux rigidus[1]

Degenerate arthritis of the first MTPJ, leading to pain and functional limitation of movement.

Causes

- Not fully determined.
- Congenital. Due to a shortened metatarsal.
- Acquired. Normally traumatic or idiopathic degeneration.

Symptoms

- Pain and swelling of the first MTPJ with profound stiffness (limited dorsiflexion).
- May irritate on shoes.
- Neurological symptoms due to pressure on the digital between osteophyte and shoe.

Investigations

AP and lateral X-rays of the foot (demonstrate osteoarthritic changes).

Treatment

- Adolescents/young. Rocker sole to relieve pain.
- Adults.
  - MTPJ replacement (rare).
  - Cheilectomy (excision of dorsal osteophyte and about 25% dorsal metatarsal head).
  - Arthrodesis.
  - Excision arthroplasty (elderly only).

References

1 ℘ http://www.blackburnfeet.org.uk/hyperbook/conditions/conditions_index.htm#hallux.
2 Coughlin MJ (1996). Hallux valgus. *J Bone Joint Surg Am* **78-A**, 932–66: [Instructional course lecture]

Arthroplasty

- The surgical reconstruction or replacement of a malformed or degenerate joint.
- The primary goal is to relieve pain.
- Increases in mobility and function are secondary aims.

Classification

- *Excision*, e.g. Keller's or Mayo at the first MTPJ.
- *Interposition*. A joint is excised and then a piece of tissue is implanted in the gap to cause a thick scar.
- *Partial (hemi-) or total replacement*. All or one-half of the articular surface is removed and replaced with other material. This has been made possible by the massive advances in both biomaterials and bioengineering, which have produced inert, sterilizable materials of acceptable strength to perform the joint functions.

Example: total hip replacement[1–3]

Indications

- Osteo- and rheumatoid arthritis when pain affects sleep, quality of life, and normal daily activities.
- Multiple joint involvement where hip is the worst.
- AVN of the head of the femur with secondary joint degeneration.

Prevention of infection

Deep infection is a potentially devastating complication of hip or any arthroplasty and its incidence should be ≤1% in all units. This is achieved by the following.

- *Ultraclean air systems and exhaust body suits*. The air in a conventional theatre is filtered so that there are >20 changes/h. By using a unidirectional laminar flow system, 300 or more changes/h with filtration can be achieved. The purpose is to make the number of colony-forming units (CFUs) in the air the minimum possible. Body suits, although cumbersome, provide the best physical barrier between the patient and the surgical team.
- *Prophylactic antibiotics*. These are given IV on the induction of anaesthesia; 10min is usually required for them to penetrate bone to an acceptable level. Broad-spectrum antibiotics are usually used, e.g. cefuroxime 1.5g, co-amoxiclav (Augmentin®) 1.2g, and gentamicin 80mg, being the most common. Two further doses at 6 and 12h post-operatively are usually given.
- *Strict theatre discipline*.

Procedure

The surgical approach exposes both the femoral head and acetabulum. The head of the femur is exposed, dislocated, and either reshaped (resurfacing arthroplasty) or more commonly, removed at the neck. The acetabulum is then deepened and reshaped to allow a cup to be placed (the new 'socket'). A cavity is then created within the cut surface of the femur, going downward to allow a stem to be placed (the new 'ball'). The stem and cup are usually 'grouted' in place with polymethylmethacrylate bone cement and the two components reduced and stability tested.

Sometimes the cup has a metal shell behind it and components can be hammered in rather than cemented and this is known as an 'uncemented hip replacement'. This is more commonly used on the younger patient in the UK, but is the implant of choice in the USA. The wound is then closed. Patients are mobilized on day 1 post-operatively, fully weight bearing, and discharged within 5–7 days usually.

Complications
Operative
- Sciatic nerve injury due to poor technique and overstretching of tissues.
- Dislocation of the prosthesis if incorrectly aligned.
- Profound hypotension can be seen with absorption of the monomer in the cement, causing cardiotoxicity.

Post-operative
- Mortality 1%. This is major surgery.
- Thromboembolic disease (DVT or PE).
- Deep infection (1%).
- Dislocation (4%). Usually due to patient non-compliance with physiotherapy guidelines.
- Aseptic loosening ('wearing out'). Most total hip replacements would be expected to have ≥90% survival rates 10y after surgery.

References
1 http://www.orthoteers.co.uk/Nrujp~ij33lm/Orththr1.htm.
2 http://www.wheelessonline.com/o14/14.htm.
3 Huo MH, Muller MS (2004). What's new in hip arthroplasty. *J Bone Joint Surg Am* **86-A**: 2341–53.

Useful reading

Online orthopaedic hyperbooks

http://www.orthoteers.co.uk (requires subscription)
http://www.wheelessonline.com (free)
http://www.blackburnfeet.org.uk (free)
http://www.eatonhand.com (free)
http://www.eradius.com (free)

Reference textbooks

Elective

Canale T, Beaty JH (Eds.) (2007). *Campbell's operative orthopaedics*, 11th edn (4 vols). Mosby, London.

Trauma

McRae R, Esser M (2008). *Practical fracture treatment*, 5th edn. Churchill Livingstone, Edinburgh.

Schatzker J, Tile M (2005). *The rationale of operative fracture care*, 3rd edn. Springer-Verlag Berlin Heidelberg.

American College of Surgeons (2008). *Advanced trauma life support (ATLS) for doctors, student manual*, 8th edn. American College of Surgeons, Chicago.

Wenger DR, Pring ME (2006). *Rang's children's fractures*, 3rd edn. Lippincott, Williams and Wilkins, Philidelphia.

Bucholz RW, Court-Brown CM, Heckman JD, Tornetta P (Eds.) (2009). *Rockwood and Green's fractures in adults*. 7th edn. Lippincott, Williams, and Wilkins, Philadelphia.

Beaty JH, Kasser JR (Eds) (2009). *Rockwood and Wilkin's fractures in children*, 7th edn. Lippincott, Williams, and Wilkins, Philadelphia.

Review

Miller M (2008). *Review of orthopaedics*, 5th edn. Saunders, Philadelphia.

Soloman L, Warwick D, Nayagam S (Eds) (2010). *Apley's system of orthopaedics and fractures*, 9th edn. Hodder Arnold, London.

Ramachandran M (2007). *Basic orthopaedic sciences: the Stanmore guide*. Hodder Arnold, London.

Surgical exposures

Hoppenfeld S, De Boer P, Buckley R (2009). *Surgical exposures in orthopaedics: the anatomic approach*, 3rd edn. Lippincott, Williams, and Wilkins, Philadelphia.

Clinical examination

Harris N, Stanley D (Eds) (2005). *Advanced examination techniques in orthopaedics*. Cambridge University Press, Cambridge.

Plastic surgery

Suturing wounds

Principles of wound closure

A wound can be closed in the following ways:
- Direct apposition of skin edges by sutures, glue, or staples;
- Skin grafts (see 📖 p. 594).
- Flaps (see 📖 p. 596).

Key facts

A correctly orientated incision, adequate haemostasis, and minimal tissue handling are prerequisites for an ideal scar. When closing wounds, bear in mind the following:

- All wounds leave scars. You must warn your patient of this.
- Hypertrophic scars are more likely on the sternum and deltoid area.
- Speed of healing depends on site. The face heals more quickly than the trunk and limbs.
- Children and young adults heal more quickly and achieve stronger scars than the elderly, the chronically ill, and those on steroids.
- Stitch marks ('tramline effect') are caused by epithelial growth into suture tracks and occur when sutures are left in longer than 7 days.
- Cross-hatching is more common when tight sutures cause ischaemia.
- If sutures are removed too early, the wound may dehisce, leaving a worse scar.

Suture techniques

- Eliminate dead space with deep sutures or a drain, but avoid suturing fat, which contributes no strength and may lead to fat necrosis.
- Consider buried, interrupted dermal sutures to reduce skin tension.
- Dermal sutures can be combined with a subcuticular running suture or skin tapes to avoid suture marks.
- Use the finest suture possible to maintain wound closure—5/0 or 6/0 for the face; 4/0 or 5/0 for the hand; 2/0 to 4/0 for the trunk.
- Evert the wound to reduce dead space and allow rapid healing.
- Approximate wound edges without strangulating the skin.
- Dressings can be used to splint a wound or immobilize a limb during healing.
- Elevation will reduce post-operative swelling, bleeding, and pain.
- In a low tension wound closure, sutures may be removed at 5–7 days on the face, 7–10 days on the arm and anterior trunk, and 14 days on the back and lower limb.
- Most wounds benefit from being splinted with skin tape after removal of sutures.

Interrupted skin suture (see Fig. 16.1(a))
- Use fine-toothed Adson forceps or a skin hook to evert the skin.
- Pass the needle perpendicular to the skin through its full thickness.
- Either remove the needle through the wound or continue in one sweep to the other side of the wound, using the forceps for counter pressure so the needle passes perpendicular to the skin on its way out.
- Tie the knot so the skin edges are just apposed, bearing in mind the wound will swell post-operatively.
- Place the sutures evenly, approximately twice as far apart as they are from the wound margins.
- The distance between the suture and the wound margin should be similar to the thickness of the skin.

Mattress suture (see Fig. 16.1(b)) Pass the needle as above across the wound, then turn it around and pass it back as if doing another interrupted suture in the opposite direction. The second pass can be along the wound from the first (a horizontal mattress) or nearer the wound margin than the first pass (a vertical mattress suture).

Deep dermal suture (see Fig. 16.1(c)) Use the forceps or skin hook to evert the skin and pass the needle from deep to superficial on the dermal surface of the wound. Move to the other side of the wound and pass the needle from superficial to deep within the dermis. Tie a knot which should be buried deep in the wound.

Continuous suture (see Fig. 16.1(d)) A combination of repeated interrupted-type sutures or interrupted, then mattress sutures.

Subcuticular suture (see Fig. 16.1(e)) The suture is passed continuously within the dermis, usually near the dermo-epidermal junction, from one end of the wound to the other, and pulled tight. It may be secured with a knot buried deeply at either end or with skin tapes laid over the suture ends and the wound surface.

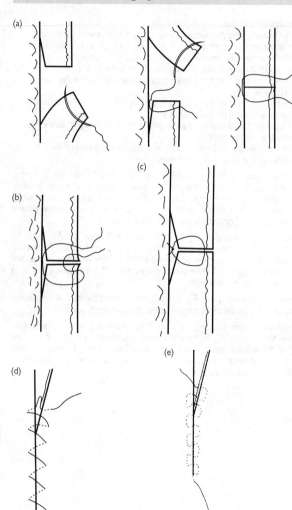

Fig. 16.1 Types of suture. (a) Interrupted suture. (b) Mattress suture.
(c) Deep dermal suture. (d) Continuous suture. (e) Subcuticular suture.

Skin grafts

Definition

A skin graft is a piece of dermis and epidermis that is completely removed from its original bodily attachment (the donor site). It is fixed to a recipient site and develops a new blood supply from the underlying tissue.

- *Autograft.* Transfer from one part of a person's body to another part.
- *Isograft.* Transfer between genetically identical individuals.
- *Allograft.* Transfer between individuals of the same species.
- *Xenograft.* Transfer between individuals of different species.

Full thickness skin grafts (Wolfe grafts) (see Table 16.1)

- Contain epidermis plus the entire thickness of dermis.
- Adnexal structures, e.g. hair, are included.
- Harvested by elliptical excision from sites of skin laxity, e.g. post-auricular skin crease, supraclavicular, preauricular, groin, or medial upper arm skin.
- Graft secured with a tie-over dressing, e.g. proflavine-soaked cotton wool, and inspected after a week.
- Donor site sutured closed.

Split thickness skin grafts (Thiersch grafts) (see Table 16.1)

- Consist of epidermis plus a variable thickness of dermis.
- Harvested by shaving off a layer of skin with a skin graft knife or dermatome. Can be taken from any area of the body (thigh skin most often used—plentiful and easy to access).
- Graft is often fenestrated (to stop blood or serous fluid collecting under it) or meshed (to expand the graft and allow it to contour to the wound bed).
- Graft secured with glue, sutures, or staples, then a non-adherent, compressive dressing. Inspected after 5 days.
- Defect heals by re-epithelialization from skin appendages.

Graft healing

Stages of graft take

- Adherence (immediate). Fibrin bond between graft and recipient bed.
- Serum imbibition (days 2–4). Graft absorbs fluid and nutrients from bed.
- Revascularization (after day 4). Blood enters the graft, either by flowing directly into the graft vessels (inoculation) or by new vessel ingrowth.

Reasons for graft failure

- Shearing. Revascularization cannot occur if the graft is mobile.
- Infection. Either of the bed or the graft tissue.
- Separation of graft from its bed. By haematoma or seroma.
- Inadequate bed, e.g. bare cortical bone; tendon without paratenon.
- Damage to the graft, e.g. poor surgical technique, excessive dressing pressure.

Table 16.1 Split thickness grafts versus full thickness grafts

	Split skin graft	Full thickness skin graft
Cosmesis	Thin, often hypertrophic skin	Good cosmesis
Contracture	Frequent	Less frequent
Availability	Plentiful; can re-harvest after 14 days	Limited by skin laxity
Take	Good—low metabolic needs	Needs optimal bed
Donor scar	Minimal—colour change only	Linear scar
Contraindications	Inadequate bed, e.g. exposed bone, tendon, cartilage (in which case flap needed) Infected bed Areas where cosmesis is paramount	Large area to be covered Inadequate bed

Vacuum dressings

These are dressings that apply negative pressure via a sponge placed in the wound cavity, covered with an airtight adhesive silicone sheet and connected to a vacuum pump. They increase the initial rate of granulation in a variety of wounds, including dehisced or infected sternotomy and laparotomy wounds, pressure sores, chronic open wounds, flaps, grafts, and burns. The dressing is changed every 48–72h. Fluid from the wound bed is collected in a disposable canister. Chronic wounds may heal by secondary intention (see 📖 p. 146) or be closed primarily.

Surgical flaps

Definition
A flap is a unit of tissue that maintains its own blood supply while being transferred from donor to recipient site.

Classification of flaps
Also see Fig. 16.2.

By blood supply
- *Random pattern.* Survive on blood vessels in dermal and subdermal plexuses which have no specific anatomical pattern. Length to breadth ratio is therefore limited to 1:1 (or 3:1 on the face).
- *Axial pattern.* Have at least one specific artery running longitudinally within the flap, so length to breadth ratio can be greatly increased.

All composite flaps and all free flaps have an axial blood supply.

By mode of transfer (for local flaps)
- *Advancement.* The base of the flap advances in the direction of the flap axis, e.g. V-Y flap of perianal skin into anal canal for anal stenosis.
- *Pivot.* Rotation or transposition. The flap rotates around a single pivot point, e.g. scalp rotation flap to cover facial defect after tumour excision.
- *Interpolation.* The flap pedicle passes over or under adjacent skin to inset the flap into a nearby defect, e.g. deltopectoral flap for head and neck reconstruction after radical tumour surgery.

Transfer of distant flaps
- *Direct.* Flap moved directly to non-adjacent area, e.g. cross finger flap.
- *Tubed.* Pedicle curled inwards to form a tube until base of flap divided, e.g. tubed flap from upper arm for nose reconstruction.
- *Free.* Artery and vein to flap are completely divided, then reattached with microvascular anastomoses to a suitable artery and vein at the recipient site, e.g. radial forearm flap to release neck scar contracture.

By composition
- *Cutaneous.* Skin and subcutaneous tissue only, e.g. groin flap.
- *Fasciocutaneous.* Includes deep fascia, making flap vascularity more reliable and allowing length to breadth ratio to be increased.
- *Fascial or adipofascial.* The fascia (and subcutaneous fat) is transferred, but the skin, still attached, is replaced on the donor site, e.g. temporalis fascial flap. The transposed flap can then be skin grafted.
- *Muscle.* Useful for infected or traumatic wounds. The flap is skin grafted, e.g. gastrocnemius flap for exposed knee prostheses.
- *Myocutaneous.* Used in reconstructive surgery. The muscle carries the blood supply to the skin, e.g. latissimus dorsi myocutaneous flap.
- *Perforator flaps.* Modified myocutaneous flaps. A single artery and vein are dissected from skin, through muscle, to the parent vessels. The muscle remains *in situ*, so its function is retained, e.g. deep inferior epigastric perforator (DIEP) flap.
- *Bone, osseocutaneous.* Bone with or without skin, e.g. fibular flap for reconstruction of mandible. Muscle may also be included.

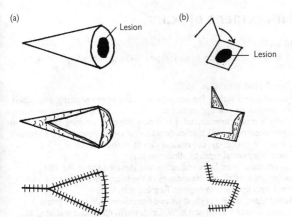

Fig. 16.2 Types of surgical flaps. (a) V-Y flap. (b) Rhomboid flap.

Management of scars

Definition
A scar is an area of fibrous connective tissue, produced by healing.

Clinical features
A normal scar is initially flat and pale, then becomes red, itchy, and raised. Over months to years, it settles back to a flat, pale, slightly shiny patch. Scarring is more pronounced if infection intervenes during healing or in the presence of foreign bodies. Scars settle more slowly in children and will improve over 2–3y, but resolve rapidly in the elderly.

There are several types of abnormal scar.
- *Hypertrophic scars.* Firm, red, itchy, and elevated above the skin surface, but within the boundaries of the injury. More common over presternal and deltoid regions. Regress with time.
- *Keloid scars.* Extend beyond wound boundaries. Do not regress spontaneously. Painful and itchy. Common in dark skins and sites as above.
- *Stretched scars.* Due to dehiscence of dermis under intact epidermis. Common on the back.
- *Scar contractures.* Common over flexor surfaces of joint. Occur when wounds heal by secondary intention, after split skin grafting, or when incisions cross a joint perpendicular to the crease.

Treatment
Treatment aims to improve poor cosmesis, relieve local symptoms (pain, itch, irritation), or reduce restriction of associated joint movement.

Medical/conservative treatment
- *Observation.* 'Benign neglect'.
- *Massage.* Scar achieves flat, pale state more quickly. Relieves itch.
- *Pressure.* Pressure garments for large areas, e.g. skin-grafted burns. Pressure devices, e.g. clip earrings for earlobe keloids. Worn continuously till scars mature. Reduce hypertrophy and contracture.
- *Silicone gel.* Either a sheet of gel tape worn on the scar or a jelly rubbed into it scar. Reduces hypertrophy and relieves itch.
- *Lasers.* Pulsed dye lasers used to reduce redness and hypertrophy. Carbon dioxide laser resurfaces depressed scars.
- *Intralesional injections.* Steroids and cytotoxics (e.g. bleomycin, 5-FU) reduce excess collagen formation; used to flatten hypertrophic and keloid scars and reduce pain and itch. Usually need repeated injections at 1–2-month intervals.
- *Radiotherapy.* Occasionally given immediately post-operatively to wounds in patients known to be prone to hypertrophic or keloid scarring.

Surgical treatment

- *Excision and closure.* For stretched scar or scar with 'tramlines'. Usually restretch to some extent. Keloid or hypertrophic scars are likely to recur if excised and may be much larger than the original scar. Keloids should only be excised in combination with a post-operative course of steroid injections.
- *Z-plasty* (see Fig. 16.3(a)). Lengthens scar. Can re-orientate scar into lines of relaxed skin tension, or break up the line of the scar and make it less noticeable.
- *W-plasty* (see Fig. 16.3(b)). Breaks up line of scar. Used on scalp to avoid a hairless linear scar.
- *Scar release and resurfacing.* Used when Z-plasty inadequate for scar release, either because there is insufficient laxity adjacent to the contracture or if adjacent skin is of poor quality. Resurfacing may include skin grafting, local flaps, or free tissue transfer.

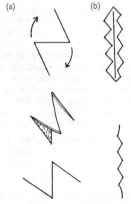

Fig. 16.3 Surgical techniques for managing scars. (a) Z-plasty. (b) W-plasty.

Excision of simple cutaneous lesions

Planning

- Under good light and before infiltration of anaesthesia, mark the borders of the lesion. Mark the appropriate margin of excision: 2–5mm for basal cell carcinoma (BCC), 4–6mm for squamous cell carcinoma (SCC), 1–2mm for biopsy of a pigmented lesion.
- Incision biopsies should include a border of the lesion and normal skin.
- For direct closure, convert the excision to an ellipse, using lines of relaxed skin tension as the long axis. Be guided by wrinkles and line of hair growth (hair generally grows in the direction of relaxed skin tension lines (RSTLs)).
- Wedge excisions are used on the borders of the ear, eyelid, and lip. Circular excisions are used where there is little skin laxity, using flaps or grafts to close the defect.

Anaesthesia

- Calculate the maximum safe dose for your patient (see 📖 p. 218).
- Consider a mixture of bupivacaine 0.25% with lidocaine 1% to provide longer acting anaesthesia. Adding sodium bicarbonate makes the injection less painful.
- Using adrenaline with the infiltration reduces intraoperative bleeding, but should not be used near anatomical 'end' arteries (e.g. the digital arteries) due to the risk of distal ischaemic necrosis.
- In the face, nerve blocks (e.g. mental, infraorbital, supraorbital, and supratrochlear) may reduce the pain of infiltration, the volume of anaesthetic needed, and distortion of the tissues by the anaesthetic fluid.
- Check the anaesthetic is working before starting excision.

Shave excision For benign, non-pigmented naevi and seborrhoeic keratoses. Use a number 10 blade to cut horizontally across the lesion at mid-dermal level.

Excision

- Be aware of underlying structures (e.g. the frontal branch of the temporal nerve when excising lesions from the temple). Ask your assistant to stretch the skin.
- Use a size 15 blade on the face; consider a larger size 10 blade on the thicker skin of the back.
- Cut the margins of the lesion perpendicular to the skin; this will aid closure.
- Cut away from the corners of the wound to avoid X-shaped overcuts. Cut the lower edge before the upper one; blood trickling down may obscure your view.
- Lift one corner of the lesion gently with a skin hook or fine-toothed (Adson's) forceps and cut along the base of the lesion in horizontal lines at the level of the subcutaneous fat. Avoid traumatic handling of the lesion, which may compromise histological analysis.
- Perform accurate haemostasis.
- Close and dress the wound.

Post-operative care

- All lesions should be sent for histological analysis, clearly labelled (if necessary with a marking stitch for orientation).
- Elevate the wound.
- Keep the wound dry until the skin is healed.
- Paracetamol, ibuprofen, and codeine are suitable analgesics; aspirin is best avoided due to risk of bleeding.
- Patients should not drive on the day of surgery.

Skin cancer

Key facts

- BCC, a neoplasm of the basal cells of the epidermis affects 20–40% Caucasians. It almost never metastasizes, but can invade deeply and may therefore be fatal.
- SCC is a malignant neoplasm of the keratinizing cells of the epidermis affecting 1 in 2000 Caucasians per year.
- Melanoma is a malignant neoplasm of melanocytes, with a lifetime risk of about 1 in 70 for Caucasians. The incidence has doubled over the past 20 y.

Clinical features

- Melanoma presents with a change in a pre-existing or new mole (naevus). Remember **A**symmetry; **B**order irregularity; **C**olour change or variegated colour; **D**iameter >6mm; **E**levation, itch, or bleeding. All these features are suspicious of melanoma.
- The typical BCC is a skin ulcer with a pearly edge and telangectasia; however, there may not be any of these features. A persistent, itchy, scaly patch in a sun-exposed area may also be a BCC.
- SCC typically presents as an ulcer with a raised, rolled edge, but also may take many forms from scaly patch to keratotic horn.

Risk factors

- Fair skin and blue eyes.
- Sun exposure, both adult and childhood, especially sunburn.
- Family history.
- Previous skin cancer.
- Immunosuppression, especially post-organ transplantation.
- Xeroderma pigmentosum.
- Pre-malignant lesions. Multiple atypical naevi and giant congenital naevi for melanoma; sebaceous naevus of Jadassohn for BCC; Bowen's disease, solar keratosis, and chronic ulcers for SCC.
- Radiotherapy.
- A variety of chemicals, e.g. arsenic and coal, predisposes to SCC and BCC.

Assessment

- History includes sun exposure, previous skin lesions, drug history, and family history.
- Examine the entire skin and palpate draining lymph nodes.
- Dermatoscopy is used to improve accuracy of clinical diagnosis of melanoma.

Management

Melanomas and SCCs are managed by skin cancer MDTs.

Melanoma

- All suspicious pigmented lesions are biopsied with a 2mm margin to include subcutaneous fat and sent for histological analysis.
- Surgery aims to cure melanoma. Radiotherapy and chemotherapy are used for palliation only. Wide local excision margins depend on the depth of invasion (Breslow thickness) of the tumour and are typically 1cm for lesions <1mm thick, 2cm for lesions 1–2cm thick, and 2–3cm for lesions >2cm thick.
- Sentinel lymph node biopsy may be considered, with lymph node dissection of the neck, axilla, or groin if positive.
- Prognosis depends on Breslow thickness, ulceration of the tumour, and lymph node involvement.

SCC

- Lesions are excised with a 4–6mm margin depending on the site; 95% of tumours are cured by this treatment.
- Moh's micrographic surgery probably gives the highest cure rate.
- Radiotherapy is used as an adjuvant treatment for metastatic tumours or as primary treatment if the tumour or the patient mean that surgery is not possible.
- Palpable lymph nodes in the draining basin are investigated by FNA, with lymphadenectomy if positive.
- Prognosis depends on diameter of lesion, depth of invasion, nerve or vessel invasion on histology

BCC

- Margins of 3–4mm are suitable for well-defined BCCs, but wider margins are used when margins are unclear and in recurrent tumours.
- Moh's micrographic surgery is also used, particularly when wide excision would leave an unacceptable defect, e.g. around the eye.
- Other treatment modalities include curettage and cautery, cryotherapy, radiotherapy, efudix, imiquimod.
- Ninety-five per cent of lesions are cured by complete excision, 99% with Moh's surgery. Radiotherapy cures 90%.

Burns: assessment

❶ Assessment and management of burns go hand in hand and are simultaneous in practice. They have been divided here only for ease of reading.

Causes Most burns are due to flame or contact with hot surfaces; scalds are more common in children and the elderly. Chemical, electrical, irradiation, and friction burns are rare.

History

• Find out the exact mechanism, including temperature of water, duration of contact, concentration of chemical, voltage.
• Record factors suggesting inhalation injury, e.g. burns in a confined space, flash burns.
• Enquire about other injuries.
• Document first aid given so far.
• Document timings of injury, first aid, and resuscitation.

Examination

Estimate area of burn Do not include areas of unblistered erythema.
• Rule of nines (see Fig. 16.4).
• Patient's hand is approximately 1% total body surface area (TBSA).
• Lund and Browder chart (see Fig. 16.5) is the most accurate method.
• Subtract % unburned skin from 100% to check calculation.
• Draw a picture, ideally filling in the Lund and Browder chart.

Estimating depth of burn

• *Epidermal*. Erythema only.
• *Superficial dermal*. Pink, wet or blistered, sensate, blanches and refills.
• *Deep dermal*. Blotchy red, wet or blistered, no blanching, insensate.
• *Full thickness*. White or charred, leathery, no blanching, insensate.

Signs of inhalation injury
• Singed nasal hair.
• Burns to face or oropharynx. Look for blistered palate.
• Sooty sputum.
• Drowsiness or confusion due to carbon monoxide inhalation.
• Respiratory effort, breathlessness, stridor, or hoarseness are signs of impending airway obstruction and require immediate intubation.

Features of non-accidental burns injury Refer to paediatric burns unit if suspected in a child. Features include:
• Delayed presentation.
• History inconsistent or not compatible with injury.
• Other signs of trauma.
• Suspicious pattern of injury, e.g. cigarette burns, bilateral 'shoes and socks' scalds.

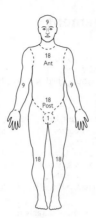

Fig. 16.4 Rule of nines.

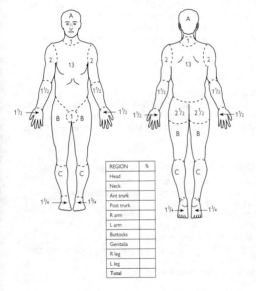

REGION	%
Head	
Neck	
Ant trunk	
Post trunk	
R arm	
L arm	
Buttocks	
Genitalia	
R leg	
L leg	
Total	

AREA	0	1	5	10	15	Adult
A = ½ of head	9½	8⅓	6½	5½	4½	3½
B = ½ of one thigh	2¾	3¼	4	3½	3½	4¾
C = ½ of one lower leg	2½	2½	2¾	3	3¼	3½

Fig. 16.5 Lund and Browder chart.

Burns: management

Immediate first aid
- Stop the burning process (do not endanger yourself).
- Cool the wound. Running water at 2–15°C for 20min (beware risk of hypothermia in infants, young children, and adults with >25% TBSA).

Resuscitation

- A. Airway maintenance with C-spine control. Intubate if suspected inhalation injury; airway oedema can be rapidly fatal.
- B. Breathing and ventilation.
- C. Circulation with haemorrhage control.
- D. Disability and neurological status.
- E. Exposure and environmental control.
- F. Fluid resuscitation: child, >10% TBSA; adult, >15% TBSA burned.

- Two large peripheral IV lines, preferably through unburned skin.
- Send blood for FBC, U&E, clotting, amylase, carboxyhaemoglobin.
- Give 3–4mL Hartmann's solution/kg/% TBSA burned. Half of this is given over the first 8h following injury, half over the next 16h.
- Children need maintenance fluid in addition.
- Monitor resuscitation with urinary catheter (aim for urine output 0.5–1mL/kg/h in adults and 1–1.5mL/kg/h in children).
- Consider ECG, pulse, BP, respiratory rate, pulse oximetry, ABGs.

Perform secondary survey.

Referral to a burns unit (see Box 16.1) Intubate before transfer if inhalation injury suspected. Give humidified 100% O_2 to all patients. Wash the burn and cover with cling film. Give IV morphine analgesia. Discuss NGT and catheter insertion with burns unit. Give tetanus prophylaxis if required.

Box 16.1 Criteria for referral to a burns unit
>10% TBSA burn in adult; >5% TBSA in child.
Burns to face, hands, feet, perineum, genitalia, major joints.
Full thickness burns >5% TBSA.
Electrical or chemical burns.
Associated inhalation injury—always intubate before transfer.
Circumferential burns of limbs or chest.
Burns in very young or old, pregnant women, and patients with significant comorbidities.
Any burn associated with major trauma.

Management of the burn wound

- Superficial dermal burns will heal without scarring within 2 weeks as long as infection does not deepen the burn.
- For small burns, outpatient treatment with simple, non-adherent dressings and twice weekly wound inspection is sufficient.
- Wash burns with normal saline or chlorhexidine.
- Debride large blisters. Elevate limbs to reduce pain and swelling.
- Dress hands in plastic bags to allow mobilization.
- Topical silver sulphadizine is used on deep burns to reduce risk of infection (but should not be applied until the patient has been reviewed by a burns unit as it makes depth difficult to assess).

Escharotomy Performed for circumferential full thickness burns to the chest that limit ventilation or to the limbs that limit circulation. Loss of pulses or sensation is a late sign. In the early stages, pain at rest or on passive movements of distal joints indicates ischaemia. Patients may also need fasciotomies.

Excision and skin grafting Performed for deep dermal or full thickness burns that are too large to heal rapidly by secondary intention.

Electrical injuries

- *Low voltage* (<1000V). Domestic electrical supply. Causes local contact wounds, but no deep injury. May cause cardiac arrest.
- *High voltage* (>1000V). High tension cables, power stations, lightning. Causes cutaneous and deep tissue damage with entry and exit wounds.
- ECG on admission for all injuries. Continuous cardiac monitoring for 24h for significant injuries.
- In high voltage injury, muscle damage may require fasciotomy.
- Myoglobinuria can cause renal failure. Urine output >75–100mL/h.

Chemical burns

Treat with copious lavage for at least 30min until all chemical has been removed and skin pH is normal.

- *Acid*. Causes coagulative necrosis; penetrates skin rapidly, but is easily removed.
- *Alkali* (includes common household chemicals and cement). Causes liquefactive necrosis so needs longer irrigation (>1h).
- *Hydrofluoric acid*. Fluoride ions penetrate burned skin, causing liquefactive necrosis and decalcification; 2% TBSA burn can be fatal.
  - Irrigate with water.
  - Trim fingernails.
  - Topical calcium gluconate gel, 10%.
  - Local injection of 10% calcium gluconate.
  - IV calcium gluconate.
  - May need urgent excision of burn.
- *Elemental Na, K, Mg, Li*. Do not irrigate initially; they ignite in water. Brush off particles and direct high pressure jet of water to wound.
- *Phosphorus*. Irrigate with water, then debride particles which will otherwise continue to burn. Apply copper sulphate which turns particles black so they are easier to identify.

- *Bitumen*. Burns by heat; treat by cooling with water. Remove cold bitumen with peanut or paraffin oil.
- *Tar*. Burns by heat. Treat by cooling with water; no need to remove tar as it gradually gets emulsified with topical ointments used for treatment.

Soft tissue hand injuries

History
- Mechanism of injury.
- Dominant hand, occupation, hobbies.
- Medical and smoking history, previous hand injuries, social history.

Examination

Use local anaesthetic block if needed for pain (check sensation first).

Look Posture of hand and digits. Site of laceration(s) and tissue loss.

Feel Perfusion of hand and digits, pulses. Sensation in distribution of radial, ulnar, median, and digital nerves. Pain over bones.

Move
- Long extensors extend MCPJs.
- EPL extends thumb dorsal to plane of hand (i.e. up off a table).
- FDP tendons flex DIPJs.
- FDS tendons flex PIPJs. Isolate FDS by holding all digits except the one under examination extended.
- Testing wrist flexors and extensors is unreliable as finger flexors and extensors may mimic function, but pain on movement suggests injury.
- Examine intrinsics, hypothenar and thenar muscles, particularly abductor pollicis brevis (supplied by median nerve) and Froment's sign (for adductor pollicis supplied by ulnar nerve).
- Check stability of joints. Pain or abnormal movement on lateral deviation suggests collateral ligament damage.

Investigations X-ray for fractures of foreign bodies. Photographs.

Treatment
- *Finger pulp injury.* Debride under tourniquet. If there is no bone exposed, it will heal by secondary intention. Exposed bone may need surgery to shorten bone or cover it with a local flap.
- *Subungual haematoma.* Painful bruise under nail. Trephine nail with sterile needle to evacuate haematoma.
- *Nailbed injury.* Often with distal phalanx (DP) fracture. Remove nail under tourniquet; irrigate wound; repair nail with absorbable 7/0 suture using loupe magnification. Replace fenestrated nail as splint for eponychial fold.
- *Mallet finger.* Immobilize in stack splint for 6–8 weeks unless large bony fragment present which may require surgical fixation.
- *Foreign bodies.* Remove organic matter and painful foreign bodies.
- *Lacerations and puncture wounds.*
  - Always explore with anaesthetic and tourniquet to determine underlying structural damage.
  - Irrigate wounds and debride as necessary.
  - Tetanus prophylaxis (see 📖 p. 175).
  - Co-amoxiclav (500mg tds PO) for bites.

- Repair tendons, ideally primarily. Post-operative regimes typically involve splints for 6 weeks and 6 more weeks without heavy lifting.
- Repair nerves under magnification. Axonal regeneration progresses at 1mm/day after 1 month from repair.
- Thoroughly irrigate open joints due to the risk of septic arthritis. Collateral ligaments may need to be repaired and are splinted for around 4 weeks post-repair.
- *Complications*. Haematoma, infection, tendon or ligament rupture, stiffness, painful scars, neuroma, complex regional pain syndrome, scar contracture, cold sensitivity.

Hand infections

Key facts

Usually follows a penetrating injury (which may seem insignificant) or a bite. Haematogenous spread of infection to the hand is rare.

- *Infecting organisms.* After penetrating injury, *Staphylococcus aureus* is the most common, followed by streptococci. Human bites are often also contaminated with *Eikenella corrodens*. Viruses (hepatitis B and C, HIV) are rarely transmitted. *Pasteurella* spp. are common in infected cat and dog bites.
- *Paronychia.* Infection of nailfold. *Candida albicans* causes chronic paronychia and may require excision of crescent of epinychium and topical antifungals. *Herpes simplex* causes whitlow with vesicles or bullae around the nail, but no pus. Avoid surgery in these cases.
- *Felon.* Finger pulp infection.
- *Palmar space infection.* There are four fascial compartments in the palm (web space, hypothenar, mid-palm, and thenar). They usually confine infection initially. Pain, swelling, and reduced movement are features. Swelling is often more prominent on the dorsal surface of hand.
- *Flexor sheath infection.* The cardinal signs are flexed posture of finger, pain on passive extension, fusiform swelling, pain along flexor sheath. Often requires continuous saline irrigation for 24–48h post-drainage.
- *Bites.* High risk of infection so always irrigate, give antibiotic prophylaxis (co-amoxiclav 500mg PO tds), and refer for surgical exploration.

Treatment

Delay can be disastrous, resulting in stiffness, contracture, and pain. Early cellulitis (24–48h after onset) may be treated by elevation, splints, and antibiotics. Any collection of pus must be drained urgently.

Initial treatment

- Tetanus prophylaxis if indicated.
- Elevation and splintage.
- IV co-amoxiclav 1g tds (unless penicillin allergy) till sensitivities known.
- Plain X-ray may be useful to exclude associated fractures, foreign bodies, underlying osteomyelitis, and evidence of gas-forming infection.

Surgical treatment

- Use a tourniquet, but elevate rather than exsanguinate the limb.
- Send pus swabs and tissue samples for culture.
- Debride and irrigate wounds; fully explore pockets of pus.
- Leave wound open for delayed primary closure.

Post-operative care

- Continue elevation.
- Daily saline soaks or irrigation of the wound.
- Splint for comfort with wrist extended, MCPJs flexed, and interphalangeal joints (IPJs) extended. Mobilize with physiotherapists.
- Antibiotics until infection resolved.

Dupuytren's disease

Key facts
A progressive thickening of the palmar and digital fascia that may lead to contractures. Aetiology is unknown, but there is a higher incidence among relatives of affected patients. Associated conditions include diabetes and epilepsy. Alcoholism, TB, HIV, hand trauma, and tobacco have all also been implicated. Incidence is 1–3% of northern Europeans, but it is uncommon in Africa and Asia. It increases with age; ♂ > ♀, approximately 7:1.

Pathogenesis
- Disease classified by Luck into three phases: proliferative, involutional, and residual.
- In the proliferative phase, immature fibroblasts, many of which are myofibroblasts, produce extracellular matrix containing type IV collagen. Resembles a healing wound histologically.
- Mechanical tension appears to play a role in contractures.

Clinical features
- Thickened palmar and digital fascia forms nodules and cords.
- Progresses to contractures of the MCPJs and PIPJs of the affected rays.
- Tends to affect digits in order: ring, little, thumb, middle, index.
- Normal fascia is referred to as bands; diseased bands are called cords.
- A spiral cord may be a feature, wrapping around the neurovascular bundle (NVB) and displacing it to the midline and superficially, putting it at risk during surgery.
- The disease affects longitudinal fascial structures; the transverse palmar fascia is never involved and provides a landmark for dissecting NVBs.

Extra-palmar manifestations
- Garrod's pads. Thickening over dorsal aspect of PIPJs.
- Peyronie's disease. Thickened plaques in the shaft of the penis.
- Ledderhose's disease. Thickened plantar fascia.

Treatment
Indications for surgery
- Over 30° fixed flexion contracture at MCPJ or any PIPJ contracture. Also any rapidly progressing contracture. Results are better for release of MCPJs than PIPJs.
- Tabletop test. Surgery indicated when hand will not lie flat on table.
- Pain in nodules or Garrod's patches. Injection with steroid or excision.

Many people with Dupuytren's disease never require surgery.

Surgical considerations

Skin

Typical incisions include the following.
- Linear incisions with Z-plasties.
- Bruner incisions.
- Multiple V to Y incisions.
- Lazy 'S' incisions.
- Transverse palmar incision with longitudinal extensions.
- Multiple short curved incisions.
- Multiple Z-plasties.

Closure may be direct with skin grafts (split or full thickness) or palm left open to heal by secondary intention.

Fascia

This may be incised (fasciotomy) or excised (fasciectomy).
- Radical fasciectomy removes the entire palmar fascia.
- Regional or limited fasciectomy removes only the diseased fascia.
- Segmental fasciectomy excises sections of the diseased cord.
- Fasciotomy via a percutaneous approach using a needle provides temporary relief from contracture.
- Dermofasciectomy. Excision of fascia with overlying skin, used for severe skin involvement and where risk of recurrence is high, e.g. surgery for recurrent disease.
- Specimens are sent for histological analysis to rule out the rare differential diagnosis of epithelioid sarcoma.

Joint contractures

Release of fascia usually resolves contracture at the MCPJ. Fixed flexion at the PIPJ is more difficult to release and contracture often recurs. Consider releasing the check-rein and accessory collateral ligaments. DIPJs are rarely involved except in recurrent disease.

Post-operative care The affected fingers are splinted in extension and active exercises begun in the first week, unless a skin graft has been used. Night splints are used for at least 3 months.

Complications

- *Early.* Damage to neurovascular structures (1–3%), PIPJ hyperextension, haemorrhage.
- *Intermediate.* Infection, skin flap necrosis.
- *Late.* Complex regional pain syndrome; recurrence (25% of patients treated surgically will need further surgery for Dupuytren's disease).

Treatment of recurrence

Recurrence may be treated by repeat surgery although this tends to be less successful and more extensive at each event. Amputation of a fixed flexed digit is occasionally an option, particularly if the digit hampers work or leisure activities.

Breast reduction

To reduce the volume and weight of the hypertrophied breast while maintaining a blood supply to the nipple and creating an aesthetically pleasing breast.

Indications

- Neck, back, or shoulder pain.
- Indentation of shoulder skin by bra straps.
- Persistent infections or soreness in the inframammary crease.
- Restriction in activity, especially sport.
- Inability to find clothes that fit.
- Psychological. Embarrassment, low self-esteem, loss of sexual appeal.

Operative considerations

Blood supply to the nipple

In order to lift the nipple, skin around it is de-epithelialized or excised. The base of the nipple is left attached to a mound of breast parenchyma (the pedicle) through which its blood supply travels. Due to the rich vascular anastamoses in the breast, numerous techniques are possible. Pedicles can be based inferiorly, superiorly, supero-medially, laterally, or centrally. Alternatively, the nipple can be removed before the breast is reduced and replaced as a full thickness graft.

Skin excision and scars

An anchor shape (Wise pattern) excision leaves an inverted 'T-shaped scar. It runs around the areola, vertically down to the inframammary fold and horizontally along the fold. Other options include periareolar incision only or periareolar incision with a vertical scar. These techniques limit the amount of breast tissue that can be resected. L-shaped and horizontal scar techniques are also possible, but more rarely used.

Post-operative care

The patient usually stays in hospital overnight or longer if drains are used. She should wear a supportive bra and avoid heavy lifting for 4–6 weeks post-operatively.

Complications

- *Early*. Haematoma, infection, altered nipple sensation, skin loss or necrosis, fat necrosis, delayed wound healing, asymmetry.
- *Late*. Unsightly scar, inability to breastfeed, pseudoptosis ('bottoming out'), recurrence (if done before breast fully grown).

However, most patients are happy with the result, even if they do suffer complications.

Breast augmentation

To enhance breast size by placing an artificial implant beneath the breast.

Indications

Performed for asymmetry, hypoplasia, and psychological reasons, e.g. self-consciousness or problems with sexual relationships. Inadequate breast volume may be due to hypoplasia or involution following childbirth or menopause.

Operative considerations

Incision

- *Inframammary fold.* Good visualization of implant pocket; visible scar.
- *Periareolar.* Semicircular incision at the border of the areolus. Scar fades well, but access is limited. More likely to alter nipple sensation.
- *Transaxillary.* Eliminates scars on breast. Limited access improved by using endoscope. Better for subpectoral implants.
- *Transumbilical.* Only used for saline-filled implants, inserted along a tunnel created superficial to rectus sheath. Endoscope confirms position of implant pocket. Implant inflated once in position.

Position of implant

- *Submammary.* Under the normal breast.
- *Subpectoral.* Under the pectoralis major (slightly less obvious upper border in the thin; have lower rates of capsular contracture, but may move when the pectoralis contracts).

Type of implant

- *Size.* Depends on patient's choice.
- *Shape.* Round implants are low or high profile (depending on how much they project forwards); anatomical implants are teardrop-shaped.
- *Shell.* Implants are made of a silicone shell that is smooth or textured. Textured implants have lower rates of capsular contracture.
- *Implant filling.* Saline-filled implants allow for fine adjustment of volume and can be filled or emptied post-operatively. Silicone gel-filled implants feel more like normal breast tissue. No current evidence to support implication of silicone in causing autoimmune diseases.

Post-operative care

- Usually an overnight stay procedure (longer if drains are used).
- A supportive bra is worn and heavy lifting avoided for 4–6 weeks.

Complications

- *Early.* Haematoma, infection, nerve injury (altering sensation to the nipple), incorrect position of implant.
- *Late.* Capsular contracture, rupture, or deflation; silicone gel bleed.
- Implants have a limited lifespan, up to about 20y. The likelihood is that they will need to be removed or replaced at some time. Patients can usually breastfeed after augmentation. Patients are warned that mammography is technically more difficult, requiring different views.

Breast reconstruction

Aims

To recreate a breast mound resembling the contralateral breast with minimal donor deficit, using a technique appropriate for the patient. After mastectomy, breast reconstruction is of psychological benefit. It is technically easier to perform it at the same time as mastectomy, rather than as a delayed procedure as there is no scarring around the breast and original landmarks are present. It also reduces the number of operations required. However, there may be logistical difficulties if a combined breast surgery/plastic surgery team is needed. Also, some patients prefer to wait.

Surgical options

Tissue expander

Placed in the subpectoral position. Inflated with saline once the wounds are healed (2–4 weeks post-operatively) via a subcutaneous port. The skin is slowly stretched until a satisfactory size is reached. The implant can later be changed for a silicone gel-filled implant.

Latissimus dorsi myocutaneous flap

A pedicled flap based on the thoracodorsal vessels. The latissimus dorsi muscle, with an ellipse of overlying skin and fat, is tunnelled under the intervening skin bridge into the breast defect. Depending on the size of the contralateral breast, an implant may be used under the flap.

Abdominal flaps

The transverse rectus abdominis myocutaneous (TRAM) flap consists of a transverse ellipse of skin on the lower abdomen, plus one of the two rectus abdominis muscles. This versatile flap may be based on either its upper (deep superior epigastric) or lower (deep inferior epigastric) vascular pedicles. The upper pedicle is used as a pedicled flap, tunnelled under the abdominal skin into the breast. The lower pedicle is used as a free tissue transfer. If a sizeable muscular perforator vessel is identified, a DIEP flap can be used, leaving the muscle behind. This flap is usually large enough not to need an implant.

Nipple reconstruction At a later stage, the reconstructed breast can be tattooed with a picture of a nipple or a nipple formed with a combination of local flaps, skin graft, and grafts from the contralateral nipple.

Surgery to the contralateral breast The opposite breast may be reduced, augmented, or lifted to improve symmetry.

Cardiothoracic surgery

Basics

Common cardiac emergencies

Atrial fibrillation (see 📖 p. 55)
- Give 10–20mmol K⁺ via central line to get serum K⁺ 4.5–5.0mmol/L.
- Give empirical 20mmol Mg⁺ via central line if none given post-op.
- Give of 300mg amiodarone IV over 1h in patients with good left ventricle, followed by 900mg amiodarone IV over 23h.
- In patient with poor left ventricular function, give digoxin in 125mcg increments IV every 20min until rate control is obtained, up to a maximum of 1500mcg in 24h.
- Synchronized DC cardioversion for unstable patients (📖 p. 189).

Bleeding (see 📖 p. 180)
- Get immediate help if bleeding is >400mL in 30min.
- Give gelofusine to get CVP 10–14 and systolic BP 80–100mmHg.
- Order further 4U of blood, 2U FFP, and 2 pools platelets.
- Send clotting and FBC, request a CXR.
- Transfuse to achieve Hb >8.0g/dL, platelets >100 x 10⁹/L, APTT <40.
- Give empirical protamine 25mg IV.
- Emergency re-exploration is indicated for excessive bleeding.

Profound hypotension
- Get immediate help.
- Quickly assess pulse, rhythm, rate, CVP, O₂ sats, and bleeding.
- Defibrillate VF or pulseless VT, treat AF as above.
- Treat bradycardia with atropine 0.3mg IV or pace.
- Give gelofusine to raise CVP to 12–16mmHg, place bed head down.
- If suspect cardiac tamponade (📖 p. 480), prepare for re-sternotomy.
- If patient warm and vasodilated, draw up 10micrograms of metaraminol into 10mL of saline and give 1mL through a central line, and flush.
- If patient still profoundly hypotensive, give 1mL 1:10 000 adrenaline IV.

Poor gases (see 📖 p. 108)
- If O₂ sats <85% and falling, get immediate help.
- Increase the FiO₂ to 100% temporarily, check the pulse oximeter.
- Look at expansion, auscultate the chest, check PaO₂.
- If you suspect tension pneumothorax, treat immediately (📖 p. 480).
- Suction the ET tube, check that the patient is not biting on it.
- Check that the drain tubing is patent and drains are on suction.
- Treat bronchospasm with salbutamol 5mg nebulizer.
- Disconnect from the ventilator and hand-ventilate the patient.
- Get a CXR: look for pneumothorax, haemothorax, atelectasis, ET tube position, and lobar collapse, and treat (see 📖 p. 108).

Poor urine output (see 📖 p. 112)
- Check that the Foley catheter is patent.
- If the patient is hypotensive, treat this first.
- Give a fluid challenge of gelofusine to raise the CVP to 14mmHg.
- If not hypotensive and CVP >14mmHg, give 20mg furosemide IV.

Key revision points: coronary artery anatomy (see Fig. 17.1)

- *The left main stem* (LMS) arises from the ostium of the left sinus of Valsalva, travels between the pulmonary trunk anteriorly and the left atrial (LA) appendage to the left atrioventricular (AV) groove, dividing after 1–2cm into left anterior descending (LAD) artery, circumflex (Cx), and occasionally a third artery (the intermediate). As it provides almost the entire blood supply to the left ventricle (LV), occlusion can be fatal; severe left main disease is known as 'the widow maker'.
- The *LAD* runs down the anterior interventricular groove to the apex of the heart, usually extending round the apex to the posterior interventricular groove. A variable number of *diagonals* are given off over the anterior surface of the LV, small branches supply the anterior surface of the right ventricle (RV), and superior *septals* are given off perpendicularly to supply the anterior two-thirds of the interventricular septum. Occlusions of the LAD result in anterior MI.
- The *circumflex* originates at 90° from the LMS and runs medially to the LA appendage for 2–3cm, continuing in the posterior left AV groove to the crux of the heart. Occlusions of the Cx result in posterior infarcts. In left dominant hearts (5–10%), the Cx turns 90° into the posterior interventricular groove to form the posterior descending artery (PDA). In 85–90% of hearts, the PDA arises from the right coronary artery (RCA) (right dominant). About 5% of hearts are co-dominant.
- A variable number of *obtuse marginals* (OMs) arise from the Cx to supply the posterior LV. The first branch of the Cx is the *AV nodal artery* in which 45% course round the LA near the AV groove.
- The *RCA* arises from an ostium in the right sinus of Valsalva, gives off an *infundibular branch* and then a branch to the *sinoatrial (SA) node*, and runs immediately into the deep right AV groove where it gives off *RV branches* to the anterior RV wall. Occlusions of the RCA result in inferior infarcts and bradycardia. The *acute marginal* is a large branch which crosses the acute margin of the heart. In right dominant hearts, the RCA reaches the crux of the hearts where it turns 90° to form the *PDA*, which runs in the posterior interventricular groove. *Inferior septals*, which supply the inferior third of the interventricular septum, arise from 90° from the PDA. The *AV node artery* is given off by the RCA in 55% at the crux.

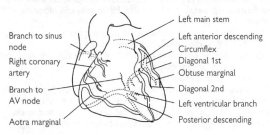

Branch to sinus node

Right coronary artery

Branch to AV node

Aotra marginal

Left main stem

Left anterior descending

Circumflex

Diagonal 1st

Obtuse marginal

Diagonal 2nd

Left ventricular branch

Posterior descending

Fig. 17.1 Coronary artery anatomy.

Principles of cardiac surgery

Key facts
- The majority of procedures are coronary artery bypass graft (CABG) operations, followed by aortic valve replacements, and mitral valve (MV) repair and replacements.
- Many patients are elderly with multiple comorbidities, but 90% should be out of ICU within a day or two, and ready to go home in a week.

Preoperative preparation
Careful preoperative work-up is essential. All investigations must be checked; small abnormalities which would not cause a problem in other specialties can have catastrophic results in cardiac surgery.
- *Full history.* Quantify symptoms, previous MI or stroke. Comorbidities (especially COPD, renal failure, peripheral vascular disease), MI <90 days (which increases mortality), drugs (aspirin, clopidogrel, and warfarin normally stopped 5 days preop to reduce bleeding), allergies, recent chest infection. Valve patients must have been cleared by dentist. Ask about previous heart surgery, varicose vein surgery.
- *Full examination.* Look for signs of heart failure. Active infection, e.g. abscess is a relative contraindication to valve replacement. Look at conduit: any evidence of varicose veins?
- All patients should have FBC, U&E, LFTs, clotting screen.
- Cross-match 2U of blood.
- ECG and CXR.
- All patients undergoing coronary artery surgery and patients >35y undergoing valve surgery should have coronary angiogram less than 1y-old.
- Patients undergoing valve surgery must have had an echo.
- Carotid duplex in any patient with history of stroke, TIA, or carotid bruits; some centres perform these routinely in patients >70y old.
- Consent by registrar or consultant.
- Sliding scale for diabetic patients (see 🕮 p. 52).

Cardiopulmonary bypass (CBP)
Any operation that involves stopping or opening the heart (valve surgery, surgery on septal defects) or great vessels (ascending and arch aortic dissection and aneurysm surgery, resection of some tumours invading great vessels, e.g. renal cell) requires CPB to maintain blood flow. This involves:
- *Heparinizing* the patient so that blood does not clot in the CPB circuit.
- Securing a 24F aortic cannula in the ascending aorta.
- Securing a 32F venous cannula in the RA or in the superior vena cava (SVC) and inferior vena cava (IVC).
- Connecting both cannulae to the bypass circuit.
- The venous return from the body is siphoned into the bypass circuit.
- The venous blood is oxygenated, filtered, and can be cooled or warmed, and is pumped back to the patient via the aortic cannula.
- At the end of bypass, heparin is reversed with protamine.

- Complications of CPB include stroke (atheromatous emboli, hypoperfusion, air, microemboli), SIRS, renal and pulmonary dysfunction (see 📖 p. 622).

Pathophysiology of CPB

CPB is unavoidable for many operations. It has a major impact on nearly every organ system and problems associated with bypass include:
- Activation of coagulation and complement cascades.
- Consumption of platelets and clotting factors, causing coagulopathy.
- Microemboli and atherosclerotic emboli from aortic cannulation which can cause stroke and peripheral limb and end-organ ischaemia.
- Increased capillary permeability.
- Renal, pulmonary, hepatic, and pancreatic dysfunction.

Cardioplegia

CPB does not stop the heart; it just bypasses the beating heart. If the surgeon wants to operate on a still heart, CPB gives the surgeon three options: fibrillate the heart, cool the patient, or use cardioplegia. Cardioplegic arrest is by far the commonest technique.
- Cardioplegia is a potassium rich solution.
- It can be based on blood or crystalloid (blood delivers O_2 better).
- It can be warm or cold (cold may reduce ischaemic injury more).
- It is delivered into the coronary arteries, either anterogradely by inserting a cannula into the aortic root which is clamped distal to the cardioplegia cannula or retrogradely via the coronary sinus vein.
- It can be given continuously or intermittently, every 20min or so.
- Cardioplegia arrests the heart and prevents myocardial ischaemia.

Post-operative management

Management of five common post-operative emergencies is outlined on 📖 p. 620. Most patients are well enough to be extubated within 6h, leave ITU within 24h, and go home within 5 days. Stable patients should have bloods, CXRs, and ECGs on days 1, 2, 4, and 6.

First 6 hours
- Myocardial function deteriorates due to ischaemia-reperfusion injury.
- Inotropic support and pacing may be required.
- Patient should be fit for extubation by 6h post-op.
- Patients should have diuresis >1mL/kg/h.
- Mediastinal bleeding should steadily decrease.
- Insulin requirements usually increase.

Days 1–2
- Inotropes and pacing weaned, invasive monitoring lines removed.
- Chest drains removed after 2h of zero drainage.
- Catheter and any epidural removed, patient mobilized.
- PCA morphine reduced to oral analgesia.
- Patient should be on aspirin, low molecular weight heparin, furosemide.
- Patient normally eating and drinking.

Days 3–5
• Temporary pacing removed if ECG satisfactory.
• Valve repair patients should undergo echocardiography.
• Physiotherapists assess exercise tolerance.
• Back to baseline weight, medications stabilized, ready for discharge.

Coronary artery disease

Coronary artery disease

Definition
Narrowing of the coronary arteries caused by atherosclerosis (see 📖 p. 152).

Incidence
Five in 1000 males over 40y have symptomatic ischaemic heart disease (IHD), 5 in 1000 heart attacks per year, 6000 coronary artery operations per year in the UK.

Aetiology
Age, male sex, smoking, ↑ BP, diabetes, hyperlipidaemia, obesity, family history, stress.

Pathology
See 📖 p. 152 for description of atherosclerotic disease. Stenoses tend progress in severity and distribution. Rate of progression is variable and regression of lesions has been observed.
- Narrowings of 50% of cross-sectional area limit coronary flow reserve (the increase in blood flow that occurs to meet increased O_2 demand).
- Coronary blood flow at rest is reduced by narrowings of 90%.
- LV function may be abnormal. In normal people, global LV systolic function improves with exercise, but in patients with coronary artery disease (CAD), it gets worse in the area supplied by the stenotic arteries.
- *Acute MI* is caused by acute total or subtotal vessel thrombotic occlusion. Patients with proximal LAD lesions are particularly at risk (see 📖 p. 54 for description of anatomic territories).

Clinical features
- *Angina and/or dyspnoea.* Severity is classified using the New York Heart Association (NYHA) score. Dyspnoea implies congestive heart failure (CCF).
- *Class I.* Symptoms only with prolonged or strenuous exertion.
- *Class II.* Symptoms causing slight limitation of ordinary activity.
- *Class III.* Symptoms with marked limitation of ordinary activity.
- *Class IV.* Angina occurring even with mild activity or at rest.

Diagnosis
- History and examination.
- ECG may show evidence of old infarcts.
- Exercise treadmill has 97% specificity for exertional angina.
- Coronary angiography is diagnostic and obligatory for planning surgery.
- Myocardial perfusion studies such as thallium scans are also useful.
- CT coronary angiography is increasingly used to screen lower risk patients, but is not helpful in evaluating lesions in high risk patients.

Indications for surgery

The options are medical and percutaneous coronary intervention (angioplasty or stent). Many large trials have been carried out to decide which groups of patients benefit most from surgery. This is currently:

* Patients with >70% LMS stenosis.
* Symptomatic patients with >70% proximal LAD stenosis.
* Symptomatic patients with >70% disease in all three vessels (three-vessel disease).
* Patients with less significant coronary disease having cardiac surgery for other reasons, e.g. valve replacement.

Coronary artery bypass surgery

Median sternotomy. A piece of conduit (saphenous vein, left internal thoracic artery (LITA), radial artery) is anastomosed to the coronary artery beyond the lesion and then to the ascending aorta. The LITA is usually anastomosed to the LAD because this combination remains patent for decades and the LAD is the most important stenosis to treat. The LITA is a branch of the left subclavian artery and runs down the inside of the rib cage 2cm lateral to the sternum. The origin from the subclavian is left intact; it does not need to be anastomosed to the aorta.

* Coronary artery bypass is mostly performed on-pump (with the use of a CPB machine) on the still heart.
* Performing on the beating heart off-pump (without CPB) is more difficult, but gives some advantages (see 📖 p. 622).

Complications

Complications (see 📖 p. 620) are more likely with advanced age, poor LV function, renal failure, COPD. Risk of mortality is scored, e.g. EUROscore.

* Death, 0–1% in low risk patients.
* Stroke, 1–2% in low risk patients.
* Re-sternotomy for bleeding or tamponade 5%.
* Chest infection, AF, wound infection, renal failure.

Prognosis

* In untreated patients with symptoms severe enough to warrant coronary angiography, 10% have an acute MI within 1y and 30% have an acute MI within 5y. Hospital mortality of MI is 7–10%.
* In three-vessel disease, the 5y survival is 50%, lower if LV function is impaired.
* LMS disease has a 2y survival of 50%.

Valvular heart disease

Mitral regurgitation (MR)
- *Incidence* Commonest valvular lesion. Prevalence 2–6%.
- *Aetiology* MV prolapse (congenital or rupture of chordae/papillary muscles), rheumatic disease, endocarditis, connective tissue disorders.
- *Clinical features* Acute MR presents with signs of CCF. Chronic MR causes exertional dyspnoea, orthopnoea. Displaced apex beat, soft S1, pansystolic murmur—loudest at apex, radiating to axilla. AF in 80%.
- *Diagnosis* CXR shows cardiomegaly. Transthoracic echocardiogram (TTE) diagnostic.
- *Indications for surgery* Acute MR, severe chronic MR.
- *Prognosis* Mortality of untreated severe MR is 5% per year. Operative mortality is 2–3% for low risk cases.

Mitral stenosis
- *Incidence* Prevalence <1% in west, commoner in Asia and Africa.
- *Aetiology* Rheumatic heart disease.
- *Clinical features* Dyspnoea, bronchitis, haemoptysis, AF, left parasternal heave, tapping apex beat, loud S1, rumbling mid-diastolic murmur at apex.
- *Diagnosis* CXR shows splaying of carina (enlarged LA). Echo diagnostic.
- *Indications for surgery* MV area <1.0cm^2 (normal valve 3–4cm^2).
- *Prognosis* Poor once symptoms of heart failure present.

Aortic stenosis
- *Incidence* Prevalence 1–2% in age over 65.
- *Aetiology* Calcific degeneration, bicuspid valve, rheumatic disease.
- *Clinical features* Triad of angina, syncope, dyspnoea. Sudden death. Slow rising and low volume pulse, heaving apex beat, reversed splitting S2, ejection systolic murmur loudest in aortic area radiating to carotids.
- *Diagnosis* ECG shows LV hypertrophy, TTE diagnostic.
- *Indications for surgery* Symptomatic aortic stenosis.
- *Prognosis* Without surgery, 50% of patients with angina are dead in 5y, 50% with syncope are dead in 3y, and 50% with dyspnoea are dead in 2y. UK perioperative mortality is 3–5%.

Aortic regurgitation (AR)
- *Incidence* Less than 1% prevalence.
- *Aetiology* Rheumatoid, endocarditis, aortic dissection, Marfan's and other connective tissue disorders, calcific degeneration, trauma.
- *Clinical features* Acute AR (endocarditis) presents with signs of left ventricular failure (LVF). Chronic AR often asymptomatic. Later, orthopnoea, fatigue, dyspnoea. Signs of wide pulse pressure, collapsing water hammer pulse, Quinke's sign (nail bed pulsation), Corrigan's sign (visible neck pulsation), De Musset's sign (head nodding), Durozier' sign (femoral diastolic murmur), hyperdynamic displaced apex beat, early diastolic murmur, Austin Flint mid-diastolic murmur due to regurgitant stream hitting anterior MV cusp.
- *Diagnosis* CXR shows cardiomegaly. TTE diagnostic.

- *Indications for surgery* Acute AR is a surgical emergency. Chronic AR is operated on before the ejection fraction <55% or LV dilates >5.5cm.
- *Prognosis* Acute AR has poor prognosis. Chronic AR has good outcome until failure occurs (50% 2y mortality). UK operative mortality is 3–5%.

Options for valve surgery

MV repair (annuloplasty and valvuloplasty)
Results of repair of the aortic valve are unpredictable so it is usually replaced. The MV is often repaired with good results.

Mechanical valves, e.g. St Jude mechanical, Carbomedics
These are made of ceramic. They can be mono- or bileaflet. Ball-and-cage like the Starr Edwards is no longer used.
- *Advantages.* Last forever so patient will not need future surgery.
- *Disadvantages.* Thromboembolic so patient must be warfarinized; patients with bleeding diatheses, women of childbearing age, professional sports players may not be suitable for long-term warfarinization.

Tissue valves (xenografts), e.g. Mosaic, Perimount
These are made of pig valves or cow or horse pericardium, usually suspended on a metal frame covered by a cloth sewing ring.
- *Advantages.* Patient does not need to be warfarinized.
- *Disadvantages.* Tissue valves last for 10–15y in the aortic position and 6–10y in the mitral position, depending on the age of the patient; younger patients (<65–70y) will often need a second operation.

Principles of valve surgery
Median sternotomy incision. MV may be approached via R thoracotomy. Valve surgery must be carried out with CPB (see 📖 p. 626).

Complications
Complications (see 📖 p. 620) are more likely with advanced age, poor LV function, renal failure, COPD, pulmonary hypertension, additional CABG.
- Death, 0–3% in low risk patients.
- Stroke, 5–10% (debris from removing calcified valve, cannulating aorta).
- Re-sternotomy for bleeding or tamponade, 5%.
- Chest infection, AF, complete heart block requiring permanent pacemaker insertion, wound infection, renal failure.
- Prosthetic endocarditis, failure, thrombosis, paravalvular leak.

Key revision points—anatomy of heart valves
- Aortic valve. Tricuspid valve, sitting within bulb of aortic root. Three dilatations called sinuses of Valsalva. Left coronary sinus gives rise to LMS, right gives rise to right coronary artery. Third known as non-coronary sinus. AV node lies between right and non-coronary cusp. Annulus (where leaflets attach to aorta) is coronal-shaped.
- MV. Bileaflet valve, lying between LA and LV. Anterior leaflet smaller than posterior leaflet. Leaflets held in place by chordae which attach to two papillary muscles of LV. Annulus is oval-shaped.

Cardiothoracic ICU

Commonly used terminology (see Table 17.1)

- Instead of referring to systolic and diastolic blood pressure, arterial pressure is usually described using single figure: the *mean arterial pressure (MAP)* which is calculated by adding a third of the difference between diastolic and systolic pressures to the diastolic pressure, e.g. the MAP of a patient with a BP 120/60mmHg is 80mmHg.
- The MAP on its own does not adequately describe cardiac function; a number of other parameters are frequently used.
- *Cardiac output.* The volume of blood ejected by the heart per minute.
- *Stroke volume.* The volume of blood ejected by the heart per beat.
- Cardiac output equals heart rate x stroke volume.
- *Cardiac index.* Is simply the cardiac output adjusted to take into account the size of the patient and is a more accurate reflection of cardiac function.

Low cardiac ouput

Much of the initial care after cardiac surgery is aimed at preventing, recognizing, and treating low cardiac output states, as these can lead to organ failure, contribute to sepsis, and cause death, even in 'straightforward' patients. Low cardiac output can be defined as a cardiac index <2.2mL/min or evidence of end-organ hypoperfusion (e.g. lactic acidosis, oliguria, low mixed venous O_2 saturations).

- Common causes of low cardiac output include:
  - Bleeding (occasionally other causes of hypovolaemia, e.g. polyuria).
  - Tamponade.
  - Arrhythmias.
  - Acidosis, hypoxia.
  - Preoperative cardiomyopathy.
  - Ischaemia and stunning (myocardial recovery from surgery).
- Hypotension can due to low cardiac output, but even a patient with a high cardiac output could be hypotensive if they were very vasodilated (most commonly due to SIRS (see 🕮 p. 138) or sepsis).
- Sometimes a number of problems may be going on at once and it is easy to miss important problems so a systematic approach to assessing post-operative cardiac surgery patients is vital.

General assessment of cardiac surgery patients

- Except in emergencies, usually you have time to evaluate every system.
- Review the history. What was the ventricular function preop? What other comorbidities? What operation was done—any problems?
- *Cardiovascular.*
  - Look at the heart rate and rhythm and check the ECG for evidence of ischaemia (ST segment changes), comparing with preop.
  - Look at the MAP and CVP. A high CVP is always concerning, suggesting tamponade, ventricular failure, or respiratory problems.
  - Look at the cardiac output, lactate, mixed venous, and feel the patient's extremities; a warm patient with good peripheral pulses cannot have a low cardiac output. What is the SVR?
  - What inotropes, vasoconstrictors, and antihypertensives are on?

- *Respiratory.* Is the patient breathing spontaneously or ventilated? Look at the O_2 saturations and a recent blood gas to check the PaO_2, $PaCO_2$, and pH. What does the CXR look like?
- *Renal.* How much urine is the patient making (ideally >1mL/kg/h)? What is the patient's fluid balance (if it is negative or low, the patient may be hypovolaemic; if it is very high, fluid overload is a concern). Check electrolytes; abnormalities can cause arrhythmias.
- *Bleeding.* Should be less than 100cm³/h in the chest tubes, with steady fall in the rate. Look at wound sites (remember groin + leg). Is the haematocrit dropping? Check coagulation.
- Assess mental status and focal neurology, analgesia.

Table 17.1 Key haemodynamic formulae and normal values

Cardiac output = SV x HR	
Cardiac index = CO/BSA	
Stroke volume index = SV/BSA	
Mean arterial pressure = DP + (SP – DP)/3	
Systemic vascular resistance = ((MAP – CVP)/CO) x 80	
Systemic vascular resistance index = SVR/BSA	
Pulmonary vascular resistance = ((PAP – PAWP)/CO) x 80	
Pulmonary vascular resistance index = PVR/BSA	

	Normal value
Cardiac output (CO)	4.5–8L/min
Stroke volume (SV)	60–100mL
Body surface area (BSA)	2–2.2m²
Cardiac index (CI)	2.0–4.0L/min/m²
Stroke volume index (SVI)	33–47mL/beat/m²
Mean arterial pressure (MAP)	70–100mmHg
Diastolic pressure (DP)	60–80mmHg
Systolic pressure (SP)	110–150mmHg
Systemic vascular resistance (SVR)	800–1200dyne-s/cm⁵
Central venous pressure (CVP)	6–12mmHg
Systemic vascular resistance index (SVRI)	400–600dyne-s/cm⁵/m²
Pulmonary vascular resistance (PVR)	50–250dyne-s/cm⁵
Pulmonary artery pressure (PAP)	20–30mmHg
Pulmonary artery wedge pressure (PAWP)	8–14mmHg
Pulmonary vascular resistance index (PVRI)	20–125dyne-s/cm⁵/m²

Lung cancer

Key facts

- Commonest cause of death from cancer in the UK.
- ↑ Incidence in females (25% of cancer-related deaths in women).

Risk factors

- Cigarette smoking. Strongly positive association with cigarette smoking (polycyclic aromatic hydrocarbons plus nicotine-related carcinogens).
- Radon exposure.
- Occupational factors. Asbestos, polycyclic aromatic hydrocarbons, arsenic, nickel, silica, coal tar, aluminium production, coal gassification, exposure to paints, chromium compounds, bischloromethal ether.
- Genetic predisposition and male sex.

Pathology

Bronchial carcinoma is classified as non-small cell or small cell.

Non-small cell lung cancer

Squamous cell carcinoma

- Twenty to thirty per cent of all lung cancers.
- Most common histological type in Europe.
- Often arising in large airways as an endobronchial mass (two-thirds).
- Slow-growing, late to metastasize.

Adenocarcinomas

- Thirty to fifty per cent of lung cancers. Incidence increasing.
- Usually peripheral tumours (approximately three-quarters).
- Moderate growth with early metastasis.

Large cell undifferentiated carcinoma:

- Fifteen per cent of all lung cancers.
- Peripheral location more common than central.
- Two subtypes. Clear cell carcinoma and giant cell carcinoma. Giant cell tumours are uncommon, <1% of lung cancers. Very poor prognosis.

Histological subtypes

- *Bronchioloalveolar tumours.* Highly differentiated adenocarcinoma; 2.5% all lung cancers.
- *Adenosquamous carcinomas.*

Small cell lung cancer

Neuroendocrine tumours

Approximately 20% of lung cancers. Aggressive tumours, not usually amenable to surgical resection. Three subtypes—pure small cell (90%), mixed small and large cell, combined small cell with areas of squamous or glandular differentiation.

Clinical features

- Proximal tumours tend to produce symptoms of major airway obstruction and irritation (haemoptysis, dyspnoea, cough, wheezing,

stridor, hoarseness, Horner's syndrome, SVC obstruction, post-obstructive pneumonia, pleural effusion, Pancoast's syndrome).
- Peripheral tumours are often asymptomatic or present with signs and symptoms of pleural or chest wall invasion or pleural effusion (pleuritic chest wall pain, progressive dyspnoea).
- May present with symptoms and signs of metastatic spread. Neurological—headache, blurred vision, nausea, diplopia, decreased consciousness, ataxia; bony pain and pathological fracture; liver and abdominal pain, anorexia, jaundice, ascites, liver failure, hepatomegaly; adrenal glands—symptoms of Addison's disease.
- Paraneoplastic syndromes.

History and examination
- *Ask about:* history of tobacco smoking (pack years), asbestos exposure, employment history, weight loss of greater than 5% body weight, recent onset of joint pains, change in voice, chest wall pain, back pain.
- *Look for:* lymphadenopathy, evidence of significant weight loss, pleural effusion, localized chest wall pain, clubbing, cutaneous lesions.

Principles of management

Non-small cell lung cancer is relatively resistant to chemotherapy. Curative resection allows best chance of long-term survival. Surgery is normally offered to all patients with stage I and stage II disease, along with specific patients with stage III disease (after chemoradiotherapy). Surgical principles of resection are:
- No spillage of cells from primary tumour during resection.
- Entire tumour must be resected by lobectomy or pneumonectomy along with intrapulmonary lymph nodes; lesser resections proven to have worse outcome, only considered in high risk patients.
- All accessible mediastinal lymph nodes should be excised or biopsied to allow complete staging and plan for any adjuvant therapy.
- Frozen section analysis of resection margins to confirm appropriate surgical resection and complete excision of primary tumour.

Survival
- Stage I, 5y survival 75%; stage II, 5y survival 40%; stage III, 5y survival <30%.
- Post-operative mortality rate. Lobectomy, 2%; pneumonectomy, 6%.

Chemotherapy

To date, no proven benefit from adjuvant therapy in patients with surgically resectable and potentially curative disease.

Radiotherapy
- *Radical.* Used in patients unfit or unwilling to undergo surgery. Also used in those with bulky stage IV disease. Survival benefit in non-surgical patients when combined with concomitant chemotherapy.
- *Adjuvant.* Also used as an adjunct to surgery or as palliation.

Pleural effusion

Key facts

Abnormal amount of fluid within the pleural space. Pleural effusions may be divided into transudates and exudates, according to Light's criteria (see Box 17.1), but the divide is not always clear.

Box 17.1 Light's criteria

An exudate is characterized by:
- Pleural fluid:serum protein >0.5.
- Pleural fluid:serum LDH >0.6.
- Pleural fluid LDH >200IU.

Causes of transudates
- Cirrhosis of the liver.
- Nephrotic syndrome.
- Glomerulonephritis.
- CCF.
- Myxoedema.
- Sarcoidosis.
- Multiple PE.

Causes of exudates
- Neoplasms. Mesothelioma, metastatic disease, primary lung cancer.
- PE.
- Chylothorax.
- Haemothorax.
- Infectious diseases. Viral and bacterial infections, fungal and parasitic infections, TB.
- Gastrointestinal disease. Pancreatitis, subphrenic abscess, intrahepatic abscess, perforated oesophagus.
- Collagen vascular disease. Systemic lupus erythematosus, Wegener's granulomatosis, Sjögren's syndrome.
- Drug-induced pleural disease.
- Mediterranean fever.
- Rheumatoid disease, sarcoidosis, yellow nail syndrome.
- Asbestos exposure, electrical burns, radiation therapy.
- Trapped lung, post-pericardiectomy.
- Uraemia, urinary tract obstruction.
- Post-myocardial syndrome, Meigs' syndrome.

Clinical presentation
- Small effusions are often asymptomatic. Larger effusions cause cough, chest pain, dyspnoea.
- Decreased ipsilateral chest expansion, dullness to percussion, decreased breath sounds over the effusion on auscultation, crepitations may be heard.

Investigations
- *Chest radiograph.* Small effusions are demonstrated by blunting of the costodiaphragmatic angles; larger effusions produce a fluid level with a meniscus.
- *Ultrasound scan.* Useful for loculated effusions, helps to localize optimal site for chest drainage.
- *CT.* Useful when looking at underlying lung and pleural lesions.
- *Pleural aspiration cytology.* May obtain diagnostic information, helpful when planning treatment.

Management
If possible, treat the underlying cause. Simple pleural effusions due to fluid overload may resolve with diuresis.
- Tube thoracostomy (see 📖 p. 200).
- Chemical pleurodesis (tetracycline, blood, talc).
- Surgical abrasion pleurodesis.
- Surgical pleurectomy (open or thoracoscopic).
- Pleuroperitoneal shunt.

Complications
- Infection and empyema.
- Treatment failure with recurrence of pleural effusion.
- Damage to underlying lung parenchyma, leading to prolonged air leak and bronchoalveolar air leak.

Empyema
This is an infected pleural fluid collection, commonly after pneumonia.
- *Stage I. Acute exudative phase.*
  - Typically occurs 2–5 days after a pneumonia.
  - Accumulation of fluid with low cellular content and viscosity.
  - Characterized by low WCC, LDH, and glucose, and a normal pH.
  - Can be successfully treated with antibiotics only.
- *Stage II. Fibrinopurulent phase.*
  - Typically occurs 5–14 days after a pneumonia.
  - Turbid or purulent fluid with heavy fibrin deposits.
  - Appearance of simple loculations and septations.
  - May have bacterial invasions and high numbers of PMNs and lymphocytes.
  - Characterized by low pH and glucose and increased LDH.
  - Antibiotics and chest tube drainage is required, may need video-assisted thoracoscopic surgery (VATS) decortication.
- *Stage III. Chronic organizing phase.*
  - Lung trapping by collagen visceral and parietal pleural peel with ingrowth of fibroblast and capillaries.
  - Antibiotics and aggressive decortications, generally by thoracotomy.
  - Bacteriology.

Pneumothorax

Key facts
The presence of air in the pleural space with secondary lung collapse.

Aetiology
- Primary spontaneous pneumothorax.
- Secondary spontaneous pneumothorax.
- Post-traumatic and iatrogenic.

Primary spontaneous pneumothorax
Commonly seen in young tall male smokers. More common on the right side. Less than 10% of cases are bilateral. Usually caused by rupture of small subpleural blebs (collections of air <2cm). Usually found at the apex of the upper lobe or the apical segment of the lower lobe. The rest of the lung parenchyma is normal. May also be caused by rupture of bullae (large air-filled spaces).

Presentation
- Dyspnoea, chest pain, cough, tachypnoea.
- Ipsilateral decreased chest wall movement, hyperresonant hemithorax to percussion, absent breath sounds on auscultation, pleural rub, tachycardia.

Investigations
- PA chest radiograph usually diagnostic.
- CT scan gives an accurate estimate of size of pneumothorax and is useful for assessment of remaining lung parenchyma and contralateral lung.

Complications
- Tension pneumothorax.
- Pneumomediastinum.
- Haemopneumothorax.
- Recurrent pneumothorax.

Conservative management
- Observation (small, <20% pneumothorax).
- Needle aspiration.
- Tube thoracostomy ± chemical pleurodesis.

Surgery
- Surgery is indicated in the following cases.
- First episode. Prolonged air leak, tension pneumothorax, haemothorax, bilateral pneumothoraces, residual collapse of lung despite non-surgical treatment, 100% pneumothorax, occupational hazard, pneumothorax secondary to giant bulla, previous contralateral pneumonectomy.
- Recurrence of pneumothorax.

The aim is to resect the blebs or bullae and obliterate the pleural space with adhesions, either using chemical or abrasion pleurodesis or parietal pleurectomy (apical or full). It may be performed through a mini-thoracotomy, axillary incision, or thoracoscopically

Recurrence rate
- Less than 2% following surgical pleurectomy via mini-thoracotomy.
- Five per cent following thoracoscopic procedures.
- Five to ten per cent following chemical pleurodesis.

Secondary spontaneous pneumothorax
Causes
- Cystic fibrosis, chronic obstructive airways disease (COAD) and other bullous disease, asthma.
- Interstitial lung disease.
- Infections, including AIDS, mycobacterial, *Pneumocystis carinii*, bacterial, parasitic, mycotic.
- Malignancy. Bronchogenic carcinoma, metastatic lung cancer (sarcoma and lymphoma).
- Collagen diseases, catamenial, Ehlers–Danlos syndrome, histiocytosis X, scleroderma, lymphangioleiomyomatosis, Marfan's syndrome.
- Rupture of the oesophagus.

Cystic fibrosis Pneumothorax found in 10% of patients. Remember these patients are possible candidates for future lung transplantation when considering management options. Full parietal pleurectomy is a contraindication to lung transplantation.
COAD The most common cause of secondary pneumothorax. Age usually >50y. Patients often have very little pulmonary reserve. They may not tolerate surgical management and single lung ventilation. Treatment options are therefore tube thoracoscopy and chemical pleurodesis or long-term tube thoracoscopy.
Infection Cavitating pulmonary lesions rupture into pleural space.
AIDS Usually secondary to *Pneumocystis carinii* and pneumonia. May be presenting feature of AIDS. Most effective treatment is surgical.
Catamenial Age 20–30y. Incidence 3–6% of women. Occurs 2–3 days following onset of menstruation. Right side more commonly affected. Usually small, presenting with dyspnoea and chest pain. Pathogenesis unclear.

Primary spontaneous pneumomediastinum
Uncommon. Males affected more frequently than females. Occurs following exertion or increased intra-abdominal pressure. Commonly associated with cocaine, marijuana, and crack cocaine usage. It is caused by rupture of alveolar sacs with air tracking along the peribronchial and perivascular spaces into the neck.

Presentation
- Sudden onset of chest pain, dyspnoea, dysphagia, cough.
- Subcutaneous emphysema over neck and chest wall, Hamman's sign.
- Chest radiograph confirms diagnosis.

Management Non-operative, treat expectantly. Emergency surgical decompression very rare.

Mediastinal disease

Pericardial effusion and cardiac tamponade

Key facts
- Pericardial effusion is abnormal fluid in the pericardial space; there is normally about 20mL of plasma ultrafiltrate.
  - Pericardial effusion may be acute or chronic.
  - Acute accumulation of fluid can cause cardiac tamponade which is a surgical emergency (see Box 17.2).
  - Effusions commonly results from pericarditis, CCF, metastatic spread to pericardium commonly from lung or breast malignancy, lymphoma or leukaemia, autoimmune disorders, chronic hepatic and renal failure, infections—specifically HIV.

Clinical features
- Very dependent on the time course. Acute accumulation of a small amount of fluid can cause life-threatening cardiac tamponade, whereas slow accumulations of large volumes of fluid may be well tolerated.
- Chronic pericardial effusion commonly may present with decreased exercise tolerance, atypical chest pain, orthopnoea, and associated signs of CCF, as well as features of cardiac tamponade.

Box 17.2 Cardiac tamponade

Suspect cardiac tamponade if the patient has a history of chest trauma.
- ↓ **BP, ↑ JVP, (Beck's triad is ↓ BP, ↑ JVP + muffled heart sounds).**
- **Pulsus paradoxus** (exaggeration of the normal ↓ BP with inspiration).
- Progressive tachycardia and dysrhythmias, including SVT, VF, and EMD.
- ↓ Urine output.
- Excessive widening of the mediastinum on CXR.
- Echo may show clot in pericardium and collapse of RV in diastole.
- Equilibration of cardiac filling pressures (at cardiac catheterization).

Management
- **Emergency pericardiocentesis** (📖 p. 204).
- **Emergency thoracotomy or sternotomy.**
- **Aggressive fluid resuscitation is a temporizing measure.**

Management
- Medical management includes diuretics and pericardiocentesis.
- Creating a hole in the pericardium or pericardial window so that fluid can drain directly into the pleura via:
  - Thoracotomy or subxiphoid approach.
  - Left VATS approach.

Thymoma

Key facts

- The thymus is a bilobar structure located in the anterior mediastinum which contains lymphoid tissue. It is the location for maturation of T-cells in early life.
- Thymoma may be benign or malignant.
- Thymectomy is the definitive treatment for myasthenia gravis.

Clinical features

- Thymoma is usually asymptomatic in adults, whereas children often present with thoracic outlet obstruction or upper airway compromise.
- Clinical features of myasthenia gravis are described on 📖 p. 63.
- Thymoma appears as a smooth mass in the upper half of the CXR.
- CT shows enlarged thymus as well as lymph node involvement.

Treatment

- Thymectomy via a median sternotomy.

Key revision points—mediastinal anatomy

- **Mediastinum** is the space between the pleural sacs, below the thoracic inlet and above the diaphragm.
- **Superior mediastinum.**
  - From thoracic inlet to the line from sternal angle to T4–5 space.
  - Contains great vessels, trachea, oesophagus, phrenic nerves, vagus nerves, thoracic duct.
- **Anterior mediastinum.**
  - Anterior to pericardium.
  - Contains sternopericardial ligaments, thymus, lymph nodes.
- **Middle mediastinum.**
  - Contains pericardial cavity, heart, great vessels, phrenic nerves.
- **Posterior mediastinum.**
  - Posterior to pericardium.
  - Contains oesphagus, descending aorta, azygous veins, thoracic duct, lymph nodes.

Peripheral vascular disease

Acute limb ischaemia

Definition Any sudden decrease in limb perfusion that causes a potential threat to viability.

Prevalence One in 6000 of the population.

Causes and features

Acute thrombosis in a vessel with pre-existing atherosclerosis (60% of cases)
- Predisposing factors are: dehydration, hypotension, malignancy, polycythaemia, or inherited prothrombotic states.
- Features suggestive of thrombosis are:
  - Previous history of intermittent claudication.
  - No obvious source of emboli (see below).
  - Reduced or absent pulses in the contralateral limb.

Emboli (30% of cases)
- Eighty per cent have a cardiac cause (AF, MI, ventricular aneurysm).
- Arterial aneurysms account for 10% of distal emboli and may be from the aorto-iliac, femoral, popliteal, or subclavian arteries.
- Rarely, acute thrombosis in pre-existing atherosclerosis (see above) will embolize.
- Commonest sites of impaction are the brachial, common femoral, popliteal, and aortic bifurcation ('saddle embolus').
- Features suggestive of embolism are:
  - No previous history of claudication.
  - Presence of AF or recent MI.

Rare causes
- Aortic dissection, trauma, iatrogenic injury, peripheral aneurysm (particularly popliteal), and intra-arterial drug use.

Symptoms and signs (any cause)
Six Ps:
- **P**ain, **p**allor, **p**ulselessness, **p**araesthesia, **p**aralysis, **p**erishingly cold.

Complications
- Death (20%).
- Limb loss (40%). Severe ischaemia leads to irreversible tissue damage within 6h.

Emergency management
Remember, patients will usually have coexisting coronary, cerebral, or renal disease.

Resuscitation
- Give 100% O_2.
- Get IV access and consider crystalloid fluid up to 1000mL if dehydrated.
- Take blood for FBC, U&E, troponin, clotting, glucose, group and save.
- Request CXR and ECG (look for dysrhythmias).

- Give opiate analgesia (5–10mg morphine IM).
- Call for senior help.

Establish degree of urgency
- Limb viability assessment. Involve senior help early.
  - *Irreversible.* Fixed mottling of skin, petechial haemorrhages in skin, woody hard muscles.
  - *Immediate treatment needed.* Muscles tender to palpation/swollen, loss of power, loss of sensation.
  - *Prompt treatment after investigation.* Pulseless, pale, cold, reduced capillary refill.

Treatment of all patients
Give heparin (5000IU unfractionated heparin IV bolus and start an infusion of 1000IU/h) if there are no contraindications (e.g. aortic dissection, multiple trauma, head injury).
- Recheck APTT in 4–6h.
- Aim for a target time of 2–2.5 x the normal range.

Definitive management
Depends on the severity of ischaemia (as above) and there are three broad categories.
- *Irreversible* (non-salvageable limb). Amputation is inevitable and urgent (but not emergency).
- *Immediate treatment needed* (to prevent the systemic complications of muscle necrosis—hyperkalaemia, acidosis, acute renal failure, and cardiac arrest). Consider amputation if ischaemic changes advanced and life-threatening. Surgery to revascularize limb and perform fasciotomies (to prevent or treat compartment syndrome).
- *Prompt treatment after investigation.* Continue heparinization. Angiogram (stop heparin 4h before) or duplex/CT angio to determine cause/location of disease. Thrombolysis, angioplasty, arterial surgery, or combination. Limb may remain viable and functional after period of heparinization alone.

Principles of embolectomy (see 📖 p. 746)

Chronic upper limb ischaemia

Key facts

Upper limb ischaemia occurs less frequently than in the lower limb.

Causes

- Previous trauma or axillary irradiation, leading to arterial stenosis.
- *Atherosclerosis.* As in the lower limb.
- *Buerger's disease.* Affects small vessels of the hands and feet, principally in smokers, associated with Raynaud's phenomenon, mostly young men, but women may be affected, presents with digital gangrene/ischaemia and may present with acute limb ischaemia in young people.
- *Subclavian steal syndrome.* Stenosis of subclavian artery proximal to vertebral artery origin; arm claudication causes reversed flow in the vertebral artery/diminished hindbrain perfusion (dizziness/syncope).
- *Takayasu's arteritis.* Uncommon in Europe; major arch/upper limb vessels affected.
- *Thoracic outlet syndrome* (see Fig. 18.1).
  - Term used to cover a spectrum of symptoms resulting from the compression of the neurovascular bundle (NVB) as it leaves the chest to enter the upper limb, in an area enclosed by the first rib, clavicle, and the scalenus anterior muscle.
  - Presents as a variable combination of neural, arterial, and venous symptoms exarcebated by elevation of the limb, with shoulder, arm, or head pain, and parasthesiae, weakness, or arm claudication. Ninety-five per cent are neurogenic and 5% are arterial or venous manifestations (arm engorgement, swelling with subclavian vein stenosis or thrombosis—Paget–Schroetter syndrome).

Clinical features

- Weakness, cramp or exercise-related pain, and digital ischaemia/gangrene.
- Examine bilateral upper limb pulses, BP in both arms (elevated/at sides), wrist Doppler pressures.
- *Roos test.* Arm abducted to 90°, hands up with elbows braced backward, chin elevated, hands serially clenched/opened for 1–2min, positive if pain or weakness in hand or forearm.
- *Adson's test.* Pulse diminishes or absent on elevation/abduction of arm with head turned to contralateral side. Reliability improved by using in conjunction with arterial duplex.
- *Allen's test.* Assesses integrity of the palmar arch and dominant vessel (radial or ulnar).
- *Tinel's test.* For carpal tunnel syndrome.

Diagnosis and investigation

- Cervical spine and thoracic outlet X-rays, wrist Doppler pressures.
- CT/MRI to look for fibrous bands/ribs and stenoses/occlusions.
- Arterial duplex or angiography to diagnose proximal arterial lesions.
- Duplex or venography for subclavian vein stenosis or occlusion.

Treatment

Thoracic outlet syndrome

- Mild neurogenic problem. Simple analgesia, physiotherapy, and advice on risk factors.
- Surgery (supraclavicular or axillary approach) has good results for those with arterial or venous symptoms/complications.
- Excision of the first rib/band will improve symptoms in over 90%.
- Careful evaluation is needed prior to surgery for pure neurological symptoms, e.g. nerve conduction studies.

Cervical sympathectomy in upper limb disease

Indications

- Palmar hyperhidrosis (less effective and infrequently used for axillary).
- Buerger's disease/small vessel disease with digital ischaemia.

Approach

- Aim is to de-innervate the second and third thoracic ganglia.
- Approach is almost universally thoracoscopic and open approaches have been largely abandoned.

Complications

- Horner's syndrome.
- Pneumothorax.
- Haemorrhage.
- Compensatory truncal hyperhidrosis.
- Frey's syndrome (gustatory sweating).

Axillary hyperhidrosis Treatment of choice is now subcutaneous botulinum toxin A injections to the axillary sweat glands, repeated as necessary, often 6-monthly.

Key revision points—anatomy of thoracic outlet

Several structures can compress the neurovascular structures.
- Cervical rib. Articulates with C7.
- Scaleneus anterior. Aberrant anatomy or scarring/swelling from trauma.
- Costoclavicular ligament.

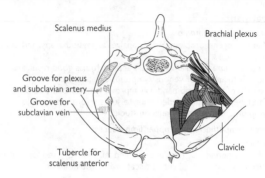

Fig. 18.1 Structures involved in thoracic outlet syndrome.

Chronic lower limb ischaemia

- Atherosclerosis is a generalized disease and has a predilection for the coronary, cerebral, and peripheral circulations (see 📖 p. 152).
- In the lower limb, it may affect the aorto-iliac, femoral or popliteal, and calf vessel levels singly or in combinations (see Fig. 18.2).
- Single-level disease usually results in intermittent claudication (IC) and two-level disease in critical limb ischaemia (CLI).

The Fontaine classification of lower limb ischaemia

- I. Asymptomatic.
- II. Intermittent claudication.
- III. Rest pain.
- IV. Ulcers/gangrene.

Grades III and IV = critical limb ischaemia.

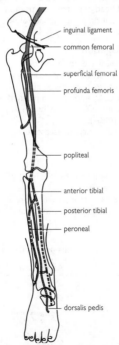

inguinal ligament

common femoral

superficial femoral

profunda femoris

popliteal

anterior tibial

posterior tibial

peroneal

dorsalis pedis

Fig. 18.2 The arterial supply to the leg. Reproduced with permission from Longmore, M. et al. (2007). *Oxford Handbook of Clinical Medicine*, 7th edn. Oxford University Press, Oxford.

Intermittent claudication

Key facts

- Affects 4% of people over 55y, mostly men.
- One-third of patients improve, one-third remain stable, and one-third deteriorate.
- Four per cent require an intervention and 2% result in amputation.
- Risk factors and association. See Table 18.1.

Clinical features

- Muscular pain on exercise of the affected limb, worsened with increasing level of exercise, relieved by rest; most commonly, calf.
- Differential diagnosis.
  - Spinal stenosis. Neurogenic pain caused by drop in distal cauda equina blood flow due to exercise, leading to neurogenic pain.
  - Osteoarthritis, especially hip joint.
  - Nerve root entrapment, e.g. sciatica.
  - Popliteal artery entrapment (rare). Due to compression of popliteal artery over medial head of gastrocnemius during exercise. Distal pulses reduced/absent on plantar flexion alone. Treated by surgical release after MRI defines anatomy.

Diagnosis and investigation

- Diagnosis is mostly clinical and not based on imaging.
- Post-exercise fall in ankle–brachial pressure index (ABPI) can be diagnostic.
- Measure BP, serum glucose, cholesterol, FBC.
- Imaging only if treatment by intervention planned. Angiography (usually digital subtraction (DSA)), may be CT angiogram, or magnetic resonance angiogram (MRA).
- Abdominal ultrasound if aneurysm disease suspected.

Treatment

Risk factor modification

- Forty per cent of peripheral vascular disease (PVD) patients have significant coronary or cerebral arterial disease; the mainstay of treatment is aggressive risk factor modification. Stop smoking, oral statin treatment, increased exercise, control of BP and serum glucose, antiplatelet therapy.

Table 18.1 Intermittent claudication—risk factors and associations

Risk factors	Associations
Hypertension	Obesity
Hyperipidaemia	Diet
Diabetes mellitus	Sedentary lifestyle
Tobacco smoking	Gender
Positive family history	Occupation

Endovascular treatment
- Angioplasty ± stent. Excellent results in the aorto-iliac segment (>90% success) and good results in the superficial femoral segment (90% success and 60–80% patency at 2y).
- Usually performed under LA percutaneously as a day case.
- Rarely performed for claudication in the popliteal and tibial segments due to high risk of occlusion.
- Most useful in short stenoses/occlusions.

Surgery
- Used for short distance claudication, severe lifestyle limitation, and failure/unsuitability of endovascular treatment in the aorto-iliac segments.
- Procedures available are:
  - *Aortobifemoral graft.* 5y patency of >90%, but carries 5–8% mortality and a risk of impotence. Used for younger patients.
  - *Femorofemoral cross-over bypass graft.* Used for isolated unilateral iliac disease; 90% 1y patency.
  - *Common femoral endarterectomy.* Used for isolated common femoral disease; good results and a low complication rate.
  - *Femoro-above knee popliteal bypass.* 80% 2y patency with vein or prosthetic graft.
  - *Femoro-below knee popliteal bypass.* 70% 2y patency with vein graft.
  - *Femoro-distal (below knee) bypass.* 5y patency <35%; usually reserved only for critical ischaemia.
- Most commonly used for long stenoses/occlusions and combined with endovascular treatment.

Critical limb ischaemia

Key facts
- Often progresses to limb loss or progressive tissue loss if it remains untreated.
- High risk condition, often occuring in high risk patients with multiple comorbidities.

Clinical features
- European consensus statement defines critical ischaemia if there is:
  - Rest pain for >2 weeks not relieved by simple analgesia; or
  - Doppler ankle pressure <50mmHg (toe pressures <30mmHg if diabetic).
  - Tissue necrosis (i.e. the presence of gangrene or ulceration).
- Rest pain typically worsens at night and during elevation of the limb and is relieved by hanging the limb dependent.
- Arterial ulceration cannot reliably be distinguished from other causes.

Diagnosis and investigation
Diagnosis is clinical. Investigation should aim to:
- Identify and treat risk factors. Treat BP, stop smoking, optimize diabetes control, reduce cholesterol (statins by choice), use antiplatelet agent (aspirin/clopidogrel by choice).
- Identify location and severity of all arterial stenoses involved. May include:
  - Colour duplex Doppler ultrasound. Zero risk, non-interventional, best for proximal vessels (iliac, common femoral).
  - Angiography (usually DSA). Interventional, carries risk of arterial injury and renal toxicity of contrast, good for popliteal and distal vessel assessment.
  - MRA. Low risk.
  - CT angiography. Low risk (radiation and contrast).

Treatment
- All efforts should be made to revascularize if possible (providing the general condition of the patient allows it).
- General principle is to deal with most proximal disease first and progress to distal disease only if critical ischaemia still present.

Medical care
- Nursing care.
- Analgesia. Opiates (e.g. Oramorph®, MST Continus®).

Endovascular treatments
Angioplasty ± stent proximal disease (aorto-iliac, common femoral, superficial femoral). Less successful in popliteal disease and distal disease.

Surgery
- Femoro-distal (e.g. to popliteal, tibioperoneal trunk, or anterior or posterior tibial arteries).

- Aorto-iliac bypass ('anatomical') or axillo-femoral or femoro-femoral ('extra-anatomical') bypass.
- Amputation.
  - Usually below knee or above knee in smoking-related atherosclerosis.
  - Distal amputations (toe, forefoot, ankle) may be appropriate in diabetic disease.
- There is little evidence of benefit from treatment with prostacyclin or sympathectomy (surgical or chemical).

Aneurysms

Key facts

- An aneurysm is an abnormal localized dilatation of a blood vessel.
- It may be associated with structural abnormalities of collagen and elastin in the vessel wall.
- Prevalence of abdominal aortic aneurysm, 4% of men aged 65, increasing with age.
- ♂:♀, 9:1.
- Associated with hypertension, tobacco smoking, and family history (all associated with atherosclerosis).

Pathological features

Types

- *True aneurysms.* Contain all three layers of artery wall. May be fusiform (symmetrical dilatation) or saccular. Underlying cause is usually atherosclerosis-related, but may be associated with infective causes ('mycotic aneurysm'), Marfan's and Ehlers–Danlos syndromes (collagen and elastin abnormalities).
- *False aneurysms.* Do not contain all three layers of vessel wall and often only lined by surrounding connective tissue or adventitia. Usually secondary to penetrating trauma, including iatrogenic injury (e.g. femoral cannulation, surgery).

Sites

Thoracic, abdominal, and peripheral (iliac, femoral, popliteal, visceral, carotid or subclavian), cerebral 'berry' aneurysms.

Clinical features

Thoraco-abdominal

- Crawford classification types I–IV (dependent on involvement of descending thoracic/abdominal aorta); managed in specialist centres.
- Often asymptomatic.
- Different clinical features to thoracic aortic dissection (acute chest pain (angina/MI), back pain, acute aortic regurgitation, or cardiac failure).
- Diagnosed by widened mediastinum on CXR or on CT/MRI.
- Rupture has high mortality and rare without prior symptoms.
- Elective surgery has up to 20% mortality and risk of paraplegia; 10% require dialysis after surgery.
- Endovascular stenting is a potential future treatment of choice due to high surgical risks.

Abdominal aortic

- Ninety-five per cent start below the origin of the renal arteries ('infrarenal').
- Fifteen per cent extend down to involve the origins of the common iliac arteries.
- Associated with other peripheral aneurysm (e.g. popliteal).
- Five to ten per cent are 'inflammatory' (have gross connective tissue changes around the aortic wall in the retroperitoneum).

- Most are asymptomatic; 40% are detected incidentally (clinical examination, ultrasound, AXR, IVU).
- A national ultrasound screening programme exists.
- Six-monthly scans for surveillance if size 4–5.4cm (1% per year risk of rupture).
- Mycotic aneurysms are rare, but have a high rupture rate.
- Risk of rupture and mortality increases with increasing aneurysm diameter.
- Surgical intervention is indicated for:
  - AP diameter >5.5cm in fit individuals.
  - Rapid increase in diameter on serial surveillance scans, e.g. >0.5cm in 6 months.

Peripheral aneurysms

- *Iliac.* Two per cent of patients >70y. Mostly common iliac and asymptomatic. Rarely palpable and rupture may be missed as acute abdomen or renal colic.
- *Femoral.* Mostly asymptomatic pulsatile groin swelling or pain. May present with lower limb ischaemia.
- *Popliteal.* Many asymptomatic and over half are bilateral. May present with acute limb ischaemia. Aneurysm thrombosis is associated with high risk of limb loss. Prophylactic bypass probably best for symptomatic, embolizing aneurysms.
- *Carotid.* Rare and may be bilateral. May present with neurological or pressure symptoms. May present simply as a pulsatile neck swelling. Rarely presents with rupture. Diagnosis with duplex scan.
- *Visceral.* Account for 1% of all aneurysms. Generally small and asymptomatic until rupture. Splenic artery most common followed by hepatic and renal arteries.

Treatment of abdominal aortic aneurysm (AAA)

Aim is to prevent death as 80% of patients with ruptured AAA will die.

Elective surgery

- Open repair by inlay synthetic graft. May be 'straight' if aneurysm confined to aorta or 'bifurcated/trouser' if there are common iliac aneurysms as well; 3–7% operative mortality.
- Laparoscopic repair may offer earlier return to normal function and reduced hospital stay.

Endovascular repairs

- *Endovascular aneurysm repair (EVAR) with a stent graft.* Percutaneous insertion of covered stent to exclude the aneurysmal segment from arterial pressure.
- *Advantages.* Percutaneous technique, reduced early mortality.
- *Disadvantages.* High early re-intervention rate, requires lifelong surveillance, no long-term survival benefits over open repair shown to date.

Ruptured abdominal aortic aneurysm

Causes and features

- Associated with hypertension (especially uncontrolled), smoking, family history, and atherosclerosis.
- Rare in patients aged <55.
- Risk of rupture relates to maximum AP diameter.
  - Less than 0.5% per year, <4.0cm diameter.
  - One per cent per year, 4–5.5cm.
  - Over 3% per year, >5.5cm.
- Patients with a 'contained leak' with initial haemodynamic stability proceed rapidly to rupture.
- Less than 50% of patients with a ruptured AAA reach hospital alive and the overall mortality of the condition may be as high as 75–95%.
- Outcome is best in the hands of an experienced vascular team (vascular surgeon, vascular anaesthetist, theatre nursing team, two assistants, and ITU) and a rapid transfer from the emergency department to theatre.

Symptoms

- Severe/sudden onset epigastric and/or back/loin pain.
- History of sudden 'collapse', often with transient hypotension.
- May have history of AAA under surveillance.

Signs

- Cardinal signs are unexplained rapid onset hypotension, pain, and sweating.
- A pulsatile abdominal mass is not always easy to feel (due to pain and abdominal wall rigidity).

Emergency management

Resuscitation

- If the diagnosis is seriously considered, call for senior surgical assistance immediately. Transfer to theatre may be required even as resuscitation continues.
- 'Permissive hypotension'. Do not 'chase' a 'normal' systolic BP to reduce the risk of worsening the rupture.
- If the patient is *critically* hypotensive, consider calling a peri-arrest cardiac emergency.
- IV access via two large bore cannulae, catheterize, cross-match blood (10U), order FFP and platelets.
- High flow O_2 via non-rebreathing mask.
- Give modest doses of analgesia (morphine 5–10mg).
- Alert anaesthetist, theatres, ITU.
- Witnessed verbal consent for surgery may be the only practical way and is acceptable here.

Establish a diagnosis

- If patient stable and diagnosis uncertain, request contrast CT.
- If going to CT, ensure blood is sent for cross-match and IV access has been established before going.

Early management

Ruptures fall into three groups:

- *Considered not a candidate for surgery.* For analgesia and palliative care. Mortality approximates to 100%. The decision is based on age, physiological status, comorbidities, expressed patient preference, family wishes.
- *Free rupture with collapse and critical condition.* All candidates for surgery require emergency transfer to theatre.
- *Contained leak.* May be stable after initial presentation, but likely to progress to free or complicated rupture unless urgently surgically treated.

Principles of surgery for rupture

- Go straight to the operating table, not anaesthetic room.
- If unstable, muscle relaxation/anaesthesia is not started until patient is prepared/draped and surgical team ready to go.
- If haemodynamically stable, central line and arterial line sited while waiting for blood to arrive and surgical team in theatre.
- Give antibiotic prophylaxis.
- Proximal neck is controlled rapidly with aortic cross-clamping. Full fluid expansion with blood can now safely begin.
- Distal outflow of aneurysm is controlled.
- The sac is opened and lumbar vessels and inferior mesenteric artery are oversewn to control back bleeding.
- Dacron/Gore-Tex® graft is sewn to proximal neck and tested.
- Distal anastomosis performed next and tested.
- Sequential reperfusion is undertaken accompanied with volume expansion to minimize post-declamping shock. Ideally the systolic BP should be maintained over 85mmHg.
- Blood products at this stage may be required to correct coagulopathy (e.g. platelets and FFP).
- The sac is closed over the graft to reduce the risk of aortoenteric fistula.

Post-operative care

- Transfer to ITU.
- Normalize core temperature.
- Correct clotting and maintain Hb >10g/dL.
- Adequate analgesia and accurate fluid balance.
- Attention to cardiac/renal/pulmonary dysfunction.

Complications

- Death (overall up to 50% of operated cases).
- MI.
- Renal failure.
- Lower limb embolism.
- Gut ischaemia/infarction.
- Abdominal compartment syndrome.

Vascular developmental abnormalities

Key facts

Classified broadly into two principal groups.

Vascular tumours (e.g. haemangiomas)

- All congenital or idiopathic.
- Mostly sporadic, but may rarely be part of a familial syndrome (e.g. von Hippel–Lindau).
- Pulmonary haemangiomas, commonly seen in hereditary haemorrhagic telangiectasia, are linked to a deficiency in endoglin (endothelial growth factor).

Vascular malformations

- Vascular malformations are histologically categorized as capillary, venous, lymphatic, arteriovenous malformations (AVM), or mixed-in type, depending on the predominant vessel type affected and subdivided into low or high flow (AVMs) varieties.
- AVMs have three main causes.
  - *Congenital.* Origin/cause unknown.
  - *Traumatic.* May follow relatively minor trauma.
  - *Iatrogenic.* Following a variety of surgical/interventional procedures.

Clinical features

- Congenital AVMs are usually evident at birth and the superficial lesion may only represent a part of the overall abnormality.
- Symptoms are dependent on the size, site, and type of vessel affected, and whether the AVMs are high or low flow.

Low flow

- May result in considerable cosmetic deformity if large (e.g. Klippel–Trenaunay—port wine stain + ipsilateral hypertrophy, usually limb).
- Pain may be a feature due to spontaneous thrombosis of some/all of the venous elements.
- Typically, the symptoms are worse after exercise when blood flow is maximized.

High flow

- These are largely asymptomatic, but there may be a detectable venous hum or bruit.
- They may result in local hyperhidrosis, heat, ulceration, or present with profuse bleeding.
- May lead to high output cardiac failure if large and untreated.

Diagnosis and investigation

- Colour duplex. Diagnoses lesion, can estimate flow rate, and is useful for follow-up monitoring.
- MRI has replaced CT as the best imaging modality and gives both the extent and related anatomy for complex lesions.
- Angiography is reserved for high flow lesions when suitability for embolization or surgery is being assessed.

Treatment

- Largely conservative.
  - Congenital AVMs frequently reduce in size with growth of the child and treatment is rarely easy with recurrence common.
  - Adult AVMs only require treatment for complications or occasionally cosmesis.

Interventional radiology

- Percutaneous or intravascular embolization using wire coils or sclerosant under radiological guidance.
- Risks include:
  - Those of percutaneous puncture (infection, false aneurysm formation, inadvertent embolization of adjacent vessels).
  - Tissue necrosis after successful lesion embolization.
  - *Post-embolization syndrome* may occur with pain at the site of embolization, accompanied by malaise, fever and leucocytosis, hyperkalaemia. This usually settles with symptomatic treatment in 24–48h. Due to tissue necrosis and cytokine release.

Surgery

- Small lesions may be excised completely.
- Obliteration of small superficial venous malformations can be undertaken by direct puncture and injecting a sclerosant such as STD (sodium tetradecyl sulphate).
- Open surgery is mostly confined to high flow lesions after preoperative embolization.

Carotid disease

Key facts

- A cerebrovascular accident (CVA) or 'stroke' is 'a rapidly developing neurological deficit lasting >24h'.
- A transient ischaemic attack (TIA) is 'an acute episode of focal (cerebral or visual) neurological deficit which resolves within 24h'.
- CVA is the third most common cause of death in UK after coronary heart disease and cancer.
- Incidence—stroke 200 per 100 000, TIA 35 per 100 000.
- Approximately 150 000 CVAs occur in the UK per year and approximately 15% of these are due to atherosclerotic disease of the carotid arteries.

Pathological features

CVA or TIA arises from disease at the origin of the internal carotid artery (ICA) and may be due to platelet or atheromatous embolization from the surface of the plaque (usually after an acute rupture or opening of the plaque surface).

Clinical features

- Several clinical variants of a classic CVA are recognized.
  - *Stroke in evolution.* Progressive neurological deficit occurring over hours/days.
  - *Completed stroke.* The stable end result of an acute stroke lasting over 24h.
  - *Crescendo TIA.* Rapidly recurring TIA with increasing frequency, suggesting an unstable plaque with ongoing platelet aggregation and small emboli.
- Carotid bruits are detectable in over 10% of patients aged >60, poor correlation with the degree of stenosis/risk of CVA, and may not arise from the ICA.
- Patients with a significant stenosis may have no audible bruit.

Neurological features

Depend on the territory supplied by the vessel affected by the embolism, the degree of collateral circulation to that territory, and the size/resolution of the embolism.

- *Amaurosis fugax.* Transient monocular visual loss (described as a curtain coming down across the eye), lasting for a few seconds or minutes—*central retinal artery (occlusion can lead to permanent blindness).*
- *Internal capsular stroke.* Dense hemiplegia, usually including the face—*striate branches of the middle cerebral artery.*
- *Hemianopia.* Loss of vision in one half of the visual field.

Prognosis of patients with TIA

Eighty per cent of TIAs are in the carotid territory. The risk of stroke following a TIA is around 18% in the first year, 10% in the first 90 days, and 4% in the first 24h.

Diagnosis and investigation
- Colour duplex scan. All patients with TIA/CVA within last 6 months.
- MRA or CT angiography (CTA). Used when duplex is inconclusive or difficult due to calcified vessels.

Treatment
Medical management
- Best medical therapy is an antiplatelet agent (e.g. aspirin, dipyridamole), smoking cessation, optimization of BP and diabetes control, and a statin (e.g. simvastatin 40mg daily) for cholesterol lowering, irrespective of baseline cholesterol.
- Acute thrombolysis in CT-proven ischaemia indicated in specialized units if detected early.

Surgery
Carotid endarterectomy (CEA)
- Offered to patients with symptomatic >70% stenosis of the ICA or >50% stenosis if recent TIA/CVA and high ABCD2 risk score (**a**ge, **B**P, **c**linical, **d**uration, diabetes).
- Urgent CEA within 2 weeks now considered for all patients presenting of acute TIA/CVA.
  - ECST (Europe) and NASCET (North America) trials demonstrated ↓ CVA in the first year following CEA from 18% with best medical therapy to 3–5% with surgery and best medical therapy. No significant benefit to symptomatic patients with <70% stenoses.
  - ACST (UK) and ACAS (North American) trials have shown some benefit of CEA to asymptomatic patients with >70% stenosis, but the numbers needed to prevent one stroke are 22 patients treated.
- Technical details.
  - Increasingly undertaken under local (LA) block.
  - Incision anterior to sternomastoid.
  - Carotid vessels controlled after dissection.
  - IV heparin prior to trial clamp (if patient awake).
  - Cerebral circulation protected in 10% of awake patients with a shunt (Pruitt/Javed) (without an intact *circle of Willis*, there is not enough collateral blood flow from the contralateral carotid).
  - Shunt in GA patients, depending on surgeon preference and cerebral monitoring (stump pressure of 50mmHg or transcranial Doppler monitoring of middle cerebral artery blood flow).
  - Patch closure of the arteriotomy common. Eversion endarterectomy technique may avoid the need for a patch.
  - Post-operatively, close monitoring of BP and neurological state.
- Complications.
  - Death or major disabling stroke, 1–2%.
  - Minor stroke with recovery, 3–6%.
  - MI.
  - Wound haematoma.
  - Damage to hypoglossal nerve (weak tongue, moves to side of damaged nerve), glossopharyngeal nerve (difficulty swallowing), facial numbness.

The diabetic foot

Key facts

Foot ulceration is the commonest endpoint of diabetic vascular complications. Diabetics are 15 times more likely to undergo major lower limb amputation than non-diabetics.

Causes and features

- Key features of the diabetic foot are:
  - Ulceration.
  - Infection.
  - Sensory neuropathy.
  - Failure to heal trivial injuries.

Ulceration

- Risk factors for ulceration include:
  - Previous ulceration.
  - Neuropathy (stocking distribution loss and 'Charcot's joints').
  - Peripheral arterial disease (more commonly affects the below-knee calf vessels (trifurcation) which are frequently highly calcified, giving rise to falsely elevated ABPI readings or incompressible vessels).
  - Altered foot shape.
  - Callus, indicating high foot pressures.
  - Visual impairment.
  - Living alone.
  - Renal impairment.
- Secondary to either large vessel or small vessel arterial occlusive disease or neuropathy or a combination of both.
- Forty-five per cent of diabetic foot ulceration are purely neuropathic in origin, 10% are purely ischaemic, 45% are of mixed neuro-ischaemic origin.

Diagnosis and investigation

Pure neuropathic ulceration

- Warm foot with palpable pulses.
- Evidence of sensory loss, leading to unrecognized repeated local trauma.
- Normal or high duplex flows.

Ischaemic/neuro-ischaemic ulceration

- Foot may be cool.
- Absent pulses.
- Ulcers commonly on toes, heel, or metatarsal head.
- Secondary infection may be present with minimal pus and mild surrounding cellulitis.
- ABPIs may be misleadingly high.
- Duplex ultrasound assessment.
- Angiography for suspected critical ischaemia.

Treatment

Prophylactic management

- Best undertaken in a specialist diabetes foot clinic with multidisciplinary input.
- Regular foot inspection for evidence of pressure/ulceration.
- Always use appropriate wide-fitting footwear.
- Attention to nail care with regular chiropody.
- Chiropodist debridement of pressure sites/callus.
- Keep away from heat and do not walk barefoot.

Established ischaemic ulceration

- Treat local or systemic infection.
  - Broad-spectrum antibiotics (local guidelines).
  - Debride obviously dead tissue, including digital amputation.
  - Drain collections of pus.
  - Take plain X-ray for signs of underlying osteomyelitis.
- Consider revascularization if appropriate.
  - Angioplasty.
  - Femoro-distal bypass grafts.
- Consider amputation for failed medical or surgical treatment.
  - Often possible to do limited distal amputations (e.g. transmetatarsal).
  - May be progressive if disease spreads.

The diabetic surgical patient

- Renal disease requires close monitoring of hydration, BP, and renal function.
- Metformin needs to be stopped for 48h before angiography to avoid lactic acidosis.
- Insulin-dependent diabetics starved for any reason require a sliding scale.
- Avoid pressure sores if immobile for any long period with foam leg troughs, heel elevation, and prompt attention to any skin breaks.

Amputations

Key facts

- Ninety per cent for arterial disease, 10% for trauma, and rarely for venous ulceration, tumour, or deformity.
- Amputation may be a very beneficial treatment for pain, to restore mobility or occasionally, to save a life in trauma or acute limb ischaemia.
- Amputation for arterial disease carries a significant mortality and a major morbidity.
- The surgical aim is to achieve a healthy stump for a suitable prosthesis and successful rehabilitation.
- Amputees are at the centre of a large team, including surgeons, nurses, physiotherapists, prosthetists, occupational therapists, pain team, counsellors, and the family.

Causes and features

- 'Dangerous': life-saving.
  - Spreading gangrene, e.g. necrotizing fasciitis, gas gangrene.
  - Extensive tissue necrosis following burns or trauma.
  - Uncontrolled sepsis (diabetic foot) with systemic infection.
  - Primary malignant limb tumours not suitable for local excision.
- 'Dead': vascular events.
  - Critical limb ischaemia with unreconstructable disease.
  - Extensive tissue necrosis.
- 'Damn nuisance': neuropathic or deformed. Failed, complicated orthopedic surgery with severely impaired gait.

Level

- The level is chosen according to:
  - Lowest level where tissue is viable for healing.
  - Include as many working major joints as possible to improve function.
  - Ideally sited between large joints to allow prosthesis fitting.
- *Above knee.* Most will heal, but only young and fit achieve walking with a prosthesis.
- *Through knee.* Fewer heal and some achieve walking.
- *Below knee.* About two-thirds heal and more achieve walking than with above-knee amputations.

Types

- *Hip disarticulation.* Rarely needed, but indicated for trauma or tissue necrosis above high thigh.
- *Above knee amputation (AKA).* Bone transected at junction of upper two-thirds and lower third of femur (12–15cm above knee joint), common in end-stage vascular disease.
- *Gritti–Stokes (supracondylar AKA).* Increasingly popular for bilateral amputees as creates a long stump; especially good for wheelchair-dependent patients.

- *Through-knee amputation (TKA)*. Produces a wide stump, which is difficult for prosthesis fit.
- *Below-knee amputation (BKA)*. Weight bearing on patellar tendon with good prosthetic fit; good knee function essential.
  - Skew flap is arguably best technique as it produces a better stump for prosthetic fitting.
  - Alternative is a posterior flap, which is bulkier and leads to longer time to mobilization.
  - The tibia is transected 8–10cm distal to the tibial tuberosity and the fibula 2cm more proximally.
  - Post-operative mobilization is early and temporary limb aids can be used when the wound is sound.
- *Symes (ankle)*. Few indications for this in vascular patients and best avoided other than in trauma or diabetics. Prosthetic fitting is difficult and a good BKA is better for walking.
- *Transmetatarsal*. Useful in diabetics or when several toes are gangrenous.
- *Ray*. Used when digital gangrene extends to forefoot, especially useful for diabetics when infection tracks up tendon sheath.
- *Digital*. Usually only for diabetic disease or local trauma.

Treatment

Preoperative care
- Restore Hb levels and correct fluid and electrolyte balance.
- Ensure good diabetes control.
- Cross-match 2U of blood.
- Adequate analgesia (epidural may reduce phantom pain).
- ECG and CXR.
- Optimize cardiac function.
- Prophylactic antibiotics to include gentamicin.
- Counselling if available.

Post-operative care
- Pain control with epidural ± PCA.
- Regular physiotherapy to prevent muscle atrophy or contractures as well as upper limb exercises.
- Early rehabilitation on temporary limb aid.
- Own wheelchair to aid early mobilization.

Complications
- Infection.
- Non-healing of stump.
- Progression of underlying disease and higher level amputation.
- Phantom limb pain. Due to hypersensitivity in divided nerves, can be helped with gabapentin, amitryptyline, or carbamazepine.
- Failed mobilization. Early regular analgesia and physiotherapy are important.
- Perioperative cardiovascular events in arteriopathic patient.

Vasospastic disorders

Key facts
Many systemic disorders have vasospasm as part of their presentation.

Causes
Rheumatological disease
Often associated with autoimmune disease.
- Systemic sclerosis.
- Systemic lupus erythematosus (SLE).
- Rheumatoid arthritis.
- Sjögren's syndrome.
- Dermatomyositis.
- Polymyositis.

Neurological disease
- Reflex sympathetic dystrophy.
- Post-traumatic vasospasm.
- Vibration white finger (due to exposure to handheld vibrating tools in miners, fitters, builders, platers).

Drug induced
α-agonist treatment (ergotamine).

Idiopathic
Raynaud's disease.
- ♂:♀, 9:1.
- Affects 20–30% of young women, with a possible familial predisposition.
- Possibly due to deficiency of a potent vasodilator (a calcitonin gene-related peptide) in the digital nerves, allowing action of unopposed cold stress-induced release of the vasoconstrictor, *endothelin*.

Features
Vasospasm of any cause results in 'Raynaud's phenomenon'.
- Intermittent attacks.
- Initiated with pallor ('white'). Due to local tissue oligaemia.
- Proceeding to cyanosis ('blue'). Due to venous stasis and deoxygenation.
- Followed by rubor ('red'). Due to reactive hyperaemia as blood flow is restored.

Diagnosis and investigations
- Stop all vasoactive treatment 24h prior to assessment.
- After local cooling to 15°C, finger Doppler pressures change (fall >30mmHg significant).
- Screen. FBC, U&E, urinalysis, thyroid function tests, plasma viscosity, rheumatoid factor, autoantibody screen.

Treatment

Medical

- Avoidance of precipitating factors (e.g. outdoor work, smoking).
- Electrically heated gloves/socks.
- Drug therapy used if symptoms are severe enough to interfere with work/lifestyle.
  - Calcium channel blockers (e.g. nifedipine 10mg/day increasing to 20mg/day tds) may help, but side effects (headache) may limit use.
  - Iloprost® (prostacyclin) infusion. Weight-related doses given IV over 48–72h, as tolerated by side effects, for severe pain or impending/actual tissue loss.

Surgical

Sympathectomy. Reserved for patients with failure to respond to medical therapy or secondary complications (e.g. digital ulceration).

- *Lumbar*. Open/laparoscopic/chemical for foot symptoms; effects are mostly short-lived.
- *Cervical*. Mostly now thoracoscopic technique; effects are poor response rate and high relapse rate.

Varicose veins

Key facts

- The venous system of the leg comprises of three groups.
  - *Superficial.* Long (great) and short (lesser) saphenous systems and tributaries.
  - *Deep.* Between the muscle compartments of the legs following the major arteries.
  - *Perforators.* Connecting the superficial and deep systems.
- Blood passes from the superficial to deep systems via perforators in the calf, and also at the saphenofemoral junction (SFJ), saphenopopliteal junction (SPJ), and mid-thigh perforators (MTP) which contain one-way valves.
- Varicose veins are tortuous and dilated segments of veins, associated with valvular incompetence.
- Affect 35% of the population.
- Males and females almost equal prevalence.

Causes and features

Classification

- *Thread veins.* Intradermal dilated veins, also called 'flare', 'starburst', or 'broken' veins.
- *Reticular veins.* Subdermal 1–2mm diameter veins.
- *Truncal veins.* The long or short saphenous systems.
- *Varicose veins.* Usually arising from the truncal veins.
- *Venous malformations.* For example, congenital (Klippel–Trenaunay syndrome).

Causes

- Congenital.
- Primary idiopathic (the majority).
- Acquired.
  - Pelvic masses (e.g. pregnancy, uterine fibroids, ovarian mass, pelvic tumour).
  - Pelvic venous abnormalities (e.g. after pelvic surgery or irradiation, previous iliofemoral DVT).

Clinical features

- *Symptoms.* Pain, aching, itching, heaviness, swelling, oedema, worse at end of day/hot weather/premenstruation, cosmetic concerns.
- *Complications.* Eczema, phlebitis, lipodermatosclerosis, ulceration, or bleeding.

Diagnosis and investigations

- *General history and examination.* Oedema, eczema, ulcers (usually medial calf), lipodermatosclerosis, atrophie blanche, healed ulceration.
- *Visible standing.* Cough impulse, thrill, or saphenovarix at SFJ.
- *Tap test.* Tap downwards over vein from SFJ, impulse should be felt lower down if valves are incompetent (outdated and unhelpful).

- *Trendelenberg test.* For competence of SFJ, MTP, and SPJ (rarely used now Doppler/duplex available).
  - With the patient supine, elevate the leg, empty veins, apply tourniquet high in the thigh, and ask patient to stand.
  - Look for venous filling and then release the tourniquet, observing filling of the veins.
  - If controlled by the tourniquet and then rapidly fill on release, the incompetent valve is above the level of the tourniquet, i.e. SFJ.
  - Then repeat twice with tourniquet just above knee and below knee to test the MTP and SPJ, respectively.
- *Handheld Doppler (HHD).* Listen over SFJ and SPJ and apply calf compression with other hand and listen for reflux lasting 1–2s. Most accurate outpatient method of diagnosis and localization of primary venous reflux disease.
- *Colour duplex.* Gold standard investigation in defining anatomy and incompetence. Can be used for all or selectively for recurrent varicose veins, suspected short saphenous vein reflux, known or suspected previous DVT, mismatch between clinical examination and HHD.

Treatment options
Medical
- Microsclerotherapy, laser sclerotherapy for thread and reticular veins.
- Foam sclerotherapy for truncal and varicose veins.
- Compression stockings.

Surgical
- Local 'stab' avulsions. Deals with varicosities.
- Saphenofemoral or saphenopopliteal disconnection.
- Long saphenous vein stripping (effectively avulses all incompetent thigh perforators). Not usually done below the knee due to risk of saphenous nerve injury.
- Endovenous laser therapy (EVLT).
- Radiofrequency ablation (endoluminal heating).
- Subfascial endoscopic perforator ligation (SEPL). For calf perforators.

Indications for treatment
- Cosmetic.
- For symptoms.
- To prevent complications.
- To reduce risk of recurrent complications.

Complications of surgery
- Bruising (virtually universal).
- Recurrence (50% cases at 10y).
- Haemorrhage (minor or, rarely, major from damaged femoral vein).
- Wound infection (commonest in groin).
- Saphenous or sural nerve damage with paraesthesia (20% numbness, 1% dysaesthesia).
- Damage to major arteries, e.g. femoral (rare).

Deep venous thrombosis

Causes and features

- Occurs due to abnormalities of the vein wall, blood flow, or constituents of blood (*Virchow's triad*).
- May be due to vein compression or stasis (immobility, trauma, mass, surgery, paralysis, long distance travel, including airline travel).
- May be due to inherited hypercoagulability (factor V Leiden, protein C, protein S, or antithrombin insufficiency).
- May be due to acquired hypercoagulability (surgery, malignancy, polycythaemia, smoking, hormone replacement therapy, oral contraceptive pill (OCP), dehydration).
- Severity may vary from isolated asymptomatic tibial/calf thrombosis to severe iliofemoral segment thrombosis with *phlegmasia caerulea dolens* (venous gangrene).

Clinical features

- Clinical manifestations may be absent.
- Local features of venous engorgement and stasis.
  - Limb swelling.
  - Pain.
  - Erythema and warmth to the touch.
  - Mild fever and tachycardia result from release of inflammatory mediators.
  - Homan's sign. Calf pain on dorsiflexion of the foot is very unreliable and should NOT be performed.
- Complications.
  - PE.
  - Venous gangrene (*phlegmasia caerulea dolens*).

Diagnosis and investigations

Aim to confirm presence and extent of thrombosis (to decide on necessity and type of treatment, risk of embolization).

- *Ascending venography.* Rarely used now.
- *Duplex scan.* Investigation of choice; visualizes anatomy, gives extent of thrombosis, and relies on flow of blood and compressibility of vein. Operator-dependent and has lower sensitivity for calf DVT.
- *VQ scan.* If suspicion of PE.
- *CT pulmonary angiography (CTPA).* Most sensitive and specific investigation for suspected PE.

Treatment

- Effective prophylaxis is better than treatment (see 📖 p. 72).
- Conservative measures. Elevation and good hydration.
- Uncomplicated DVT. Low molecular weight heparin (LMWH), initially in hospital, may be as an outpatient via a dedicated DVT clinic. Subsequent treatment is with oral anticoagulation with warfarin for 3–6 months.
- Complicated DVT. Initially with IV unfractionated heparin (UFH) or LMWH whilst converting to oral anticoagulation with warfarin.

- Thrombolysis or surgical thrombectomy are reserved for severe thrombosis with venous gangrene.
- Vena caval filter. Percutaneously inserted via jugular or femoral vein into infrarenal IVC to catch thromboemboli and prevent PE.
  - Used for patients with recurrent PE despite treatment, at risk of major central PE and anticoagulation contraindicated, requiring urgent or major surgery (so cannot be anticoagulated), major DVT with concomitant CNS injury or major fractures.
  - Risks include air embolism, arrhythmias, pneumo/haemothorax, IVC obstruction, renal vein thrombosis, retained, misplaced, migrating, eroding, embolizing or broken catheters/sheaths, complications of insertion (e.g. bleeding).

Chronic venous insufficiency Severe forms are often secondary to extensive or recurrent lower limb DVT (post-phlebitic limb).

Clinical features
- Leg/ankle oedema.
- Varicose/eczema, pigmentation, lipodermatosclerosis.
- Venous ulceration (medial more common than lateral).
- Venous claudication (rare).

Assessment
- Many (80%) venous disease alone, others mixed with arterial disease.
- History of proven/suspected DVT is common.
- Ulcers present in many patients and 70% are recurrent.

Investigations
- Handheld Doppler pressures (e.g. arterial disease ABPI <0.85).
- Venous duplex to detect DVT or deep venous incompetence and to look for superficial venous disease.

Treatment
- Elevation, bed rest, and elevation of foot of bed.
- Four layer bandaging (Charing Cross) if ulceration present and ABPI >0.85. Up to 75% ulcer healing at 12 weeks.
- Graduated compression hosiery (when ulcers healed).
  - *Class I.* Ankle pressure <25mmHg, prophylaxis.
  - *Class II.* Ankle pressure 25–35mmHg, marked varicose veins and chronic venous insufficiency.
  - *Class III.* Ankle pressure 35–45mmHg, chronic venous insufficiency.
  - *Class IV.* Ankle pressure 45–60mmHg, lymphoedema.

Surgery
- Skin grafts (split skin and pinch skin grafts).
- Ulcer bed clearance of slough/infection (physical, chemical, larval—maggots, vacuum debridement).
- Surgery for superficial venous disease only (as for varicose veins surgery).
- Role in mixed superficial and deep venous disease is controversial.
- May need arterial revascularization.

Thrombolysis

Key facts

- Introduced over 30y ago.
- Use diminishing over last 5y due to up to 5% risk of major haemorrhage or stroke.
- Usually administered as a low dose intra-arterial infusion or as an adjunct to surgery intraoperatively.

Agents

- *Urokinase.* Expensive, rarely used in UK other than for dialysis catheters.
- *Streptokinase.* Cheap, but has systemic effects and 27min half-life. Has side effects of anaphylaxis, fever, and antibody resistance, limiting repeated use. Widely used for treatment of MI.
- *Recombinant tissue plasminogen activator (tPA).* Powerful clot affinity, lower systemic effects and bleeding complications, and half-life <6min.

Indications

- Treatment of acute limb ischaemia with viable limb due to *in situ* thrombosis or embolism not suitable for surgery or extensive distal (calf) thrombosis.
- Treatment of acute surgical graft complications, e.g. prosthetic graft occlusion <2 weeks duration.
- Treatment of residual thromboembolic disease during reconstructive surgery (intraoperatively).
- Thrombosed popliteal artery aneurysm (allows clearance of distal calf vessels).
- Venous thrombosis (axillary/femoral) may be treatable by venous or arterial lysis, but need to balance risk of haemorrhage and stroke.

Regimen

- Administered via arterial catheter and simultaneous heparin via catheter sheath.
- Regular clinical assessment and coagulation checks are needed with clear protocols. Half-hourly temperature, pulse rate, and BP as well as foot observations.
- Regular review with repeat angiography.
- Increased complication rate after 24–36h of infusion.

Contraindications

- Increased risk of bleeding (haemorrhagic disorders, current peptic ulcer, recent haemorrhagic stroke, recent major surgery, or multiple puncture sites).
- Evidence of muscle necrosis as may result in reperfusion syndrome and multi-organ failure.
- Urgent cases because threatened limb viability if lysis takes too long to work.

Complications

- *Minor*. Allergic, catheter problems (leak, occlusion), bruising, 15% risk of minor haemorrhage.
- *Major*. Five per cent risk of major haemorrhage or stroke.

Complications in vascular surgery

Complications may occur in the perioperative, early, or late post-operative periods. In general, vascular patients are older and have increased cardiac, cerebral, pulmonary, and renal comorbidities. This is due to the associated risk factors of hypertension, diabetes mellitus, hypercholesterolaemia, and smoking.

General

Cardiac (see 📖 p. 106)
- Atherosclerosis is a systemic disease with a predilection for the cerebral, coronary, peripheral arterial, and renal circulations.
- Forty per cent of patients with PVD have at least two other circulations affected.
- Twenty per cent of patients undergoing non-cardiac vascular surgery have evidence of silent myocardial ischaemia.
- Seventy per cent of the mortality associated with aortic surgery is attributable to perioperative cardiac dysfunction.

Pulmonary (see 📖 p. 108)
- Worsened by pre-existing pulmonary disease, smoking, and obesity.
- Ensure adequate analgesia with PCA or epidural and good physiotherapy and early mobilization.

Haemorrhage (see 📖 p. 102)
- *Perioperative.* Bleeding from uncontrolled blood vessels.
- *Post-operative.* May be due to breakdown of vascular anastomoses. Recognized by acute hypotension, shock, abdominal swelling, and pain. Return to the operating theatre.

Renal failure
- Many vascular patients have pre-existing renal impairment due to renovascular disease, drug treatments, or surgery.
- Acute perioperative risks include dehydration, use of IV contrast, use of NSAIDs, or nephrotoxic antibiotics.

Infection
- Wound infections reduced by prophylactic antibiotics.
- MRSA easy to prevent (hand hygiene), but difficult and expensive to treat.
- *Clostridium difficile* enteritis (hand washing prevents) associated with antibiotic mis/overuse in inpatients.

Specific

Post-declamp shock (reperfusion syndrome)
- Ischaemic extremities during surgery reperfused into circulation.
- Features of acute haemodynamic instability due to release of toxins (potassium, myoglobin).
- Prevented by controlled gradual reperfusion with fluid resuscitation and vasopressor treatment to maintain a good perfusion pressure to the coronary, cerebral, and renal circulations.
- Mannitol often used as a free radical scavenger.

Trash foot
- Embolization of debris to the skin of feet or buttocks after aorto-iliac surgery.
- Avoided by careful surgical technique and distal vessel clamping first.

Swollen limb
- Most are due to reperfusion injury of previously ischaemic limbs.
- Consider investigations for DVT.

Lymphocoele
- Occurs mostly after groin surgery.
- Presents as a fluctuant, non-tender swelling.
- Most will settle spontaneously, although larger collections may be aspirated under STRICT aseptic conditions.
- Rarely require further surgery to oversew the lymphatics.

Gut ischaemia
- May follow aortic surgery (ischaemic colitis); 2.5% after ruptured AAA surgery and <1% of elective aortic aneurysm surgery due to loss of gut blood supply.
- May present as vague abdominal pain or bloodstained diarrhoea.
- Sigmoidoscopy usually confirms the diagnosis.
- If there is no evidence of peritonitis, then fluids to rehydrate and close observation are required.
- If there is evidence of peritonitis, then an urgent laparotomy is needed with resection of the ischaemic bowel.

Impaired sexual function
Due to damage to the peri-aortic or hypogastric plexus and underlying vascular disease of the blood supply to the pelvis.

Late complications
Graft occlusion
- *Early failure (<30 days)*. Technical cause; recognized by acute deterioration in symptoms or acute limb ischaemia.
- *Late failure*. Usually due to intimal hyperplasia, continued smoking, or disease progression; recognized by progressively worsening symptoms, falling ABPI, or duplex scanning showing graft stenosis.

False aneurysm
Usually secondary to infection or occasionally, fatigue of graft material (long-term). Further surgery is usually required.

Graft infection
- Mostly gut bacteria or coagulase-negative staphylococci; MRSA an increasing problem.
- Can be minimized by prophylactic antibiotics, meticulous technique, and infection control policies on vascular wards.
- Once infected, the graft usually has to be removed and alternative reconstruction required.
- Recognized by signs of low grade or chronic sepsis (↑ CRP, ↓ Hb, fever).

Aortoenteric fistula
- Rare, usually fatal if not treated.
- Usually follows aortic grafting. Can be years later.
- Presents with small, often overlooked, GI bleeds or anaemia.
- Diagnosis difficult. CT can be helpful; often all other causes of bleeding are negative.
- Treatment by open surgery or endovascular exclusion and antibiotics.

Transplantation

Basic transplant immunology

Allorecognition

Allorecognition is the identification of antigen as 'non-self'. It is a function mainly of the adaptive immune response, but is dependent on priming by an inflammatory response from the innate immune system; such a response occurs in transplantation, both from the inflammatory response to surgery and ischaemia-reperfusion injury in the graft.

Allorecognition depends on two main processes. First, alloantigen must be taken up and complexed with surface major histocompatibility complex (MHC) molecules on antigen-presenting cells (APCs) that include dendritic cells and macrophages. *Direct recognition* occurs when donor APCs within the allograft perform this function whereas *indirect recognition* is the term used when host APCs do this. Secondly, antigen-specific host T-cell receptors must bind to the peptide fragments of alloantigen complexed with the MHC molecules on APCs. This T-cell binding only activates a response if there is also co-stimulatory signal from the APC.

B- and T-cell diversity

Lymphocytes are able to identify non-self by the presence of both T-cell receptors (TCR) and B-cell receptors (BCRs) specific for each alloantigen. The production of a huge number of receptors (approximately 2.5×10^7), each specific to a particular peptide fragment, is possible because of the millions of potential combinations of the thousands of TCR and BCR gene segments. The TCR gene segments are located in chromosomes 14 and 7; the BCR gene fragments are on chromosome 14.

T-cell activation

When the TCR binds to antigen complexed with MHC molecules, a chain of reactions between intracellular signalling molecules leads to cell apoptosis unless a co-stimulatory signal from the APC also occurs. Binding of the TCR as well as CD and co-stimulatory molecules with the MHC leads to T-cell activation, differentiation, and clonal expansion. This results in the rapid production of large numbers of cells able to coordinate and effect destruction of tissues bearing the specific alloantigen; this manifests clinically as rejection.

Rejection

There are several types of rejection:

- Hyperacute rejection is mediated by preformed antibodies that bind to antigens of ABO blood groups, non-self HLA, causing immediate tissue oedema, haemorrhage, and thrombosis, which can produce a severe systemic reaction like an ABO-incompatible blood transfusion.
- Acute rejection is mediated either by T-cells ('cellular rejection') or newly formed antibodies ('humoral rejection') and results in tissue destruction over days to many months after transplant.
- Chronic rejection is a poorly understood vasculopathy associated with fibrosis of small blood vessels that occurs over years. It is a chronic inflammatory condition which probably has an alloreactive component.

A basic glossary of terms in transplant immunology

- **Adaptive immunity.** Learned response to specific non-self antigens.
- **Allo-.** Tissue from genetically different member of same species. *Alloantigen.* Antigen from genetically different member of same species. *Allogenicity.* Ability of tissue to provoke an immune response when transplanted into genetically different member of same species. **Allorecognition.** Recognition of alloantigen as non-self.
- **Antigen.** Cell surface glycoproteins.
- **Antibody.** Specific proteins produced by B-cells in response to non-self antigen, consisting of two light and two heavy chain proteins composing a constant and a variable region. The variable chain region binds with the antigen that triggered the response and the constant region coordinates the cellular response.
- **APC (antigen-presenting cells).** These cells ingest and process antigen, then present it bound to surface MHC to T-cells. APCs are most commonly dendritic cells or macrophages, but other cells can act as APCs.
- **B-cells.** These cells mature in bone marrow. They produce antibodies, but can also present antigen. In response to antigen, they undergo clonal expansion, triggered and coordinated by T helper cells.
- **Cellular immunity.** Adaptive immunity mediated by lymphocytes.
- **CD.** Cellular differentiation molecule (followed by a number, e.g. CD4).
- **Clonal expansion.** Production of large numbers of identical cells.
- **Co-stimulatory molecules.** Molecule receptors that must be activated, in addition to a main receptor, for a process to happen.
- **Direct recognition.** Donor APCs present alloantigen to host T-cells.
- **HLA (human leucocyte antigen).** Human MHC.
- **Humoral immunity.** Immunity mediated by non-cellular components of the immune system such as antibodies or complement.
- **Indirect recognition.** Host APCs present alloantigen to host T-cells.
- **Innate immunity.** Rapid inbuilt response to certain non-self proteins.
- **MHC (major histocompatibility complex).** Glycoproteins expressed on the surface of all cells, coded for by the MHC genes on chromosome 6. Alloantigen must be bound to MHC for T-cells to recognize it. There are two classes of MHC. Class I (HLA molecules A, B, and C) is present on all cell membranes. Class II (HLA molecules DP, DQ, and DR), also known as minor histocompatibility complex, is present on only certain cell types. Class II is less allogeneic.
- **Rejection.** Injury to tissue by host immune response.
- **T-cells.** These cells mature in the thymus. T-cells that bind to thymic tissue (self) are destroyed. **T helper cells** that are CD4 +ve coordinate and **T cytotoxic cells** (CD8 +ve) effect the response. **Regulatory T-cells** are also CD4 +ve and reduce the alloreactive response.
- **Tolerance.** A condition of lack of immune response to alloantigen where such a response is expected or has occurred previously.
- **Xenograft.** Tissue transplanted between species.

Immunosuppression and rejection

The goal of immunosuppression is to inhibit the immune response to alloantigen, while preserving the immune response to infection and malignancy. Immunosuppression consists of a short, intense induction phase followed by a maintenance phase in which immunosuppression dosage is tapered. A careful balance is maintained between therapeutic and toxic doses of immunosuppression; this is generally achieved by combining drugs with different mechanisms of action (see Box 19.1).

Acute rejection

Diagnosis

Clinical features depend on the organ transplanted and are generally manifested by clinical and biochemical evidence of impaired organ function or organ injury (such as elevated transaminase levels in liver transplantation). Systemic immune symptoms are less common and include low grade fever, malaise, and tenderness over the graft. Blood tests may reveal a lymphocytosis. Diagnosis is made by biopsy, which will also determine whether rejection is T-cell mediated or humoral, and can identify other causes of graft dysfunction.

The immunosuppression may mask symptoms until rejection is quite advanced, so routine surveillance may be undertaken, especially for those organs where loss of function would be catastrophic. When required, optimal surveillance is by 'protocol biopsies' taken at predetermined time points such as at 7–10 days after transplantation, with repeat biopsies taken at intervals. Percutaneous imaging-guided biopsy is typically used in liver and renal transplantation, endoscopic biopsy in small bowel and lung transplantation, and transjugular biopsy in heart transplants or liver transplants with uncorrectable coagulopathy.

Management

- Asymptomatic mild rejection may be monitored in some organs, but is always treated in renal transplants as kidneys are very immunogenic.
- The main form of treatment is increased immunosuppression.
- Up to 3 days IV methylprednisolone 500–1000mg/day is typically given as initial treatment for acute rejection.
- Repeat biopsy is performed if no improvement, followed by repeat steroid course if ongoing rejection, or give rescue therapy if severe.
- Rescue protocols include administration of anti-T-cell antibodies.
- Plasmapheresis to remove antibody may be required in humoral rejection, diagnosed by positive CD4 staining.
- Retransplantation is occasionally performed after graft loss due to refractory rejection, but is not performed for certain organs, such as the heart and lung, as results are extremely poor.

Chronic rejection

Chronic rejection is a chronic inflammatory process associated with intimal hyperplasia with dependent ischaemia and fibrosis. The cause is unknown, but appears related to the severity of acute inflammatory processes at the time of transplantation, such as ischaemia-reperfusion injury and acute rejection.

The intimal hyperplasia and dependent ischaemia affect the organs in different ways, such as coronary artery disease in heart, glomerulosclerosis in kidneys, and vanishing bile ducts in livers.

The term 'chronic rejection' is not widely used at present, with a variety of different names used according to the affected organ such as cardiac allograft vasculopathy (heart), bronchiolitis obliterans (lung), and chronic allograft nephropathy (kidney).

There is no specific treatment available for chronic rejection at the present time, with retransplantation as the only effective option.

Side effects of immunosuppression

Opportunistic infection

Cytomegalovirus (CMV) can cause life-threatening infection in transplant recipients and is especially common in the first 6 months. Examples are CMV pneumonitis and CMV colitis. Diagnosis is by quantitative polymerase chain reaction (PCR) and treatment by oral valganciclovir or IV ganciclovir for severe infections. Recipients felt to be at risk based on donor and recipient serology are given prophylactic valganciclovir for 100–200 days.

Pneumocystis jiroveci (*P. carinii*) infection can lead to a severe atypical pneumonia in immunosuppressed patients. It is generally prevented by prophylactic co-trimoxazole for the first 3 months.

BK virus infection is generally asymptomatic, but is a possible cause of failure of renal transplants.

Malignancy

Immunosuppression reduces immune surveillance of tumours, so some are more common in transplant recipients and others can be more aggressive than would otherwise be the case. Virally-mediated tumours and squamous cell carcinoma of the skin are especially common.

Post-transplant lymphoproliferative disorder (PTLD) is a condition of B-cell proliferation which may extend to B-cell lymphoma and is due to inhibition by immunosuppressant drugs of the IL2-dependent mechanism by which T-cells regulate the B-cell proliferation occurring in Epstein–Barr virus infection.

Although not a complication of immunosuppression per se, malignancy can also be transmitted from transplant donors to recipients and so must be excluded as far as possible with potential donors.

Box 19.1 Immunosuppressive agents

Corticosteroids

Corticosteroids inhibit the immune response at many levels. They decrease production of γ-interferon and interleukins that would normally cause up-regulation of the lymphocyte response and reduce macrophage function.

Calcineurin inhibitors (CNI)

Ciclosporin and tacrolimus are calcineurin inhibitors: they inhibit the production of IL-2 by T helper cells, selectively reducing the cytotoxic T-cell response. Nephrotoxicity is a major side effect, but they also impair glucose tolerance and affect lipid metabolism.

Mammalian target of rapamycin (mTOR) inhibitors

Sirolimus (rapamycin) and everolimus both inhibit the production of IL-2 by T-cells and thus stops their clonal expansion in a manner similar to the calcineurin inhibitors. mTOR inhibitors are not themselves nephrotoxic, but they appear to potentiate the nephrotoxicity of CNIs if given together.

Mycophenolic acid

Mycophenolic acid inhibits purine synthesis in lymphocytes, reducing clonal expansion and lymphocyte counts. It can cause severe GI side effects which are reduced by administration as enteric-coated tablets or as the pro-drug, mycophenolate mofetil (MMF).

Azathioprine

Azathrioprine reduces lymphocyte production by suppression of purine synthesis. Allopurinol inhibits the metabolism of azathioprine. Bone marrow suppression and pancreatitis are common adverse reactions.

Basiliximab

Monoclonal antibody that binds to the IL-2 receptor of T-cells and thus prevent clonal expansion of T-cells. Usually given as induction agent.

Anti-thymocyte globulin (ATG)

Derived from rabbits or horses immunized with T-cells; primarily directed against the T-cell receptor. Systemic inflammatory reactions occur due to cytokine release from T-cells when the receptor bound.

Alemtuzumab (Campath)

Monoclonal antibody binding to CD52 receptor, leading to depletion of T-cells, B-cells, natural killer cells, lymphocyte precursors, dendritic cells, and macrophages. It thus reduces all the cells involved in antigen presentation, cellular rejection, and humoral rejection. Usually used as an induction agent. Side effects include bleeding and sepsis.

Belatacept

A new drug which blocks co-stimulation of T-cells by antigen presenting cells. Not nephrotoxic or diabetogenic. Long-term effect unknown.

Transplant recipients

Indications for transplantation

Cardiac transplantation
- End-stage heart disease with a life expectancy of 12–18 months.
- NYHA class III or IV heart failure, refractory to medical or surgical therapy.
- Cardiomyopathy and congenital heart disease.

Lung transplantation End-stage lung disease where conventional therapy is not likely to provide acceptable benefits or satisfactorily improve life expectancy.

Renal transplantation All patients with end-stage renal failure should be considered for renal transplant unless there are specific contraindications.

Liver transplantation
- Unacceptable quality of life because of liver disease.
- Anticipated 1y mortality >9% without transplant.

Pancreas transplantation
- Usually with or after kidney transplantation for diabetic nephropathy.
- Can be done alone for hypoglycaemic unawareness (consider islets).

Small bowel transplantation (often part of multivisceral)
- Congenital extensive atresia.
- Life-threatening complications of TPN in patients with intestinal failure.
- Loss of central venous access sites in patients with intestinal failure.

Absolute contraindications to transplantation
- Predicted life expectancy <5y due to comorbidity.
- Inability to comply with immunosuppression.
- Chronic current systemic infection.
- Continued abuse of alcohol or other drugs.
- Irreversible secondary organ failure not appropriate for combined transplant.
- Severe cerebrovascular disease.
- Active malignancy.
- Other life-threatening medical condition.

Relative contraindications to transplantation
- HIV (controversial), hepatitis B/C (except in liver transplants).
- COPD with FEV_1 <50%, PVR >4 Wood units in heart transplants.
- Chronic renal impairment with GFR >50mL/min, unless candidate for renal transplant, including combined transplants with kidney.
- Diabetes with target organ damage (heart).
- Lipid disorders refractory to diet or therapy (heart).
- Severe osteoporosis.
- Amyloidosis.
- Continued smoking (heart or lung).

Routine investigations in transplant assessment

- A full history and clinical examination.
- CXR, ECG.
- Functional cardiopulmonary assessment if indicated, e.g. CPEX.
- Cardiac catheterization and coronary angiography if indicated.
- Lung function tests.
- MSU, urinalysis, nose swab, and MRSA screen.
- Blood group antibody screen.
- FBC and coagulation profile.
- U&E, calcium, phosphate, LFTs, fasting blood glucose, and lipids.
- Serology for hepatitis B/C, HIV, syphilis, rubella, EBV, herpes varicella and zoster, CMV, toxoplasma.
- HLA typing, lymphotoxic antibody screen.
- Assessment of compliance; may include interview with social worker.
- Further organ-specific tests as indicated.

Accepting a patient on to the transplant list

Accepting a patient for transplantation is a multidisciplinary process which varies from organ to organ. Potential kidney and/or pancreas transplant recipients are typically initially assessed by their nephrologist and then referred to a transplant surgeon. Potential recipients of liver, small bowel, heart, or lung transplants are usually discussed in a multidisciplinary meeting of transplant surgeons, anaesthetists, physicians, transplant coordinators, and specialist nurses. The patient is informed of the decision and receives:

- A detailed explanation of the waiting list procedures (including their responsibility to be within contact and available for potential transplant at all times and duty to inform the transplant team of any changes in their health; planned holidays can be permitted by temporary suspension from the list).
- A booklet describing this in more detail and explaining what to do when called for surgery, the operation, post-operative care, and follow-up arrangements.

Transplant donors

Availability of organs for transplantation

The increasing success of organ transplantation as a modality of treatment for end-stage organ disease has increased demand, a problem further exacerbated by widening the criteria for which patients can be considered suitable candidates for transplantation. This has lead to an increasing national shortage of organs despite efforts to increase donation.

A national Organ Donation Task Force was set up in the UK in 2006 and issued fourteen recommendations in 2008 for increasing organ availability. The final phase of their implementation commenced in 2010.

Deceased donation

Deceased donors form the majority of organ donors in the UK. Traditionally, the majority have been heart-beating donors after brainstem death (DBD), but increasingly non-heart-beating donors after circulatory death (DCD) are being used. Potential donors undergo a review of their history and clinical examination, ECG, CXR, ABGs, ABO typing, testing for HIV, hepatitis C/B, and CMV, and tests of organ function (e.g. U&E, LFTs, echo).

Criteria for cadaveric organ donation

- Signed donor card, registration as organ donor, or agreement by next of kin.
- Haemodynamic stability without high dose inotropic support.
- Absence of septicaemia, extracerebral malignancy, HIV, hepatitis B/C, viral encephalitis, use of human growth hormone, and new variant CJD.
- Brainstem death testing performed twice by two senior doctors after essential preconditions met and apnoea test performed (for DBD donors) (see Box 19.2).
- Organ-specific criteria include the following.
  - *Kidney*. Age 1–90y with acceptable renal function.
  - *Heart*. Age 1 month–60y with no known cardiac disease.
  - *Heart–lung*. As above; no pulmonary disease or trauma; PO_2, pCO_2 levels acceptable on less than 50% inspired oxygen.
  - *Liver*. Age 1 month–70y. No known liver disease, drug addiction, or hepatitis B.
  - *Pancreas*. Age 10–60y with no diabetes.

Box 19.2 Brainstem death testing (UK code)

Essential preconditions

The patient must be in an apnoeic coma, i.e. unresponsive and dependent on a mandatory ventilation mode, following irreversible structural brain damage due to a 'disorder which may cause brain death'.

Drug intoxication, hypothermia, and metabolic or endocrine disturbances must be excluded before brainstem death testing as these may mimic brainstem death clinically.

Apnoea test

Confirmation of apnoeic coma is performed by ventilator disconnection, with lack of spontaneous respiratory effort despite rising arterial carbon dioxide tension. Care must be taken to avoid hypoxia which could potentially cause further brain injury in a patient who might not yet be brainstem dead.

- Ensure systolic BP >90mmHg and adequate intravascular volume.
- Preoxygenate with 100% O_2 for 10min.
- Check $PaCO_2$ is at least 5.3kPa (40mmHg). If not, give 95% O_2/5% CO_2 until $PaCO_2$ >5.3kPa.
- Disconnect ventilator and insufflate 100% O_2 at 6L/min via an intratracheal catheter passed to the level of the carina.
- Continue disconnection until $PaCO_2$ >6.65kPa (50mmHg), which should occur within 8min.

Apnoea testing should be abandoned if there are cardiac arrhythmias, hypotension, or arterial desaturation. In the UK, apnoea testing must be attempted again before brainstem death is diagnosed.

Clinical tests

The brainstem reflexes should be tested by two experienced doctors, one of whom must be a consultant and neither of whom is a member of the transplant team. They may perform the tests together or independently and must repeat all the tests after a period of at least 2h.

- No pupillary response to light (both direct and indirect reflexes).
- No corneal reflex.
- No vestibulo-ocular reflex. No eye movement on irrigation of tympanic membrane with 20–50mL ice-cold water.
- No cranial nerve motor responses, e.g. grimacing to pain.
- No gag or cough reflex on deep bronchial suctioning.
- No oculocephalic reflex ('doll's eyes test').

Management of brainstem-dead organ donors (DBD)

Resuscitation of organ donors requires early recognition and assiduous support. Brain death is associated with a variety of sequelae, which include haemodynamic instability, hypothermia, coagulopathy, fall in T_3 and T_4, myocardial depression, and diabetes insipidus.

Therapeutic intervention must be continued up to and throughout the donation procedure. Unnecessary delays should be avoided and the retrieved organs must be in optimal condition.

Monitoring
- ECG.
- Radial artery line (MAP 60–70mmHg).
- Urine output (>100mL/h).
- CVP (greater than or equal to 12cmH$_2$O).
- Temperature (over 35.5°C).

Cardiovascular support
Noradrenaline (norepinephrine) is used for refractory hypotension. Dopamine may exacerbate any polyuria and cause vasoconstriction with end-organ damage. Dobutamine may exacerbate hypotension.

Hormone replacement therapy
- T$_3$. Bolus of 4 micrograms, then infusion of 3 micrograms/h.
- Diabetes insipidus. Replace urine loss with 5% dextrose and water via NGT. Vasopressin may exacerbate vasoconstriction, so its analogue, desmopressin (DDAVP), is generally used instead. The aim is to achieve 1.5–3mL urine/kg/h output.

Respiratory support Respiratory support requires meticulous asepsis. Oxygen delivery is optimized to achieve a normal PaCO$_2$. High PEEP should be avoided to minimize lung injury.

Haematological support Coagulopathies are treated with FFP and platelets, guided by the local laboratory.

Management of donors after circulatory death (DCD)
Most DCD are controlled donors, where life-prolonging treatment is withdrawn after a decision that the overall prognosis means that such treatment is felt to be futile. As such donors are living patients until the time of cardiac arrest and generally lack capacity to consent due to being unconscious, they can only be treated in line with their best interests under common law, restricting the interventions possible to optimize the condition of the transplanted organs.

Uncontrolled DCD following failed resuscitation for cardiac arrest cannot, by definition, be optimized prior to cardiac arrest, but basic measures to improve organ viability after death but prior to consent for donation are allowed under the Human Tissue Act and can include femoral cannulation to start aortic perfusion and peritoneal cooling.

Principles of cadaveric organ retrieval
The aim is to minimize ischaemic times of all organs. Retrieval of multiple organs is common, so a coordinated approach is needed. Inotropic, volume, and respiratory support is continued until the retrieval teams are ready to start cold perfusion.
- A midline incision from sternal notch to pubis is made.
- IV heparin 200U/kg is given.
- A diagnostic laparotomy is performed to assess for any undiagnosed disease, especially malignancy.

- Organs are carefully examined for evidence of trauma and disease. The aim is to retain adequate vascular and visceral cuffs to facilitate later anastomosis. Variant vascular anatomy to the liver is common and can affect retrieval of liver and pancreas, so this must be carefully assessed.
- As soon as both the abdominal and thoracic teams have completed their assessment and are ready for cold perfusion, the supracoeliac aorta is cross-clamped, ventilator stopped, cold perfusion established through aortic cannulae, and ice slush poured into the abdomen and the thorax. The organs are then dissected out and removed once cold.

Retrieval of organs from donors after circulatory death is different as cardiac arrest has already occurred, so the first priority is to start cold perfusion, with assessment of anatomy and disease done in the cold phase prior to organ retrieval.

Organ preservation

The key to minimizing ischaemic injury remains minimizing ischaemic time, but use of appropriate perfusion solutions reduces the severity of ischaemic injury. A variety of storage solutions are used at temperatures of 4–10°C. Two categories exist: extracellular solutions characterized by high Na^+ and low K^+ such as Bretschneider (HTK) and intracellular solutions characterized by high K^+ and low Na^+ such as University of Wisconsin solution (UW) or St Thomas's cardioplegia solution.

Machine perfusion

Organs are usually stored in ice slush once perfused, but are sometimes stored in a machine providing continuous perfusion of the organ. This is especially common for DCD kidneys using a cold perfusion circuit, which can also allow assessment of viability by measurement of pressure-flow characteristics and biochemical markers of ischaemic injury.

Warm perfusion using oxygenated perfusion solutions to assess and treat ischaemic injury prior to implantation has been used experimentally and may enter clinical practice in the near future.

Living donors

These are generally relatives or from genetically unrelated, but emotionally connected individuals (mostly commonly spouses), though undirected living donation to complete strangers is also allowed ('altruistic donation'). Living donation requires meticulous preparation to minimize risk to the donor and exclude coercion or financial reward; potential altruistic donors must also be psychologically assessed.

Kidneys are the most common transplants from living donors. Donation of a liver lobe is also possible due to the large functional reserve of the liver and its ability to regenerate by hypertrophy; left lobe liver donation from adults to children is especially common.

Living donation of lung lobes is also possible, but requires two donors for each recipient. Living pancreas donation using a distal pancreatectomy has been described, but is not widely used due to the potential risks to the donor of diabetes or pancreatic duct leakage.

- All donors undergo blood grouping, tissue typing, and assessment of viral status for hepatitis B/C, HIV, and CMV.

- Tests of organ function, such as isotope split GFR for kidneys, are needed to ensure adequate post-operative function for both donor and recipient.
- General tests of donor fitness are also essential to minimize risk.

ABO-incompatible living donors (see Tables 19.1 and 19.2)

Although ABO incompatibility is normally an absolute contraindication to transplantation as the preformed antibodies will lead to hyperacute rejection, it is possible to desensitize the potential recipient by a preoperative course of plasma exchanges or immunoadsorption to remove the antibody preceded by an infusion of the anti-B-cell antibody, rituximab, to prevent antibody regeneration. This treatment is only feasible for living donor transplants as these are planned operations.

Similar treatment can also be given to desensitize patients with preformed antibodies directed against the HLA type of their potential donor (such antibodies can be formed after sensitizing events, such as previous transplants or blood transfusions).

To prevent resensitization, care must be taken to avoid accidentally transfusing anti-ABO antibodies when administering blood products after the transplant. Red cell and platelets transfusions should use washed cells of recipient blood group. FFP and cryoprecipitate transfusions must be donor-type if the transplant is donor group A or B to recipient group O or type AB if the transplant is between A and B; alternatively, recipient-type blood products can be used if screened for low antibody activity.

Where recipient desensitization is not possible, paired exchange may be an alternative where the donor from each pair donates to the recipient of the other pair. Paired exchange requires a large pool of donor-recipient pairs to be successful and is only feasible for kidney transplants.

Table 19.1 ABO compatibility for transplants

Recipient blood group	Donor blood group			
	A	**B**	**AB**	**O**
A	Yes	No	No	Yes
B	No	Yes	No	Yes
AB	Yes	Yes	Yes	Yes
O	No	No	No	Yes

Table 19.2 Paired exchange to avoid ABO incompatibility

Donor Mr Smith (group A)	donates a transplant to	Recipient Mr Jones (group A)
Recipient Mrs Smith (group B)	receives a transplant from	Donor Mrs Jones (group B)

Heart and lung transplantation

Cardiac transplantation

Matching donor to recipient

- *ABO compatibility.* Donor and recipient must be ABO-compatible; hyperacute rejection occurs in ABO-incompatible patients. Children under 1y can be transplanted despite ABO incompatibility.
- *HLA typing.* Although heart is amongst the least allogeneic organs and a HLA mismatch is not a contraindication to transplantation, HLA-A$_2$ or -A$_3$ mismatch has been associated with chronic rejection and some centres choose to avoid this.
- *Size match.* Important; up to 30% undersize acceptable if normal PVR, oversize if high PVR.

Technique of transplantation

Orthotopic heart transplantation involves transplanting the donor organ into the space vacated by the recipient heart. There are several techniques of orthotopic heart transplantation.

- The most commonly used is the *bicaval anastomosis* technique. The donor cavae are attached directly to the recipient cavae. This results in less tricuspid regurgitation and better haemodynamic performance.
- In the *original technique*, right and left atria of donor and recipient are preserved; anastomosing atria to atria is technically less demanding than bicaval anastomosis.
- In the *total anastomotic technique*, each pulmonary vein is individually anastomosed.
- In *heterotopic transplantation*, used in 2.5% of heart transplants, the donor heart is retained and the transplanted heart is anastomosed so that it acts to bypass the left heart. The technique is reserved for severe pulmonary hypertension.

Post-operative care Monitoring for rejection is done via transvenous endomyocardial biopsy.

Complications

- Infections (nosocomial, opportunistic, or acquired).
  - Bacterial (common nosocomial (see 📖 pp. 104, 174) and opportunistic infections include *Pneumocystis carinii, Mycobacterium* spp.).
  - Viral (CMV, HBV, HIV may be transmitted from graft).
  - Fungal (*Candida albicans, Aspergillus*).
- Rejection (📖 pp. 676, 678) and graft ischaemic heart disease.
- Hyperlipidaemia and diabetes secondary to immunosuppression.
- Renal failure (similar risk factors to heart failure, perioperative hypoperfusion, nephrotoxic immunosuppression regimes).
- Hypertension. Aetiology poorly understood.
- Malignancy. Decrease in the T-cell response to EBV as a result of immunosuppression.

Results of cardiac transplantation
- UK 30-day mortality is 4%.
- 1y survival is 82%; 5y survival is 65%; 10y is 50%.

Lung and heart–lung transplantation

Matching donor to recipient
- *ABO compatibility*. Donor and recipient must be ABO-compatible; hyperacute rejection occurs in ABO-incompatible patients.
- *HLA typing*. Although a HLA mismatch is not a contraindication to transplantation, improved graft survival is associated with matching HLA-B, HLA-A, and HLA-DR loci.
- *Size match*. Important.

Technique of transplantation
- *Single lung transplant* is performed where the remaining native lung will not compromise graft function or present a hazard; emphysema, asthma, and sarcoid require single lung transplants.
- *Double lung* transplants are performed via a clam-shell incision for cystic fibrosis and bronchiectasis.
- Because of donor organ shortages, *heart–lung transplants* are performed less often with an increase in the use of lung transplants.
- *Domino heart–lung transplants*, where a heart–lung transplant was performed for septic lung disease and the healthy explanted heart then transplanted into a second recipient, is now rarely performed.

Post-operative care
Early post-operative management centres around maintaining a balance between adequate perfusion and gas exchange, while minimizing fluid load, cardiac work, and barotrauma. Cardiovascular management and complications are very similar to those outlined on 📖 p. 622. Monitoring for rejection is done by transbronchial biopsy and bronchoalveolar lavage.

Complications
- Infections (nosocomial, opportunistic, or acquired).
  - Bacterial (common nosocomial (see 📖 p. 174) and opportunistic infections include *Pneumocystis carinii*, *Mycobacterium* sp.).
  - Viral (CMV, HBV, HIV may be transmitted from graft).
  - Fungal (*Candida albicans*, *Aspergillus* sp.).
- Vascular stenoses. Arterial stenosis results in pulmonary oligaemia and venous stenosis in pulmonary oedema.
- Tracheal stenoses.
- Tracheal ischaemia may result in leak and mediastinitis.
- Infection with *Pseudomonas* sp. is common in cystic fibrosis patients. CMV infection is dangerous.

Results of lung transplantation
- 1y survival is 61%.
- 5y survival is 40%.

Kidney transplantation

Kidney transplantation is the commonest form of organ transplant. A total of 2739 were performed in the UK in 2009–10, of which 1038 were kidneys from living donors.

Matching donor to recipient
- *ABO compatibility.* Donor and recipient must normally be ABO-compatible; hyperacute rejection occurs in ABO-incompatible patients unless desensitization treatment has been performed preoperatively.
- *HLA typing.* Graft survival is better if there is no more than one mismatch for HLA-A and/or HLA-B and no mismatches for HLA-DR.
- *Children.* Given priority; even small children can take adult kidneys.

Technique of transplantation
The kidney is normally placed extraperitoneally into the iliac fossa. Both the left and right kidneys can be placed into either iliac fossa, but the right is easier as the external iliac vein is more accessible.
- The renal vessels are anastomosed to the external iliac vessels. The common or internal iliac artery can be used if the external is diseased.
- The ureter is anastomosed to the bladder, usually over a stent.
- Preoperative native nephrectomy is only occasionally needed for continued/recurrent urinary infection, TB of the kidney, or massive polycystic kidney disease.

Post-operative care
Early post-operative management centres around maintaining a balance between adequate renal perfusion and BP control.
- Graft function is monitored by serial creatinine measurements (this is especially useful if these are plotted on an inverse creatinine chart).
- Early graft failure is usually due to lack of perfusion following an arterial or venous thrombosis, so graft perfusion should be assessed by DTPA scan or Doppler ultrasound if there is not immediate graft function.
- Delayed graft function with oliguria or anuria is common early after transplantation, especially if there has been ischaemic injury prior to organ retrieval or a prolonged cold ischaemic time.
- Intermittent haemodialysis may be needed if there is delayed function.
- Polyuria is common once the kidney starts to function until renal tubular function recovers; fluid needs to be replaced to prevent pre-renal failure of the graft.
- Biopsy to confirm suspected rejection is done percutaneously under ultrasound guidance.

Complications
- Infection.
- Rejection (see 📖 p. 678).
- Renal vein or artery thrombosis may result in loss of the kidney.
- Ureteric stenosis. Treated by ureteroplasty and a stent or surgery.
- Urinary leak often can be managed by urinary catheterization for 6 weeks followed by cystogram to confirm healing.

- Lymphocoele is managed by percutaneous drainage or by laparoscopic or open marsupialization into the peritoneum.

Results of kidney transplantation
- For cadaveric kidney transplantation. 1y survival is 88%; 2y survival is 81%; 5y survival is 71%.
- For living donor kidney transplantation. 1y survival is 94%; 2y survival is 93%; 5y survival is 84%.

Pancreas and islet transplantation

Pancreatic transplantation is performed for insulin-dependent diabetes. It is either performed alone (rare) or in conjunction with kidney transplantation for diabetics in end-stage renal failure. A total of 160 combined kidney and pancreas transplants were performed in the UK in 2009–10.

Pancreas transplantation

The transplant operation

The pancreas is usually retrieved as the whole organ with the duodenum attached. It is transplanted either intraperitoneally or extraperitoneally into the right iliac fossa using similar techniques to those of renal transplantation.

The dual arterial supply of the pancreas, based on the splenic artery and superior mesenteric artery branches, is provided by forming an arterial Y graft from a length of common, internal, and external iliac arteries retrieved from the donor. The venous drainage is from the portal vein attached to the pancreas, which is generally anastomosed to the recipient's external iliac vein or vena cava; some centres anastomose the vein to a portal vein tributary, but this is technically challenging and requires a vein extension graft formed from donor iliac vein.

The drainage of exocrine function is by anastomosis of the attached duodenum either to the bladder or to a loop of small intestine. Most complications arise from the unwanted exocrine function of the graft. Bladder-drained exocrine secretions can cause chemical cystitis, requiring later conversion to enteric drainage in up to 25%. Exocrine anastomotic leakage may occur, giving rise to local inflammation, peritonitis, or pseudoaneurysm of the iliac artery.

Post-operative management

Immunosuppression is as for kidney transplantation although higher levels of immunosuppression, including use of induction antibody therapy such as alemtuzumab or ATG, is common.

Bladder-drained graft function may be monitored by assay of urinary amylase; this should be sampled from a 24h urine collection as there is diurnal variation in amylase secretion. Bicarbonate supplementation is required for bladder-drained pancreas transplants.

Enteric-drained pancreas transplants may be monitored by serial serum amylase and lipase levels. Immunological damage to the pancreas is advanced before changes in blood sugar are recognized.

When the pancreas is transplanted with a kidney, the kidney may be biopsied if rejection is suspected as it usually affects both organs or the kidney alone if only one organ is rejected.

Thrombosis of the venous drainage of the pancreas is common, so some centres routinely anticoagulate pancreas transplant recipients.

Fungal infections are a major problem, so antifungal prophylaxis with oral fluconazole is administered for the first week to 10 days or until the drains have been removed.

Islet cell transplantation

To avoid the complications associated with the exocrine secretions of the pancreas, transplantation of the pancreatic islets alone is an attractive option. The islets are isolated from the retrieved pancreas and prepared as an infusion to be embolized into the liver via a portal venous catheter inserted by an interventional radiologist.

Islet cell retrieval is especially feasible from donors with high BMI as the steatotic pancreas often has a large number of functioning islets, but the pancreas is infiltrated with fat and tolerates ischaemia poorly, leading to severe pancreatitis after reperfusion.

Islet cell transplantation only leads to insulin independence in a minority of patients, but it usually does improve glycaemic control and hypoglycaemia is rare. It is therefore an especially good option for diabetics with hypoglycaemic unawareness.

Complications of islet cell transplantation include portal vein thrombosis and bleeding. Transient elevation of liver enzymes is commonly seen. Acute rejection does occur, but is impossible to diagnose. Recurrent infections can increase levels of antibodies, reducing success rates.

Liver transplantation

Approximately 700 liver transplants are performed each year in the UK, but around 14% of patients listed die before being transplanted. The liver can be split into right and left lobes for transplantation into an adult and child simultaneously or to allow living donor liver transplants.

Diseases suitable for transplantation

- Hepatitis C cirrhosis.
- Alcoholic liver disease (6 months abstinence before consideration).
- Primary biliary cirrhosis.
- Primary sclerosing cholangitis (excluding cholangiocarcinoma).
- Hepatocellular carcinoma (HCC) in a cirrhotic liver (selected cases).
- Fulminant hepatic failure (e.g. acute viral hepatitis, drug reactions, or paracetamol overdose).

Clinical indications (also see Table 19.3)

- Acute fulminant liver failure (see Table 19.4).
- *Category 1.* Expected 1y mortality >9% without liver transplant.
- *Category 2.* HCC within 'Milan criteria' (see Box 19.3).
- *Category 3.* Variant syndromes affecting quality of life.
  - Persistent and intractable pruritus.
  - Diuretic-resistant ascites.
  - Hepatorenal syndrome.
  - Hepatopulmonary syndrome.
  - Chronic hepatic encephalopathy.

The transplant procedure

The liver is transplanted on an urgent basis, ideally within 12h of retrieval. The recipient undergoes removal of the native liver, may be placed on veno-venous bypass, and then the new liver is implanted in an orthotopic position, restoring the normal vascular anatomy with the biliary drainage via an end-to-end choledocho-choledochostomy or a Roux-en-Y hepatico-jejunostomy if the recipient bile duct is diseased.

If the recipient has accessory hepatic arteries, the common hepatic artery may be insufficient to perfuse the liver and so arterial conduits can be fashioned from the donor iliac arteries retrieved with the liver.

Post-operative management

Most commonly, immunosuppression is achieved using combination of tacrolimus, azathioprine, and steroids. The liver is less prone to acute rejection than other organs, so immunosuppression can be fairly rapidly tapered after the immediate post-operative phase.

Hepatic artery thrombosis (HAT) is a common complication, usually requiring immediate retransplantation, and usually presents as metabolic acidosis with rising serum lactate levels. Doppler ultrasound scanning is done as soon as possible after the operation to detect HAT at an early stage. Administration of platelet transfusions increases the risk of HAT. Graft survival is 80% at 1y and 60% at 5y.

Table 19.3 Monitoring disease progression using a Child–Pugh score. Patients in class C should be referred for transplantation

- Child–Pugh class B, 5–6 points.
- Child–Pugh class B, 7–9 points.
- Child–Pugh class C, 10–15 points.

	1 point	2 points	3 points
Bilirubin (µmol/L)	<34	34–51	>51
Albumin (g/L)	>35	28–35	<28
Prothrombin time (seconds prolonged)	1–3	4–6	>6
Ascites	None	Slight	Moderate
Encephalopathy grade	None	1–2	3–4

Table 19.4 King's College criteria for transplantation for acute liver failure

Paracetamol overdose	Other causes
Arterial pH <7.3; OR	PT >100s; OR
All three of:	Any three of:
PT >100s;	Bilirubin >300µmol/L;
Creatinine >300µmol/L;	Encephalopathy within 7 days;
Grade III/IV encephalopathy.	PT >50s;
	Age <10 or >40;
	Drug toxicity.

Box 19.3 The Milan criteria for transplantation for hepatocellular carcinoma (HCC)

- Child's class B or C cirrhosis; and
- Single tumour <5cm or up to three tumours <3cm; and
- Absence of macrovascular portal vein invasion.

Small bowel transplantation

Small bowel transplantation is rarely performed compared with other organs, with around 10 per year in the UK. Small bowel may be performed alone, in combination with a liver transplant, or as part of a multivisceral transplant.

The results of small bowel transplantation were previously very poor, but have improved dramatically in recent years. Graft survival at 1y increased from 52% to 75% between 1997 and 2005, with 1y patient survival increasing from 57% to 80% over the same time period.

Indications

The main indication is short bowel syndrome with permanent requirement for parental nutrition; long-term TPN is often associated with liver failure, so many small bowel transplants are combined with a liver transplant.

Indications for small bowel transplantation are chronic intestinal failure (most commonly due to Crohn's in adults) with one or more of:

- Loss of two or more central venous access sites.
- Loss of single venous access site from infection after appropriate attempts to salvage with aggressive line-conserving treatment.
- Early cholestatic liver disease or portal hypertension.

Successful small bowel transplantation is dependent on adequate central venous access being available, so potential candidates need to be referred before loss of all access sites.

Small bowel transplantation may also be considered in patients with chronic intestinal failure due to disease conditions where survival on long-term TPN is expected to be poor such as for chronic obstruction, extremely short bowel (<50cm), and end-jejunostomy without colon.

Combined liver and small bowel transplantation is appropriate for patients who would be candidates for small bowel transplantation, but also have advanced liver disease.

Small bowel transplantation is cost-effective, with lower maintenance costs compared with home TPN and additionally, recipients can normally resume full normal activities with potential return to employment. Quality of life is also better than home TPN.

Post-operative management

- Feeding tube inserted to introduce early enteral nutrition.
- Serial video zoom endoscopy to assess mucosa. Villous atrophy is early sign of acute rejection.
- Endoscopic protocol biopsies to exclude early acute rejection.
- Diarrhoea is main presenting symptom of graft dysfunction, whether due to rejection, infection, or ischaemia and is investigated by endoscopy and biopsy.

Acute rejection remains a major concern. It is common as there is a high population of immune cells in the gut compared with other organs. It is problematic as acute rejection reduces gut wall barrier function, leading to sepsis, especially in the context of augmented immunosuppression to treat rejection. Rejection is still associated with high risks, both of graft loss and death, so early diagnosis is the key.

In the long term, most foods can be tolerated although foods high in simple carbohydrates and soluble fibre may cause dumping syndrome symptoms.

Chapter 20

Surgery in tropical diseases

Medicine in the tropics

Key facts

Although the principles of surgical care are the same in the tropics as in developed countries, there are important differences as resources are limited in the tropics.

- There are major transport problems.
- Treatment is often complicated by underlying disease such as anaemia and malnutrition.
- There are differences in cultural attitudes to disease, for example:
  - Stomas are often considered an intolerable burden in some societies for religious or cultural reasons.
  - Sexually-transmitted diseases may carry greater a stigma than in the UK.

Treatment

Surgery on tropical diseases requires flexibility in both clinical management and surgical techniques. Doctors, irrespective of where they work, should be knowledgeable about common tropical diseases and be aware of the possibility of seeing an imported disease in a patient, with the concomitant risks to the patient and the community.

Spending time in tropical medicine

- Find out about where you are going to, the conditions you will work under, and the local diseases. Be prepared for these conditions. Visit an occupational service before you go to plan antimalarials and vaccinations. Discuss with them options for post-exposure HIV prophylaxis.
- When you arrive, listen to local health care workers. They always know more than you do.
- Your elective is the perfect time to develop a research mind—look and ask why things are being done. Develop a relationship with a more senior doctor and find questions relevant to his/her practice. However, do not expect to get an awful lot done or make any major breakthroughs in just a few weeks.
- Beware 'getting in a bit of practice'. An elective is not designed to allow you to get in a bit of practice doing things to 'the natives' that you are not allowed to do at home. This is a real risk when Western medical students go to under-resourced tropical hospitals. By all means, expand your horizons and use your skills to their limit, but know your limits and always work within them wherever you are.
- You will always be advised to eat only cooked or peeled food. This is clearly impossible. However, when the diarrhoea starts, do not sit on it as you might in more temperate climes. We have twice had to put up drips on medical students who arrived to spend time working with us, having had diarrhoea for several days.
- In regions where dengue or malaria occurs, a fever lasting more than a day requires a visit to a doctor for a blood film and FBC, despite apparently focal signs such as diarrhoea. Again, don't sit out a fever in the tropics. ICUs are not the best places to spend electives.
- The most dangerous time during your time in the tropics is likely to be time spent travelling. Think before you get on bus, boat, or plane. Ask yourself: is this a safe form of transport? Can I minimize the risk in any way? Do not feel ashamed for stopping your journey and getting out of the vehicle if you realize the risk is significant. You might meet someone fascinating…
- Lastly, show respect for the local culture. It is often difficult to appreciate some things and easy to hark back to good things at home. Careless expression of such thoughts can cause great distress to people proud of what they have accomplished.

Typhoid

Key facts

- Caused by *Salmonella (S.) typhi* or *S. paratyphi* (Gram –ve bacilli), ingested via contaminated food or water (faecal-oral or urine-oral routes from infected patients or chronic carriers).
- Approximately 33 million cases per year.
- Endemic in whole regions due to inadequate sewage disposal and contaminated water supplies.
- There are two clinical forms, typhoid and paratyphoid fever, collectively known as enteric fever.

Clinicopathological features

- Following ingestion, the bacilli penetrate the intestinal mucosa and multiply within the mesenteric lymph nodes.
- Re-entry into the bloodstream after about 10–14 days causes a bout of 'typhoid fever'.
- Systemic complications ensue due to haematogenous spread.
- Re-infection of the gut occurs through bile or bacteraemic spread and the bacilli localize in Peyer's patches in the lower ileum which become swollen and red.
- Infection of the bone marrow may cause neutropenia.

Complications of typhoid fever

- Paralytic ileus.
- Intestinal haemorrhage.
- Cholecystitis with perforation. Bacilli in the bile can produce a carrier state which can cause isolated outbreaks of typhoid fever ('typhoid Mary' was the cook who infected food wherever she worked).
- Infected aortic aneurysm.
- Phlebitis, especially of the left common iliac vein.
- Intestinal perforation along the anti-mesenteric border of the ileum at the site of Peyer's patches in the long axis of the gut.
- Genitourinary typhoid.
- Bone and joint infection.
- Myositis and myalgia.
- Parotitis.
- Laryngitis.
- Sinus bradycardia.

Clinical features

- Disease affects older children and young adults with an incubation period of about 10–14 days.
- Onset is gradual with high fever, headache, abdominal discomfort, cough, malaise, and anorexia.
- Characteristic stepwise increase in fever occurs over several days and pea-soup diarrhoea is a feature.
- In severe cases, mental changes can occur with change in conscious level and psychiatric features. Meningism is also a feature, but meningitis is rare.

- Maculopapular ('rose spot') rash may appear during the second or the third week, usually on the upper abdominal and lower chest. It fades within 2–3 days.

Diagnosis
- Widal test (serology).
- Stool culture with selective enrichment media (e.g. McConkey or DCA agar).

Treatment
- Chloramphenicol is extremely effective, cheap, and readily available in the tropics, but complications are not uncommon. Works by destroying the organisms responsible for the production of vitamin B complex.
- Alternative antibiotics are amoxicillin, trimethoprim, ciprofloxacin (less available in the tropics and more expensive).
- Treatment of intestinal perforation is surgical, with lavage and closure of the perforation and IV chloramphenicol.

Prevention Immunization—intradermal or intramuscular doses of killed/attenuated organism. Often given with parathyphoid immunization. Finite period of protection may require re-inoculation every 2y.

Amoebiasis and amoebic liver abscess

Key facts Amoebic liver abscess is a complication of amoebic hepatitis secondary to amoebic dysentery.

Pathological features

- Caused by *Entamoeba histolytica* protozoal infection.
- Cysts ingested from infected water or food.
- Amoebae enter ileal and colonic wall, especially in the ascending colon, multiply, and enter the portal venous circulation.
- Amoebae that traverse the liver enter the general circulation and systemic effects may occur.
- Amoebae in the liver destroy liver tissue directly with little or no tissue reaction (no abscess 'rim'). Secondary infection may occur. The central 'pus' is characteristically chocolate-coloured due to liver cell liquefaction and usually also contains staphylococci, streptococci, *Escherichia coli*, and *Entamoeba histolytica*.

Complications

- Infected individuals may be asymptomatic and act as 'carriers'.
- Intestinal amoebiasis producing dysentery and dysenteric colitis and/or amoebic appendicitis. Complications include:
  - Perforation and generalized peritonitis.
  - Haemorrhage, bloody diarrhoea, chronic anaemia of blood loss.
  - Intussusception.
- Hepatic amoebiasis and liver 'abscess'. Complications include:
  - Intraperitoneal rupture with peritonitis.
  - Intrapleural rupture with amoebic empyema.
  - Rupture into an attached loop of bowel.
  - Rupture into the pericardium.
- Extraintestinal amoebiasis may be hepatic or cutaneous.

Clinical features

Intestinal amoebiasis

- Fever, anorexia, weight loss.
- Acute or acute-on-chronic diarrhoea (may be bloody).

Hepatic amoebiasis

- Additional night sweats, rigors.
- Fever, anorexia, weight loss.
- Right upper quadrant and lower chest rigidity and tenderness.
- Right shoulder tip pain and right-sided basal changes, including a pleural rub may also occur.
- Hepatomegaly.

Diagnosis and investigations

- Microscopy and culture of fresh hot stool for amoebae.
- Liver ultrasound to assess number, size, and distribution of abscesses and allow aspiration of pus.

Treatment

Medical
- Emetine 40mg IM for 7 days and metronidazole 800mg tds for 7–10 days.
- Repeated abscess aspirations.

Surgical
- Open drainage of abscess that fails to respond.
- Excision of perforated viscera or for uncontrollable haemorrhage.

Anaemias in the tropics

Key facts

- The main causes of anaemias are iron deficiency or secondary to infections and infestations.
- Others causes include:
  - Glucose-6-phosphate dehydrogenase deficiency.
  - Thalassaemias.
  - Sickle cell anaemia.

Sickle cell anaemia

Pathological features

- Substitution of valine for glutamic acid at sixth position of the haemoglobin gamma chain. Leads to sickle cell anaemia if both genes are affected (homozygotes) or sickle cell trait in single gene carriers (heterozygotes).
- Sickle cell S-haemoglobin forms crescent-shaped rods when in the reduced state (deoxygenated).
- High incidence in Africa is because heterozygous carriers are more resistant than normal to *Plasmodium falciparum* malaria during early childhood and hence have a degree of 'natural selection' for survival and passing on their genes.

Clinical features

- Vaso-occlusive episodes precipitated by low O_2 tension in tissues.
- The abnormally shaped red cells cannot pass through arterioles and capillaries. Infarction, pulmonary emboli, recurrent infections, and arthralgia are common. These episodes of vaso-occlusion may also result from GA.
- Patients with a sickle cell trait have no clinical disabilities, but may suffer from sickling episodes when at altitude or flying in unpressurized aircraft. Sickling tendency may lead to splenic infarction.

Complications

Susceptibility to infection, in particular, pneumococcal infection, meningitis, and salmonella. Several types of crisis can occur:
- Painful crisis. Typically affects extremities, bones, and joints.
- Organ infarction, e.g. spleen, renal, brain.
- Sequestration crisis. When sickled erythrocytes are sequestered in the liver and the spleen, leading to a massive drop in blood volume.
- Aplastic crisis. Loss of red cell production.

Diagnosis and investigations

At-risk patients must be identified before surgical procedures to ensure adequate oxygenation during GA and to prevent dehydration.
- Carry out a 'sickling test' on suspected patients. Add a reducing agent, e.g. carbon dioxide (CO_2), to an unstained drop of blood. Homozygote blood sickles in a few hours. Heterozygote blood takes up to 24h.
- If the sickling test is positive, ensure adequate oxygenation during GA and prevent dehydration.

Treatment

- During a crisis, the main objective is to keep tissue oxygen tension high and preventing slow flow in vessels, which promotes sickling. This is achieved by:
  - Providing analgesia.
  - Keeping the patient fully hydrated.
  - Keeping the patient warm (especially the peripheries).
  - Giving supplemental O_2 (high flow or even hyperbaric) if possible.
  - Giving antibiotics to prevent secondary infection.
- Following a crisis, give the patient folic acid (5mg per day) to ensure red cell production is not inhibited by inadequate levels.

Malaria

Key facts

- Endemic in Africa, South East Asia, and South America.
- Attempts to eradicate it have been unsuccessful because of economic factors and the development of resistance to drugs.

Malaria can present as an acute abdomen with pain, pyrexia, and vomiting. Consider it when other causes of abdominal pain have been excluded, especially in patients who have recently returned from the tropics who have not taken antimalarial prophylaxis.

Pathological features

- The causal organisms are:
  - *Plasmodium (P.) falciparum*. Malignant tertian malaria.
  - *P. vivax*. Benign tertian malaria.
  - *P. ovale*. Benign tertian malaria.
  - *P. malariae*. Quartan malaria.
- Transmission is by the anopheline mosquito, the female alone of which bites. The mouthpiece (full of organisms) inoculates the skin by repeated bites.
- Parasites enter into red blood cells and divide.
- The incubation period is 10–14 days before multiplying organisms enter the bloodstream and cause clinical disease.
- Organisms may be cleared from the circulation by the immune system, but eradication of those within the red cells is rarely possible without drug treatment and repeated episodes of systemic infection are characteristic of all forms of malaria (e.g. every 3 days = 'tertian'; every 4 days = 'quartan').
- Chronic carriage of organisms may occur with repeated episodes of illness, eventually causing immunosuppression and debility.
- Infected red cells may be removed from circulation by the spleen and liver, which may carry a particularly heavy load of organisms.

Clinical features

The fever of malaria is characteristically:
- Intermittent.
- Associated with sweating, chills, and rigors.
- Followed by an afebrile period.

Complications

Complications are more likely with more virulent species, especially *P. falciparum*.
- Increased blood viscosity during attacks/'crises' may lead to microvascular infarction of organs such as:
  - Brain (cerebral malaria).
  - Kidney (renal failure with haemoglobinuria—'blackwater fever').
  - Liver (jaundice and even acute hepatic failure).
- Increased haemolysis of infected red cells leading to:
  - Haemolytic anaemia.
  - Haemoglobinuria.

Diagnosis and investigations

This is based on a history of exposure (e.g. tourists) and the clinical features with microscopy of bloodstained smear which increases the chance of finding parasites.

- Microscopy and culture of fresh hot stool for amoebae.
- Liver ultrasound to assess number, size, and distribution of abscesses and allow aspiration of pus.

Treatment

Medical

Prophylaxis

All visitors to areas of endemic disease *must* be advised to take full prophylaxis. The recommended regimen depends on the predominant species and the presence of resistant strains.

Uncomplicated malaria

A 3-day course of the antimalarial drug, chloroquine 600mg PO, immediately followed by 300mg PO qds for 3 days, then 300mg PO daily for 2 days.

Complicated malaria

- Should always be managed in a hospital with experience and appropriate facilities, if possible.
- Begin active rehydration immediately (IV crystalloid).
- Quinine hydrochloride 600mg IV over 10min every 8h for 7–10 days.
- Blood transfusion for anaemia.
- IV steroids for cerebral malaria.
- Monitor renal function.

Prognosis Untreated vivax malaria subsides in 10–30 days, but may recur intermittently. Intercurrent infection worsens the prognosis. Untreated falciparum malaria is frequently fatal.

Schistosomiasis (bilharziasis)

Key facts Endemic in many parts of north Africa, the Middle East, and South East Asia.

Pathological features

- Caused by the helminths, *Schistosoma (S.) haematobium*, *S. mansoni* (Africa), or *S. japonicum* (Asia).
- Infestation occurs from standing in infected water. The intermediate host is a snail (bullinus contortus) that inhabits slow running water.
- Multiplication of the larvae occurs in the snail; they then become free swimming and enter the human victim. After shedding their tails, they are swept by the bloodstream to all parts of the body. The worms have a particular preference for some sites according to their species.
- *S. haematobium* has an affinity for the vesical plexus, i.e. are mostly found in the urinary bladder and ureter. *S. mansoni* and *S. japonicum* have an affinity for the mesenteric veins and biliary tree, i.e. cause intestinal disease.
- Those that reach the liver develop into male and female worms, living in erythrocytes and when they mature, they leave the liver via the bloodstream to reach the vesical venous plexuses. The worms mate and the ova pass into the urine and faeces where they pass out and infect new water (especially stagnant). After hatching, the larvae enter the snail within 24h.

Clinical features and complications

- Intestinal worms cause:
  - Intestinal ulcers with bleeding, leading to abdominal pain and distension (due to ascites).
  - Perforation with peritonitis.
  - Pseudopolyps and inflammation, leading to bloody diarrhoea;
  - Chronic malabsorption and malnutrition.
  - Liver fibrosis (periportal), leading to portal hypertension.
- Systemic infection may affect:
  - Brain, causing malaise and fever.
  - Lungs, causing dyspnoea.
  - Spinal cord, causing paralysis.
- Bladder worms produce:
  - Inflammation of mucosa and slough (dysuria, frequency, haematuria).
  - Obstruction of the urinary tract (hydronephrosis).
  - Squamous carcinoma of the bladder is associated with long-term carriage.

Diagnosis and investigations

- Microscopic examination of an early morning urine or faecal specimen can demonstrate the presence of living eggs.
- Histological examination of a biopsy from the bladder or rectal mucosa can also provide confirmation of infection.

Treatment

Medical
Antimony preparations may be used in the early stages. Metrifonate and praziquantel are the most effective. It can take many months before the dead worms are expelled.

Surgical
Surgical intervention is necessary when complications such as portal hypertension, urethral stricture, or peritonitis after perforation develop.

Filariasis

Key facts

- Caused by a range of nematode worms, including *Wuchereria bancrofti*, *Onchocercia volvulus*, and *Brugia malayi*.
- Widespread in tropical and subtropical areas (India, Africa, China, the West Indies, and Australia).

Clinicopathological features

- Transmitted to humans by the bite of many genera of mosquitoes.
- Wuchererial worms enter the lymphatic system and cause:
  - Acute lymphangitis. Acute, swollen, painful lymphatics and nodes.
  - Chronic lymphadenitis and lymphatic obstruction. Especially of the lower limbs and genitalia—'elephantiasis'.
- Onchocercial worms may reach the eye (especially in African disease) and cause disruption of the intraocular tissues—'river blindness'.

Diagnosis Is usually clinical.

Treatment

Acute lymphadenitis

- Rest the affected part.
- Antibiotics (ampicillin 500mg by IM injection bd for 10 days) are used to treat secondary infection caused by beta-haemolytic streptococcus and *Staphylococcus aureus*.
- Specific antifilarial drugs, diethylcarbamazine citrate (Hetrazan®, Banocide®), start at 1mg/kg orally tds for 3 weeks.
- Surgical drainage of abscesses when they occur.

Chronic lymphoedema ('elephantiasis')

There is no satisfactory operation. Abnormal subcutaneous tissue can be excised and the affected part covered with a split skin graft. One variation is to excise the skin of the leg in long strips and then excise the subcutaneous tissue and apply skin to the denuded tissue. Apply a plaster of Paris dressing. The results are satisfactory, but certainly not cosmetic.

Hydatid disease

Key facts Occurs in sheep- and cattle-raising areas of the world, e.g. rural Wales, New Zealand, and not just the tropics.

Clinicopathological features

Pathological features

- Caused by the larval forms of the cestode worms, *Echinococcus granulosus* and *Echinococcus multinodularis*.
- Dogs are usually the primary host, eating infected sheep or cow offal, and the echinococcus parasite, about 1cm long, develops in the dog's intestine.
- It consists of a head and three segments, the last of which contains hundreds of ova. These are passed on to grass, for example, by defecation.
- Sheep and cattle ingest the ova to complete the normal life cycle. Humans are an incidental 'dead end' host, but the ova penetrate the small intestine and enter the portal circulation.
- Eighty per cent of the ova thrive in the liver with the development of hydatid cysts.
- They may also enter the general circulation, forming cysts elsewhere (e.g. kidneys, lungs, brain).

Clinical features/complications

- Infection is usually contracted in childhood, but produces symptoms and signs in adult life.
- Commonest presentation is of a liver cyst (either found as a palpable mass, incidentally on CT scanning, or during abdominal surgery).
- Compression of the intrahepatic bile ducts may produce jaundice.
- Rupture of a cyst into the peritoneal cavity causes peritonitis and shock. Cyst fluid also causes a severe allergic reaction with urticaria and eosinophilia if it enters the circulation (either by spontaneous rupture or surgical intervention).
- The prognosis is poor.

Diagnosis

- Casoni's test (serum antigen) is positive in 80%, but gives many false positives.
- Indirect haemagglutination tests are most accurate.
- Ultrasound and CT scanning may be used to localize cysts.
- ERCP may demonstrate connections with or compression of the bile ducts.

Treatment

Medical

Mebendazole 400mg tds for 30 days.

Intraperitoneal rupture

- Treat shock.
- Carry out peritoneal toilet.
- Give hydrocortisone before, during, and after surgery.

Surgical

Excision or aspiration of the cyst(s).

- Extreme caution must be taken to prevent peritoneal contamination. Black packs soaked in hypochlorite are placed around the liver to show up any daughter cysts or scolices.
- The cyst is partially aspirated and partially refilled with hypertonic saline which is scolicidal. It is then carefully separated from the liver and the cavity closed or drained.
- Give mebendazole post-operatively.

Prevention Community hygiene projects to reduce the risk of humans being exposed to infected dog faeces in areas of endemic disease.

Ascariasis

Key facts

- Caused by the nematode roundworm, *Ascaris lumbricoides*.
- Common in eastern and south eastern Africa, Sri Lanka, southern and south eastern India, and Bangladesh.
- The incidence of the condition is related to the state of development of the sewage systems.

Clinicopathological features

- Oral infection may occur in children or adults.
- Worms cross the intestinal wall and remain in the GI tract.
- Entry into the circulation may lead to systemic spread to other organs, e.g. liver, lungs, upper aerodigestive tract, blood.
- Intestinal infection causes:
  - Abdominal colicky pain and indigestion.
  - Diarrhoea.
  - Obstructive appendicitis.
  - Intestinal obstruction due to inflammation and impaction of a 'worm mass' or intussusception that may present as a mobile abdominal mass.
  - Protein-losing enteropathy with hypoproteinaemia and bleeding, leading to anaemia.
- Lung infestation may cause severe pneumonitis.
- Bile duct or pancreatic infestation may cause:
  - Bile duct strictures.
  - Liver abscess.
  - Cholangitis and empyema of the gall bladder.

Diagnosis

- Ova are demonstrated by examination of hot fresh stools.
- A plain AXR or barium meal may demonstrate radiolucent lines within a dense shadow, which represent individual worms.

Treatment

Medical

- Piperazine, one dual dose sachet repeated after 14 days (adults), one-third sachet (age 3–12 months), two-thirds sachet (age 1–6y), 1 sachet (age >6y). Causes flaccid paralysis of roundworms and threadworms and permits their expulsion by peristalsis.
- Mebendazole, 100mg bd for 3 days (adults and children >2y). Immobilizes the worms by disrupting their transport systems.

Surgical

- Abdominal surgery is only indicated for obstruction or peritonitis.
- If intestines are not inflamed, the worm load is squeezed into the caecum and colon where it will be removed by peristalsis. Alternatively, remove it via an enterostomy. Any non-viable gut is resected.
- Biliary infestation may be treated by antispasmodics to allow the sphincter to relax and then kill the worm load with antihelminthics or removal by ERCP or laparotomy.

Leishmaniasis

Key facts A spectrum of diseases caused either by the direct effects of infestation by protozoans of the *Leishmania* group or the type IV delayed hypersensitivity to the presence of the organisms.

Clinicopathological features

- The common route of infection is by bites from infected sand flies.
- The organisms spend their life cycle in the cytoplasm of circulating macrophages.
- Causative organisms include:
  - *Leishmania (L.) donovani.* Visceral leishmaniasis ('kala-azar', Indian subcontinent).
  - *L. tropicana, braziliensis, mexicana.* Cutaneous leishmaniasis.
  - *L. brasiliensis brasiliensis, tropica Ethiopia.* Mucocutaneous leishmaniasis ('espundia', South America and Africa).

Cutaneous leishmaniasis

- May be a simple sore at the site of fly bite with primary healing.
- May become a systemic infection if immune response poor.
- Severe type IV hypersensitivity reaction causes multiple skin ulcers ('recidiva').

Visceral leishmaniasis (kala-azar)

- An infection of the reticuloendothelial system with enlargement of the liver, spleen, and lymph nodes.
- May cause splenomegaly and pancytopenia if there is marrow infection.
- Secondary dermoid leishmaniasis occurs in failing immunity and is highly infectious.

Mucocutaneous leishmaniasis

- Affects the skin and subsequently the mucous membranes of the mouth and nose, causing nodules and ulceration.
- Large ulcers on the skin of the face and destruction of skin and cartilage are referred to as 'Chiclero's ear'.

Diagnosis

- Bone marrow aspiration.
- FNA of the spleen or liver.
- Complement fixation test.
- Leishmania skin test (Montenegro).

Treatment

- Cutaneous leishmaniasis often heals spontaneously, but when skin lesions are extensive, treat with sodium stibogluconate, an antimony compound in a dose of 20mg/kg/day by IM or IV injection for 20 days.
- Treat skin lesions for 10 days.
- Use amphotericin in unresponsive cases (AmBisome® 1–3mg/kg daily for 10–21 days). Cautions include hepatic impairment and pregnancy.

Trypanosomiasis

Key facts
- Caused by infection with flagellate protozoa of the *Trypanosoma* group.
- Two main sites of infection are South America and Africa.

Clinicopathological features
- Causative organisms are:
  - *Trypanosoma (T.) brucei rhodensiense* (east African). 'Sleeping sickness'.
  - *T. brucei gambiense* (west African). 'Sleeping sickness'.
  - *T. cruzi* (South American). 'Chagas' disease'.
- Transmission is by bites of infected tsetse flies in sleeping sickness or from infected faeces from small 'bedbugs' entering the mouth or eye in Chagas' disease.

Sleeping sickness
- Bite site develops primary chancre/ulcer.
- Parasitaemia results in acute lymphadenitis (often cervical—'Winterbottom's sign').
- Progressive waves of parasitaemia cause successively less effective immune responses with IgM and eventual failure of the immune response with widespread systemic parasite infestation.
- CNS infection leads to:
  - Spasm and tremor.
  - Discoordination.
  - Spastic and flaccid paralysis.
  - Unrousable sleep, progressing to coma and eventually death.

Chagas' disease
- Acute flu-like illness following infection. Lymphadenopathy and splenomegaly may occur.
- Eventual systemic parasite infection has a predilection for autonomic and neural crest derived nervous tissue, for example:
  - Enteric nervous system destruction leads to 'megaoesophagus' and 'megacolon'.
  - Myocardial infection causes myocarditis.
  - Cardiac conducting system destruction leads to ventricular aneurysm formation, dysrhythmias, and sudden death syndrome.

Diagnosis
- Wet blood film showing viable parasites.
- FNAC of lymph nodes and/or lumbar puncture may reveal organisms.

Treatment
Medical
- Suramin 0.1–0.2g initially. If there is no renal impairment, 1g every 5–7 days to a maximum of 10g.
- Pentamidine 3–4mg/kg daily for 10 days.

Surgical Rarely required for complications of Chagas' disease (e.g. cardiac or intestinal surgery).

Tuberculosis in the tropics

Key facts

- Caused by *Mycobacterium tuberculosis*.
- In the tropics, chronic malnutrition and associated immunosuppression lead to more acute illness, more rapid advancement of disease, and presentation at a much more advanced stage.
- Intestinal TB is much more common in tropical presentations.

Clinicopathological features

Infection routes include:
- Infection from food contaminated with the bacilli.
- Swallowed sputum containing bacilli.
- Bacteraemic phase of primary lung infection.

Features of intestinal disease
- May affect the terminal ileum, mesenteric lymph nodes, omentum, peritoneum, and solid organs related to the GI tract.
- Low grade fever with night sweats, malaise, anorexia, and weight loss.
- Dull abdominal pain and abdominal distension.
- Ascites.
- Rectal examination may reveal fistulas or fissures.

Pathological types
- *Ulcerative.* Deep, transversely placed ulcers in the direction of the lymphatics that may cause perforation and peritonitis.
- *Hyperplastic.* Fibroplastic reaction, resulting in thickening of the bowel wall along the mesentery and affecting the lymph nodes and the omentum, which may lead to malabsorption.
- *Sclerotic.* Associated with strictures in the small intestine, leading to intestinal obstruction.

Diagnosis
- FBC. ↑ WCC (lymphocytosis).
- Barium meal and follow-through may show intestinal strictures or ulcers that may be indistinguishable from those of Crohn's disease as seen in temperate climates.
- Ultrasound and CT scanning may suggest inflammatory masses (typically in the right iliac fossa).
- Intestinal tissue biopsies may demonstrate caseating granulomas.

Treatment
Medical
Antituberculous therapy:
- Streptomycin, 15–20mg/kg IM daily (unlicensed in UK).
- Isoniazid, 7–10mg/kg daily for 12 months.
- Rifampicin, 10mg/kg for 6 months.

Surgical Laparotomy for peritonitis due to perforation, obstruction, or unresolving inflammatory masses.

Leprosy ('Hansen's disease')

Key facts
- Endemic in much of Africa, Southern Asia, the Far East, and South America.
- Affects about 15 million people.

Clinicopathological features
- Caused by the acid-alcohol fast bacillus, *Mycobacterium leprae*.
- Commonly contracted in late childhood or adolescence, the likely source of infection being nasal discharge from infected patients (rather than open skin lesions).
- Infiltration of nasal membranes leads to very slow systemic spread (incubation period of 3–5y).
- Bacilli eventually infiltrate areas of the body at lower than normal temperatures (especially dermis, upper respiratory tract, and peripheral nerves), although central organs (e.g. liver, bone marrow, kidneys, and spleen) may be involved, especially later in the disease.
- Patterns of disease depend on the degree of host cell-mediated immune (CMI) reaction:
  - *Poor CMI.* Lepromatous leprosy (LL). Highly infectious; open ulcerating lesions contain macrophages loaded with bacilli.
  - *Modest CMI.* Dimorphous/indeterminate leprosy (BB). Features of both types (loss of CMI leads to LL, but treatment produces TT-type disease).
  - *Good CMI.* Tuberculoid leprosy (TT). Pronounced lymphocytic infiltration of lesions causing scarring; nerve damage is prominent feature.

Clinical features
Consider the diagnosis of leprosy in any patient who presents with a combination of neural and dermatological disorders.
- Lepromatous leprosy.
  - Dermal changes. Typically widespread hypopigmented and erythematous rash affecting the face, limbs, and trunk.
  - Generalized malaise, fever, and arthralgia.
  - Neural lesions. Often widespread neuritis followed by nerve thickening and progressive neuropathic tissue injury and ulceration due to anaesthesia.
  - Associated iritis is common.
  - Systemic amyloidosis may occur.
- Tuberculoid leprosy.
  - Dermal changes. Typically focal destruction of melanocytes (hypopigmentation), hair follicles, sweat and sebaceous glands (dry, hairless, anaesthetic plaques of tissue).
  - Neural lesions. Isolated, thickening of nerves (e.g. ulnar, peroneal), with late and relatively limited deformity.

Diagnosis

Diagnosis is based on:
- A history of contact.
- The clinical findings.
- Histological confirmation of *Mycobacterium leprae*.

In practical terms, infected tissue is usually obtained by taking a smear with a scalpel blade inserted into the pinched skin of an affected eyebrow or earlobe. The tissue fluid obtained is stained with a modified Ziehl–Nielsen stain.

Treatment

Medical
- Dapsone (diaminodiphenysulphone) 50–100mg daily.
- Combination chemotherapy is often used to reduce the incidence of dapsone resistance, for example:
  - Rifampicin 600mg once per month.
  - Dapsone 100mg daily.
  - Clofazimine 50mg daily + 300mg once per month.
- Continue treatment for at least 2y and often required for life.
- Contacts receive BCG vaccination or prophylactic dapsone.

Surgical
Surgical treatment is indicated to correct deformities which may be:
- *Primary*. Caused directly by the disease, e.g. thickening of the skin, paralysis of the eyelids, paralysis of the hands and feet.
- *Secondary*. Due to neuropathic injury. Education of the patient in avoidance of injury and self-care is vital to prevent progressive injury since damaged nerves may be permanently anaesthetic.

Severely damaged limbs may require amputation.

Guinea worm infestation

Key facts This freshwater-borne disease is common in the Middle East, South East Asia, certain parts of Africa, and India.

Clinicopathological features

- Contracted from drinking fresh water contaminated by the arthropod, Cyclops, which contains the larva of the guinea worm (*Dracunculus mediensis*).
- Stomach and upper small bowel lining is infected with the larvae.
- Direct spread occurs to the connective tissue of the abdominal wall where larvae mature and mate.
- Females then migrate to the areas of the body likely to be submerged in water, such as the lower leg, where the eggs are laid.
- The worm produces a proteolytic toxin, which leads to blister formation. When the blister bursts, the worm physically extrudes to allow the cycle of water re-infection to complete.

Clinical features Usually present as blistering rash on the legs with visible worm in the base.

Complications

- The subcutaneous worms may cause cellulitis, abscess, and sinus formation.
- Systemic infection can result in allergic conjunctivitis, osteomyelitis, or arthritis.

Diagnosis When the worms die, they may be visible as calcified areas in the subcutaneous tissue of the soles of the feet, legs, groin, scrotum, and back.

Treatment

The worms must be removed from their subcutaneous cavities slowly. A sudden pull will break the worm and leave the remaining part needing surgical removal.

Slow, progressive winding of the exposed worm around a small stick over several days is usually successful.

Threadworms

Key facts Endemic in tropical and temperate climates.

Clinicopathological features

- Caused by infestation by the round nematode, *Enterobius vermicularis*.
- Caught by ingestion of food or water infected by worm ova.
- Typically spreads throughout a family, especially one with young children.
- Worms live in the lumen of the lower colon and rectum and often migrate to the anal margin at night.

Clinical features

- There is chronic, and sometimes severe, anal irritation with associated excoriation of the perianal skin. It may be confused with other perianal disease and should be considered, particularly in children.
- Vaginitis and urethritis are associated complications.

Diagnosis

- Proctoscopy and sigmoidoscopy often reveal the worms in the colonic mucosa.
- A mucosal smear can be taken, but is usually unnecessary once the worms have been visualized. This is done using a wooden spatula to the end of which adhesive tape has been applied, adhesive surface outwards. The skin or mucosa is touched with the tape and smeared on to a slide, thus enabling the diagnosis to be made.

Treatment

Treat the whole family.

- Piperazine, one dual dose sachet repeated after 14 days orally for adults, one-third sachet (3 months–1y), two-thirds sachet (1–6y), one sachet (>6y); or
- Mebendazole 100mg orally repeated after 2–3 weeks (>2y).

Mycetoma (madura foot)

Key facts
- Caused by a subcutaneous fungal infection.
- May be caused by different species with different colours of spores, but the clinical picture is remarkably uniform.

Clinicopathological features
- The first sign is a painless swelling in the foot that gradually develops multiple sinuses and sometimes discharges purulent material containing the grains of the fungus.
- Local spread may occur if the primary infection is not treated, leading to deep tissue infection, e.g. fungal osteomyelitis.
- Systemic fungal infection is rare.

Diagnosis Microscopy of the discharge shows fungal hyphae.

Treatment

Medical treatment Dapsone, co-trimoxazole, streptomycin, and rifampicin are used either alone or in combination.

Surgical treatment
- All the affected area, including all sinuses, must be excised once treatment has begun.
- Amputation is occasionally necessary if deep osteomyelitis has occurred.

Common operations

Diagnostic laparoscopy

Indications (typical)

Acute/emergency
- Lower abdominal pain with suspected acute appendicitis (see 📖 p. 298) or ruptured ovarian cyst.
- Upper abdominal pain with suspected perforated peptic ulcer (see 📖 p. 284).

Elective
- Investigation of subfertility.
- Investigation of chronic abdominal pain.
- To perform biopsy (e.g. omental or lymph node) in suspected malignancy.

Pre-theatre preparation
- Always GA, therefore NBM 2h and fluids only 4h preop.
- Group and save required.
- Ensure consent is obtained for proceeding to other procedures if they are anticipated.

Positioning and theatre set-up
- *Urethral catheterization.* Usual, especially if lower abdominal pathology/ assessment likely, to ensure the bladder is decompressed.
- *NGT.* NOT required unless the patient is vomiting or gastric distension/surgery is likely.
- *Table positioning.* Supine. It is always best to have the patient in leg extensions. They allow the perineum to be accessed if vaginal manipulation or lower GI endoscopy is needed and they help to secure the patient on the table if head downtilt or lateral role is required.
- *Monitor/stack position.* Depends on the expected pathology.

Steps of surgery
- *Incision.* Periumbilical; usually curved infra-umbilical although supra-umbilical is also used. Vertical infra-umbilical can be used, especially where conversion to a midline laparotomy is anticipated.
- *Exposure of the linea alba.* By sharp dissection.
- *Incision of linea alba.* Elevate with forceps and incision with scalpel (no. 11 or 15).
- *Open trochar insertion.* Elevate linea alba with forceps, blunt scissor opening of pre-umbilical fat pad and peritoneum and placement of trochar (blunt) or:
- *Blunt trochar insertion.* Elevate linea alba with forceps without a small initial incision, insert trochar (blunt or with visual assistance using laparoscope inside the port) or:
- *Verres needle insertion.* Elevate linea alba with forceps, insert Verres needle using only thumb and finger pressure until 'clink' felt, test for intraperitoneal placement with saline 'drop' test.

- *Insufflation.* CO_2 typical pressure between 12–15mmHg; use slow flow initially, check for low pressure flow before increasing flow rate.
- *Assessment.* Inspect area beneath insertion port for signs of visceral injury or bleeding, assess anterior abdominal wall for availability of further port sites, inspect viscera sequentially.

Closure

Port sites 10mm and above require musculofascial closure, 5mm ports do not.

Post-operative care and instructions

- Remove catheter unless required for post-operative fluid balance observation.
- Antibiotics. Only required for pathology found.
- Oral diet. Normal as soon as tolerated.

Complications (specific to the procedure)

- Port site infection, <5%.
- Port site herniation, <2% if closed.
- Visceral injury during port insertion/basic laparoscopy and assessment, <1%.

Principles of laparotomy

Laparotomy is the term for any open access to the peritoneal cavity and includes midline incisions as well as paramedian and oblique approaches. It is the traditional method of access for most visceral surgery. It is still the approach of choice for some trauma, many emergency presentations, and some extensive surgery.

Pre-theatre preparation

- All, but smaller lower abdominal incisions which may be performed under regional or field block LA, require GA.
- Group and save or cross-match, depending on procedure.
- Ensure consent is obtained for other procedures if anticipated.

Positioning and theatre set-up

- Urethral catheterization. Usual, especially if lower abdominal pathology/assessment likely, to ensure the bladder is decompressed.
- NGT. Usual for upper intestinal obstruction (to reduce risk of aspiration at induction).
- Table positioning. Several are possible (see 📖 p. 76).
  - *Supine.* Most common for open visceral surgery (e.g. small and large bowel, gastric and major arterial).
  - *Lloyd Davis* (supine with hips slightly flexed and abducted). Used where access is required to the peritoneal cavity and the perineum/anorectum.
  - *Lateral.* For combined approaches to the retroperitoneal structures.

Steps of surgery

- *Skin incision.* Scalpel or cutting diathermy with needle point electrode.
- *Fat incision.* Blend diathermy to reduce risk of bleeding.

Midline access (see 📖 p. 82)

- *Midline fascia (linea alba) incision.* At or above the umbilicus (pre-peritoneal fat reduces the risk of underlying bowel injury). The midline can be identified by the presence of oblique crossing/interleaved fascial fibres. Expose fascia, elevated with clips to generate negative intra-abdominal pressure and sharply incised.
- *Access extension.* With blend diathermy in the midline.

Paramedian access

- *Rectus sheath fascia incision.* Vertical with blend diathermy.
- *Rectus muscle.* Fibres separated with minimum muscle division.
- *Peritoneal incision.* Elevated between clips and sharply incised.
- *Access extension.* With blend diathermy vertically.

Oblique access (e.g. gridiron, subcostal)

- *Rectus sheath fascia incision.* Oblique with blend diathermy.
- *Muscle.* For small incisions, fibre separation may achieve adequate access; this may be multiple layers (e.g. gridiron) or single (e.g. mini-subcostal). For larger incisions, muscle division with coagulation diathermy is required (e.g. full subcostal).

Basic procedures

- *Assessment of 'non-target' viscera*. Traditionally performed, but less important with preoperative imaging (especially CT scanning). Done in logical progression, e.g. central (small bowel, omentum, transverse colon), left upper quadrant (LUQ) (spleen, stomach), right upper quadrant (RUQ) (liver, gall bladder), right flank (right colon, right kidney), pelvis (bladder, uterus, ovaries, rectum), left flank (left colon/ kidney).
- *Assessment of 'target' organ(s)*. Depends on pathology expected, but consider these issues—'resectability' (tethering/involvement of vital, non-resectable structures), extent of resection (length or additional organs/structures to remove), mobility (adequate approximation of structures to be joined).

Specimens

- *Ascites* (free fluid). Send for M,C,&S; send for cytology if suspected malignancy.
- *Pus*. Send for M,C,&S (as liquid specimen if possible) or swab.
- *Peritoneal tissue*. Excise or biopsy peritoneal tissue nodules (parietal or visceral).

Key principles of emergency laparotomy

- *Bleeding*. Control by pressure (packs) initially rather than direct closure (clips or sutures); remove packs, starting with those least likely to cover bleeding sites; allow anaesthetic 'catch up time'.
- *Multiple visceral injuries*. 'Close and control' rather than 'restore and join'. Preventing contamination and visceral leakage are required, but restoration of anatomy/physiology can be deferred to subsequent procedures.
- *Contamination*. Seek out and treat all areas of pus/contamination. Frequently overlooked areas are subphrenic, subhepatic, interloop ileal, pelvic. Wash should be warm, copious, and repeated sequential dilutions rather than a single large washout. Large calibre drains for heavily soiled areas (likely to recollect), consider repeat ('re-look') surgery in 24–48h.

Closure

- *Peritoneum*. Should be approximated where possible (reduces risk of adhesions to exposed muscle) with absorbable suture; may be included with musculo-fascial closure (e.g. mass closure).
- *Muscle fibres*. Where parted—will usually re-approximate without sutured closure; where slit—may require absorbable sutures.
- *Fascia*. Always closed, usually heavy absorbable sutures, but may be non-absorbable.
- *Skin*. Sutures (subcuticular or interrupted) or clips.

Complications (specific to the procedure)

- Wound infection, 2–30%, depending on pathology.
- Incisional hernia, up to 30%; affected by sepsis, malnutrition, age.

Cholecystectomy

Simple cholecystectomy (removal of gall bladder and proximal cystic duct) is restricted to benign disease.

Open approach (elective) is usually only indicated for common bile duct exploration where laparoscopic exploration is not possible.

Indications (typical)

- Symptomatic proven gallstones.
- Symptomatic congenital abnormalities of the gall bladder.
- Previous acalculous cholecystitis.
- Very rarely indicated for prophylaxis in individuals at risk of cholecystitis (congenital heart disease, immunosuppressed).

Pre-theatre preparation

- Always GA, therefore NBM 2 h and fluids only 4h preop.
- Group and save required.
- Ensure consent is obtained for proceeding to other procedures if they are anticipated (e.g. common bile duct exploration).
- Check LFTs and any previous ERCP/MRCP imaging has been reviewed.

Positioning and theatre set-up

- Urethral catheterization; NGT NOT required.
- Table positioning. Supine. Some surgeons prefer to stand between the legs for the dissection (requires the patient in leg extensions).
- Monitor/stack position. LUQ.
- Patient may be placed slightly head up and left side down to improve RUQ exposure.

Steps of surgery

- Establish laparoscopy (see 🕮 p. 730) if appropriate.
- Incision for open surgery. Right subcostal ('Kocher's') with (partial) division of upper right rectus muscle.
- Expose gall bladder neck, cystic duct and common bile duct ('Calot's triangle')—fundal traction. *Tip: if exposure is poor, try adding further 5mm ports for retraction and ask for another assistant.*
- Identify cystic duct origin from gall bladder neck by blunt dissection.
- Identify cystic artery by blunt dissection.
- Clip (or tie if open) cystic duct (2 distal, 1 or 2 proximal on gall bladder neck) and divided. Repeat for cystic artery.
- Dissect gall bladder from liver 'bed' by retrograde dissection (i.e. from neck to fundus). Dissection is carried out close to the gall bladder wall.
- Gall bladder retrieved (usually in a waterproof bag if laparoscopic via epigastric port).
- Check haemostasis.

Closure

- Port sites (see Fig. 21.1). See laparoscopy (see 🕮 p. 730).
- Open. Usually closed in layers (peritoneum, (musculo)fascial, and skin).

Post-operative care and instructions

- Remove catheter unless required for post-operative fluid balance observation.
- Antibiotics. Only required for pathology found (e.g. cholecystitis).
- Oral diet. Normal as soon as tolerated.

Complications (specific to the procedure)

- Port site infection, <5%.
- Bleeding, 2%.
- Conversion to open surgery (if laparoscopic), 2% (depends on gender, age, sex, previous inflammatory episodes, previous abdominal surgery).
- Visceral injury during port insertion/basic laparoscopy and assessment, 1%.
- Common bile duct injury, 1 in 300.

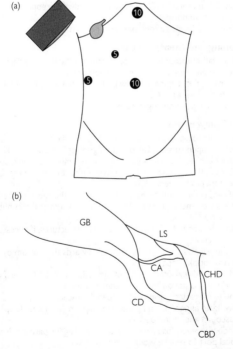

Fig. 21.1 (a) Ports sites for laparoscopic cholecystectomy. (b) View of Calot's triangle after dissection prior to structure division. (Borders: LS, liver surface; CHD, common hepatic duct; CD cystic duct. Other structures: GB, gall bladder; CBD, common bile duct; CA, cystic artery.)

Appendicectomy

Most surgeons prefer the laparoscopic approach for suspected or proven appendiceal pathology. Open right iliac fossa (RIF) incisions offer less exposure with greater tissue trauma. Consider a lower midline laparotomy if there is a large appendix mass, the patient is elderly, and other pathology is suspected.

Indications (typical)
- Acute appendicitis (see 📖 p. 298).
- Acute abdominal pain where diagnostic laparoscopy has revealed no other cause (not always performed).
- Previous resolved appendicitis ('interval appendicectomy').
- Appendix mass or mucocele (usually discovered on CT imaging).

Pre-theatre preparation
- Always GA, therefore NBM 2h and fluids only 4h preop.
- Group and save normal.
- Check the CT imaging if one has been performed.

Positioning and theatre set-up
- Urethral catheterization. Aids port placement safety, especially in females, by ensuring the bladder is decompressed.
- Table positioning. Supine; it is always best to have the patient in leg extensions (see 📖 p. 76).
- Monitor/stack position. Right caudal.

Steps of surgery
- Establish laparoscopy (see 📖 p. 730) if appropriate.
- Incision for open surgery, RIF oblique ('gridiron'). Incision of skin, open external oblique, internal oblique, and transversus abdominis, splitting the fibres in the direction of their travel without cutting them. Open the peritoneum between clips.
- Identify appendix from the base attachment to the caecum (the base lies reliably on the inferomedial pole of the caecum at the confluence of the taenia coli, the tip is variable in position).
- Mobilize the appendix from all surrounding structures, if necessary, by blunt dissection.
- Open the appendix mesentery from tip towards the caecum by diathermy (hook if laparoscopic).
- Identify appendiceal artery by blunt dissection and clip (or tie if open) (2 proximal, 1 distal on appendix side) and divide.
- Complete mesenteric division to appendiceal-caecal angle.
- Doubly ligate appendix stump close to caecum (with Endoloop® if laparoscopic) and divide between.
- Appendix retrieved (usually in a waterproof bag if laparoscopic via umbilical port to reduce wound infection risk).
- The appendix stump is now rarely buried with a purse-string suture at open appendicectomy; there is no evidence that it reduces stump complications.

Closure

- Port sites (see Fig. 21.2). See laparoscopy (see 🕮 p. 730).
- Open. Usually closed in layers (peritoneum, (musculo)fascial for each layer of the oblique muscles, and skin).

Post-operative care and instructions

- Antibiotics. Five-day course if acute appendicitis with perforation.
- Oral diet. Normal as soon as tolerated.

Complications (specific to the procedure)

Wound/port site infection, <5% (greater if open and perforated).

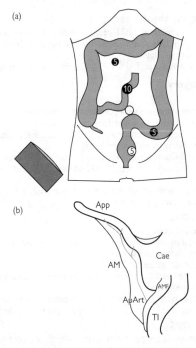

Fig. 21.2 (a) Port sites for laparoscopic appendicectomy—main ports sites in black; alternative layout for 2 × 5mm port sites in white. Monitor usually right side, caudal. (b) View of appendix and mesentery prior to dissection/division. (App, appendix; AM, appendix mesentery; AppArt, appendiceal artery; Cae, caecum; AMF, antemesenteric fat of terminal ileum; TI, terminal ileum.)

Inguinal hernia repair

Open approach is still very popular, especially for LA/regional anaesthetics, but laparoscopic approaches (transabdominal pre-peritoneal surgery (TAPS) or totally extra-peritoneal surgery (TEPS) are also widely used, especially for bilateral hernias (see 📖 p. 338).

Indications (typical)
- Symptomatic inguinal hernia.
- Asymptomatic inguinal hernia with high risk of complications or patient at high risk if complications develop.

Pre-theatre preparation
May be GA, LA (± sedation), or regional block (e.g. spinal).

Positioning and theatre set-up
- Urethral catheterization. NOT usually required for open unless the patient is at high risk of acute retention, but used for TEPS/TAPS.
- Table positioning. Supine.
- Monitor/stack position (TAPS/TEPS). Caudal end, same side as hernia.

Steps of surgery
Open
- Identify external oblique aponeurosis and cord at the superficial ring.
- Open aponeurosis, identify cord and deep ring.
- *Direct hernia*. Separate cord from sac, reduce sac, and plicate transversalis fascia to hold sac reduced.
- *Indirect hernia*. Open cord, separate sac from cord structures, sac may be reduced and the deep ring plicated or sac ligated and excised at the deep ring.
- Polypropylene mesh placed to cover from pubic tubercle to lateral to the deep ring; usually sutured in place.

Laparoscopic TAPS
- Establish laparoscopy (see 📖 p. 730).
- Open parietal peritoneum above hernia (e.g. hook diathermy) and dissect to groin structures.
- Identify testicular vessels and vas deferens.
- Reduce sac intraperitoneally where possible (part reduce and excise apex where necessary).
- Polypropylene mesh placed to cover from pubic tubercle to lateral to the deep ring; usually secured with laparoscopic tacking device.

Laparoscopic TEPS
- Open cut down to pre-peritoneal space via umbilical port access; opening the peritoneum is avoided.
- Open the pre-peritoneal space from umbilicus to groin (usually with assistance from a balloon dissecting device), then as for TAPS step 3.

Closure
- Port sites 10mm and above require musculo-fascial closure.
- Open, layers with absorbable sutures.

Post-operative care and instructions
Remove catheter (once fully mobile if open op with risk of ARU).

Complications (specific to the procedure)
- Groin wound infection, <5%.
- Recurrence, 3% lifetime.
- Groin haematoma, 2%.
- Painful scar/chronic groin pain, 1–2%.
- Injury to testicular vessels (causing ischaemia), <1%.

Perforated peptic ulcer repair

Traditionally by an open approach, but now frequently done by laparoscopy since this offers complete abdominal assessment prior to proceeding and may allow a targeted long or lower midline laparotomy if other pathology is found.

Indications (typical)

Suspected perforated peptic ulcer from history ± CT imaging findings (see 📖 p. 284).

Pre-theatre preparation

• Always GA, therefore NBM 2h and fluids only 4h preop.
• Group and save required.
• Ensure consent is obtained for proceeding to other procedures (e.g. bowel resection since other pathologies may be found).

Positioning and theatre set-up

• Urethral catheterization. Fluid balance chart required post-operatively.
• NGT. Not indicated.
• Table positioning. Supine, but well secured to allow for head uptilt.
• Monitor/stack position. Right cranial.

Steps of surgery

• Open incision. Mini-vertical supra-umbilical laparotomy (may be extended).
• Laparosopic. Establish laparoscopy (see 📖 p. 730).
• Confirm diagnosis and identify site of perforation (duodenal, prepyloric or gastric).
• Assess pathology. If suspicion of underlying malignancy in perforated gastric ulcer, consider if excision or partial gastrectomy may be required (senior help).

Repair is by patch closure of the ulcer wherever possible using omental tissue and not by sutured apposition closure of the defect (see Fig. 21.3).

• Dissect a broad 'tongue' of omentum using diathermy (at least 5cm wide x 10cm long).
• Three sutures placed through each edge of the ulcer, but not tied.
• Omental strip laid under and secured in place by sutures (snug, but not tight).
• Copious intra-abdominal lavage (all quadrants); drainage rarely required.

Closure

• Port sites. See laparoscopy (see 📖 p. 730 and Fig. 21.1a).
• Incision. See laparotomy (see 📖 p. 732).

Post-operative care and instructions

• Antibiotics. Not required for simple peptic ulcer perforation.
• Oral diet. Start liquid diet as soon as tolerated .

Complications (specific to the procedure)
Leakage at closure site, 5% (worst in immunosuppressed or advanced malignancy).

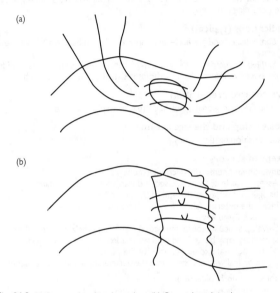

Fig. 21.3 (a) Sutures placed in ulcer edges. (b) Omental patch in place.

Haemorrhoid surgery

Surgical treatment is usually reserved for failed outpatient treatment (see 📖 p. 412) although the choice to go to surgery depends on symptoms, patient preference, and anatomy of the haemorrhoids.

Haemorrhoid de-arterialization procedures (blind or ultrasound-guided) are becoming more popular.

Indications (typical)
- *'Conventional' haemorrhoidectomy.* Intero-external haemorrhoids (one or more).
- *'Stapled haemorrhoidectomy'.* Circumferential, prolapsing haemorrhoids, or extensive internal haemorrhoids resistant to outpatient treatment.

Pre-theatre preparation
May be GA or regional anaesthesia (e.g. low spinal or caudal).

Positioning and theatre set-up
Table positioning. Lithotomy.

Steps of surgery
Conventional haemorrhoidectomy (see Fig. 21.4)
- Assess pedicle(s) to be excised and clarify which mucocutaneous bridges will be left at the end of the procedure.
- Incise the external (skin) margin (caution to not over-excise; the skin defects enlarge easily!).
- Develop subcutaneous/submucosal plane (superficial to internal sphincter); may be assisted with weak adrenaline solution injection.
- 'Cone' mucosal excision to apex of the pedicle.
- Ligate or seal with energy source the pedicle origin and vascular supply.

Stapled haemorrhoidectomy
- Determine anorectal mucosal 'ring' to be excised.
- Anal dilatation with circular dilator and rotating 'windowed' retractor.
- Circumferential running purse-string suture into mucosa and submucosa, avoiding circular smooth muscle (internal sphincter).
- Placement of staple-gun anvil 'head' above the purse-string level and tightening-tying of purse-string.
- Stapling device closed onto plicated mucosal ring, avoiding inclusion of anal canal lining by gentle eversion during closure.
- Excision of anorectal mucosal plicated ring by stapling device and check of homeostasis.

Closure
- No closure required.
- Anal pack not usually required.
- LA to conventional haemorrhoidectomy wounds.

Post-operative care and instructions
- *Laxatives.* If prone to constipation.
- *Antibiotics.* No proven benefit in reducing post-operative pain.

Complications (specific to the procedure)

- Bleeding (requiring intervention), <5%.
- Painful anal wound, 2%.
- Anorectal leakage, 2–3%.
- Anal stenosis, 1% (worse in conventional haemorrhoidectomy).

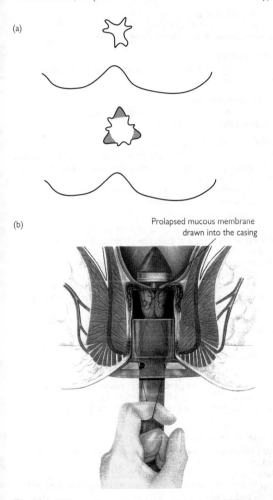

Fig. 21.4 (a) Extent of conventional haemorrhoidectomy. (b) Correct positioning of anorectal mucosal plication and stapling device.

Pilonidal sinus excision (Bascom II)

Different options exist for excision and primary closure of a non-acutely infected pilonidal sinus (see 🕮 p. 408)—Bascom I, Bascom II, Karayadakis, rhomboid flap, rotational flap. Principles of all primary closure procedures are:

- Excision/extirpation of sinus disease.
- Obliteration (elevation) of natal cleft.
- Asymmetric closure of natal cleft (scar off the midline).

Indications (typical)

Symptomatic pilonidal sinus disease with unilateral or limited bilateral secondary cutaneous openings.

Pre-theatre preparation

- Usually under GA, therefore NBM 2h and fluids only 4h preop.
- Single dose antibiotics on induction.

Positioning and theatre set-up

- Usually prone, sometimes with slight prone flexion at the hip. Buttocks may initially be taped laterally to aid retraction (should be released for final mobilization and closure).
- May be performed in left or right lateral jackknife position, but symmetrical buttock position is hampered.

Steps of surgery (Bascom II) (see Fig. 21.5)

- Asymmetrical, semi-elliptical excision of sinus pit origins.
  - Choice of lateral extent usually determined by the site of any lateral tracks.
  - 'Rat's tail' extension of cutaneous incision on the 'short side' to prevent final dig ear closure.
- Excision of skin and pits only with preservation of subcutaneous fat.
- Curettage, excision, and diathermy obliteration of all sinus tracks and lateral tracks.
- Mobilization of cutaneous skin flap of 'long side' of the incision.
- Mobilization of edge of skin flap of 'short side' of the incision.
- Scrupulous haemostasis and wound wash-out.
- Sutured closure apposition of natal cleft fat.

Closure

- Closure of skin flaps (interrupted mattress sutures—removable monofilament or dissolvable subcuticular suture).
- Small calibre low pressure suction drain occasionally used for larger flaps.

Post-operative care and instructions

- Remove catheter unless required for post-operative fluid balance observation.
- Antibiotics. Only required for pathology found.
- Oral diet. Normal as soon as tolerated unless indicated by further procedure performed.

Complications (specific to the procedure)

- Wound infection, 5%.
- 'Recurrent' sinus formation (wound sinus formation or wound non-healing), 3–5%.
- Painful scar, 2%.

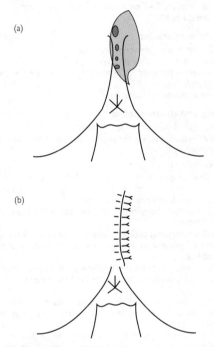

(a)

(b)

Fig. 21.5 (a) Typical incision for midline pits (shown in dark grey) with extent of skin removal (shown in light grey). (b) Fat and flap closure to achieve natal cleft obliteration and para-midline scar.

Femoral embolectomy

Femoral embolectomy should only be undertaken where there are facilities for further vascular surgical exploration or procedures since underlying occlusive vascular disease and alternative diagnoses are common

Indications (typical)

Strongly suspected or proven acute embolic occlusion of the distal superficial femoral artery (SFA) or popliteal artery with acute critical limb ischaemia (see 📖 p. 642).

Pre-theatre preparation

- May be GA or, more commonly, under LA.
- Group and save and clotting required.
- Ensure consent is obtained for proceeding to other procedures if they are anticipated.
- Single dose antibiotics on induction.

Positioning and theatre set-up

- Operating table should be X-ray compatible.
- NGT. NOT required unless the patient is vomiting or gastric distension/surgery is likely.

Steps of surgery (see Fig. 21.6)

- Incision. Oblique groin over the common femoral artery.
- Expose and control all inflow and outflow vessels (common femoral, superficial femoral, and profunda femoris).
- 3 or 4 FG Fogarty catheter is passed proximally and distally, and embolus retrieved.
- If good inflow and good backflow achieved, then close with interrupted 6/0 prolene sutures and confirm return of distal pulses or reperfused limb.
- Completion angiography may be undertaken on table (senior help).
- On table, thrombolysis may be required if there is residual thrombus (senior help).
- Surgical reconstruction or bypass may be necessary if there is *in situ* thrombosis on an underlying critical stenosis instead of simply embolism (senior help).
- Consider fasciotomies (up to four compartments) if there is suspicion of a post-operative compartment syndrome (muscles are tense or tender or prolonged ischaemia >6h).

Closure

Subcuticular suture.

Post-operative care and instructions

- Monitor pulse, BP, distal limb perfusion, pain, and pulses closely post-operatively.
- IV heparin infusion—24 000IU over 24h by pump and check APTT at 4–6h and daily after. Also repeat APTT 4h after every change in dosage, keeping APTT at 2–2.5 times the normal range.
- Start warfarinization at 48h.

Complications (specific to the procedure)

- Haematoma formation, 5%.
- False aneurysm formation, <1%.
- Distal limb compartment syndrome.

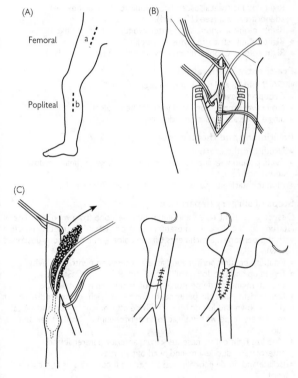

Fig. 21.6 Vessel exposure and control. (A) Incisions for femoral and popliteal artery exposure. (B) Control of femoral artery and its branches. (C) Femoral embolectomy and closure without and with a vein prosthetic patch.

Right hemicolectomy

Usually performed by laparoscopy although open access may be indicated for large or locally extensive tumours, previous abdominal surgery, inability to tolerate pneumoperitoneum. Laparoscopy may be multi- or single port.

Indications (typical)
- Right colonic (caecal, ascending colonic, or hepatic flexure) adenocarcinoma (see 📖 p. 404).
- Right colonic adenomas too extensive for endoscopic excision.
- Right colonic stricture (symptomatic).
- Right colonic Crohn's disease (symptomatic) (see 📖 p. 394).

Pre-theatre preparation
- GA (NBM 2h and fluids only 4h preop).
- Group and save required.
- No bowel preparation usual for right hemicolectomy.
- Single dose antibiotics on induction.

Positioning and theatre set-up
- Urethral catheterization.
- Table positioning. Supine, well secured to allow for head up/down tilt and lateral role.
- Monitor/stack and ports positions. Right side (see Fig. 21.7).

Steps of surgery (laparoscopic)
Dissection of right colon and ileum may be done from medial to lateral (starting at the ileocolic mesentery) or from lateral to medial (starting with the peritoneal attachments off the colon—one method is described below).
- Establish pneumoperitoneum, assess access and peritoneal cavity.
- (Head up and left down roll) Open and divide right gastrocolic omentum and divide peritoneum above the hepatic flexure.
- Divide right paracolic peritoneum and reflect right colon medially.
- (Head down and left down roll) Divide attachment of ileal and caecal mesentery to pelvic brim/iliac fossa peritoneum and reflect caecum superiorly.
- Mobilize right colon mesentery from anterior pararenal fascia, anterolateral duodenum, and head of pancreas.
- Isolate and divide ileocolic vessels and right colic vessels at mesenteric root.
- Divide transverse colic and terminal ileal mesenteries.
- Divide terminal ileum and proximal transverse colon (linear stapler).
- Deliver specimen via (peri)umbilical incision and form ileocolic anastomosis (extracorporeal).

Closure
- Mass closure to (peri)umbilical wound.
- Port sites. See laparoscopy (see 📖 p. 730) (see Fig. 21.7).

Post-operative care and instructions

Enhanced recovery programme usual. Oral fluids day 1, light diet day 2.

Complications (specific to the procedure)

- Conversion to open procedure, (up to) 20%.
- Anastomotic leak, 2–5% (see 📖 p. 420).
- Temporary stoma formation, 2% (see 📖 p. 750).
- Intra-abdominal bleeding, 5%.
- Port site infection, <5%.

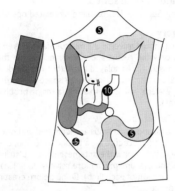

Fig. 21.7 Typical port sites and monitor position and extent of resection.

Stoma formation

Indications (typical) (see 📖 p. 84).

Pre-theatre preparation
- GA if done as part of other procedures or if laparoscopically formed; may be LA/regional if isolated loop stoma formation.
- Group and save required.
- Ideal sites for proposed stomas should be marked by stoma specialist preoperatively unless emergency surgery.
- Single dose antibiotics.

Positioning and theatre set-up
Table positioning. Supine unless required by related operation.

Steps of surgery
Ideally, any stoma should traverse the musculo-fascial layers of the abdominal wall (commonly the rectus abdominis); incisions in the fascia placed vertically with muscle fibres splayed apart (but not divided unless where necessary) to allow the stoma adequate space without 'pinching', but reduce the longer-term risk of herniation (a major problem especially in long-term stomas).

Loop ileostomy formation
- Ensuring proximal and distal limbs are identified and orientated (if done as an isolated procedure via a trephine incision, this is difficult; the only reliable indicator is the antemesenteric fat 'stripe' leading onto the surface of the caecum; much more reliably done laparoscopically for direct visualization of each limb). Done before creating defect if laparoscopic procedure.
- Opening of the antemesenteric wall of the loop (slightly oblique towards the distal limb).
- Placement of sutures (untied) to 'spout' the proximal limb (see Fig. 21.8).
- Placement and tying of sutures across the posterior wall of the loop and around the distal limb.
- Tying the proximal limb sutures and spouting the proximal limb.

A bridge is almost never necessary.

Closure
Port sites. As per laparoscopy.

Post-operative care and instructions
Oral diet. Normal as soon as tolerated unless indicated by further procedure performed.

Complications (specific to the stoma formation)
- Stomal oedema, ~30% (common and usually requires no treatment).
- Stomal ischaemia, <5% (serious and requires prompt treatment).
- Intestinal obstruction (due to tight musculo-fascial opening), 5%.

- Stoma retraction (usually due to inadequate mobilization), <5%.
- Stoma prolapse, <5%.
- Stomal/parastomal hernias (rare acutely), up to 50% long term.

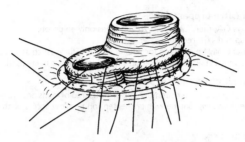

Fig. 21.8 Suture placement for spouting of proximal limb of loop ileostomy.

Wide local excision—breast

Indications (typical)

Carcinoma of the breast. Preferred to mastectomy for all, but large, tumours in small breasts, multifocal carcinomas, or those with multifocal DCIS and central tumours.

Pre-theatre preparation

- Always GA, therefore NBM 2h and fluids only 4h preop.
- Group and save required.
- Consent may be required for additional procedures (such as axillary node surgery), especially if sentinel node detection is being used.

Positioning and theatre set-up

- *Radiography.* Ensure mammograms or other radiographs are available.
- *Table positioning.* Supine with arm extension to allow access to the axilla.

Steps of surgery

- Skin incision according to breast folds and skin lines. Skin excision only required for superficial tumours with skin changes.
- Dissection carried out in a column or wide sphere of normal breast tissue margin down to fascia of pectoralis major.
- Haemostasis. Scrupulous care required.

Closure

Dissolvable sutures to fascia and skin.

Post-operative care and instructions

- The specimen requires orientation with marking (by sutures or clips) to mark three out of the six 'surfaces': anterior, inferior, and medial surfaces—'AIM'.
- Drains not usually required but if so, remove once output.

Complications (specific to the procedure)

Breast haematoma, 5%.

Below knee amputation

Indications (typical)
- Unreconstructible peripheral vascular disease of distal limb with critical ischaemia (involving vessels below the popliteal artery).
- Acute unsalvageable distal limb ischaemia (involving vessels below the popliteal artery).
- Unreconstructible trauma below the mid-tibia.
- Tumours of the soft tissue or bone of the distal limb (some).
- Unreconstructible congenital deformities of the foot with complications.

Pre-theatre preparation
- May be GA; spinal or regional common in vascular disease.
- Group and save required, may need cross-match for 2U.

Positioning and theatre set-up
- Table positioning. Supine.
- Ensure angiograms/limb CT scans available if appropriate.

Steps of surgery (see Fig. 21.9)
Two approaches are commonly used—'long posterior flap' and 'skewed symmetrical flaps'. 'Long posterior' flap is more common, especially in ischaemia.

Long posterior flap
- Mark flaps. Anterior flap slightly convex 10cm (in adults) below tibial tuberosity, just over hemicircumference of the calf skin. Posterior flap at least twice the length of the anterior flap. Opening of skin to fascia.
- Opening and division of fascia, then muscles of anterior and lateral compartments with diathermy.
- Identify anterior tibial neurovascular bundle; separate vessels and ligate; divide nerve under tension (promotes nerve retraction). Same for peroneal bundle.
- Fibular, then tibial divisions (flexible, wire, or powered saw); division of fibula high; bevel front of tibia at 45°.
- Stripping of posterior compartment muscles off tibia and interosseous septum below level of the division to the extent of the posterior flap.
- Identify posterior tibial neurovascular bundle; separate vessels and ligate; divide nerve under tension (promotes nerve retraction).
- Trimming soleus and gastrocnemius to reduce bulk of posterior flap to allow comfortable coverage of bony stump.
- Suturing of muscle/fascia to tibial peritosteum.

Closure
- Skin and fascia. interruptible sutures.
- Drain usually placed deep to myocutaneous flap.

Post-operative care and instructions
Early physiotherapy to knee joint to promote range of movements.

Complications (specific to the procedure)
- Flap necrosis, <5%.
- Haematoma.

Skew flap

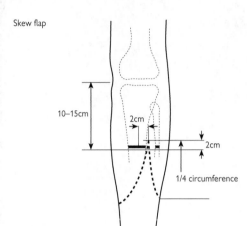

10–15cm

2cm

2cm

1/4 circumference

Burgess flap   'Rule of thirds'

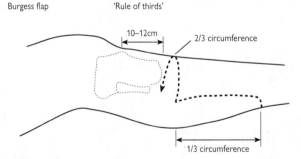

10–12cm

2/3 circumference

1/3 circumference

Fig. 21.9 Flaps used of below knee amputation. (a) Long posterior flap. (b) Skewed symmetrical flaps.

Eponymous terms and rarities

Acanthosis nigricans Pigmentation of the axillary skin associated with breast or gastric cancer.

Achondroplasia Familial dwarfism in which growth of the long bones and skull is defective.

Adenomyomatosis, gall bladder Thickening of the gall bladder wall with occasional intramural sinuses that may partially occlude the gall bladder lumen.

Adiposa dolorosa Multiple lipomas, usually on the arms and trunks, that are occasionally painful.

Adrenogenital syndrome A condition, usually autosomal recessive inheritance, affecting 1 in 5000 to 1 in 15 000 births, characterized by cortisol and/or aldosterone deficiency due to an enzymatic defect in cortisol synthesis, which results in secondary adrenal hyperplasia through loss of feedback on the pituitary gland. Diversion of precursors into the synthesis of other steroids, particularly androgens, results in virilization and ambiguous genitalia (through clitoral hypertrophy) of the female fetus and pseudoprecocious puberty in the male. Early closure of the epiphyseal plates leads to short stature. Impaired aldosterone secretion can cause a salt-losing state that requires replacement therapy.

Aerocele The collection of air in one or more tissue layers of the cranium due to injured or inflamed cranial air sinuses.

Albers–Schönberg disease See osteopetrosis.

Albright's hereditary osteodystrophy An X-linked form of pseudohypoparathyroidism characterized by mental retardation, low serum calcium, cataracts, and tetany. Patients tend to be of short stature and have short first, fourth, and fifth metacarpals. Metastatic calcification of the basal ganglia is a feature.

Albright's syndrome/polyostotic fibrous dysplasia A condition thought to be due to disordered bony development, featuring fibrodysplastic bony changes, patchy skin pigmentation, and precocious puberty in girls. Affected bones become soft and deformed from childhood onwards.

Allen's test This assesses the adequacy of the collateral circulation to the hand. Digital pressure is applied to both the radial and ulnar arteries at the wrist and the patient repeatedly clenches a fist. Adequate collateral supply exists if there is complete palmar flushing with 15s of release of each vessel in turn.

Amastia Absence of both breast and nipple. Ninety per cent of patients with unilateral amastia have absent or hypoplastic pectoral muscles.

Amaurosis fugax Episodes of transient blindness due to central retinal artery embolization from carotid vessel disease/proximal vessel atherosclerosis.

Amazia Congenital absence of breast tissue, but not the nipple. It is now known as hypoplasia of the breast, to differentiate it from amastia.

Angiodysplasia Vascular lesions of unknown aetiology, most frequently found in the right colon, occasionally associated with cutaneous and oral lesions. They occur with increasing age and present with bleeding that may be torrential, but more often as a series of small bleeds.

Angiomyoneuroma (glomus tumour) A small, painful, benign tumour of blood vessels, rarely larger than a few mm in size, mainly found in the extremities. Half arise in the digits, predominantly subungally. They are exquisitely painful and tender and appear blue-purple in colour. Treat by excision with a wide margin.

Angiosarcoma A soft tissue tumour of young men and women, producing a hot, bulky tumour with a tendency to bleed and metastasize to the lungs.

Ankyloglossia Also known as tongue-tie, it is due to a short lingual frenulum. It rarely affects speech, but frenectomy is recommended when food control and oral hygiene are a problem.

Antibioma A hard, oedematous swelling containing sterile pus following the treatment of an abscess with long-term antibiotics, rather than incision and drainage.

Aortoenteric fistula A connection between the aorta and small intestine, resulting in haemorrhage that becomes increasingly frequent and may culminate with exsanguinations; most commonly due to infection of a prosthetic graft rather than primary spontaneous fistula.

Apert's syndrome Occurs in 1 in 160 000 births. Thirty per cent of cases are autosomal dominant. Skull is 'tower-shaped' (oxycephaly) with premature fusion of all the sutures. Mild face aplasia and syndactyly of the middle three fingers occur. Other associations include oesophageal atresia, renal and congenital heart anomalies.

Aphthous ulcers The most common disorder affecting the oral mucosal membranes. Of unknown aetiology. They are painful, recurrent, and occur most commonly in childhood, rarely in the edentulous. Large ulcers, present for 3 months or more, may mimic carcinomas and should be biopsied if doubt exists.

Arnold–Chiari malformation A hindbrain abnormality where the cerebellum and medulla are found to lie below the level of the foramen magnum. Compression of the foramen of Magendie results in obstructive hydrocephalus in 80–90% of cases. Syringomyelia and spina bifida are commonly associated.

Askanazy cell tumour/Hurtle cell adenoma, thyroid A tumour consisting of featureless granular cells of varying size distributed in the fibrous stroma of the thyroid. They are difficult to differentiate from malignant tumours, but are regarded as benign.

Asplenia Absence of the spleen, associated with cardiac anomalies, including situs inversus.

Athelia Absence of the nipple. It is exceedingly rare.

Baker's cyst A central swelling of the popliteal fossa, most evident when the patient stands. It represents a synovial membrane diverticulum, almost always associated with knee joint pathology such as arthritis or torn meniscus.

Balanitis xerotica obliterans A disease of unknown aetiology characterized by keratotic lesions with inflammatory changes, leading to phimosis and occasional meatal stenosis. It has the appearance of a white stenotic band at the end of the foreskin and minor trauma often results in haemorrhage.

Ballance's sign Fixed dullness in the left flank with shifting dullness best appreciated in the right flank, resulting from intraperitoneal and extraperitoneal bleeding following splenic rupture.

Barrett's oesophagus The presence of columnar lined mucosa in the anatomical oesophagus; may be due to acid or biliary reflux. It is found in 10% of patients undergoing endoscopy for reflux symptoms. Strictures, ulceration, bleeding, dysplasia, and malignant transformation may occur.

Battle's sign Bruising over the mastoid process following a base of skull fracture that involves the petrous temporal bone.

Bazin's disease See erythrocyanosis frigida.

Beckwith–Wiedemann syndrome A congenital defect of the anterior abdominal wall associated with macroglossia, gigantism, and transient hypoglycaemia episodes.

Bezoars Masses of ingested human hairs (trichobezoars) or indigestible vegetable matter and fibre (bezoars) that form in the stomach and interfere with digestion or may migrate into the small bowel and cause intestinal obstruction.

Bier spots The presence of white patches amongst the mottled blue–purple appearance of an acutely ischaemic limb that has been in a warm environment for several hours.

Blind loop syndrome Malabsorption due to colonization of a blind-ending segment of bowel by abnormal bacteria that prevent the digestion and absorption of food. Causes include congenital abnormalities (e.g. small bowel diverticula), strictures, or, more commonly, surgical construction of small bowel anastomoses and loops.

Blue naevus Results when embryonic melanocyte migration from the neural crest is arrested in the dermis.

Bochdalek hernia A posterior diaphragmatic hernia where the septum transversum fails to unite with the intercostal part of the diaphragm. It occurs in infants and is characterized by gross herniation of abdominal contents and associated lung hypoplasia.

Boehaave's syndrome Spontaneous oesophageal rupture following an episode of intense vomiting or retching, characterized by severe upper abdominal and chest pain, tachycardia, tachypnoea, and subcutaneous emphysema.

Bornholm disease (epidemic pleurodynia) Coxsackie B4 virus infection of pleura and peritoneum characterized by severe upper abdominal and chest pain (worse on movement and respiration) associated with dyspnoea, pleuritic pain, headache, and sore throat.

Bowen's disease An irregular, reddish brown cutaneous plaque, occasionally ulcerated and commonly found on the trunk. It is an intra-epidermal carcinoma *in situ* and may develop into squamous cell carcinoma.

Branham's test When a pneumatic tourniquet is inflated around the root of a limb with a suspected arteriovenous malformation, a significant fall in the pulse rate suggests a significant arteriovenous shunt.

Budd–Chiari syndrome Post-hepatic venous obstruction that may result from spontaneous thrombosis, extrinsic compression by tumour, or a web in the vena cava.

Buschle–Lowenstein tumour A rare benign penile 'tumour' caused by human papilloma virus infection with giant tumour growth, but only local tissue destruction; may result in urethral fistula formation.

Cloquet's (Callisen's) hernia A deep femoral hernia that cannot protrude from the saphenous opening as it lies deep to the femoral vessels.

Calot's triangle An essential landmark in laparoscopic cholecystectomy surgery. Its boundaries are the common hepatic duct, cystic duct, and inferior border of the liver.

Campbell de Morgan spots Small, red spots that commonly occur on the trunk in middle age and do not blanch. They are of no significance.

Cancer en cuirasse Multiple malignant nodules on the chest wall in breast cancer that mimic the breast plate on a suit of armour.

Caput medusa Engorged veins radiating from the periumbilical region, resulting from extrahepatic portosystemic shunting from portal hypertension.

Carbuncle Multiple, adjacent follicular infections with *Staphylococcus aureus*, commonly seen in diabetics. Treat with flucloxacillin and surgical drainage as required.

Cardiac myxoma A rare primary cardiac tumour, commonly arising in the left atrium, which can present either with obstruction mimicking mitral stenosis or tumour emboli.

Carnett's test Determines whether an abdominal lump lies intraperitoneally or within the abdominal wall. The patient lies flat and raises his extended legs off the couch. An intraperitoneal lump disappears whereas one in the abdominal wall persists.

Caroli's disease An anatomical abnormality characterized by intrahepatic cystic changes with an increased risk of bile duct cancer.

Carr's concretions Microscopic calculi within the papilla of the kidney thought to be involved in the pathogenesis and propagation of renal calculi.

Charcot's triad Fever, rigors, and jaundice characteristic of acute cholangitis. Right hypochondrial pain is often an additional feature. This is a serious and potentially fatal condition, caused by ascending infection of the biliary tree associated with partial biliary obstruction.

Chemodectoma A carotid body tumour extending from the carotid bifurcation that presents with a solitary or bilateral lump(s) anterior and deep to sternocleidomastoid. Characteristically, they can be displaced laterally, but not vertically, and are associated with bruits and thrills in 20% of cases. The risk of malignancy increases with size.

Chopart's amputation An amputation made through the tarsal bones.

Churg–Strauss syndrome Affects young and middle-aged adults, often with a history of atopy, asthma, and allergic rhinitis, in which there is a marked eosinophilia. Clinical manifestations include peripheral neuropathy, cardiac involvement (heart failure and myocardial infarction), and vascular involvement that affects the stomach, small bowel, kidneys, and CNS due to aneurysm formation, thrombosis, and infarction.

Chvostek's sign Hyperexcitability of the facial nerve to local percussion over the parotid gland in patients with a reduced serum calcium concentration. It can also occur in 10% of normal people.

Chylothorax The accumulation of lymphatic fluid (which can have the appearance of pus) within the pleural cavity following thoracic duct trauma (blunt and penetrating injuries or surgical procedures), obstruction by malignant disease (particularly lymphomas and carcinomas of the lung and breast), and congenital defects (usually also associated with ascites).

Codman's triangle Radiographic evidence of periosteal elevation found with osteosarcomas.

Contrecoup injury Injury to the brain on the opposite side of the initial injury, due to the transmitted movements of the cerebral tissue within the skull.

Cooper's hernia A rare multilocular deep femoral hernia that enters the thigh via deep investing fascia.

Corrigan's pulse A collapsing pulse found in the presence of an arteriovenous fistula.

Courvoisier's law A palpable distended gall bladder in a jaundiced patient is more likely to be due to malignant disease obstructing the bile ducts than gall stones (where the gall bladder tends to be fibrotic and contracted).

Craniocleidodysostosis An autosomal dominant disease characterized by partial or complete clavicular aplasia, vertebral and digital deformities, and patent fontanelles.

Craniofacial dysostosis/Crouzon's syndrome A condition characterized by stenotic cranial sutures, maxillary hypoplasia and prognathism, beaked nose, exophthalmos, and mental retardation.

Crigler–Najjar syndrome Pre-hepatic jaundice due to an inability to conjugate bilirubin within the liver. There are two types, autosomal recessive (type I) and autosomal dominant (type II).

Cronkhite–Canada syndrome A triad of GI polyps, alopecia, and fingernail atrophy. The changes are not neoplastic, but due to an unidentified deficiency state.

Crueveilhier's sign (saphena varix) It is positive if an impulse is felt at the saphenofemoral junction when the patient stands and coughs.

Cullen's sign Periumbilical bruising seen in acute severe necrotizing pancreatitis or other form of severe intraperitoneal bleed, i.e. ectopic pregnancy, abdominal trauma.

Curling's ulcer Acute gastroduodenal ulceration associated with severe burns.

Curtis–Fitz–Hugh syndrome Severe right hypochondrial pain due to perihepatitis due to *Chlamydia trachomatis* infection.

Cushing's ulcer Acute gastroduodenal ulceration associated with stress, such as severe haemorrhage, myocardial infarct, multiple trauma, and in critically ill patients.

Dandy–Walker syndrome Congenital absence of the foramen of Magendie, resulting in marked ventricular dilatation. The lateral sinuses appear higher than normal on X-ray because of cerebellar hemisphere widening and the higher attachment of the tentorium cerebelli.

DeQuervain's disease Inflammation around the extensor pollicis brevis and abductor pollicis longus tendons, often associated with thickening of the extensor retinaculum. This results in pain on movement of the thumb and tenderness where the tendons cross the radial styloid.

DeQuervain's thyroiditis Self-limiting viral inflammation of the thyroid gland, which usually follows a recent upper respiratory tract infection, characterized by giant cell infiltration.

Dermatomyositis A condition of insidious onset characterized by proximal muscular weakness, pain, and tenderness. There is a characteristic purple skin rash that affects the cheeks and light-exposed areas. Association with occult malignancies of the colon, lung, breast, and genitourinary tract.

Desmoid tumour A locally expanding tumour of mesenchymal tissue often found in the infra-umbilical abdominal wall muscles or intra-abdominal mesenchymal tissue. It commonly affects middle-aged females and requires wide excision. Associated with familial adenomatous polyposis.

Dietl's crisis The passage of large volumes of urine following acute intermittent hydronephrosis. Classically, there is ureteric colic and a palpable, distended kidney. Both resolve after the passage of urine.

Dysplastic naevus (famm) syndrome Dysplastic naevi are considered precursors of malignant melanoma when there is a family history.

Solitary lesions in the absence of a family history are not. All patients should avoid excessive sunlight.

Ectopia vesicae (bladder exstrophy) Occurs in 1 in 30 000 live births, more commonly in males. There is an open bladder and defective anterior abdominal wall associated with separated pubic bones and penile epispadias or bifid clitoris. Associated with glandular metaplasia and the risk of squamous carcinoma of the bladder remnant.

Ehlers–Danlos syndrome A rare collagen disorder characterized by the development of saccular or dissecting aneurysms.

Emphysematous cholecystitis A rapidly progressive infection of the gall bladder due to anaerobic organisms, characterized by air in the wall of the gall bladder and a high risk of perforation.

Empyema—gall bladder A pus-filled gall bladder, resulting from impaction of a gallstone in the neck of the gall bladder.

Encephalocele The protrusion of cranial meninges, cerebrospinal fluid, and brain tissue through an opening in the skull.

Epidermal naevus syndrome The presence of extensive light brown warty lesions in association with skeletal and CNS developmental abnormalities.

Epiplocele A hernial sac containing omentum.

Epispadias A rare condition characterized by failure of development of the anterior wall of the lower urogenital tract, affecting the glans and penis alone (1 in 120 000) or the whole urinary tract when it is commonly associated with bladder exstrophy (1 in 30 000). It most commonly affects males and is characterized by the urethra exiting from the dorsal penile surface at varying sites.

Epithelioma of Malherbe Another term for a pilomatrixoma, a red/ white subepidermal nodule, frequently calcified and found on the upper body.

Erythrocyanosis frigida Also known as Bazin's disease. It affects healthy females with fat and often hairless legs. Capillary dilatation alongside arteriolar constriction results in dusky red/purple blotches that blanch on pressure and rapidly refill. They can be painful. Ulceration and persistent oedema may occur in severe cases.

Erythromelalgia A condition characterized by erythema and pain in the dependent extremities, relieved by elevation. The inappropriate release of local vasodilators has been implicated..

Erythroplasia of Queryat A reddish brown, irregular lesion found on the glans penis, which may ulcerate and crust. It is regarded as a carcinoma *in situ* and nearly always occurs in uncircumcised patients.

Exophthalmos Proptosis (sticking out of the globe of the eye), lid retraction, conjunctival oedema, and, in severe cases, ophthalmoplegia or optic nerve damage. Affects 2–3% of patients with Graves' disease.

Extradural haematoma The formation of a haematoma in the extradural space, most commonly following a fracture of the parietal or temporal bones with rupture of the middle meningeal artery or its branches that traverses them.

FAP (familial adenomatous polyposis) Autosomal dominant syndrome characterized by multiple colorectal and intestinal polyps as well as other intestinal and mesenchymal lesions.

Fallot's tetralogy Congenital cyanotic heart disease with four features: (1) ventriculoseptal defect, (2) pulmonary stenosis, (3) overriding aorta, (4) right ventricular hypertrophy. The infant becomes cyanosed on exertion and adopts a classical squatting position which raises their systemic vascular resistance, thereby increasing pulmonary blood flow.

Felty's syndrome An association between rheumatoid arthritis, splenomegaly, and granulocytopenia, which may be complicated by leg ulcers and recurrent infections.

Finkelstein's test Used to identify cases of stenosing tenosynovitis. The patient places his thumb in his palm and clenches a fist. The examiner pushes the hand into ulnar deviation and, if positive, pain is felt at the radial styloid, radiating down the forearm.

Foster Kennedy syndrome Optic atrophy of one eye and papilloedema in the other, which is due to a frontal tumour blocking the subarachnoid space on the ipsilateral side, but causing papilloedema on the other side because of raised intracranial pressure.

Fournier's gangrene A form of necrotizing fasciitis involving the perineal or scrotal skin, leading to subcutaneous necrosis. Synergy appears to occur between normal non-pathogenic organisms, leading to local vascular thrombosis and necrosis. Associated with uncontrolled diabetes mellitus.

Frey syndrome Gustatory sweating of the cheek following accidental or surgical trauma of the parotid region. It results from cross-regeneration of the transected sympathetic and parasympathetic fibres and develops over about 12 months.

Froment's sign Weakness of the adductor pollicis, following a high ulnar nerve palsy, leads to compensatory overaction of the flexor pollicis longus (innervated by the median nerve) when the patient is asked to squeeze a sheet of paper between thumb and index finger.

Galactocele A cystic lesion containing breast milk, occurring in women who suddenly stop breastfeeding.

Gamekeeper's thumb A sprain of the metacarpophalangeal joint of the thumb, leading to rupture of the ulnar collateral ligament. Non-healing leads to chronic instability and weakened pinch grip.

Gardner's syndrome Variant of FAP, involving an association between multiple epidermal cysts, intestinal polyposis, desmoid tumours, and osteomas.

Garrod's pad Subcutaneous tissue thickening over the proximal interphalangeal joints that are histologically similar to those found in Dupuytren's disease.

Gaucher's disease A genetic abnormality leading to active storage of abnormal glucocerebrosides in the spleen, resulting in massive childhood splenomegaly.

Gilbert's syndrome Congenitally acquired mild jaundice due to a failure of transport of bilirubin to the liver, which can be precipitated by episodes of starvation. There is an absence of urinary bilirubin although faecal and urinary urobilinogen levels are increased. It is of little clinical significance.

Glomus tumour See angiomyoneuroma.

Glucagonoma A tumour of the pancreatic islet cells characterized by mid-maturity onset diabetes, an erythematous rash that tends to blister and crust, glossitis, and raised glucagon levels.

Gluteal hernia A very rare type of hernia where visceral contents pass through the greater sciatic notch. It is often only discovered during laparotomy for the relief of intestinal obstruction of no obvious cause. Rarely, swelling around the buttock and pain referred along the sciatic nerve occur.

Grawitz tumour Adenocarcinoma of the kidney.

Grey–Turner sign Bruising in the flanks resulting from retroperitoneal haemorrhage (e.g. haemorrhagic pancreatitis).

Gynaecomastia The benign growth of breast tissue in males. The breast is uniformly enlarged and soft. May be physiological (e.g. maternal oestrogens, oestrogen-androgen imbalance of puberty), hypogonadism (pituitary disorders, androgen blockade), neoplasms (adrenal/gonadotrophic tumours, bronchogenic, renal cell, etc.), systemic disease (hepatic failure, renal dialysis, hypothyroidism), and drug-induced (androgen blockers, oestrogens, cimetidine, spironolactone, ketoconazole, methyldopa, metoclopramide, etc.).

Hamartoma Overgrowths of one (or more) cell type(s) normally found within the organ from which they arise, e.g. neurofibromas.

Hammer toe Hyperextension of the metatarsophalangeal joint and distal interphalangeal joint with flexion of the proximal interphalangeal joint. This can lead to the development of bursae and calluses. Frequently associated with hallux valgus, overcrowded toes, and diabetic neuropathy.

Hand–Schüller–Christian disease Multiple visceral and lytic skeletal lesions, characteristically also involving the skull, that are associated with diabetes insipidus and exophthalmos.

Hangman's fracture Traumatic disruption of the pars interarticularis of the atlas (C2) following a hyperextension injury.

Hashimoto's disease A diffusely enlarged, painless thyroid gland due to lymphocyte infiltration. Rubbery in nature and often mimicking a multinodular goitre. If enlargement is asymmetrical, other causes must be excluded. Clinically, the patient is euthyroid or mildly hyperthyroid.

Henle–Coenen sign If an arteriovenous fistula is occluded and the distal vessels still pulsate, this indicates that the fistula can be safely treated by ligation.

Hereditary osteodystrophy An X-linked form of pseudohypoparathyroidism characterized by hypoparathyroidism, low serum calcium, mental retardation, cataracts, and tetany. Metastatic calcification of the basal ganglion is also a feature.

Hesselbach's hernia A rare form of external femoral hernia that enters the thigh lateral to the deep epigastric and main femoral vessels.

Hibernoma A lipoma consisting of brown fat cells.

Hidradenitis suppurativa A chronic recurrent deep-seated skin infection of the axilla or perineum.

Housemaid's knee Chronic bursitis of the prepatellar bursa from the trauma of repeated kneeling (as in scrubbing floors).

Howship–Romberg sign Pain referred to the inner aspect of the knee via the genicular branch of the obturator nerve, which may arise from an obturator hernia that strangulates.

Hunner's ulcer Stellate white ulcers within the bladder, resulting from chronic inflammation, that open up on distension and bleed on decompression. Aetiology is unknown and women are more frequently affected. Bladder capacity is reduced and symptoms include urinary frequency and pain on distension, relieved by micturition.

Hydatid of Morgagni Also known as the appendix testis. Remnant of the Müllerian duct found at the upper pole of the testis, situated in the groove between the testis and epididymis; may undergo torsion.

Hyperhidrosis Excessive sweating of the axilla, palms, and feet, which can be socially embarrassing and distressing.

Hyperostosis frontalis interna (Morgagni's hyperostosis) Increased density and projection of the frontal bones, affecting the inner table only. Aetiology is unknown. Patients are often asymptomatic.

Hypersplenism A combination of splenomegaly, anaemia, leucopenia, and/or thrombocytopenia with bone marrow hyperplasia. Splenectomy may be required.

Inspissated bile syndrome Inspissation of bile in the common bile duct during early infancy (usually from haemolysis), resulting in proximal bile duct and gall bladder dilatation.

Insulinoma A rare tumour of pancreatic islet beta-cells, characterized by hypoglycaemic attacks that are both unpredictable and worsen in severity with time. Diagnosis is based on Whipple's triad.

Intraperitoneal rupture of bladder Usually traumatic in origin, from surgical instrumentation or abdominal trauma in the presence of a full bladder.

Jansen's disease An inherited autosomal dominant form of metaphyseal dysostosis, characterized by deafness and extreme dwarfism.

Jefferson's (burst) fracture Disruption of the ring of atlas (C2) following traumatic injury to the neck. Spinal column damage is uncommon as the fragments tend to open outwards.

Kalokerino's sign A filling defect of the fundus of the stomach that mimics a neoplasm. It arises when part of the fundus to the left of the cardio-oesophageal junction is about to herniate through it.

Kanavel's sign Is due to an infected ulnar bursa. Greatest tenderness is elicited in the transverse palmar crease on the ulnar side.

Kantor's string sign Is indicative of Crohn's disease. Involvement of the terminal ileum leads to structuring of the lumen. This gives the radiological appearance of a thread-like structure on barium follow-through.

Kaposi's sarcoma Painless red-brown macules on the limbs and anal and oral mucosa. Occasionally, they may ulcerate. They can be found in the elderly, endemically (e.g. in Africa), and in immunosuppressed patients (e.g. transplant patients, HIV).

Kartagener's syndrome Bronchiectasis and sterility resulting from abnormal ciliary action.

Kehr's sign Left shoulder pain referred from splenic injury and rupture.

Kenaway's sign A venous hum that is louder on inspiration (on auscultation with the bell of the stethoscope below the xiphisternum), associated with splenomegaly in patients with bilharzial cirrhosis of the liver.

Keratoacanthoma See molluscum sebaceum.

Killian's dehiscence The weak point between the cricopharyngeal and thyropharyngeal muscles through which pharyngeal mucosa can herniate, leading to the formation of a pharyngeal pouch.

'Kiss' cancer Cancer implanted in one area by local contact from another affected site, e.g. cancer of the lip, vulval labium.

Klein's sign Right iliac fossa pain that moves to the left when the patient turns on to his left side. It can be associated with mesenteric lymphadenitis and Meckel's diverticulum.

Klippel–Trenaunay syndrome A condition of the lower limb characterized by congenital varicose veins, deep vein abnormalities, bony and soft tissue deformity, limb elongation, and capillary naevi.

Köhler's disease Osteochondritis of the navicular bone. This can be one of the causes of a painful limp in a child under 5y of age.

Krukenberg tumour An ovarian tumour arising from transcoelomic spread of a primary gastric carcinoma.

Ladd's bands Persistent fibrous bands between the small bowel mesentery and liver, which can lead to obstruction of the second part of the duodenum. They are commonly associated with incomplete rotation of the bowel.

Laugier's hernia A rare form of femoral hernia that enters the thigh through a defect in the pectineal part of the inguinal ligament.

Li–Fraumeni syndrome An inherited predisposition to cancer thought to be due to mutation of the *p53* tumour suppressor genes.

Linitis plastica Also known as leather bottle stomach. Submucosal proliferation of fibrous tissue secondary to carcinoma of the stomach leads to gastric wall thickening and a reduction in stomach volume and plasticity. Because it spreads readily along the mucosa plane and presents late, its prognosis is poor.

Lipodystrophy Excessive fat deposition in the legs that may be mistaken for oedema.

Livedo reticularis Cyanotic skin mottling due to vasospasm of the arterioles with concomitant capillary dilatation.

McBurney's point Lies one-third of the way along a line drawn from the right anterior superior iliac spine to the umbilicus. It is the classical point of maximal tenderness in acute appendicitis and the centre point for the gridiron (McBurney's) incision used in open appendicectomy.

McMurray's test This is used to identify medial meniscal tears. With the patient supine, the knee is flexed and foot rotated medially and laterally while bringing the knee to 90° of flexion. Discomfort or a click is noted in the presence of a tear.

Madelung's deformity Dorsal subluxation of the lower end of the ulna that is congenital or traumatic in origin.

Maisonneuve's fracture The triad of a medial malleolar fracture, spiral fracture of the neck of fibula, and separation of the distal tibiofibular joint found in severe ankle trauma.

Malgaigne's bulges Bulges seen above the inguinal ligament in thin individuals on coughing or straining. They are variants of normal and do not represent inguinal hernias.

Mallory–Weiss syndrome/tear Haematemesis resulting from prolonged violent vomiting, leading to mucosal tears in the cardia of the stomach.

Marble bone syndrome See osteopetrosis.

Marfan's syndrome A rare inherited collagen disorder characterized by tall stature, arachnodactyly (webbed fingers), lens subluxation, and the development of saccular and dissecting aneurysms, particularly of the thoracic aorta. Aortic regurgitation may occur due to aortic root dilatation.

Marion's disease A rare cause of bladder outflow obstruction in young men due to narrowing of the bladder neck.

Marjolin's ulcer A longstanding venous ulcer that fails to heal in which squamous cell carcinoma develops.

Maydl's hernia The presence of a double loop of bowel within the neck of a hernia, 'W' in shape, where strangulation of the middle loop can occur.

Medullary sponge kidney Is due to dilatation of the terminal collecting ducts of the kidney, which predisposes to the formation of renal calculi.

Meigs' syndrome Ascites and pleural effusions associated with benign ovarian tumours.

Meleney's gangrene A form of necrotizing fasciitis mostly seen after abdominal surgery.

Ménétrier's disease Hypertrophy of the gastric mucosa, most typically proximally, resulting in hypochlorhydria and hypersecretion of gastric juices, leading to protein loss. Patients may present with epigastric discomfort and peripheral oedema. There is no associated increased risk of gastric cancer.

Meralgia paraesthetica Numbness and hyperalgesia around the lateral thigh following entrapment of the lateral cutaneous nerve of the thigh as it passes beneath the inguinal ligament.

Mesentericoparietal hernia of Waldeyer An internal paraduodenal hernia that lies medially and inferior to the third part of the duodenum. It may present with recurrent episodes of abdominal pain and vomiting due to small bowel obstruction.

Meyer–Weigert's law In patients with complete ureteric duplication, it is the lower pole ureter that refluxes because its mucosal tunnel through the bladder wall is shorter.

Milia Small, white, superficial facial spots derived from hair follicles. They appear in newborn babies and following skin grafting and dermabrasion and are treated by expression.

Mills' manoeuvre When the forearm is pronated while holding the elbow straight, pain over the common extensor origin is consistent with extensor tenosynovitis (tennis elbow).

Milroy's disease Lymphoedema, presenting from adulthood onwards, resulting from congenital aplasia of the lymphatic trunk.

Mirrizi's syndrome Obstructive jaundice resulting from impaction of a gallstone in the cystic duct, which presses against the common hepatic duct, causing extrinsic compression.

Molluscum contagiosum Small, pale, firm nodules with a characteristic central depression that follow infection with the pox virus. They tend to regress with time although they can be treated by curettage.

Molluscum sebaceum A solitary skin tumour that grows rapidly over 6–8 weeks and involutes over about 6 months to leave a residual scar. It has the appearance of a dome-shaped lesion with a central keratin-filled crater and can be mistaken both clinically and histologically for a well-differentiated squamous cell carcinoma.

Mondor's disease of the breast Superficial thrombophlebitis affecting the veins of the breast. Initially, there may be tenderness which is followed by fibrosis and contraction, resulting in skin dimpling.

Morgagni hernia A congenital diaphragmatic hernia that presents in early adult life with dyspnoea or as an incidental mediastinal mass. Abdominal contents expand into the anterior mediastinal compartment through a persistent defect in the anterior diaphragm.

Morgagni's syndrome See hyperostosis frontalis interna.

Murphy's sign Pain and tenderness in the right upper quadrant directly beneath the ninth costal upon deep inspiration while the examiner's fingers rest over the edge of the lower thoracic margin at this point. It is due to an inflamed gall bladder and the patient may be unable to fully inspire because of the pain.

Myositis ossificans Ectopic bone formation arising within haematoma in muscle following soft tissue injury.

Nail–patella syndrome An inherited condition characterized by radial head subluxation, small patellae, and absent or deformed nails.

Narath's hernia A rare form of femoral hernia that extends anterior to the femoral artery beneath its investing fascia.

Nelson's syndrome The presence of skin hyperpigmentation and accelerated growth of a pituitary tumour following bilateral adrenalectomy for pituitary-dependent Cushing's. It results from loss of pituitary feedback.

Nutcracker oesophagus Alternative name for diffuse oesophageal spasm—the presence of long-duration, high-intensity peristaltic contractions in the oesophagus, which may be associated with chest pains and dysphagia.

Obturator sign The aggravation of right iliac fossa pain upon passive internal rotation of the right hip in patients with appendicitis where the appendix lies adjacent to obturator internus.

Osteogenesis imperfecta An inherited collagen disorder, resulting in fragile bones that fracture easily, blue sclera, deafness, and soft teeth.

Osteopetrosis (Albers–Schönberg disease, marble bone disease) An inherited disorder of bone, resulting in increased bone density, fractures, and anaemia. The recessive form is less severe than the autosomal dominant form.

Osteopoikilosis Infantile, patchy, long bone sclerosis (found radiologically) associated with yellow skin lesions. It has autosomal dominant inheritance and is of no clinical significance.

Oxycephaly An autosomal dominant condition characterized by stenotic sutures, resulting in a tower-shaped skull, prominent nose, and a lateral squint. Facial deformities are also common. Mental retardation, optic atrophy, and deafness can also occur.

Painful arc syndrome Shoulder pain occurring between 70° and 110° of abduction due to the passage of an inflamed supraspinatus tendon between the acromion process and head of humerus. The subacromial space is narrowest at this point, leading to impingement.

Pancreas divisum Arises when the ventral and dorsal pancreatic buds fail to fuse during embryological development. Consequently, the main pancreatic duct drains via an accessory ampulla. The vast majority of patients are asymptomatic although it may be one of the causes of chronic pancreatitis.

Panda sign Bilateral black eyes following a head injury, suggestive of a base of skull fracture involving the anterior cranial fossa.

Parkes–Weber syndrome Bony and soft tissue limb overgrowth resulting from multiple arteriovenous fistulas. Lipodermatosclerosis, ulceration, and high cardiac output failure may also occur.

Paterson–Brown Kelly syndrome The association of a pharyngeal web with dysphagia and iron deficiency anaemia. There is an increased risk of post-cricoid carcinoma.

Peau d'orange Localized oedema found in breast cancer where the skin of the breast has the pitted appearance of an orange skin.

Pendred syndrome Familial association of deafness and goitre with peroxidase deficiency (involved in the synthesis of thyroxine).

Phalen's test The reproduction of discomfort and paraesthesia of the fingers in the distribution of the median nerve (lateral three and half fingers) when the wrist is held in flexion. It is due to compression of the median nerve as it passes beneath the flexor retinaculum through the carpal tunnel.

Phlegmasia alba dolens A swollen, white, oedematous limb, occasionally seen in patients with severe iliofemoral venous thrombosis. Progression to phlegmasia caerulea dolens may occur.

Phlegmasia caerulea dolens A blue, swollen, oedematous limb following severe proximal venous thrombosis. This may progress to venous gangrene as circulatory congestion and stasis occur.

Plagiocephaly Development of an asymmetrical skull arising from the early closure of sutures on one side of the skull.

Plummer–Vinson syndrome See Paterson–Brown Kelly syndrome.

Pneumatosis cystoides intestinalis Gas-filled cysts within the intestinal and mesenteric walls, most commonly affecting the small intestine. These can be seen on plain abdominal X-rays.

Pneumaturia The passage of flatus in urine, which can arise from a colovesical fistula (e.g. diverticular disease, carcinoma, inflammatory bowel disease) or urinary tract infection in diabetics where the glucose is fermented by the infecting organism.

Poland's syndrome An association between pectoral muscle abnormality, absence or hypoplasia of the breast, and characteristic hand deformity of hypoplasia of the middle phalanges and skin webbing (synbrachydactyly).

Pott's carcinoma of scrotum Squamous cell carcinoma of the scrotum, associated with chronic exposure of the scrotal skin to aromatic carcinogens in coal-derived chimney soot. Now more commonly associated with exposure to heavy metals and mineral oils, particularly the ones used in the cotton industry.

Pott's disease of the spine Tuberculosis of the spine, leading to bony destruction and vertebral collapse which leads to kyphosis and spinal compression.

Pott's peculiar tumour A large trichilemmal cyst, commonly occurring on the scalp, which can ulcerate and resembles a squamous carcinoma (both clinically and histologically). They are benign, but may recur after excision. They rarely undergo malignant transformation.

Pott's puffy tumour Osteomyelitis of the skull bones following untreated frontal sinusitis. This results in overlying scalp inflammation and swelling.

Proctalgia fugax Severe recurrent rectal pain in the absence of any organic disease. Attacks may occur at night, after bowel actions, or following ejaculation. Anxiety is said to be an associated feature.

Pseudomyxoma peritonei Disseminated mucinous tumour within the peritoneal cavity. Commonly due to ruptured ovarian or appendiceal mucinous neoplasms. Locally recurrent and potentially fatal, even with heroic surgery and chemotherapy.

Ranula A saliva-containing cyst in the floor of the mouth that has a soft, bluish submucosal appearance.

Raspberry tumour A tender, granulomatous mass arising from the posterior urethral meatus.

Redcurrant jelly stool A description attributed to the bloodstained stool found in intussusception.

Reidel's thyroiditis Thyroiditis characterized by a marked fibrotic reaction, leading to a hard, non-tender thyroid gland. Thyroid function tends to be normal and differentiation from malignant disease can be difficult as fine needle aspirates tend to be acellular.

Reinke's oedema The presence of generalized oedema of the upper vocal cords in response to noxious stimuli.

Reiter's syndrome The triad of polyarthritis, conjunctivitis, and urethritis as a result of venereal infection, usually chlamydia. The initial attack lasts for 4–6 weeks although some patients develop chronic symptoms.

Rendu–Osler–Weber syndrome Hereditary haemorrhagic telangiectasia; a rare autosomal dominant condition characterized by the presence of haemangiomas affecting the lips, buccal cavity, nasopharynx, and whole GI tract. These may bleed, resulting in episodes of harmatemesis, haematuria, melaena, epistaxis, or anaemia that are self-limiting.

Richter's hernia A form of strangulated hernia in which only part of the bowel lumen becomes strangulated, leading to incomplete intestinal obstruction with ischaemia and gangrene of the strangulated part.

Rovsing's sign Pain and tenderness in the right iliac fossa produced by palpation of the left iliac fossa. It may be found in acute appendicitis.

Sabre tibia Occurs in late syphilis where new formation of subperiosteal bone results in bowing.

Saint's triad The association between cholelithiasis (gallstones), hiatus hernia, and diverticular disease.

Scheie's syndrome An autosomal recessive skeletal disorder associated with corneal clouding, cardiac anomalies, and epiphyseal dysplasia.

Scheuermann's disease A disease that predominantly affects young adolescent males where vertebral growth plates are affected by osteochondrosis or aseptic necrosis, resulting in back pain and progressive kyphosis.

Schmorl's node A lucent area with surrounding new bone formation in a vertebral body, resulting from extrusion of the nucleus pulposus into the vertebral body.

Sever's disease Osteochondritis of the posterior epiphysis of the os calcis near the insertion of Achilles tendon.

Shoveller's fracture A stable cervical injury resulting from fracture of the spinous process of C7 due to either trauma or muscular contraction.

Sinding–Larsen's disease Osteochondritis of the distal part of the patella.

Sister Joseph's nodule The appearance of umbilical nodules in the presence of advanced intra-abdominal carcinoma, typically stomach, but also large bowel, ovarian, or occasionally, breast.

Sjögren's syndrome The presence of keratoconjunctivitis sicca, salivary gland involvement (leading to xerostomia, i.e. dry mouth), and rheumatoid arthritis or other mixed connective tissue disorders. Primary Sjögren's is characterized by the first two features whereas secondary Sjögren's has all three.

Spigelian hernia A rare type of hernia due to defects within the internal oblique aponeurosis as it interdigitates with the anterior and posterior rectus sheath. Peritoneum and visceral contents may herniate through these small defects.

Stevens–Johnson syndrome Also known as erythema multiforme, characterized by ulceration that has a characteristic target appearance and results from drug allergies (particularly to sulphonamides and barbiturates), mycoplasmal infections, or idiopathically. The lesions may be associated with conjunctivitis, tracheitis, and dysphagia.

Stewart–Treves syndrome The development of angiosarcoma in a chronically lymphoedematous limb, in this particular case, following radical mastectomy for breast cancer.

Sump syndrome Due to the collection of stones and debris in the distal common bile duct following choledochoduodenostomy, resulting in epigastric pain, cholangitis, and pancreatitis.

Thrombophlebitis migrans Increased coagulability of blood associated with visceral cancers, particularly adenocarcinomas.

Tietze's disease Also known as costochondritis. Affects the costal cartilages, resulting in chest pain that can be reproduced by pressure to the affected cartilages.

Tinel's sign Transient finger paraesthesia that follows percussion of the median nerve proximal to the wrist in patients with median nerve compression due to carpal tunnel syndrome.

Treacher Collins syndrome Also known as mandibulofacial dysostosis. An autosomal dominant condition characterized by symmetrical external and middle ear, zygoma, and mandibular hypoplasia, parrot-beaked nose, absence of medial lower eyelashes, dental crowding, and abnormal palpebral fissures.

Trichobezoars See bezoars.

Troisier's sign Enlargement of the left supraclavicular lymph node due to advanced metastatic gastric carcinoma.

Trousseau's sign Phlebothrombosis of the superficial leg veins associated with gastric cancer.

Umbolith An umbilical concretion of desquamated skin, which can lead to infection.

Ureterocele A cystic dilatation of the intravesical submucosal ureter. It is often associated with other congenital anomalies, including duplicated ureters.

VACTERL syndrome The association of vertebral (V), anorectal (A), cardiovascular (C), tracheo-oesophageal (TE), renal (R), and limb (L) anomalies. Progesterone and oestrogen intake during early pregnancy have been implicated.

Vermooten's sign Digital rectal examination reveals a doughy, displaced, or absent prostate in the presence of an intrapelvic rupture of the prostatic urethra.

von Hippel–Lindau disease An inherited disorder characterized by cerebellar and spinal cord haemangioblastomas, retinal angiomas, and an increased risk of visceral cancers, particularly renal cell carcinoma.

von Recklinghausen's disease (neurofibromatosis type I) Autosomal dominant inherited nodular thickening of nerve trunks, associated with patchy skin pigmentation (*café-au-lait spots*). Malignant transformation of these neurofibromas tends to occur only in this particular subgroup of patients and their prognosis is poor.

von Rosen's sign Congenital dislocation of the hip. Results in a click when the hip is flexed and adducted, then flexed and abducted, as this causes the femoral head to dislocate and relocate.

Waldenström disease Necrosis of the articular cartilage of the head of femur following a slipped femoral epiphysis. This leads to stiffness or complete loss of movement in that hip.

Waterhouse–Friderichsen syndrome Bilateral adrenal cortical necrosis due to septicaemia (meningococcal, pneumococcal, streptococcal), haemorrhage, or burns.

Whipple's triad Fasting hypoglycaemic attacks with blood glucose less than 2.5mmol/L, relieved by glucose, and associated raised insulin levels. These are characteristic of an insulinoma.

Whitaker test Can be used to assess the degree of ureteric obstruction. Saline is perfused into the kidney via a renal puncture at a rate of 10mL/min and the pressure gradient measured across the ureteric–vesical junction. Ureteric obstruction is indicated by a pressure difference greater than 20cmH$_2$O. Less than 15cmH$_2$O is normal.

Youssef's syndrome A ureterovesical fistula that presents with monthly episodes of haematuria.

Zenker's diverticulum A pharyngeal pouch that occurs though the dehiscence of Killian, between cricopharyngeus and inferior constrictors of the pharynx. There is usually a history of food sticking and regurgitation. Progressive weight loss, dysphagia, and aspiration pneumonia can also occur.

Zollinger–Ellison syndrome Intractable duodenal ulceration due to elevated levels of circulating gastrin levels. There is an association with men type I. Diagnosis is confirmed by acid secretion tests which show elevated resting levels. Secretin challenge elevates gastrin levels in G-cell hyperplasia, but not G-cell tumours.

Anatomy and physiology key revision points index

Index

Common perioperative care

Bowel prep KleenPrep® 4 sachets over 8h the day preop *or* CitragMag® 2 sachets over 4h the night preop.

Thromboprophylaxis

Low risk, e.g. day or fully ambulatory cases: TEDS only.

Medium risk, e.g. major surgery without risk factors or past history of DVT: TEDS + Clexane® 30mg SC od or Fragmin® 2500U SC od.

High risk, e.g. pelvic surgery, malignancy, obesity, past history of DVT: TEDS + Clexane® 30mg SC bd or Fragmin® 5000U SC od.

Diabetic perioperative regimens

Minor surgery (e.g. day surgery)

Oral controlled: give normal regimen.

Insulin controlled: omit preop insulin on day of surgery; monitor blood sugar (BS) every 4h; restart normal insulin once oral diet established.

Major surgery

Oral controlled: omit long-acting hypoglycaemics preoperatively; monitor BS every 4h. If BS > 15mmol/L start IV insulin regimen.

Insulin controlled: commence on IV insulin sliding scale preoperatively once NBM and continue until normal diet re-established. Check BS 4-hourly. Restart normal insulin regimen (initially at half dose) once oral diet established.

Typical IV sliding scale (Actrapid® with 5% dextrose):

BS < 4mmol/L: infusion 0.5U/h;

BS 4–15mmol/L, infusion 2.0U/h;

BS 15–20mmol/L, infusion 4.0U/h;

BS > 20mmol/L, infusion 4.0U/h plus consult diabetology team. Consider treatment as for ketoacidosis.

Fluid balance

$$\text{Fluid depletion} = ((PCV_1 - PCV_2)/PCV_1) \times 0.7 \times \text{weight in kg}$$

where PCV_1 = normal haematocrit and PCV_2 = current haematocrit.

Fluid maintenance regimen (correct for age and losses)

Fluid volume	Na$^+$	K$^+$
100mL/kg for 1st 10kg of weight + 150mL/kg for next 10kg of weight + 20mL/kg for every kg of weight thereafter	2mmol/kg/24h	1mmol/kg/24h

Managing oliguria

Check catheter not blocked.

Check fluid balance status—try bolus crystalloid with frequent reviews.

Check drug chart for possible drug toxicity.

Managing post-operative hypotension

Check fluid balance status first. If in doubt assume it is hypovolaemia.

Check epidural status. Check drug chart for possible drug toxicity.